CLINICIAN'S POCKET DRUG REFERENCE 2011

EDITORS

Leonard G. Gomella, MD, FACS

Steven A. Haist, MD, MS, FACP

Aimee G. Adams, PharmD

www.eDrugbook.com
www.thescutmonkey.com

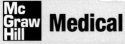 **Medical**

New York Chicago San Francisco Lisbon
London Madrid Mexico City Milan New Delhi
San Juan Seoul Singapore Sydney Toronto

Clinician's Pocket Drug Reference 2011

Copyright © 2011 by Leonard G. Gomella. Published by The McGraw-Hill Companies, Inc. All rights reserved. Printed in Canada. Except as permitted under the United States Copyright Act of 1976, no part of this publication may be reproduced or distributed in any form or by any means, or stored in a data base or retrieval system, without the prior written permission of the PUBLISHER.

1 2 3 4 5 6 7 8 9 0   TRA/TRA   14 13 12 11 10

ISBN 978-0-07-163788-6
MHID 0-07-163788-5
ISSN 1540-6725

Notice

Medicine is an ever-changing science. As new research and clinical experience broaden our knowledge, changes in treatment and drug therapy are required. The authors and the publisher of this work have checked with sources that are believed to be reliable in their efforts to provide information that is complete and generally in accord with the standards accepted at the time of publication. However, in view of the possibility of human error or changes in medical sciences, neither the authors nor the publisher nor any other party who has been involved in the preparation or publication of this work warrants that the information contained herein is in every respect accurate or complete, and they disclaim all responsibility for any errors or omissions or for the results obtained from use of the information contained in this work. Readers are encouraged to confirm the information contained herein with other sources. For example and in particular, readers are advised to check the product information sheet included in the package of each drug they plan to administer to be certain that the information contained in this work is accurate and that changes have not been made in the recommended dose or in the contraindications for administration. This recommendation is of particular importance in connection with new or infrequently used drugs.

The book was set in Times by Glyph International.
The editors were Lindsey Zahuranec and Harriet Lebowitz.
The production supervisor was Sherri Souffrance.
Project management was provided by Gita Raman, Glyph International.
Transcontinental was printer and binder.

This book is printed on acid-free paper.

CONTENTS

EDITORS

Leonard G. Gomella, MD, FACS
The Bernard W. Godwin, Jr., Professor
Chairman, Department of Urology
Jefferson Medical College
Associate Director of Clinical Affairs
Kimmel Cancer Center
Thomas Jefferson University
Philadelphia, Pennsylvania

Steven A. Haist, MD, MS, FACP
Clinical Professor
Department of Medicine
Drexel University College of Medicine,
Philadelphia, Pennsylvania

Aimee G. Adams, PharmD
Clinical Pharmacist Specialist, Ambulatory Care
Adjunct Assistant Professor
College of Pharmacy and Department of Internal Medicine
University of Kentucky HealthCare
Lexington, Kentucky

ASSOCIATE EDITORS

George A. Davis, PharmD, BCPS
Clinical Pharmacist Specialist,
Therapeutic Drug Monitoring/
Internal Medicine
Associate Adjunct Professor
College of Pharmacy
University of Kentucky HealthCare
Lexington, Kentucky

Daniel A. Lewis, PharmD, BCPS
Clinical Pharmacist Specialist,
Therapeutic Drug Monitoring/
Internal Medicine
Assistant Adjunct Professor
College of Pharmacy
University of Kentucky HealthCare
Lexington, Kentucky

PREFACE

We are pleased to present the 9th edition of the *Clinician's Pocket Drug Reference*. This book is based on the drug presentation style used since 1983 in the *Clinician's Pocket Reference*, popularly known as the Scut Monkey Book. Our goal is to identify the most frequently used and clinically important medications, including branded, generic, and OTC products. The book includes over 1200 medications and is designed to represent a cross-section of commonly used products in medical practices across the United States.

Our style of presentation includes key "must-know" facts of commonly used medications, essential for both the student and practicing clinician. The inclusion of common uses of medications rather than just the official FDA-labeled indications are based on the uses of the medication supported by publications and community standards of care. All uses have been reviewed by our editors and editorial board.

It is essential that students and residents in training learn more than the name and dose of the medications they prescribe. Certain common side effects and significant warnings and contraindications are associated with prescription medications. Although health-care providers should ideally be completely familiar with the entire package insert of any medication prescribed, such a requirement is unreasonable. References such as the *Physician's Desk Reference* and the drug manufacturer's Web site make package inserts readily available for many medications, but may not highlight clinically significant facts or key data for generic drugs and those available over the counter.

The limitations of difficult-to-read package inserts were acknowledged by the Food and Drug Administration in 2001, when it noted that physicians do not have time to read the many pages of small print in the typical package insert. Newer medications are now providing more user-friendly package insert summaries that highlight important drug information for easier practitioner reference. Although useful, these summaries do not commingle with similarly approved generic or "competing" similar products.

The editorial board and contributors have analyzed the information on both brand and generic medications and have made this key prescribing information available in this pocket-sized book. Information in this book is meant for use by health-care professionals who are already familiar with these commonly prescribed medications.

This 2011 edition has been completely reviewed and updated by our editorial board and technical contributors. Regular readers will note that we did not publish a 2010 edition due to timing issues that occasionally plague an annual publication.

More than 70 new drugs and formulations have been added, and dozens of changes in other medications based on FDA actions have been incorporated, including deletions of discontinued brand names and compounds and multiple black box updates. Where appropriate, emergency cardiac care (ECC) guidelines are provided based on the latest recommendations from the American Heart Association (*Circulation*, Volume 112, Issue 24 Supplement; December 13, 2005) with the ECC emergency medication summary in the back of the book for rapid reference.

Editions of this book are also available in a variety of electronic or eBook formats. Visit www.eDrugbook.com for a link to the electronic versions currently available. Additionally, this web site has enhanced content features such as a comprehensive listing of "look alike–sound alike" medications that can contribute to prescribing errors. Nursing versions of this book with a section of customized Nursing interventions is available and updated annually. An EMS guide based on this book with enhanced content specifically for the field provider and emergency medical practitioners was released in 2010. Information on these related topics are available on the web site.

We express special thanks to our spouses and families for their long-term support of this book and the entire Scut Monkey project (www.thescutmonkey.com). The Scut Monkey Project is designed to provide new medical students and other health professional students with the basic tools needed when entering the world of hands-on patient care.

The contributions of the members of the editorial board, in particular the long term support and dedication of Harriet Lebowitz at McGraw-Hill, are deeply appreciated. Your comments and suggestions are always welcome. Improvements to this and all our books would be impossible without the interest and feedback of our readers. We hope this book will help you learn some of the key elements in prescribing medications and allow you to care for your patients in the best way possible.

Leonard G. Gomella, MD, FACS
Philadelphia, Pennsylvania
Leonard.Gomella@jefferson.edu

Steven A. Haist, MD, MS, FACP
Philadelphia, Pennsylvania

Aimee G. Adams, PharmD
Lexington, Kentucky

MEDICATION KEY

Medications are listed by prescribing class and the individual medications are then listed in alphabetical order by generic name. Some of the more commonly recognized trade names are listed for each medication (in parentheses after the generic name) or if available without prescription, noted as OTC (over-the-counter).

Generic Drug Name (Selected Common Brand Names) [Controlled Substance] BOX: Summarized/paraphrased versions of the "Black Box" precautions deemed necessary by the FDA. These are significant precautions, warnings and contraindications concerning the individual medication. **Uses:** This includes both FDA-labeled indications bracketed by ** and other "off-label" uses of the medication. Because many medications are used to treat various conditions based on the medical literature and not listed in their package insert, we list common uses of the medication in addition to the official "labeled indications" (FDA approved) based on input from our editorial board **Acts:** How the drug works. This information is helpful in comparing classes of drugs and understanding side effects and contraindications. *Spectrum:* Specifies activity against selected microbes for antimicrobials **Dose:** *Adults.* Where no specific pediatric dose is given, the implication is that this drug is not commonly used or indicated in that age group. At the end of the dosing line, important dosing modifications may be noted (i.e., take with food, avoid antacids, etc) **Caution:** [pregnancy/fetal risk categories, breast-feeding (as noted below)] cautions concerning the use of the drug in specific settings **CI:** Contraindications **Disp:** Common dosing forms **SE:** Common or significant side effects **Notes:** Other key useful information about the drug.

CONTROLLED SUBSTANCE CLASSIFICATION

Medications under the control of the US Drug Enforcement Agency (Schedules I–V controlled substances) are indicated by the symbol [C]. Most medications are "uncontrolled" and do not require a DEA prescriber number on the prescription. The following is a general description for the schedules of DEA-controlled substances:

Schedule (C-I) I: All nonresearch use forbidden (e.g., heroin, LSD, mescaline).
Schedule (C-II) II: High addictive potential; medical use accepted. No telephone call-in prescriptions; no refills. Some states require special prescription form (e.g., cocaine, morphine, methadone).
Schedule (C-III) III: Low to moderate risk of physical dependence, high risk of psychologic dependence; prescription must be rewritten after 6 months or 5 refills (e.g., acetaminophen plus codeine).
Schedule (C-IV) IV: Limited potential for dependence; prescription rules same as for schedule III (e.g., benzodiazepines, propoxyphene).
Schedule (C-V) V: Very limited abuse potential; prescribing regulations often same as for uncontrolled medications; some states have additional restrictions.

FDA FETAL RISK CATEGORIES

Category A: Adequate studies in pregnant women have not demonstrated a risk to the fetus in the first trimester of pregnancy; there is no evidence of risk in the last two trimesters.
Category B: Animal studies have not demonstrated a risk to the fetus, but no adequate studies have been done in pregnant women.

or

Animal studies have shown an adverse effect, but adequate studies in pregnant women have not demonstrated a risk to the fetus during the first trimester of pregnancy, and there is no evidence of risk in the last two trimesters.
Category C: Animal studies have shown an adverse effect on the fetus, but no adequate studies have been done in humans. The benefits from the use of the drug in pregnant women may be acceptable despite its potential risks.

or

No animal reproduction studies and no adequate studies in humans have been done.
Category D: There is evidence of human fetal risk, but the potential benefits from the use of the drug in pregnant women may be acceptable despite its potential risks.
Category X: Studies in animals or humans or adverse reaction reports, or both, have demonstrated fetal abnormalities. The risk of use in pregnant women clearly outweighs any possible benefit.
Category ?: No data available (not a formal FDA classification; included to provide complete dataset).

BREAST-FEEDING CLASSIFICATION

No formally recognized classification exists for drugs and breast-feeding. This shorthand was developed for the *Clinician's Pocket Drug Reference.*

+   Compatible with breast-feeding
M   Monitor patient or use with caution
±   Excreted, or likely excreted, with unknown effects or at unknown concentrations
?/–   Unknown excretion, but effects likely to be of concern
–   Contraindicated in breast-feeding
?   No data available

ABBREVIATIONS

✓: check, follow, or monitor
↓: decrease/decreased
↑: increase/increased
Ab: antibody, abortion
Abd: abdominal
ABMT: autologous bone marrow transplantation
ac: before meals (*ante cibum*)
ACE: angiotensin-converting enzyme
ACH: acetylcholine
ACIP: American College of International Physicians
ACLS: advanced cardiac life support
ACS: acute coronary syndrome, American Cancer Society, American College of Surgeons
ACT: activated coagulation time
Acts: Action(s)
ADH: antidiuretic hormone
ADHD: attention-deficit hyperactivity disorder
ADR: adverse drug reaction
AF: atrial fibrillation
AHA: American Heart Association
AKA: also known as
ALL: acute lymphocytic leukemia
ALT: alanine aminotransferase
AMI: acute myocardial infarction
AML: acute myelogenous leukemia
amp: ampule
ANA: antinuclear antibody
ANC: absolute neutrophil count
APACHE: Acute physiology and chronic health evaluation
APAP: acetaminophen [*N*-acetyl-*p*-aminophenol]
aPTT: activated partial thromboplastin time
ARB: angiotensin II receptor blocker
ARDS: adult respiratory distress syndrome
ARF: acute renal failure
AS: aortic stenosis
ASA: aspirin (acetylsalicylic acid)
ASAP: as soon as possible
AST: aspartate aminotransferase
ATP: adenosine triphosphate
AUC: area under the curve
AUB: abnormal uterine/vaginal bleeding
AV: atrioventricular
AVM: arteriovenous malformation
BCL: B-cell lymphoma
BBB: bundle branch block
BPM: beats per minute
bid: twice daily
bili: bilirubin
BM: bone marrow, bowel movement
↓BM: bone marrow suppression, myelosuppression
BMD: bone mineral density
BMT: bone marrow transplantation
BOO: bladder outlet obstruction
BP: blood pressure
↓BP: hypotension
↑BP: hypertension
BPH: benign prostatic hyperplasia
BSA: body surface area
BUN: blood urea nitrogen
Ca: calcium
CA: cancer
CABG: coronary artery bypass graft

CAD: coronary artery disease

CAP: community-acquired pneumonia

caps: capsule

cardiotox: cardiotoxicity

CBC: complete blood count

CCB: calcium channel blocker

CDC: Centers for Disease Control and Prevention

CF: cystic fibrosis

CFC's: chlorofluorocarbons

CFU: colony forming units

CHD: coronary heart disease

CHF: congestive heart failure

CI: contraindicated

CIDP: Chronic inflammatory polyneuropathy

CK: creatinine kinase

CLL: chronic lymphocytic leukemia

CML: chronic myelogenous leukemia

CMV: cytomegalovirus

CNS: central nervous system

combo: combination

comp: complicated

conc: concentration

cont: continuous

COPD: chronic obstructive pulmonary disease

COX: cyclooxygenase

CP: chest pain

CPP: central precocious puberty

CR: controlled release

CRPC: castrate resistant prostate cancer

CrCl: creatinine clearance

CRF: chronic renal failure

CSF: cerebrospinal fluid

CV: cardiovascular

CVA: cerebrovascular accident, costovertebral angle

CVH: common variable hypergammaglobulinemia

CXR: chest x-ray

CYP: cytochrome P450 enzyme

÷ : divided

D: diarrhea

d: day

DA: dopamine

DBP: diastolic blood pressure

D/C: discontinue

DDP-4: Dipeptidyl peptidase-4

derm: dermatologic

D$_5$LR: 5% dextrose in lactated Ringer solution

D$_5$NS: 5% dextrose in normal saline

D$_5$W: 5% dextrose in water

DHT: dihydrotestosterone

DI: diabetes insipidus

DIC: disseminated intravascular coagulation

Disp: dispensed as; how the drug is supplied

DKA: diabetic ketoacidosis

dL: deciliter

DM: diabetes mellitus

DMARD: disease-modifying antirheumatic drug; drugs in randomized trials to decrease erosions and joint space narrowing in rheumatoid arthritis (e.g., D-penicillamine, methotrexate, azathioprine)

DN: diabetic nephropathy

DOT: directly observed therapy

DR: delayed release

d/t: due to

DVT: deep venous thrombosis

Dz: disease

EC: enteric coated

ECC: emergency cardiac care

ECG: electrocardiogram

ED: erectile dysfunction

EGFR: epidermal growth factor receptor

EIB: exercise induced bronchoconstriction

ELISA: enzyme-linked immunosorbent assay

EL.U.:ELISA

EMG: electromyelogram

EMIT: enzyme-multiplied immunoassay test

epi: epinephrine

EPS: extrapyramidal symptoms (tardive dyskinesia, tremors and rigidity, restlessness [akathisia], muscle contractions [dystonia], changes in breathing and heart rate)

ER: extended release

ESA: erythropoiesis-stimulating agents

ESRD: end-stage renal disease

ET: endotracheal

EtOH: ethanol

extrav: extravasation

FAP: familial adenomatous polyposis

Fe: iron

FSH: follicle-stimulating hormone

5-FU: fluorouracil

fam: family

Fxn: function

g: gram

GABA: gamma-aminobutyric acid

GBM: Glioblastoma multiforme

G-CSF: granulocyte colony-stimulating factor

GC: gonorrhea

gen: generation

GERD: gastroesophageal reflux disease

GF: growth factor

GFR: glomerular filtration rate

GHB: gamma-hydroxybutyrate

GI: gastrointestinal

GIST: Gastrointestinal stromal tumor

GM-CSF: granulocyte-macrophage colony-stimulating factor

GnRH: gonadotropin-releasing hormone

G6PD: glucose-6-phosphate dehydrogenase

gtt: drop, drops (*gutta*)

GU: genitourinary

GVHD: graft-versus-host disease

h: hour(s)

H1N1: swine flu strain

HA: headache

HAE: hereditary angioedema

HBsAg: hepatitis B surface antigen

HBV: hepatitis B virus

HCL: hairy cell leukemia

HCM: hypercalcemia of malignancy

Hct: hematocrit

HCTZ: hydrochlorothiazide

HD: hemodialysis

HDL-C: high density lipoprotein cholesterol

hep: hepatitis

hepatotox: hepatotoxicity

HFA: hydrofluroalkane chemicals; propellant replacing CFC's in inhalers

Hgb: hemoglobin

HGH: human growth hormone

HIT: heparin-induced thrombocytopenia

HITTS: heparin-induced thrombosis-thrombocytopenia syndrome

HIV: human immunodeficiency virus

HMG-CoA: hydroxymethylglutaryl coenzyme A

HP: high potency

HPV: human papillomavirus

HR: heart rate

↑ HR: increased heart rate (tachycardia)

hs: at bedtime (*hora somni*)

HSV: herpes simplex virus
5-HT: 5-hydroxytryptamine
HTN: hypertension
Hx: history of
IBD: irritable bowel disease
IBS: irritable bowel syndrome
IBW: ideal body weight
ICP: intracranial pressure
IFIS: intraoperative floppy iris
   syndrome
Ig: immunoglobulin
IGF: insulin-like growth factor
IHSS: idiopathic hypertropic
   subaortic stenosis
IL: interleukin
IM: intramuscular
impair: impairment
in: inches
Inf: infusion
Infxn: infection
Inh: inhalation
INH: isoniazid
inhib: inhibitor(s)
Inj: injection
INR: international normalized ratio
Insuff: insufficiency
Intravag: intravaginal
Int: international
IO: intraosseous
IOP: intraocular pressure
IR: immediate release
ISA: intrinsic sympathomimetic
   activity
IT: intrathecal
ITP: idiopathic thrombocytopenic
   purpura
Int units: international units
IUD: intrauterine device
IV: intravenous
JME: juvenile myoclonic epilepsy
JRA: juvenile rheumatoid arthritis
K/K$^+$: potassium

LA: long-acting
LABA: long-acting beta2-adrenergic
   agonists
LAIV: live attenuated influenza
   vaccine
LDL: low-density lipoprotein
LFT: liver function test
LH: luteinizing hormone
LHRH: luteinizing hormone-
   releasing hormone
liq: liquid(s)
LMW: low molecular weight
LP: lumbar puncture
LVD: left ventricular dysfunction
LVEF: left ventricular ejection
   fraction
LVSD: left ventricular systolic
   dysfunction
lytes: electrolytes
MAC: *Mycobacterium avium*
   complex
maint: maintenance dose/drug
MAO/MAOI: monoamine oxidase/
   inhibitor
max: maximum
mcg: microgram(s)
mcL: microliter(s)
MDD: major depressive disorder
MDI: multidose inhaler
MDS: myelodysplasia syndrome
meds: medicines
mEq: milliequivalent
met: metastatic
mg: milligram(s)
Mg^{2+}: magnesium
MI: myocardial infarction, mitral
   insufficiency
mill: million
min: minute(s)
mL: milliliter(s)
mo: month(s)
MoAb: monoclonal antibody

mod: moderate
MRSA: methicillin-resistant
  Staphylococcus aureus
msec: millisecond(s)
MS: multiple sclerosis,
  musculoskeletal
MSSA: methicillin-sensitive
  Staphylococcus aureus
MTT: monotetrazolium
MTX: methotrexate
MyG: myasthenia gravis
N: nausea
NA: narrow angle
NAG: narrow angle glaucoma
NCI: National Cancer Institute
nephrotox: nephrotoxicity
neurotox: neurotoxicity
ng: nanogram(s)
NG: nasogastric
NHL: non-Hodgkin lymphoma
NIAON: nonischemic arterial optic
  neuritis
nl: normal
NO: nitric oxide
NPO: nothing by mouth (*nil per os*)
NRTI: nucleoside reverse transcriptase
  inhibitor
NS: normal saline
NSAID: nonsteroidal anti-
  inflammatory drug
NSCLC: non-small cell lung cancer
N/V: nausea and vomiting
N/V/D: nausea, vomiting, diarrhea
NYHA: New York Heart Association
OA: osteoarthritis
OAB: overactive bladder
obst: obstruction
OCD: obsessive compulsive disease
OCP: oral contraceptive pill
OD: overdose
ODT: orally disintegrating tablets
OK: recommended

oint: ointment
op: operative
ophthal: ophthalmic
OSAHS: obstructive sleep apnea/
  hypopnea synd
OTC: over the counter
ototox: ototoxicity
oz: ounces
PAT: paroxysmal atrial tachycardia
pc: after eating (*post cibum*)
PCa: cancer of the prostate
PCI: percutaneous coronary
  intervention
PCN: penicillin
PCP: *Pneumocystis jiroveci* (formerly
  carinii) pneumonia
PCWP: pulmonary capillary wedge
  pressure
PDE5: phosphodiesterase type 5
PDGF: platelet-derived growth factor
PE: pulmonary embolus, physical
  examination, pleural effusion
PEA: pulseless electrical activity
PEG: polyethylene glycol
PFT: pulmonary function test
pg: picogram(s)
PGE-1: prostaglandin E-1
PGTC: primary generalized tonic-
  clonic (PGTC)
Ph: Philadelphia chromosome
photosens: photosensitivity
PI: product insert (package label)
PID: pelvic inflammatory disease
PKU: phenylketonuria
plt: platelet
PMDD: premenstrual dysphoric
  disorder
PML: progressive multifocal
  leukoencephalopathy
PMS: premenstrual syndrome
PO: by mouth (*per os*)
PPD: purified protein derivative

PPI: proton pump inhibitor
PR: by rectum
PRG: pregnancy
PRN: as often as needed (*pro re nata*)
PSA: prostate-specific antigen
PSVT: paroxysmal supraventricular
   tachycardia
pt: patient
PT: prothrombin time
PTCA: percutaneous transluminal
   coronary angioplasty
PTH: parathyroid hormone
PTSD: post-traumatic stress disorder
PTT: partial thromboplastin time
PUD: peptic ulcer disease
pulm: pulmonary
PVD: peripheral vascular disease
PVC: premature ventricular
   contraction
PWP: pulmonary wedge pressure
Px: prevention
pyelo: pyelonephritis
q: every (*quaque*)
q_h: every _ hours
q day: every day
qh: every hour
qhs: every hour of sleep
   (before bedtime)
qid: four times a day (*quater in die*)
q other day: every other day
RA: rheumatoid arthritis
RAS: renin-angiotensin system
RBC: red blood cell(s) (count)
RCC: renal cell carcinoma
RDA: recommended dietary allowance
RDS: respiratory distress syndrome
rec: recommends
resp: respiratory
RHuAb: recombinant human antibody
RIA: radioimmune assay
RLS: restless leg syndrome

R/O, r/o: rule out
RR: respiratory rate
RSI: rapid sequence intubation
RSV: respiratory syncytial virus
RT: reverse transcriptase
RTA: renal tubular acidosis
Rx: prescription or therapy
Rxn: reaction
s: second(s)
SAD: Social anxiety disorder or
   seasonal affective disorder
SAE: serious adverse event
SBE: subacute bacterial endocarditis
SBP: systolic blood pressure
SCr: serum creatinine
SCLC: small cell lung cancer
SDV: single-dose vial
SE: side effect(s)
SIADH: syndrome of inappropriate
   antidiuretic hormone
sig: significant
SIRS: systemic inflammatory response
   syndrome/capillary leak syndrome
SJS: Stevens Johnson Syndrome
SL: sublingual
SLE: systemic lupus erythematosus
SLUDGE: mnemonic for: Salivation,
   Lacrimation, Urination,
   Diaphoresis, GI motility, Emesis
SMX: sulfamethoxazole
SNRIs: serotonin-norepinephrine
   reuptake inhibitors
SOB: shortness of breath
soln: solution
sp: species
SPAG: small particle aerosol
   generator
SQ: subcutaneous
SR: sustained release
SSRI: selective serotonin reuptake
   inhibitor

SSS: sick sinus syndrome
S/Sxs: signs & symptoms
stat: immediately (*statim*)
STD: sexually transmitted disease
supl: supplement
supp: suppository
susp: suspension
SVT: supraventricular tachycardia
SWSD: shift work sleep disorder
synth: synthesis
Sx: symptom
Sz: seizure
tab/tabs: tablet/tablets
TB: tuberculosis
TCA: tricyclic antidepressant
TFT: thyroid function test
TIA: transient ischemic attack
TID: three times a day (*ter in die*)
TIV: trivalent influenza vaccine
TKI: tyrosine kinase inhibitors
TMP: trimethoprim
TMP—SMX: trimethoprim—
    sulfamethoxazole
TNF: tumor necrosis factor
tox: toxicity
TPA: tissue plasminogen activator
TRALI: transfusion related acute
    lung injury
TSH: thyroid stimulation hormone
tri: trimester
TTP: thrombotic thrombocytopenic
    purpura
TTS: transdermal therapeutic system

Tx: treatment
UGT: uridine 5′
    diphosphoglucuronosyl transferase
UC: ulcerative colitis
ULN: upper limits of normal
uncomp: uncomplicated
URI: upper respiratory infection
US: United States
UTI: urinary tract infection
V: vomiting
VAERS: Vaccine Adverse Events
    Reporting System
Vag: vaginal
VLDL: very low density lipoprotein
VEGF: vascular endothelial growth
    factor
VF: ventricular fibrillation
vit: vitamin
VOD: venoocclusive disease
vol: volume
VPA: valproic acid
VRE: vancomycin-resistant
    Enterococcus
VT: ventricular tachycardia
WBC: white blood cell(s) (count)
Wgt: weight
WHI: Women's Health Initiative
wk: week(s)
WNL: within normal limits
WPW: Wolff-Parkinson-White
    syndrome
XR: extended release
ZE: Zollinger-Ellison (syndrome)

CLASSIFICATION (Generic and common brand names)

ALLERGY

Antihistamines

Azelastine (Astelin, Optivar)
Cetirizine (Zyrtec, Zyrtec D)
Chlorpheniramine (Chlor-Trimeton)
Clemastine Fumarate (Tavist)
Cyproheptadine (Periactin)
Desloratadine (Clarinex)
Diphenhydramine (Benadryl)
Fexofenadine (Allegra)
Hydroxyzine (Atarax, Vistaril)
Levocetirizine (Xyzal)
Loratadine (Alavert, Claritin)

Miscellaneous Antiallergy Agents

Budesonide (Rhinocort, Pulmicort)
Cromolyn Sodium (Intal, NasalCrom, Opticrom)
Montelukast (Singulair)
Phenylephrine, oral (Sudafed PE, SudoGest PE, Nasop, Lusonal, AH-chew D, Sudafed PE quick dissolve)

ANTIDOTES

Acetylcysteine (Acetadote, Mucomyst)
Amifostine (Ethyol)
Atropine, systemic (AtroPen Auto-injector)
Atropine/pralidoxime (DuoDote)
Charcoal (SuperChar, Actidose, Liqui-Char Activated)
Deferasirox (Exjade)
Dexrazoxane (Totect, Zinecard)
Digoxin Immune Fab (Digibind, DigiFab)
Flumazenil (Romazicon)
Hydroxocobalamin (Cyanokit)
Ipecac Syrup (OTC Syrup)
Mesna (Mesnex)
Naloxone (generic)
Physostigmine (Antilirium)
Succimer (Chemet)

1

ANTIMICROBIAL AGENTS

Antibiotics

AMINOGLYCOSIDES

Amikacin (Amikin)
Gentamicin (Garamycin, G-Mycitin)
Neomycin sulfate (Neofradin, generic)
Streptomycin
Tobramycin (Nebcin)

CARBAPENEMS

Doripenem (Doribax)
Ertapenem (Invanz)
Imipenem-Cilastatin (Primaxin)
Meropenem (Merrem)

CEPHALOSPORINS, FIRST GENERATION

Cefadroxil (Duricef, Ultracef)
Cefazolin (Ancef, Kefzol)
Cephalexin (Keflex, Panixine DisperDose)
Cephradine (Velosef)

CEPHALOSPORINS, SECOND GENERATION

Cefaclor (Ceclor, Raniclor)
Cefotetan (Cefotan)
Cefoxitin (Mefoxin)
Cefprozil (Cefzil)
Cefuroxime (Ceftin [oral], Zinacef [parenteral])

CEPHALOSPORINS, THIRD GENERATION

Cefdinir (Omnicef)
Cefditoren (Spectracef)
Cefixime (Suprax)
Cefoperazone (Cefobid)
Cefotaxime (Claforan)
Cefpodoxime (Vantin)
Ceftazidime (Fortaz, Ceptaz, Tazidime, Tazicef)
Ceftibuten (Cedax)
Ceftizoxime (Cefizox)
Ceftriaxone (Rocephin)

CEPHALOSPORINS, FOURTH GENERATION

Cefepime (Maxipime)

FLUOROQUINOLONES

Ciprofloxacin (Cipro, Cipro XR, Proquin XR)
Gemifloxacin (Factive)
Levofloxacin (Levaquin)
Moxifloxacin (Avelox)
Norfloxacin (Noroxin, Chibroxin ophthalmic)
Ofloxacin (Floxin)

MACROLIDES

Azithromycin (Zithromax)
Clarithromycin (Biaxin, Biaxin XL)

Erythromycin (E-Mycin, E.E.S., Ery-Tab, EryPed, Ilotycin)

Erythromycin & Sulfisoxazole (Eryzole, Pediazole)

KETOLIDE

Telithromycin (Ketek)

PENICILLINS

Amoxicillin (Amoxil, Polymox)
Amoxicillin & Clavulanic Acid (Augmentin, Augmentin 600 ES, Augmentin XR)
Ampicillin (Amcill, Omnipen)
Ampicillin-Sulbactam (Unasyn)
Dicloxacillin (Dynapen, Dycill)

Nafcillin (Nallpen, Unipen)
Oxacillin (Bactocill, Prostaphlin)
Penicillin G, Aqueous (Potassium or Sodium) (Pfizerpen, Pentids)
Penicillin G Benzathine (Bicillin)

Penicillin G Procaine (Wycillin, others)
Penicillin V (Pen-Vee K, Veetids, others)
Piperacillin (Pipracil)
Piperacillin-Tazobactam (Zosyn)
Ticarcillin/Potassium Clavulanate (Timentin)

TETRACYCLINES

Doxycycline (Adoxa, Periostat, Oracea, Vibramycin, Vibra-Tabs)

Minocycline (Dynacin, Minocin, Solodyn)
Tetracycline (Achromycin V, Sumycin)

Tigecycline (Tygacil)

Miscellaneous Antibiotic Agents

Aztreonam (Azactam)
Clindamycin (Cleocin, Cleocin-T, others)
Fosfomycin (Monurol)
Linezolid (Zyvox)
Metronidazole (Flagyl, MetroGel)

Mupirocin (Bactroban, Bactroban Nasal)
Neomycin topical (see Bacitracin, Neomycin, & Polymyxin B, Topical [Neosporin Ointment], Bacitracin,

Neomycin, Polymyxin B, & Hydrocortisone, Topical [Cortisporin], Bacitracin, Neomycin, Polymyxin B, & Lidocaine, Topical [Clomycin])

Nitrofurantoin (Furadantin, Macrodantin, Macrobid)

Quinupristin-Dalfopristin (Synercid)

Rifaximin (Xifaxan)

Retapamulin (Altabax)

Telavancin (Vibativ)

Trimethoprim (Primsol, Proloprim)

Trimethoprim (TMP)–Sulfamethoxazole

(SMX) [Co-Trimoxazole, TMP-SMX] (Bactrim, Septra)

Vancomycin (Vancocin, Vancoled)

Antifungals

Amphotericin B (Amphocin, Fungizone)

Amphotericin B Cholesteryl (Amphotec)

Amphotericin B Lipid Complex (Abelcet)

Amphotericin B Liposomal (AmBisome)

Anidulafungin (Eraxis)

Caspofungin (Cancidas)

Clotrimazole (Lotrimin, Mycelex, others OTC)

Clotrimazole & Betamethasone (Lotrisone)

Econazole (Spectazole)

Fluconazole (Diflucan)

Itraconazole (Sporanox)

Ketoconazole, oral (Nizoral)

Ketoconazole, topical (Extina, Kuric, Xolegel, Nizoral AD Shampoo) [Shampoo–OTC]

Miconazole (Monistat 1 combo, Monistat 3,

Monistat 7) [OTC] (Monistat-Derm)

Nystatin (Mycostatin)

Oxiconazole (Oxistat)

Posaconazole (Noxafil)

Sertaconazole (Ertaczo)

Terbinafine (Lamisil, Lamisil AT)

Triamcinolone & Nystatin (Mycolog-II)

Voriconazole (VFEND)

Antimycobacterials

Dapsone, oral

Ethambutol (Myambutol)

Isoniazid (INH)

Pyrazinamide (generic)

Rifabutin (Mycobutin)

Rifampin (Rifadin)

Rifapentine (Priftin)

Streptomycin

Antiparasitics

Benzyl Alcohol (Ulesfia)

Lindane (Kwell, others)

Antiprotozoals

Artemether & Lumefantrine (Coartem)

Atovaquone (Mepron)

Atovaquone/Proguanil (Malarone)

Nitazoxanide (Alinia)

Tinidazole (Tindamax)

Antiretrovirals

Abacavir (Ziagen)
Daptomycin (Cubicin)
Darunavir (Prezista)
Delavirdine (Rescriptor)
Didanosine [ddI] (Videx)
Efavirenz (Sustiva)
Efavirenz/emtricitabine/
tenofovir (Atripla)
Etravirine (Intelence)
Fosamprenavir (Lexiva)
Indinavir (Crixivan)

Lamivudine (Epivir,
Epivir-HBV, 3 TC
[many combo
regimens])
Lopinavir/Ritonavir
(Kaletra)
Maraviroc (Selzentry)
Nelfinavir (Viracept)
Nevirapine (Viramune)
Raltegravir (Isentress)
Ritonavir (Norvir)

Saquinavir (Fortovase,
Invirase)
Stavudine (Zerit)
Tenofovir (Viread)
Tenofovir/Emtricitabine
(Truvada)
Zidovudine (Retrovir)
Zidovudine &
Lamivudine
(Combivir)

Antivirals

Acyclovir (Zovirax)
Adefovir (Hepsera)
Amantadine (Symmetrel)
Atazanavir (Reyataz)
Cidofovir (Vistide)
Emtricitabine (Emtriva)
Enfuvirtide (Fuzeon)
Famciclovir (Famvir)
Foscarnet (Foscavir)

Ganciclovir (Cytovene,
Vitrasert)
Interferon Alfa-2b &
Ribavirin Combo
(Rebetron)
Oseltamivir (Tamiflu)
Palivizumab (Synagis)
Peg Interferon Alfa 2a
(Peg Intron)

Penciclovir (Denavir)
Ribavirin (Virazole,
Copegus)
Rimantadine
(Flumadine)
Telbivudine (Tyzeka)
Valacyclovir (Valtrex)
Valganciclovir (Valcyte)
Zanamivir (Relenza)

Miscellaneous Antiviral Agents

Daptomycin (Cubicin)
Pentamidine (Pentam
300, NebuPent)

Trimetrexate
(NeuTrexin)

ANTINEOPLASTIC AGENTS

Alkylating Agents

Altretamine (Hexalen)
Bendamustine (Treanda)
Busulfan (Myleran,
Busulfex)
Carboplatin (Paraplatin)

Cisplatin (Platinol,
Platinol AQ)
Oxaliplatin (Eloxatin)
Procarbazine (Matulane)
Tapentadol (Nucynta)

Thiotriethylene-
phosphoramide
(Thiotepa, Thioplex,
Tespa, TSPA)

NITROGEN MUSTARDS

Chlorambucil (Leukeran)
Cyclophosphamide
(Cytoxan, Neosar)

Ifosfamide (Ifex,
Holoxan)
Mechlorethamine
(Mustargen)

Melphalan [L-PAM]
(Alkeran)

NITROSOUREAS

Carmustine [BCNU]
(BiCNU, Gliadel)

Streptozocin (Zanosar)

Antibiotics

Bleomycin Sulfate
(Blenoxane)
Dactinomycin
(Cosmegen)

Daunorubicin
(Daunomycin,
Cerubidine)
Doxorubicin
(Adriamycin, Rubex)

Epirubicin (Ellence)
Idarubicin (Idamycin)
Mitomycin (Mutamycin)

Antimetabolites

Clofarabine (Clolar)
Cytarabine [ARA-C]
(Cytosar-U)
Cytarabine Liposome
(DepoCyt)
Floxuridine (FUDR)
Fludarabine Phosphate
(Flamp, Fludara)
Fluorouracil [5-FU]
(Adrucil)

Fluorouracil, Topical
[5-FU] (Efudex)
Gemcitabine (Gemzar)
Mercaptopurine [6-MP]
(Purinethol)
Methotrexate
(Rheumatrex Dose
Pack, Trexall)
Nelarabine (Arranon)
Pemetrexed (Alimta)

Pralatrexate (Folotyn)
Romidepsin (Istodax)
6-Thioguanine [6-TG]
(Tabloid)

Hormones

Anastrozole (Arimidex)
Bicalutamide (Casodex)
Degarelix (Firmagon)
Estramustine Phosphate
(Emcyt)
Exemestane (Aromasin)
Flutamide (Eulexin)

Fulvestrant (Faslodex)
Goserelin (Zoladex)
Leuprolide (Lupron,
Lupron DEPOT,
Lupron DEPOT-Ped,
Viadur, Eligard)

Megestrol Acetate
(Megace, Megace-ES)
Nilutamide (Nilandron)
Tamoxifen
Triptorelin (Trelstar
3.75, Trelstar 11.25,
Trelstar 22.5)

Mitotic Inhibitors (Vinca alkaloids)

Etoposide [VP-16]
(VePesid, Toposar)
Vinblastine (Velban,
Velbe)

Vincristine (Oncovin,
Vincasar PFS)
Vinorelbine (Navelbine)

Monoclonal Antibodies

Bevacizumab (Avastin)
Cetuximab (Erbitux)
Erlotinib (Tarceva)

Gemtuzumab
Ozogamicin
(Mylotarg)
Lapatinib (Tykerb)

Ofatumumab (Arzerra)
Panitumumab (Vectibix)
Trastuzumab (Herceptin)

Proteasome inhibitor

Bortezomib (Velcade)

Taxanes

Cabazitaxel (Jevtana)
Docetaxel (Taxotere)

Paclitaxel (Taxol,
Abraxane)

Tyrosine Kinase Inhibitors (TKI)

Dasatinib (Sprycel)
Everolimus (Afinitor)
Gefitinib (Iressa)
Imatinib (Gleevec)

Nilotinib (Tasigna)
Pazopanib hydrochloride
(Votrient)
Sorafenib (Nexavar)

Sunitinib (Sutent)
Temsirolimus (Torisel)

Miscellaneous Antineoplastic Agents

Aldesleukin
[Interleukin-2, IL-2]
(Proleukin)
Aminoglutethimide
(Cytadren)
L-Asparaginase (Elspar,
Oncaspar)
BCG [Bacillus Calmette-
Guérin] (TheraCys,
Tice BCG)
Cladribine (Leustatin)

Dacarbazine (DTIC)
Hydroxyurea (Hydrea,
Droxia)
Irinotecan (Camptosar)
Ixabepilone Kit
(Ixempra)
Letrozole (Femara)
Leucovorin
(Wellcovorin)
Mitoxantrone
(Novantrone)

Panitumumab (Vectibix)
Pemetrexed (Alimta)
Rasburicase (Elitek)
sipuleucel-T (Provenge)
Thalidomide(Thalomid)
Topotecan (Hycamtin)
Tretinoin, Topical
[Retinoic Acid]
(Retin-A, Avita,
Renova, Retin-A
Micro)

CARDIOVASCULAR (CV) AGENTS

Aldosterone Antagonist

Eplerenone (Inspra)

Spironolactone
(Aldactone)

Alpha₁-Adrenergic Blockers

Doxazosin (Cardura,
Cardura XL)

Prazosin (Minipress)
Terazosin (Hytrin)

Angiotensin-Converting Enzyme (ACE) Inhibitors

Benazepril (Lotensin)
Captopril (Capoten,
others)
Enalapril (Vasotec)
Fosinopril (Monopril)

Lisinopril (Prinivil,
Zestril)
Moexipril (Univasc)
Perindopril Erbumine
(Aceon)

Quinapril (Accupril)
Ramipril (Altace)
Trandolapril (Mavik)

Angiotensin II Receptor Antagonists/Blockers

Amlodipine/Olmesartan
(Azor)
Amlodipine/Valsartan
(Exforge)

Candesartan (Atacand)
Eprosartan (Teveten)
Irbesartan (Avapro)
Losartan (Cozaar)

Telmisartan (Micardis)
Valsartan (Diovan)

Antiarrhythmic Agents

Adenosine (Adenocard)
Amiodarone (Cordarone,
Nexterone, Pacerone)
Atropine, systemic
(AtroPen Auto-
injector)
Digoxin (Digitek,
Lanoxin, Lanoxicaps)
Disopyramide (Norpace,
Norpace CR)

Dronedarone (Multaq)
Dofetilide (Tikosyn)
Esmolol (Brevibloc)
Flecainide (Tambocor)
Ibutilide (Corvert)
Lidocaine, systemic
(Xylocaine, others)
Mexiletine (Mexitil)

Procainamide (Pronestyl,
Pronestyl SR,
Procanbid)
Propafenone (Rythmol)
Quinidine (Quinidex,
Quinaglute)
Sotalol (Betapace,
Betapace AF)

Beta-Adrenergic Blockers

Acebutolol (Sectral)
Atenolol (Tenormin)

Atenolol &
Chlorthalidone
(Tenoretic)

Betaxolol (Kerlone)
Bisoprolol (Zebeta)

Carvedilol (Coreg, Coreg CR)
Labetalol (Trandate, Normodyne)
Metoprolol succinate (Toprol XL),
Metoprolol tartrate (Lopressor)
Nadolol (Corgard)
Nebivolol (Bystolic)
Penbutolol (Levatol)
Pindolol (Visken)
Propranolol (Inderal)
Timolol (Blocadren)

Calcium Channel Antagonists/Blockers (CCB)

Amlodipine (Norvasc)
Amlodipine/Olmesartan (Azor)
Amlodipine/Valsartan (Exforge)
Clevidipine (Cleviprex)
Diltiazem (Cardizem, Cardizem CD,
Cardizem LA, Cardizem SR, Cartia XT, Dilacor XR, Diltia XT, Taztia XT, Tiamate, Tiazac)
Felodipine (Plendil)
Isradipine (DynaCirc)
Nicardipine (Cardene)
Nifedipine (Procardia, Procardia XL, Adalat CC)
Nimodipine (Nimotop)
Nisoldipine (Sular)
Verapamil (Calan, Caover HS, Isoptin, Verelan)

Centrally Acting Antihypertensive Agents

Clonidine, oral (Catapres)
Clonidine, transdermal (Catapres TTS)
Methyldopa (Aldomet)

Combination Antihypertensive Agents

Amlodipine/Valsartan/ HCTZ (Exforge HCT)
Lisinopril and hydrochlorothiazide (Prinzide, Zestoretic, generic)

Diuretics

Acetazolamide (Diamox)
Amiloride (Midamor)
Bumetanide (Bumex)
Chlorothiazide (Diuril)
Chlorthalidone (Hygroton, others)
Furosemide (Lasix)
Hydrochlorothiazide (HydroDIURIL, Esidrix, others)
Hydrochlorothiazide & Amiloride (Moduretic)
Hydrochlorothiazide & Spironolactone (Aldactazide)
Hydrochlorothiazide & Triamterene (Dyazide, Maxzide)
Indapamide (Lozol)
Mannitol (various)
Metolazone (Zaroxolyn)
Spironolactone (Aldactone)
Torsemide (Demadex)
Triamterene (Dyrenium)

Inotropic/Pressor Agents

Digoxin (Digitek, Lanoxin, Lanoxicaps)
Dobutamine (Dobutrex)
Dopamine (Intropin)
Epinephrine (Adrenalin, Sus-Phrine, EpiPen, EpiPen jr, others)

Inamrinone [Amrinone] (Inocor)
Isoproterenol (Isuprel)
Milrinone (Primacor)
Nesiritide (Natrecor)
Norepinephrine (Levophed)

Phenylephrine, systemic (Neo-Synephrine)

Lipid-Lowering Agents

Colesevelam (WelChol)
Colestipol (Colestid)
Cholestyramine (Questran, Questran Light, Prevalite)
Ezetimibe (Zetia)
Fenofibrate (TriCor, Antara, Lofibra, Lipofen, Triglide)

Fenofibric acid (Trilipix)
Gemfibrozil (Lopid)
Niacin (Nicotinic acid) (Niaspan, Slo-Niacin, Niacor, Nicolar) [OTC forms]
Niacin and Lovastatin (Advicor)

Niacin and Simvastatin (Simcor)
Omega-3 fatty acid [fish oil] (Lovaza)

Statins

Atorvastatin (Lipitor)
Fluvastatin (Lescol)
Lovastatin (Mevacor, Altoprev)

Pitavastatin (Livalo)
Pravastatin (Pravachol)
Rosuvastatin (Crestor)
Simvastatin (Zocor)

Lipid-Lowering/Antihypertensive Combos

Amlodipine/Atorvastatin (Caduet)

Vasodilators

Alprostadil [Prostaglandin E$_1$] (Prostin VR)
Epoprostenol (Flolan)
Fenoldopam (Corlopam)
Hydralazine (Apresoline, others)

Iloprost (Ventavis)
Isosorbide Dinitrate (Isordil, Sorbitrate, Dilatrate-SR)
Isosorbide Mononitrate (Ismo, Imdur)
Minoxidil, oral

Nitroglycerin (Nitrostat, Nitrolingual, Nitro-Bid Ointment, Nitro-Bid IV, Nitrodisc, Transderm-Nitro, NitroMist, others)

Nitroprusside (Nipride, Nitropress)
Tolazoline (Priscoline)

Treprostinil Sodium (Remodulin, Tyvaso)

Miscellaneous Cardiovascular Agents

Aliskiren (Tekturna)
Aliskiren/ Hydrochlorothiazide (Tekturna HCT)

Ambrisentan (Letairis)
Conivaptan (Vaprisol)
Prasugrel hydrochloride (Effient)

Ranolazine (Ranexa)
Sildenafil (Viagra, Revatio)

CENTRAL NERVOUS SYSTEM AGENTS

Antianxiety Agents

Alprazolam (Xanax, Niravam)
Buspirone (BuSpar)
Chlordiazepoxide (Librium, Mitran, Libritabs)

Diazepam (Diastat, Valium)
Doxepin (Sinequan, Adapin)
Hydroxyzine (Atarax, Vistaril)

Lorazepam (Ativan, others)
Meprobamate (various)
Oxazepam

Anticonvulsants

Carbamazepine (Tegretol XR, Carbatrol, Epitol, Equetro)
Clonazepam (Klonopin)
Diazepam (Diastat, Valium)
Ethosuximide (Zarontin)
Fosphenytoin (Cerebyx)
Gabapentin (Neurontin)
Lacosamide (Vimpat)

Lamotrigine (Lamictal)
Levetiracetam (Keppra)
Lorazepam (Ativan, others)
Magnesium sulfate (various)
Oxcarbazepine (Trileptal)
Pentobarbital (Nembutal, others)

Phenobarbital
Phenytoin (Dilantin)
Rufinamide (Banzel)
Tiagabine (Gabitril)
Topiramate (Topamax)
Valproic Acid (Depakene, Depakote)
Vigabatrin (Sabril)
Zonisamide (Zonegran)

Antidepressants

Amitriptyline (Elavil)
Bupropion hydrobromide (Aplenzin)
Bupropion hydrochloride (Wellbutrin, Wellbutrin SR, Wellbutrin XL, Zyban)

Citalopram (Celexa)
Desipramine (Norpramin)
Desvenlafaxine (Pristiq)
Doxepin (Adapin)
Duloxetine (Cymbalta)
Escitalopram (Lexapro)

Fluoxetine (Prozac, Sarafem)
Fluvoxamine (Luvox)
Imipramine (Tofranil)
Milnacipran(Savella)
Mirtazapine (Remeron, Remeron SolTab)
Nefazodone (Serzone)

Nortriptyline (Pamelor)
Paroxetine (Paxil, Paxil CR, Pexeva)
Phenelzine (Nardil)

Selegiline transdermal (Emsam)
Sertraline (Zoloft)
Trazodone (Desyrel)

Venlafaxine (Effexor, Effexor XR)

Antiparkinson Agents

Amantadine (Symmetrel)
Apomorphine (Apokyn)
Benztropine (Cogentin)
Bromocriptine (Parlodel)
Carbidopa/Levodopa (Sinemet, Parcopa)
Entacapone (Comtan)

Pramipexole (Mirapex)
Rasagiline mesylate (Azilect)
Rivastigmine transdermal (Exelon Patch)
Ropinirole (Requip)

Selegiline (Eldepryl, Zelapar)
Tolcapone (Tasmar)
Trihexyphenidyl

Antipsychotics

Aripiprazole (Abilify, Abilify Discmelt)
Asenapine maleate (Saphris)
Chlorpromazine (Thorazine)
Clozapine (Clozaril, FazaClo)
Haloperidol (Haldol)
Iloperidone (Fanapt)
Lithium Carbonate (Eskalith, Lithobid, others)

Molindone (Moban)
Olanzapine (Zyprexa, Zyprexa Zydis)
Paliperidone (Invega)
Perphenazine (Trilafon)
Pimozide (Orap)
Prochlorperazine (Compazine)
Quetiapine (Seroquel, Seroquel XR)
Risperidone, oral (Risperdal, Risperdal

Consta, Risperdal M-Tab)
Risperidone, parenteral (Risperdal Consta)
Thioridazine (Mellaril)
Thiothixene (Navane)
Trifluoperazine (Stelazine)
Ziprasidone (Geodon)

Sedative Hypnotics

Chloral Hydrate (Aquachloral, Supprettes)
Diphenhydramine (Benadryl OTC)
Estazolam (ProSom)
Eszopiclone (Lunesta)
Flurazepam (Dalmane)

Hydroxyzine (Atarax, Vistaril)
Midazolam (various) [C-IV]
Pentobarbital (Nembutal, others)
Phenobarbital
Propofol (Diprivan)

Secobarbital (Seconal)
Temazepam (Restoril)
Triazolam (Halcion)
Zaleplon (Sonata)
Zolpidem (Ambien IR, Ambien CR, Edluar, ZolpiMist)

Stimulants

Armodafinil (Nuvigil)
Atomoxetine (Strattera)
Lisdexamfetamine
(Vyvanse)
Methylphenidate, oral
(Concerta, Metadate

CD, Methylin Ritalin,
Ritalin LA, Ritalin
SR, others)
Methylphenidate,
Transdermal
(Daytrana)

Modafinil (Provigil)
Sibutramine (Meridia)

Miscellaneous CNS Agents

Donepezil (Aricept)
Galantamine (Razadyne)
Interferon beta 1a
(Rebif)
Meclizine (Antivert)
(Bonine, Dramamine
OTC)

Memantine (Namenda)
Natalizumab (Tysabri)
Nimodipine (Nimotop)
Rizatriptan (Maxalt,
Maxalt MLT)
Sodium Oxybate
(Xyrem)

Tacrine (Cognex)

DERMATOLOGIC AGENTS

Acitretin (Soriatane)
Acyclovir (Zovirax)
Adapalene & Benzoyl
Peroxide (Epiduo Gel)
Alefacept (Amevive)
Anthralin (Anthra-Derm)
Amphotericin B
(Amphocin,
Fungizone)
Bacitracin, Topical
(Baciguent)
Bacitracin & Polymyxin
B, Topical
(Polysporin)
Bacitracin, Neomycin, &
Polymyxin B, Topical
(Neosporin Ointment)
Bacitracin, Neomycin,
Polymyxin B, &
Hydrocortisone,
Topical (Cortisporin)

Bacitracin, Neomycin,
Polymyxin B, &
Lidocaine, Topical
(Clomycin)
Botulinum Toxin Type A
[OnabotulinumtoxinA]
(Botox, Botox
Cosmetic, Myobloc,
Dysport)
Calcipotriene (Dovonex)
Calcitriol ointment
(Vectical)
Capsaicin (Capsin,
Zostrix, others)
Ciclopirox (Loprox,
Penlac)
Ciprofloxacin (Cipro,
Cipro XR, Proquin
XR)
Clindamycin (Cleocin,
Cleocin T, others)

Clotrimazole &
Betamethasone
(Lotrisone)
Dapsone Topical
(Aczone)
Dibucaine (Nupercainal)
Doxepin, Topical
(Zonalon, Prudoxin)
Econazole (Spectazole)
Erythromycin, Topical
(A/T/S, Eryderm,
Erycette, T-Stat)
Erythromycin & Benzoyl
Peroxide
(Benzamycin)
Finasteride (Propecia)
Fluorouracil, Topical
[5-FU] (Efudex)
Gentamicin, Topical
(Garamycin,
G-Mycitin)

Imiquimod Cream, 5% (Aldara)

Isotretinoin [13-*cis* Retinoic acid] (Accutane, Amnesteem, Claravis, Sotret)

Ketoconazole (Nizoral)

Kunecatechins [sinecatechins] (Veregen)

Lactic Acid & Ammonium Hydroxide [Ammonium Lactate] (Lac-Hydrin)

Lindane (Kwell, others)

Metronidazole (Flagyl, MetroGel)

Miconazole (Monistat 1 Combo, Monistat 3, Monistat 7)[OTC] (Monistat-Derm) Miconazole/

zinc oxide/petrolatum (Vusion)

Minocycline (Dynacin, Minocin, Solodyn)

Minoxidil, topical (Theroxidil, Rogaine) [OTC]

Mupirocin (Bactroban, Bactroban Nasal)

Naftifine (Naftin)

Nystatin (Mycostatin)

Oxiconazole (Oxistat)

Penciclovir (Denavir)

Permethrin (Nix, Elimite)

Pimecrolimus (Elidel)

Podophyllin (Podocon-25, Condylox Gel 0.5%, Condylox)

Pramoxine (Anusol Ointment, ProctoFoam-NS)

Pramoxine & Hydro-cortisone (Enzone, ProctoFoam-HC)

Selenium Sulfide (Exsel Shampoo, Selsun Blue Shampoo, Selsun Shampoo)

Silver Sulfadiazine (Silvadene, others)

Steroids, Topical (Table 3, page 266)

Tacrolimus [FK506] (Prograf, Protopic)

Tazarotene (Tazorac, Avage)

Terbinafine (Lamisil, Lamasil AT [OTC])

Tolnaftate (Tinactin, others [OTC])

Tretinoin, Topical [Retinoic Acid] (Avita Retin-A, Retin-A Micro, Renova)

Ustekinumab (Stelara)

Vorinostat (Zolinza)

DIETARY SUPPLEMENTS

Calcium Acetate (Calphron, Phos-Ex, PhosLo)

Calcium Glubionate (Neo-Calglucon)

Calcium Salts [Chloride, Gluconate, Gluceptate]

Cholecalciferol [Vitamin D_3] (Delta D)

Cyanocobalamin [Vitamin B_{12}] (Nascobal)

Ferric Gluconate Complex (Ferrlecit)

Ferrous Gluconate (Fergon [OTC], others)

Ferrous Sulfate

Ferumoxytol (Feraheme)

Fish Oil (Lovaza, others OTC)

Folic Acid

Iron Dextran (Dexferrum, INFeD)

Iron Sucrose (Venofer)

Magnesium Oxide (Mag-Ox 400, others [OTC])

Magnesium Sulfate (various)

Multivitamins, oral [OTC] (Table 12, page 283)

Phytonadione [Vitamin K] (Aqua-MEPHYTON, others)

Potassium Supplements (See Table 6, page 276)

Pyridoxine [Vitamin B_6]

Sodium Bicarbonate [NaHCO$_3$]

Thiamine [Vitamin B_1]

EAR (OTIC) AGENTS

Acetic Acid &
  Aluminum Acetate
  (Otic Domeboro)
Benzocaine &
  Antipyrine (Auralgan)
Ciprofloxacin, otic
  (Cetraxal)
Ciprofloxacin &
  dexamethasone, Otic
  (Ciprodex Otic)
Ciprofloxacin &
  hydrocortisone, Otic
  (Cipro HC Otic)

Neomycin, Colistin, &
  Hydrocortisone
  (Cortisporin-TC Otic
  Drops)
Neomycin, Colistin,
  Hydrocortisone, &
  Thonzonium
  (Cortisporin-TC Otic
  Suspension)
Ofloxacin otic (Floxin
  Otic, Floxin Otic
  Singles)

Polymyxin B &
  Hydrocortisone
  (Otobiotic Otic)
Sulfacetamide &
  Prednisolone
  (Blephamide, others)
Triethanolamine
  (Cerumenex [OTC])

ENDOCRINE SYSTEM AGENTS

Antidiabetic Agents

Acarbose (Precose)
Bromocriptine mesylate
  (Cycloset)
Chlorpropamide
  (Diabinese)
Exenatide (Byetta)
Glimepiride (Amaryl)
Glimepiride/pioglitazone
  (Duetact)
Glipizide(Glucotrol,
  Glucotrol XL)

Glyburide (DiaBeta,
  Micronase, Glynase)
Glyburide/Metformin
  (Glucovance)
Insulins, injectable
  (Table 4, page 269)
Metformin (Glucophage,
  Glucophage XR)
Miglitol (Glyset)
Nateglinide (Starlix)
Pioglitazone (Actos)

Pioglitazone/Metformin
  (ACTOplus Met)
Repaglinide (Prandin)
Rosiglitazone (Avandia)
Sitagliptin/Metformin
  (Janumet)
Tolazamide (Tolinase)
Tolbutamide (Orinase)

DPP-4 INHIBITORS

Saxagliptin (Onglyza)
Sitagliptin (Januvia)

Sitagliptin/Metformin
  (Janumet)

Hormone & Synthetic Substitutes

Calcitonin (Fortical,
  Miacalcin)
Calcitriol (Rocaltrol,
  Calcijex)

Cortisone Systemic and
  Topical (See Tables
  2 p 265 and 3 p 266)
Desmopressin (DDAVP,
  Stimate)

Dexamethasone,
  systemic and topical
  (Decadron)
Fludrocortisone Acetate
  (Florinef)

Fluoxymesterone
   (Halotestin, Androxy)
Glucagon
Hydrocortisone Topical
   & Systemic (Cortef,
   Solu-Cortef)

Methylprednisolone
   (Solu-Medrol)
Prednisolone
Prednisone
Testosterone (AndroGel,
   Androderm, Striant,
   Testim)

Vasopressin [Antidiuretic
   Hormone, ADH]
   (Pitressin)

Hypercalcemia/Osteoporosis Agents

Alendronate (Fosamax,
   Fosamax Plus D)
Denosumab (Prolia)
Etidronate Disodium
   (Didronel)
Gallium Nitrate (Ganite)

Ibandronate (Boniva)
Pamidronate (Aredia)
Raloxifene (Evista)
Risedronate (Actonel,
   Actonel w/calcium)
Teriparatide (Forteo)

Zoledronic acid (Zometa,
   Reclast)

Obesity

Orlistat (Xenical, Alli
   [OTC])

Sibutramine (Meridia)

Thyroid/Antithyroid

Levothyroxine
   (Synthroid, Levoxyl,
   others)
Liothyronine (Cytomel,
   Triostat, T_3)

Methimazole (Tapazole)
Potassium Iodide [Lugol
   Soln] (SSKI, Thyro-
   Block, Thyro Safe,
   ThyroShield)

Propylthiouracil [PTU]

Miscellaneous Endocrine Agents

Cinacalcet (Sensipar)
Demeclocycline
   (Declomycin)

Diazoxide (Proglycem)

EYE (OPHTHALMIC) AGENTS
Glaucoma Agents

Acetazolamide (Diamox)
Apraclonidine (Iopidine)
Betaxolol, Ophthalmic
   (Betoptic)

Brimonidine
   (Alphagan P)
Brimonidine/Timolol
   (Combigan)

Brinzolamide (Azopt)
Carteolol (Ocupress,
   Carteolol Ophthalmic)
Dipivefrin (Propine)

Dorzolamide
  (Trusopt)
Dorzolamide & Timolol
  (Cosopt)

Echothiophate Iodine
  (Phospholine
  Ophthalmic)
Latanoprost (Xalatan)

Levobunolol (A-K Beta,
  Betagan)
Timolol, Ophthalmic
  (Timoptic)

Ophthalmic Antibiotics

Azithromycin
  Ophthalmic
  1%(AzaSite)
Bacitracin, Ophthalmic
  (AK-Tracin
  Ophthalmic)
Bacitracin & Polymyxin
  B, Ophthalmic (AK-
  Poly-Bac Ophthalmic,
  Polysporin
  Ophthalmic)
Bacitracin, Neomycin, &
  Polymyxin B (AK
  Spore Ophthalmic,
  Neosporin
  Ophthalmic)
Bacitracin, Neomycin,
  Polymyxin B, &
  Hydrocortisone,
  Ophthalmic (AK
  Spore HC Ophthalmic,
  Cortisporin
  Ophthalmic)
Besifloxacin (Besivance)
Ciprofloxacin,
  Ophthalmic (Ciloxan)
Erythromycin,
  Ophthalmic (Ilotycin
  Ophthalmic)

Gentamicin, Ophthalmic
  (Garamycin, Genoptic,
  Gentacidin, Gentak,
  Others)
Gentamicin &
  Prednisolone,
  Ophthalmic (Pred-G
  Ophthalmic)
Levofloxacin ophthalmic
  (Quixin, Iquix)
Moxifloxacin ophthalmic
  (Vigamox
  Ophthalmic)
Neomycin, Polymyxin,
  & Hydrocortisone
  (Cortisporin
  Ophthalmic & Otic)
Neomycin &
  Dexamethasone (AK-
  Neo-Dex Ophthalmic,
  NeoDecadron
  Ophthalmic)
Neomycin, Polymyxin
  B, & Dexamethasone
  (Maxitrol)
Neomycin, Polymyxin
  B, & Prednisolone
  (Poly-Pred
  Ophthalmic)

Norfloxacin ophthalmic
  (Chibroxin
  ophthalmic)
Ofloxacin ophthalmic
  (Ocuflox Ophthalmic)
Silver Nitrate (Dey-
  Drop, others)
Sulfacetamide
  (Bleph-10, Cetamide,
  Sodium Sulamyd)
Sulfacetamide &
  Prednisolone
  (Blephamide, others)
Tobramycin ophthalmic
  (AKTob, Tobrex)
Tobramycin &
  Dexamethasone
  ophthalmic
  (TobraDex)
Trifluridine
  ophthalmic(Viroptic)

Miscellaneous Ophthalmic Agents

Artificial Tears (Tears
  Naturale [OTC])
Atropine, ophthalmic
  (Isopto Atropine,

generic) Cromolyn
  Sodium (Opticrom)
Bepotastine besilate
  (Bepreve)

Cyclopentolate
  ophthalmic (Cyclogyl,
  Cyclate)

Cyclopentolate with phenylephrine (Cyclomydril)

Cyclosporine Ophthalmic (Restasis)

Dexamethasone, Ophthalmic (AK-Dex Ophthalmic, Decadron Ophthalmic)

Diclofenac ophthalmic (Voltaren ophthalmic)

Emedastine (Emadine)

Epinastine (Elestat)

Ketotifen Ophthalmic (Alaway, Zaditor) [OTC]

Ketorolac Ophthalmic (Acular, Acular LS, Acular PF)

Levocabastine (Livostin)

Lodoxamide (Alomide)

Naphazoline (Albalon, Naphcon, others),

Naphazoline & Pheniramine Acetate (Naphcon A, Visine A)

Nepafenac (Nevanac)

Olopatadine ophthalmic (Patanol, Pataday)

Pemirolast (Alamast)

Phenylephrine, ophthalmic (Neo-Synephrine Ophthalmic, AK-Dilate, Zincfrin [OTC])

Ranibizumab (Lucentis)

Rimexolone (Vexol Ophthalmic)

Scopolamine ophthalmic

GASTROINTESTINAL AGENTS

Antacids

Alginic Acid + Aluminum Hydroxide & Magnesium Trisilicate (Gaviscon) [OTC] Aluminum Hydroxide (Amphojel, AlternaGEL, Dermagran) [OTC] Aluminum Hydroxide + Magnesium Carbonate (Gaviscon Extra Strength, Liquid) [OTC] Aluminum Hydroxide with Magnesium Hydroxide (Maalox)

Aluminum Hydroxide with Magnesium Hydroxide & Simethicone (Mylanta, Mylanta II, Maalox Plus) [OTC] Aluminum Hydroxide + Magnesium Trisilicate (Gaviscon, Regular Strength) [OTC] Calcium Carbonate (Tums, Alka-Mints) [OTC]

Magaldrate (Riopan-Plus) [OTC]

Simethicone (Mylicon, others) [OTC]

Antidiarrheals

Bismuth Subsalicylate (Pepto-Bismol) [OTC]

Diphenoxylate with Atropine (Lomotil, Lonox)

Lactobacillus (Lactinex Granules) [OTC]

Loperamide (Diamode, Imodium) [OTC]

Octreotide (Sandostatin, Sandostatin LAR)

Paregoric [Camphorated Tincture of Opium]

Antiemetics

Aprepitant (Emend)
Chlorpromazine (Thorazine)
Dimenhydrinate (Dramamine, others) [OTC]
Dolasetron (Anzemet)
Dronabinol (Marinol)
Droperidol (Inapsine)
Fosaprepitant (Emend, Injection)

Granisetron (Kytril)
Meclizine (Antivert, Bonine, Dramamine [OTC])
Metoclopramide (Reglan, Clopra, Octamide)
Nabilone (Cesamet)
Ondansetron (Zofran, Zofran ODT)
Palonosetron (Aloxi)

Prochlorperazine (Compazine)
Promethazine (Phenergan)
Scopolamine (Scopace, Transderm-Scop)
Thiethylperazine (Torecan)
Trimethobenzamide (Tigan)

Antiulcer Agents

Bismuth Subcitrate/ Metronidazole/ Tetracycline (Pylera)
Cimetidine (Tagamet, Tagamet HB 200 [OTC])
Dexlansoprazole (Dexilant, Kapidex)
Esomeprazole (Nexium)

Famotidine (Pepcid, Pepcid AC [OTC])
Lansoprazole (Prevacid, Prevacid IV)
Nizatidine (Axid, Axid AR [OTC])
Omeprazole (Prilosec, Prilosec OTC)

Omeprazole and sodium bicarbonate (Zegerid, Zegerid OTC)
Pantoprazole (Protonix)
Rabeprazole (AcipHex)
Ranitidine (Zantac, Zantac OTC)
Sucralfate (Carafate)

Cathartics/Laxatives

Bisacodyl (Dulcolax [OTC])
Docusate Calcium (Surfak)
Docusate Potassium (Dialose)
Docusate Sodium (DOSS, Colace)
Glycerin Suppository
Lactulose (Constulose, Generlac, Chronulac, Cephulac, Enulose, others)

Magnesium Citrate (Citroma, others) [OTC]
Magnesium Hydroxide (Milk of Magnesia) [OTC]
Mineral Oil [OTC]
Mineral Oil Enema (Fleet Mineral Oil) [OTC]
Polyethylene Glycol (PEG)-Electrolyte Solution (GoLYTELY, CoLyte)

Polyethylene Glycol [PEG] 3350 (MiraLAX)
Psyllium (Metamucil, Serutan, Effer-Syllium)
Sodium Phosphate (Visicol)
Sorbitol (generic)

Enzymes

Pancrelipase (Pancrease,
Cotazym, Creon,
Ultrase)

Miscellaneous GI Agents

Apriso (Salix)
Alosetron (Lotronex)
Alvimopan (Entereg)
Budesonide oral
(Entocort EC)
Balsalazide (Colazal)
Certolizumab Pegol
(Cimzia)
Dexpanthenol (Ilopan-
Choline Oral, Ilopan)
Dibucaine
(Nupercainal)
Dicyclomine (Bentyl)
Hydrocortisone, Rectal
(Anusol-HC
Suppository,
Cortifoam Rectal,
Proctocort, others)
Hyoscyamine (Anaspaz,
Cystospaz, Levsin,
others)

Hyoscyamine, Atropine,
Scopolamine, &
Phenobarbital
(Donnatal, others)
Infliximab (Remicade)
Lubiprostone (Amitiza)
Mesalamine (Asacol,
Canasa, Lialda,
Pentasa, Rowasa)
Methylnaltrexone
bromide (Relistor)
Metoclopramide
(Reglan, Clopra,
Octamide)
Mineral Oil-Pramoxine
HCl-Zinc Oxide (Tucks
Ointment) [OTC]
Misoprostol (Cytotec)
Neomycin Sulfate (Neo-
Fradin, generic)
Olsalazine (Dipentum)

Pramoxine (Anusol
Ointment,
ProctoFoam-NS,
others)
Pramoxine with
Hydrocortisone
(Enzone,
ProctoFoam-HC)
Propantheline
(Pro-Banthine)
Starch, topical, rectal
(Tucks Suppositories)
[OTC]
Sulfasalazine
(Azulfidine,
Azulfidine EN)
Vasopressin [Antidiuretic
Hormone, ADH]
(Pitressin)
Witch Hazel (Tucks
Pads, others [OTC])

HEMATOLOGIC AGENTS

Anticoagulants

Antithrombin,
recombinant (Atryn)
Argatroban (Acova)
Bivalirudin (Angiomax)

Dalteparin (Fragmin)
Enoxaparin (Lovenox)
Fondaparinux (Arixtra)
Heparin

Lepirudin (Refludan)
Protamine (generic)
Tinzaparin (Innohep)
Warfarin (Coumadin)

Antiplatelet Agents

Abciximab (ReoPro)
Aspirin (Bayer, Ecotrin,
St. Joseph's [OTC])
Clopidogrel (Plavix)

Dipyridamole
(Persantine)
Dipyridamole & Aspirin
(Aggrenox)
Eptifibatide (Integrilin)

Prasugrel hydrochloride
(Effient)
Ticlopidine (Ticlid)
Tirofiban (Aggrastat)

Antithrombotic Agents

Alteplase, Recombinant
[tPA] (Activase)
Aminocaproic Acid
(Amicar)

Anistreplase (Eminase)
Dextran 40 (Gentran 40,
Rheomacrodex)
Reteplase (Retavase)

Streptokinase (Streptase,
Kabikinase)
Tenecteplase (TNKase)
Urokinase (Abbokinase)

Hematopoietic Stimulants

Darbepoetin Alfa
(Aranesp)
Eltrombopag (Promacta)
Epoetin Alfa
[Erythropoietin, EPO]
(Epogen, Procrit)

Filgrastim [G-CSF]
(Neupogen)
Oprelvekin (Neumega)
Pegfilgrastim (Neulasta)
Plerixafor (Mozobil)
Romiplostim (Nplate)

Sargramostim [GM-
CSF] (Leukine)

Volume Expanders

Albumin (Albuminar,
Albutein Buminate)

Dextran 40 (Gentran 40,
Rheomacrodex)
Hetastarch (Hespan)

Plasma Protein Fraction
(Plasmanate, others)

Miscellaneous Hematologic Agents

Antihemophilic Factor
VIII (Monoclate)
Antihemophilic Factor
(Recombinant)
(Xyntha)

Decitabine (Dacogen)
Desmopressin (DDAVP,
Stimate)
Fibrinogen concentrate,
human (Riastap)

Lenalidomide (Revlimid)
Pentoxifylline (Trental)

IMMUNE SYSTEM AGENTS

Immunomodulators

Interferon Alfa
(Roferon-A, Intron A)

Interferon Alfacon-1
(Infergen)

Interferon Beta-1a
(Rebif)

Interferon Beta-1b
(Betaseron, Extavia)
Interferon Gamma-1b
(Actimmune)
Natalizumab (Tysabri)
**Peginterferon Alfa-2b
[Pegylated interferon]
(PegIntron)**

Peginterferon Alfa-2a
[Pegylated interferon]
(Pegasys)
**Immunomodulators:
disease-modifying
antirheumatic drugs
(DMARDs)**
Abatacept (Orencia)

Adalimumab (Humira)
Anakinra (Kineret)
Certolizumab Pegol
(Cimzia)
Etanercept (Enbrel)
Golimumab (Simponi)
Iinfliximab (Remicade)

Immunosuppressive Agents

Azathioprine (Imuran)
Basiliximab (Simulect)
Cyclosporine
(Sandimmune,
Gengraf, Neoral)
Daclizumab (Zenapax)
Everolimus (Zortress)
Lymphocyte Immune
Globulin
[Antithymocyte
Globulin, ATG]
(Atgam)

Muromonab-CD3
(Orthoclone OKT3)
Mycophenolic Acid
(Myfortic)
Mycophenolate Mofetil
(CellCept)
Sirolimus [Rapamycin]
(Rapamune)
Steroids, Systemic
(Table 2, page 265)

Tacrolimus [FK506]
(Prograf, Protopic)

Vaccines/Serums/Toxoids

Cytomegalovirus
Immune Globulin
[CMV-IG IV]
(CytoGam)
Diphtheria & Tetanus
Toxoids (Td)(Decavac
– for > 7 y)
Diphtheria & Tetanus
Toxoids (DT)(generic
only – for < 7 y)
Diphtheria, Tetanus
Toxoids, & Acellular
pertussis adsorbed
(DTaP) (ages < 7 y)
(Daptacel, Infanrix,
Tripedia)

Diphtheria, Tetanus
Toxoids, & Acellular
pertussis adsorbed
(Tdap) (ages > 10-11y)
(Boosters: Adacel,
Boostrix)
Diphtheria, Tetanus
Toxoids, & Acellular
pertussis adsorbed,
Hep B (Recombinant),
& Inactivated
Poliovirus Vaccine
[IPV] combined
(Pediarix)

Haemophilus B
Conjugate Vaccine
(ActHIB, HibTITER,
PedvaxHIB, Prohibit,
TriHIBit, others)
Hepatitis A (Inactivated)
& Hepatitis B
Recombinant Vaccine
(Twinrix)
Hepatitis A Vaccine
(Havrix, Vaqta)

Hepatitis B Immune Globulin (HyperHep, HepaGam B, Nabi-HB, H-BIG)

Hepatitis B Vaccine (Engerix-B, Recombivax HB)

Human Papillomavirus Recombinant Vaccine (Cervarix [Types 16, 18], Gardasil, [Types 6, 11, 16, 18])

Immune Globulin, IV (Gamimune N, Gammaplex, Gammar IV, Sandoglobulin, others)

Immune Globulin, Subcutaneous (Vivaglobin)

Influenza Vaccine, Inactivated, trivalent [TIV] (Afluria, Agriflu, Fluarix, FluLaval, Fluvirin, Fluzone)

Influenza Virus Vaccine Live, Intranasal [LAIV] (FluMist)

Measles, Mumps, & Rubella Vaccine Live [MMR] (M-M-R II)

Measles, Mumps, Rubella, and Varicella

Virus Vaccine Live [MMRV] (ProQuad)

Meningococcal conjugate vaccine [quadrivalent, MCV4] (Menactra)

Meningococcal polysaccharide vaccine [MPSV4] (Menomune A/C/Y/ W-135)

Pneumococcal 7-Valent Conjugate Vaccine (Prevnar)

Pneumococcal Vaccine, Polyvalent (Pneumovax-23)

Rotavirus Vaccine, live, oral, monovalent (Rotarix)

Rotavirus Vaccine, live, oral, pentavalent (RotaTeq)

Smallpox Vaccine (Dryvax)

Tetanus Immune Globulin

Tetanus Toxoid (TT)

Varicella Immune Globulin (VarZIG)

Varicella Virus Vaccine (Varivax)

Zoster vaccine, live (Zostavax)

MUSCULOSKELETAL AGENTS

Antigout Agents

Allopurinol (Zyloprim, Lopurin, Aloprim)

Colchicine

Febuxostat (Uloric)

Probenecid (Benemid, others)

Sulfinpyrazone

Muscle Relaxants

Baclofen (Lioresal Intrathecal, generic)
Carisoprodol (Soma)
Chlorzoxazone (Paraflex, Parafon Forte DSC, others)
Cyclobenzaprine (Flexeril)

Cyclobenzaprine, extended release (Amrix)
Dantrolene (Dantrium)
Diazepam (Diastat, Valium)
Metaxalone (Skelaxin)

Methocarbamol (Robaxin)
Orphenadrine (Norflex)

Neuromuscular Blockers

Atracurium (Tracrium)
Pancuronium (Pavulon)
Rocuronium (Zemuron)

Succinylcholine (Anectine, Quelicin, Sucostrin, others)

Vecuronium (Norcuron)

Miscellaneous Musculoskeletal Agents

Edrophonium (Tensilon, Reversol)
Leflunomide (Arava)

Methotrexate (Rheumatrex Dose Pack, Trexall)

Sulfasalazine (Azulfidine, Azulfidine EN)

OB/GYN AGENTS

Contraceptives

Copper IUD Contraceptive (ParaGard T 380A)
Estradiol Cypionate & Medroxyprogesterone Acetate (Lunelle)
Ethinyl Estradiol & Norelgestromin (Ortho Evra)
Etonogestrel Implant (Implanon)

Etonogestrel/Ethinyl Estradiol vaginal insert (NuvaRing)
Levonorgestrel intrauterine device (IUD) (Mirena)
Medroxyprogesterone (Provera, Depo Provera, Depo-Sub Q Provera)

Oral Contraceptives (see page 193 and Table 5 p 270)

Emergency Contraceptives

Levonorgestrel (Plan B)

Estrogen Supplementation

ESTROGEN ONLY

Estradiol oral
(Delestrogen,
Estrace, Femtrace,
others)
Estradiol gel (Divigel)
Estradiol gel (Elestrin)
Estradiol, spray
(Evamist)

Estradiol, transdermal
(Estraderm, Climara,
Vivelle Dot)
Estradiol, vaginal
(Estring, Femring,
Vagifem)
Estrogen, Conjugated
(Premarin)

Estrogen, Conjugated-
Synthetic (Cenestin,
Enjuvia)
Esterified Estrogens
(Estratab, Menest)
Ethinyl Estradiol
(Estinyl, Feminone)

COMBINATION ESTROGEN/PROGESTIN

Esterified Estrogens with
Methyltestosterone
(Estratest, Estratest
HS, Syntest DS, HS)
Estrogen,
Conjugated with
Medroxyprogesterone
(Prempro,
Premphase)
Estrogen, Conjugated
with Methyl

progesterone
(Premarin with Methyl
progesterone)
Estrogen, Conjugated
with Methyltestos-
terone (Premarin with
Methyltestosterone)
Estradiol/Levonorgestrel,
transdermal
(Climara Pro)

Estradiol/
Medroxyprogesterone
(Lunelle)
Estradiol/Norethindrone
acetate (FemHRT,
Activella)
Norethindrone acetate/
ethinyl Estradiol
(Femhrt, Activella)

Vaginal Preparations

Amino-Cerv pH 5.5
Cream
Miconazole (Monistat 1
Combo, Monistat 3,
Monistat 7) [OTC]
(Monistat-Derm

Nystatin (Mycostatin)
Terconazole (Terazol 7)
Tioconazole (Vagistat)

Miscellaneous Ob/Gyn Agents

Dinoprostone (Cervidil
Vaginal Insert,
Prepidil Vaginal Gel,
Prostin E2)
Gonadorelin (Factrel)
Leuprolide (Lupron)

Lutropin Alfa (Luveris)
Lysteda (tranexamic
acid)
Magnesium Sulfate
(various)

Medroxyprogesterone
(Provera, Depo
Provera, Depo-Sub Q
Provera)
Methylergonovine
(Methergine)

Mifepristone [RU 486] (Mifeprex)

Oxytocin (Pitocin)

Terbutaline (Brethine, Bricanyl)

PAIN MEDICATIONS

Local Anesthetics (Table 1, page 264)
Benzocaine (Americaine, Lanacaine, Hurricane, various [OTC])
Benzocaine & Antipyrine (Auralgan)
Bupivacaine (Marcaine)
Capsaicin (Capsin, Zostrix, others [OTC])

Cocaine
Dibucaine (Nupercainal)
Lidocaine, Lidocaine with epinephrine (Anestacon Topical, Xylocaine, Xylocaine Viscous, Xylocaine MPF, others)

Lidocaine, powder intradermal injection system (Zingo)
Lidocaine & Prilocaine (EMLA, LMX)
Pramoxine (Anusol Ointment, ProctoFoam-NS, others)

Migraine Headache

Acetaminophen with Butalbital w/ & w/o Caffeine (Fioricet, Medigesic, Repan, Sedapap-10, Two-Dyne, Triaprin, Axocet, Phrenilin Forte)

Almotriptan (Axert)
Aspirin & Butalbital Compound (Fiorinal)
Aspirin with Butalbital, Caffeine, & Codeine (Fiorinal with Codeine)
Eletriptan (Relpax)

Frovatriptan (Frova)
Naratriptan (Amerge)
Sumatriptan (Imitrex)
Sumatriptan and Naproxen Sodium (Treximet)
Zolmitriptan (Zomig)

Narcotic Analgesics

Acetaminophen with Codeine (Tylenol No. 2 3, 4)
Alfentanil (Alfenta)
Aspirin with Codeine (Empirin No. 2, 3, 4)
Buprenorphine (Buprenex)
Butorphanol (Stadol)
Codeine
Fentanyl (Sublimaze)

Fentanyl iontophoretic transdermal system (Ionsys)
Fentanyl, Transdermal (Duragesic)
Fentanyl, Transmucosal System (Actiq, Fentora)
Hydrocodone & Acetaminophen (Lorcet, Vicodin, Hycet, others)

Hydrocodone & Aspirin (Lortab ASA, others)
Hydrocodone & Ibuprofen (Vicoprofen)
Hydromorphone (Dilaudid, Dilaudid HP)
Levorphanol (Levo-Dromoran)
Meperidine (Demerol, Meperitab) [C–II]

Methadone (Dolophine, Methadose) [C-II]
Morphine (Avinza XR, Astramorph/PF, Duramorph, Infumorph, MS Contin, Kadian SR, Oramorph SR, Roxanol) [C-II]
Morphine, Liposomal (DepoDur)
Nalbuphine (Nubain)
Oxycodone [Dihydro hydroxycodeinone] (OxyContin, Roxicodone)

Oxycodone & Acetaminophen (Percocet, Tylox)
Oxycodone & Aspirin (Percodan)
Oxycodone/Ibuprofen (Combunox)
Oxymorphone (Opana, Opana ER)
Pentazocine (Talwin, Talwin Compound, Talwin NX)
Propoxyphene (Darvon)
Propoxyphene & Acetaminophen (Darvocet)

Propoxyphene & Aspirin (Darvon Compound-65, Darvon-N with Aspirin)

Nonnarcotic Analgesics

Acetaminophen [APAP, N-acetyl-p-aminophenol] (Acephen, Tylenol, other generic)
Acetaminophen + Butalbital ± Caffeine (Fioricet, Medigesic, Repan, Sedapap-10, Two-Dyne, Triapin, Axocet, Phrenilin Forte)

Aspirin (Bayer, Ecotrin, St. Joseph's [OTC])
Tramadol (Ultram, Ultram ER)
Tramadol/ Acetaminophen (Ultracet)

Nonsteroidal Anti-inflammatory Agents (NSAIDs)

Celecoxib (Celebrex)
Diclofenac (Arthrotec, Cataflam, Flector, Flector patch, Voltaren, Voltaren XR, Voltaren gel)

Diflunisal (Dolobid)
Etodolac
Fenoprofen (Nalfon)
Flurbiprofen (Ansaid, Ocufen)

Ibuprofen, oral (Motrin, Rufen, Advil)
Ibuprofen, parenteral (Caldolor)
Indomethacin (Indocin)

Ketoprofen (Orudis, Oruvail)
Ketorolac (Toradol)
Meloxicam (Mobic)
Nabumetone (Relafen)
Naproxen (Aleve [OTC], Anaprox, Naprosyn)
Oxaprozin (Daypro, Daypro ALTA)
Piroxicam (Feldene)
Sulindac (Clinoril)
Tolmetin (Tolectin)

Miscellaneous Pain Medications

Amitriptyline (Elavil)
Imipramine (Tofranil)
Pregabalin (Lyrica)
Tapentadol (Nucynta)
Tramadol (Ultram, Ultram ER)
Ziconotide (Prialt)

RESPIRATORY AGENTS

Antitussives, Decongestants, & Expectorants

Acetylcysteine (Acetadote, Mucomyst)
Benzonatate (Tessalon Perles)
Codeine
Dextromethorphan (Benylin DM, Delsym, Mediquell, PediaCare 1, others) [OTC]
Guaifenesin (Robitussin, others)
Guaifenesin & Codeine (Robitussin AC, Brontex, others)
Guaifenesin & Dextromethorphan (many OTC bands)
Hydrocodone & Guaifenesin (Hycotuss Expectorant)
Hydrocodone & Homatropine (Hycodan, Hydromet, others)
Hydrocodone & Pseudoephedrine (Detussin, Histussin-D, others)
Hydrocodone, Chlorpheniramine, Phenylephrine, Acetaminophen, & Caffeine (Hycomine compound)
Potassium Iodide [Lugol Soln] (SSKI, Thyro-Block, ThyroSafe, ThyroShield)
Pseudoephedrine (Sudafed, Novafed, Afrinol, others [OTC])

Bronchodilators

Albuterol (Proventil, Ventolin, Volmax)
Albuterol & Ipratropium (Combivent, DuoNeb)
Aminophylline
Arformoterol (Brovana)
Ephedrine
Epinephrine (Adrenalin, Sus-Phrine, EpiPen, EpiPen Jr, others)
Formoterol Fumarate (Foradil, Performist)
Isoproterenol (Isuprel)
Levalbuterol (Xopenex, Xopenex HFA)
Metaproterenol (Alupent, Metaprel)
Pirbuterol (Maxair)
Salmeterol (Serevent, Serevent Diskus)
Terbutaline (Brethine, Bricanyl)
Theophylline (Theo24, Theochron)

Respiratory Inhalants

Acetylcysteine (Acetadote, Mucomyst)
Beclomethasone nasal (Beconase AQ)
Beclomethasone (QVAR)
Beractant (Survanta)
Budesonide (Rhinocort Aqua, Pulmicort)
Budesonide/Formoterol (Symbicort)
Calfactant (Infasurf)
Ciclesonide, Inhalation (Alvesco)
Ciclesonide, Nasal (Omnaris)
Cromolyn Sodium (Intal, NasalCrom, Opticrom, others)

Dexamethasone, Nasal (Dexacort Phosphate Turbinaire)
Flunisolide (AeroBid, Aerospan, Nasarel)
Fluticasone Furoate, Nasal (Veramyst)
Fluticasone Propionate, Nasal (Flonase)
Fluticasone Propionate, Inhalation (Flovent HFA, Flovent Diskus)
Fluticasone Propionate & Salmeterol Xinafoate (Advair Diskus, Advair HFA)
Formoterol Fumarate (Foradil Aerolizer, Perforomist)

Ipratropium (Atrovent HFA, Atrovent Nasal)
Mometasone and formoterol (DULERA)
Olopatadine Nasal (Patanase)
Phenylepherine, nasal (Neo-Syenphrine Nasal OTC)
Tiotropium (Spiriva)
Triamcinolone (Azmacort)

Miscellaneous Respiratory Agents

Alpha$_1$-Protease Inhibitor (Prolastin)
Dornase Alfa (Pulmozyme, DNase)

Montelukast (Singulair)
Omalizumab (Xolair)
Zafirlukast (Accolate)

Zileuton (Zyflo, Zyflo CR)

Erectile Dysfunction

Alprostadil, Intracavernosal (Caverject, Edex)
Alprostadil, Urethral Suppository (Muse)

Sildenafil (Viagra, Revatio)
Tadalafil (Cialis)
Vardenafil (Levitra, Stayxn)

Yohimbine (Yocon, Yohimex)

Bladder Agents (Overactive Bladder, Other Anticholinergics)

Belladonna & Opium Suppositories (B & O Supprettes)

Bethanechol (Duvoid, Urecholine, others)

Butabarbital-
Hyoscyamine
Hydrobromide-
Phenazopyridine
(Pyridium Plus)
Darifenacin (Enablex)
Fesoterodine Fumarate
(Toviaz)
Flavoxate (Urispas)
Hyoscyamine (Anaspaz,
Cystospaz, Levsin)

Hyoscyamine, Atropine,
Scopolamine, &
Phenobarbital
(Donnatal, others)
Methenamine Hippurate
(Hiprex)
Methenamine Mandelate
(Uroquid-Acid No. 2)
Oxybutynin (Ditropan,
Ditropan XL)
Oxybutynin Transdermal
System (Oxytrol)

Phenazopyridine
(Pyridium,
Azo-Standard,
Urogesic, many
others)
Solifenacin (Vesicare)
Tolterodine (Detrol,
Detrol LA)
Trospium Chloride
(Sanctura,
Sanctura XR)

Urolithiasis

Potassium Citrate
(Urocit-K)
Potassium Citrate &
Citric Acid
(Polycitra-K)

Sodium Citrate/Citric
Acid (Bicitra, Oracit)
Trimethoprim (Trimpex,
Proloprim)

Benign Prostatic Hyperplasia

Alfuzosin (Uroxatral)
Doxazosin (Cardura,
Cardura XL)
Dutasteride (Avodart)

Dutasteride and
tamsulosin (Jalyn)
Finasteride (Propecia,
Proscar, generic)

Silodosin (Rapaflo)
Tamsulosin (Flomax,
generic)
Terazosin (Hytrin)

Miscellaneous Urology Agents

Ammonium Aluminum
Sulfate [Alum [OTC]]
Atropine, Benzoic Acid,
Hyoscyamine Sulfate,
Methenamine,
Methylene Blue,
Phenyl Salicylate
(Urised)

Dimethyl Sulfoxide
[DMSO] (Rimso-50)
Neomycin-Polymyxin
Bladder Irrigant
[Neosporin GU
Irrigant]

Nitrofurantoin
(Furadantin,
Macrodantin,
Macrobid)
Pentosan Polysulfate
Sodium (Elmiron)

WOUND CARE

Becaplermin (Regranex
Gel)

Silver Nitrate
(Dey-Drop, others)

MISCELLANEOUS THERAPEUTIC AGENTS

Acamprosate (Campral)
Alglucosidase Alfa (Myozyme)
C1 Esterase Inhibitor, Human (Berinert)
Cilostazol (Pletal)
Drotrecogin Alfa (Xigris)
Ecallantide (Kalbitor)
Eculizumab (Soliris)
Lanthanum Carbonate (Fosrenol)
Megestrol Acetate (Megace, Megace-ES)
Mecasermin (Increlex, Iplex)

Naltrexone (Depade, ReVia, Vivitrol)
Nicotine Gum (Nicorette, others)
Nicotine Nasal Spray (Nicotrol NS)
Nicotine Transdermal (Habitrol, Nicoderm CQ [OTC], others)
Palifermin (Kepivance)
Potassium Iodide [Lugol Solution] (SSKI, Thyro-Block, Thyrosafe, Thyroshield)

Sevelamer HCl (Renagel)
Sevelamer carbonate (Renvela)
Sodium Polystyrene Sulfonate (Kayexalate)
Talc (Sterile Talc Powder)
Varenicline (Chantix)

NATURAL AND HERBAL AGENTS

Black Cohosh
Chamomile
Cranberry (*Vaccinium macrocarpon*)
Dong Quai (*Angelica polymorpha, sinensis*)
Echinacea (*Echinacea purpurea*)
Ephedra/Ma Huang
Evening Primrose Oil
Feverfew (*Tanacetum parthenium*)
Fish Oil Supplements (Omega-3 polyunsaturated fatty acid)

Garlic (*Allium sativum*)
Ginger (*Zingiber officinale*)
Ginkgo Biloba
Ginseng
Glucosamine Sulfate (Chitosamine) & Chondroitin Sulfate
Kava Kava (Kava Kava Root Extract, *Piper methysticum*)
Melatonin
Milk Thistle (*Silybum marianum*)
Saw Palmetto (*Serenoa repens*)

St. John's Wort (*Hypericum perforatum*)
Valerian (*Valeriana officinalis*)
Yohimbine (*Pausinystalia yohimbe*) Yocon, Yohimex

GENERIC AND SELECTED BRAND DRUG DATA

Abacavir (Ziagen) **BOX:** Allergy (fever, rash, fatigue, GI, resp) reported; stop drug immediately & do not rechallenge; lactic acidosis & hepatomegaly/steatosis reported **Uses:** *HIV Infxn* **Acts:** NRTI **Dose:** *Adults.* 300 mg PO bid or 600 mg PO daily *Peds.* 8 mg/kg bid/300 mg bid max **Caution:** [C, –] CDC rec: HIV-infected mothers not breast-feed (transmission risk) **Disp:** Tabs 300 mg; soln 20 mg/mL **SE:** See Box, ↑ LFTs, fat redistribution **Notes:** Many drug interactions; HLA-B*5701 ↑ risk for fatal hypersens Rxn, genetic screen before use

Abatacept (Orencia) **Uses:** *Mod/severe RA w/ inadequate response to one or more DMARDs, juvenile idiopathic arthritis* **Acts:** Selective costimulation modulator, ↓ T-cell activation **Dose:** *Adults.* Initial 500 mg (<60 kg), 750 mg (60–100 kg); 1 g (>100 kg) IV over 30 min; repeat at 2 and 4 wk, then q4wk *Peds 6–17 y:* 10 mg/kg (<75 kg), 750 mg (75–100 kg), IV × 1 wk 0, 2, 4, then q4wk (>100 kg, adult dose) **Caution:** [C; ?/–] w/ TNF blockers; COPD; Hx predisposition to Infxn; w/ immunosuppressants **CI:** w/ Live vaccines w/in 3 mo of D/C abatacept **Disp:** IV powder 250 mg/10 mL **SE:** HA, URI, N, nasopharyngitis, Infxn, malignancy, Inf Rxns/hypersens (dizziness, HA, HTN), COPD exacerbations, cough, dyspnea **Notes:** Screen for TB before use

Abciximab (ReoPro) **Uses:** *Prevent acute ischemic comps in PTCA*, MI **Acts:** ↓ Plt aggregation (glycoprotein IIb/IIIa inhib) **Dose:** *Unstable angina w/ planned PCI w/in 24 h of dose (ECC 2005):* 0.25 mg/kg bolus, then 10 mcg/min cont Inf × 18–24 h, stop 1 h after PCI; *PCI:* 0.25 mg/kg bolus 10–60 min pre-PTCA, then 0.125 mcg/kg/min (max = 10 mcg/min) cont inf for 12 h **Caution:** [C, ?/–] **CI:** Active/recent (w/in 6 wk) internal hemorrhage, CVA w/in 2 y or CVA w/ sig neuro deficit, bleeding diathesis or PO anticoagulants w/in 7 d (unless PT <1.2 × control), ↓ plt (<100,000 cells/mcL), recent trauma or major surgery (w/in 6 wk), CNS tumor, AVM, aneurysm, severe uncontrolled HTN, vasculitis, dextran use w/ PTCA, murine protein allergy, w/ other glycoprotein IIb/IIIa inhib **Disp:** Inj 2 mg/mL **SE:** ↓ BP, CP, allergic Rxns, bleeding, ↓ plt **Notes:** Use w/ heparin/ASA

Acamprosate (Campral) **Uses:** *Maintain abstinence from EtOH* **Acts:** ↓ Glutamatergic transmission; modulates neuronal hyperexcitability; related to GABA **Dose:** 666 mg PO tid; CrCl 30–50 mL/min: 333 mg PO tid **Caution:** [C; ?/–] **CI:** CrCl <30 mL/min **Disp:** Tabs 333 mg EC **SE:** N/D, depression, anxiety, insomnia **Notes:** Does not eliminate EtOH withdrawal Sx; continue even if relapse occurs

Acarbose (Precose) **Uses:** *Type 2 DM* **Acts:** α-Glucosidase inhib; delays carbohydrate digestion to ↓ glucose **Dose:** 25–100 mg PO tid w/ 1st bite each meal; 50 mg tid (<60 kg); 100 mg tid (>60 kg); usual maint 50–100 mg PO tid **Caution:** [B, ?] w/ CrCl <25 mL/min; can affect digoxin levels **CI:** IBD, colonic ulceration, partial intestinal obst; cirrhosis **Disp:** Tabs 25, 50, 100 mg **SE:** Abd pain, D, flatulence, ↑ LFTs, hypersens Rxn **Notes:** OK w/ sulfonylureas; ✓ LFTs q3mo for 1st y

Acebutolol (Sectral) **Uses:** *HTN, arrhythmias* chronic stable angina **Acts:** Blocks β-adrenergic receptors, β₁, & ISA **Dose:** *HTN:* 400–800 mg/d; *Arrhythmia:* 400–1200 mg/d 2 ÷ doses; ↓ w/ CrCl <50 mL/min or elderly; elderly initial 200–400 mg/d; max 800 mg/d **Caution:** [B, D in 2nd & 3rd tri, +] Can exacerbate ischemic heart Dz, do not D/C abruptly **CI:** 2nd-, 3rd-degree heart block **Disp:** Caps 200, 400 mg **SE:** Fatigue, HA, dizziness, ↓ HR

Acetaminophen [APAP, N-acetyl-p-Aminophenol] (Acephen, Tylenol, Other Generic) [OTC] **Uses:** *Mild-mod pain, HA, fever* **Acts:** Nonnarcotic analgesic; ↓ CNS synth of prostaglandins & hypothalamic heat-regulating center **Dose:** *Adults.* 650 mg PO or PR q4–6h or 1000 mg PO q6h; max 4 g/24 h **Peds** *<12 y:* 10–15 mg/kg/dose PO or PR q4–6h; max 2.6 g/24 h. Administer q6h if CrCl 10–50 mL/min & q8h if CrCl <10 mL/min **Caution:** [B, +] Hepatotoxic in elderly & w/ EtOH use w/ >4 g/d; EtOH liver Dz, G6PD deficiency; liver damage in children w/ > 5 suppositories in 24 H **CI:** Hypersens **Disp:** Tabs melt away/dissolving 160 mg; tabs: 325, 500, 650 mg; chew tabs 80, 160 mg; liq 100 mg/5 mL, 120 mg/2.5 mL, 120 mg/5 mL, 160 mg/5 mL, 167 mg/5 mL, 325 mg/5 mL, 500 mg/15 mL, 80 mg/0.8 mL; *Acephen* supp 80, 120, 125, 325, 650 mg **SE:** OD hepatotoxic at 10 g; 15 g can be lethal; Rx w/ N-acetylcysteine **Notes:** No anti-inflammatory or plt-inhibiting action; avoid EtOH

Acetaminophen + Butalbital ± Caffeine (Fioricet, Medigesic, Repan, Sedapap-10, Two-Dyne, Triaprin, Axocet, Phrenilin Forte) [C-III] **Uses:** *Tension HA*, mild pain **Acts:** Nonnarcotic analgesic w/ barbiturate **Dose:** 1–2 tabs or caps PO q4–6h PRN; ↓ in renal/hepatic impair; 4 g/24 h APAP max **Caution:** [C, D, +] Alcoholic liver Dz, G6PD deficiency **CI:** Hypersens **Disp:** Caps *Dolgic Plus:* butalbital 50 mg, caffeine 40 mg, APAP 750 mg; Caps *Medigesic, Repan, Two-Dyne:* butalbital 50 mg, caffeine 40 mg, APAP 325 mg; Caps *Axocet, Phrenilin Forte:* butalbital 50 mg + APAP 650 mg; Caps: *Esgic-Plus, Zebutal:* butalbital 50 mg, caffeine 40 mg, APAP 500 mg; Liq. *Dolgic LQ:* butalbital 50 mg, caffeine 40 mg, APAP 325 mg/15 mL. Tabs *Medigesic, Fioricet, Repan:* butalbital 50 mg, caffeine 40 mg, APAP 325 mg; *Phrenilin:* butalbital 50 mg + APAP 325 mg; *Sedapap-10:* butalbital 50 mg + APAP 650 mg **SE:** Drowsiness, dizziness, "hangover" effect, N/V **Notes:** Butalbital habit forming; avoid EtOH

Acetaminophen + Codeine (Tylenol No. 2, 3, No. 4) [C-III, C-V] **Uses:** *Mild–mod pain (No.2–3); mod–severe pain (No .4)* **Acts:** Combined APAP & narcotic analgesic **Dose:** *Adults.* 1–2 tabs q3–4h PRN or 30–60 mg/ codeine q4–6h based on codeine content (max dose APAP = 4 g/d). *Peds.* APAP

10–15 mg/kg/dose; codeine 0.5–1 mg/kg dose q4–6h (guide: 3–6 y, 5 mL/dose; 7–12 y, 10 mL/dose) max 2.6 g/d if <12 y; ↓ in renal/hepatic impair **Caution:** [C, +] Alcoholic liver Dz; G6PD deficiency **CI:** Hypersens **Disp:** Tabs 300 mg APAP + codeine(No. 2 = 15 mg, No. 3 = 30 mg, No. 4 = 60 mg); caps 325 mg APAP + codeine; susp (C-V) APAP 120 mg + codeine 12 mg/5 mL **SE:** Drowsiness, dizziness, N/V

Acetazolamide (Diamox) **Uses:** *Diuresis, drug and CHF edema, glaucoma, prevent high-altitude sickness, refractory epilepsy*, metabolic alkalosis **Acts:** Carbonic anhydrase inhib; ↓ renal excretion of hydrogen & ↑ renal excretion of Na$^+$, K$^+$, HCO$_3^-$, & H$_2$O **Dose:** **Adults.** *Diuretic:* 250–375 mg IV or PO q24h *Glaucoma:* 250–1000 mg PO q24h in ÷ doses *Epilepsy:* 8–30 mg/kg/d PO in ÷ doses *Altitude sickness:* 250 mg PO q8–12h or SR 500 mg PO q12–24h start 24–48 h before & 48 h after highest ascent *Metabolic alkalosis:* 250 mg IV q6h × 4 or 500 mg IV × 1 **Peds.** *Epilepsy:* 8–30 mg/kg/24 h PO in ÷ doses; max 1 g/d Diuretic: 5 mg/kg/24 h PO or IV *Alkalinization of urine:* 5 mg/kg/dose PO bid-tid *Glaucoma:* 8–30 mg/kg/24 h PO in 3 ÷ doses; max 1 g/d; ↓ dose w/ CrCl 10–50 mL/min; avoid if CrCl <10 mL/min **Caution:** [C, +] **CI:** Renal/hepatic/ adrenal failure, sulfa allergy, chloremic acidosis **Disp:** Tabs 125, 250 mg; ER caps 500 mg; Inj 500 mg/vial, powder for recons **SE:** Malaise, metallic taste, drowsiness, photosens, hyperglycemia **Notes:** Follow Na$^+$ & K$^+$; watch for metabolic acidosis; ✓ CBC & plts; SR forms not for epilepsy

Acetic Acid & Aluminum Acetate (Otic Domeboro) **Uses:** *Otitis externa* **Acts:** Anti-infective **Dose:** 4–6 gtt in ear(s) q2–3h **Caution:** [C, ?] **CI:** Perforated tympanic membranes **Disp:** 2% otic soln **SE:** Local irritation

Acetylcysteine (Acetadote, Mucomyst) **Uses:** *Mucolytic, antidote to APAP hepatotox/OD* adjuvant Rx chronic bronchopulmonary Dzs & CF* prevent contrast-induced renal dysfunction **Acts:** Splits mucoprotein disulfide linkages; restores glutathione in APAP OD to protect liver **Dose:** **Adults & Peds.** *Nebulizer:* 3–5 mL of 20% soln diluted w/ equal vol of H$_2$O or NS tid-qid *Antidote:* PO or NG: 140 mg/kg load, then 70 mg/kg q4h × 17 doses (dilute 1:3 in carbonated beverage or OJ), repeat if emesis w/in 1 h of dosing *Acetadote:* 150 mg/kg IV over 60 min, then 50 mg/kg over 4 h, then 100 mg/kg over 16 h *Prevent renal dysfunction:* 600–1200 mg PO bid × 2 d **Caution:** [B, ?] **Disp:** Soln, inhaled and oral 10%, 20%; Acetadote IV soln 20% **SE:** Bronchospasm (inhaled), N/V, drowsiness, anaphylactoid Rxns w/ IV **Notes:** Activated charcoal adsorbs PO acetylcysteine for APAP ingestion; start Rx for APAP OD w/in 6–8 h

Acitretin (Soriatane) **BOX:** Not to be used by females who are PRG or who intend to become PRG during/for 3 y following drug D/C; no EtOH during/2 mo following D/C; no blood donation for 3 y following D/C; hepatotoxic **Uses:** *Severe psoriasis*; other keratinization Dz (lichen planus, etc) **Acts:** Retinoid-like activity **Dose:** 25–50 mg/d PO, w/ main meal; ↑ if no response by 4 wk to 75 mg/d **Caution:** [X, −] Renal/hepatic impair; in women of reproductive potential **CI:** See

Box; ↑ serum lipids; w/ MTX or tetracyclines **Disp:** Caps 10, 25 mg **SE:** Hyperesthesia, cheilitis, skin peeling, alopecia, pruritus, rash, arthralgia, GI upset, photosens, thrombocytosis, ↑ triglycerides, ↑ Na, K, PO₄ **Notes:** ✓ LFTs/lytes/ lipids; response takes up to 2–3 mo; informed consent & FDA guide w/ each Rx required

Acyclovir (Zovirax) Uses: *Herpes simplex* (HSV) (genital/mucocutaneous, encephalitis, keratitis), *Varicella zoster*, *Herpes zoster* (shingles) Infxns* **Acts:** Interferes w/ viral DNA synth **Dose:** *Adults.* Dose on IBW if obese (>125% IBW) *PO: Initial genital HSV:* 200 mg PO q4h while awake (5 caps/d) × 10 d or 400 mg PO tid × 7–10 d *Chronic HSV suppression:* 400 mg PO bid *Intermittent HSV Rx:* As initial, except Rx × 5 d, or 800 mg PO bid, at prodrome *Topical: Initial herpes genitalis:* Apply q3h (6×/d) for 7 d *HSV encephalitis:* 10 mg/kg IV q8h × 10 d *Herpes zoster:* 800 mg PO 5×/d for 7–10 d *IV:* 5–10 mg/kg/dose IV q8h **Peds.** *Genital HSV:* **3 mo–2 y:** 15 mg/kg/d IV ÷ q8h × 5–7 d, 60 mg/kg/d max **2–12 y:** 1200 mg/d PO ÷ q8h × 7–10 d *>12 y:* 1000–1200 mg PO ÷ q8h × 7–10 d *HSV encephalitis:* **3 mo–12 y:** 60 mg/kg/d IV ÷ q8h × 10 d *>12 y:* 30 mg/kg/d IV ÷ q8h × 10 d *Chickenpox:* ≥2 y: 20 mg/kg/dose PO qid × 5 d *Shingles:* <12 y: 30 mg/kg/d PO or 1500 mg/m²/d IV ÷ q8h × 7–10 d; ↓ w/ CrCl <50 mL/min **Caution:** [B, +] **CI:** Component hypersens **Disp:** Caps 200 mg/ tabs 400, 800 mg; susp 200 mg/5 mL; Inj 500 & 1000 mg/vial; Inj soln 25 mg/mL, 50 mg/mL oint 5% and cream 5% **SE:** Dizziness, lethargy, malaise, confusion, rash, IV site inflammation; transient ↑ Cr/BUN **Notes:** PO better than topical for herpes genitalis

Adalimumab (Humira) BOX: Cases of TB have been observed; ✓ TB skin test prior to use; hep B reactivation possible, invasive fungal, and other opportunistic Infxns reported; lymphoma/other cancer possible in children/adolescents Uses: *Mod–severe RA w/ an inadequate response to one or more DMARDs, psoriatic arthritis (PA), juvenile idiopathic arthritis (JIA), plaque psoriasis, ankylosing spondylitis (AS), Crohn Dz* **Acts:** TNF-α inhib **Dose:** *RA, PA, AS:* 40 mg SQ q other wk; may ↑ 40 mg qwk if not on MTX. JIA 15–30 kg 20 mg q other wk *Crohn Dz:* 160 mg d 1, 80 mg 2 wk later, then 2 wk later start maint 40 mg q other wk **Caution:** [B, ?/–] See Box do not use w/ live vaccines **CI:** None **Disp:** Prefilled 0.4 mL (20 mg) & 0.8 mL (40 mg) syringe **SE:** Inj site Rxns, anaphylaxis, cytopenias, demyelinating Dz, new onset psoriasis **Notes:** Refrigerate prefilled syringe, rotate Inj sites, OK w/ other DMARDs

Adapalene & Benzoyl Peroxide (Epiduo Gel) Uses: *Acne vulgaris* **Action:** Retinoid-like, modulates cell differentiation, keratinization, and inflammation w/ antibacterial **Dose:** *Adults & Peds > 12 yo.* Apply 1 × daily to clean/dry skin **Caution:** [C, ?] Bleaching effects, photosensitivity **CI:** Component sensitivity **Disp:** Topical gel adapalene 0.1% and benzoyl peroxide 2.5% (45g) **SE:** Local irritation, dryness **Notes:** Vit A may ↑ SE

Adefovir (Hepsera) BOX: Acute exacerbations of hep seen after d/c Rx (monitor LFTs); nephrotoxic w/ underlying renal impair w/ chronic use (monitor renal Fxn); HIV resistance/untreated may emerge; lactic acidosis & severe hepatomegaly w/ steatosis reported **Uses:** *Chronic active hep B* **Acts:** Nucleotide analog **Dose:** CrCl >50 mL/min: 10 mg PO daily; CrCl 20–49 mL/min: 10 mg PO q48h; CrCl 10–19 mL/min: 10 mg PO q72h; HD: 10 mg PO q7d postdialysis; adjust w/ CrCl <50 mL/min **Caution:** [C, −] **Disp:** Tabs 10 mg **SE:** Asthenia, HA, Abd pain; see Box **Notes:** ✓ HIV status before use

Adenosine (Adenocard) **Uses:** *PSVT*; including w/ WPW **Acts:** Class IV antiarrhythmic; slows AV node conduction **Dose:** *Adults.* 6 mg over 1–3 s, then 20 mL NS bolus, elevate extremity; repeat 12 mg in 1–2 min PRN, max single dose 12 mg *(ECC 2005)* **Peds** *<50 kg:* 0.05–0.1 mg/kg IV bolus; may repeat q1–2min to 0.3 mg/kg max **Caution:** [C, ?] Hx bronchospasm **CI:** 2nd-/3rd-degree AV block or SSS (w/o pacemaker); A flutter, AF, V tachycardia, recent MI or CNS bleed **Disp:** Inj 3 mg/mL **SE:** Facial flushing, HA, dyspnea, chest pressure, ↓ BP **Notes:** Doses >12 mg not OK; can cause momentary asystole w/ use; caffeine, theophylline antagonize effects

Albumin (Albuminar, Buminate, Albutein) **Uses:** *Plasma vol expansion for shock* (e.g., burns, hemorrhage) **Acts:** Maintain plasma colloid oncotic pressure **Dose:** *Adults.* Initial 25 g IV; then based on response; 250 g/48 h max **Peds.** 0.5–1 g/kg/dose; Inf at 0.05–0.1 g/min; max 6 g/kg/d max **Caution:** [C, ?] Severe anemia; cardiac, renal, or hepatic Insuff d/t protein load & hypervolemia **CI:** CHF, severe anemia **Disp:** Soln 5%, 25% **SE:** Chills, fever, CHF, tachycardia, ↓ BP, hypervolemia **Notes:** Contains 130–160 mEq Na⁺/L; may cause pulm edema

Albuterol (Proventil, Ventolin, Volmax) **Uses:** *Asthma, COPD, prevent exercise-induced bronchospasm* **Acts:** β-Adrenergic sympathomimetic bronchodilator; relaxes bronchial smooth muscle **Dose:** *Adults. Inhaler:* 2 Inh q4–6h PRN; 1 Rotacaps inhaled q4–6h *PO:* 2–4 mg PO tid-qid *Nebulizer:* 1.25–5 mg (0.25–1 mL of 0.5% soln in 2–3 mL of NS) tid-qid *Prevent exercise-induced asthma:* 2 puffs 5–30 min prior to activity **Peds.** *Inhaler:* 2 Inh q4–6h *PO:* 0.1–0.2 mg/ kg/dose PO; max 2–4 mg PO tid *Nebulizer:* 0.05 mg/kg (max 2.5 mg) in 2–3 mL of NS tid-qid *2–6 y.* 12 mg/d max, 6–12 y 24 mg/d max **Caution:** [C, +] **Disp:** Tabs 2, 4 mg; XR tabs 4, 8 mg; syrup 2 mg/5 mL; 90 mcg/dose metered-dose inhaler; soln for nebulizer 0.083, 0.5% **SE:** Palpitations, tachycardia, nervousness, GI upset

Albuterol & Ipratropium (Combivent, DuoNeb) **Uses:** *COPD* **Acts:** Combo of β-adrenergic bronchodilator & quaternary anticholinergic **Dose:** 2 Inh qid; nebulizer 3 mL q6h; max 12 Inh/24 h or 3 mL q4h **Caution:** [C, +] **CI:** Peanut/ soybean allergy **Disp:** Metered-dose inhaler, 18 mcg ipratropium & 103 mcg albuterol/ puff (contains ozone-depleting CFCs; will be gradually removed from US market); nebulization soln (DuoNeb) ipratropium 0.5 mg & albuterol 2.5 mg/3 mL 0.042%, 0.21% **SE:** Palpitations, tachycardia, nervousness, GI upset, dizziness, blurred vision

Aldesleukin [IL-2] (Proleukin) **BOX:** High dose associated w/ capillary leak synd w/ hypotension and ↓ organ perfusion; ↑ Infxn d/t poor neutrophil activity; D/C w/ mod–severe lethargy, may progress to coma **Uses:** *Met RCC &

melanoma* **Acts:** Acts via IL-2 receptor; many immunomodulatory effects **Dose:** 600,000 Int Units/kg q8h × 14 doses days 1–5 and days 15–19 of 28-d cycle (FDA-approved dose/schedule for RCC); other schedules (e.g., "high dose" 24 × 10⁶ Int Units/m² IV q8h on days 1–5 & 12–16) **Caution:** [C, ?/–] Organ allografts **Disp:** Powder for recons 22 × 10⁶ Int Units, when reconstituted 18 mill Int Units/mL = 1.1 mg/mL **SE:** Flu-like synd (malaise, fever, chills), N/V/D, ↑ bili; capillary leak synd; ↓ BP, tachycardia, pulm & edema, fluid retention, & wgt gain; renal & mild hematologic tox (↓ Hgb, plt, WBC), eosinophilia; cardiac tox (ischemia, atrial arrhythmias); neurotox (CNS depression, somnolence, delirium, rare coma); pruritic rashes, urticaria, & erythroderma common.

Alefacept (Amevive) **BOX:** Monitor CD4 before each dose; w/hold if <250; D/C if <250 × 1 mo **Uses:** *Mod/severe chronic plaque psoriasis* **Acts:** Fusion protein inhib **Dose:** 7.5 mg IV or 15 mg IM once/wk × 12 wk **Caution:** [B, ?/–] PRG registry; associated w/ serious Infxn **CI:** Lymphopenia, HIV **Disp:** 15-mg powder for recons **SE:** Pharyngitis, myalgia, Inj site Rxn, malignancy, Infxn **Notes:** IV/IM different formulations; may repeat course 12 wk later if CD4 OK

Alendronate (Fosamax, Fosamax Plus D) **Uses:** *Rx & prevent osteoporosis male & postmenopausal female, Rx steroid-induced osteoporosis, Paget Dz* **Acts:** ↓ nl & abnormal bone resorption, ↓ osteoclast action **Dose:** *Osteoporosis:* Rx: 10 mg/d PO or 70 mg qwk; Fosamax plus D 1 tab qwk *Steroid-induced osteoporosis:* Rx: 5 mg/d PO, 10 mg/d postmenopausal not on estrogen *Prevention:* 5 mg/d PO or 35 mg qwk *Paget Dz:* 40 mg/d PO **Caution:** [C, ?] Not OK if CrCl <35 mL/min, w/ NSAID use **CI:** Esophageal anomalies, inability to sit/stand upright for 30 min, ↓ Ca²⁺ **Disp:** Tabs 5, 10, 35, 40, 70 mg, soln 70 mg/75 mL *Fosamax plus D*: Alendronate 70 mg w/ cholecalciferol (vit D₃) 2800 or 5600 Int Units **SE:** Abd pain, acid regurgitation, constipation, dyspepsia, musculoskeletal pain, jaw osteonecrosis (w/ dental procedures, chemo) **Notes:** Take 1st thing in AM w/ H₂O (8 oz) >30 min before 1st food/beverage of day; do not lie down for 30 min after. Use Ca²⁺ & vit D supl w/ regular tab; may ↑ atypical subtrochanteric femur fractures

Alfentanil (Alfenta) [C-II] **Uses:** *Adjunct in maint of anesthesia; analgesia* **Acts:** Short-acting narcotic analgesic **Dose:** *Adults & Peds >12 y:* 3–75 mcg/kg (IBW) IV Inf; total depends on duration of procedure **Caution:** [C, +/–] ↑ ICP, resp depression **Disp:** Inj 500 mcg/mL **SE:** ↓ HR, ↓ BP arrhythmias, peripheral vasodilation, ↑ ICP, drowsiness, resp depression, N/V/constipation

Alfuzosin (Uroxatral) **BOX:** May ↑ QTc interval **Uses:** *symptomatic BPH* **Acts:** α-Blocker **Dose:** 10 mg PO daily immediately after the same meal **Caution:** [B, –]w/any hx ↓ BP; use w/ PDE5 inhibitors may ↓ BP **CI:** w/ CYP3A4 inhib; mod–severe hepatic impair; protease inhibitors for HIV **Disp:** Tabs 10 mg ER **SE:** Postural ↓ BP, dizziness, HA, fatigue **Notes:** Do not cut or crush; ↓ ejaculatory disorders compared w/ similar drugs

Alginic Acid + Aluminum Hydroxide & Magnesium Trisilicate (Gaviscon) [OTC] **Uses:** *Heartburn*; hiatal hernia pain **Acts:** Protective layer blocks gastric acid **Dose:** Chew 2–4 tabs or 15–30 mL PO qid followed by H_2O **Caution:** [B, –] Avoid w/ renal impair or Na^+-restricted diet **Disp:** Chew tabs, susp **SE:** D, constipation

Alglucosidase Alfa (Myozyme) BOX: Life-threatening anaphylactic Rxns seen w/ Inf; medical support measures should be immediately available **Uses:** *Rx Pompe DZ* **Acts:** Recombinant acid α-glucosidase; degrades glycogen in lysosomes **Dose:** *Peds 1 mo–3.5 y* 20 mg/kg IV q2wk over 4 h (see PI) **Caution:** [B, ?/–] Illness at time of Inf may ↑ Inf Rxns **Disp:** Powder 50 mg/vial **SE:** Hypersens, fever, rash, D,V, gastroenteritis, pneumonia, URI, cough, resp distress/failure, Infxns, cardiac arrhythmia w/ general anesthesia, ↑/↓ HR, flushing, anemia

Aliskiren (Tekturna) BOX: May cause injury and death to a developing fetus; D/C immediately when PRG detected **Uses:** *HTN* **Acts:** 1st direct renin inhib **Dose:** 150–300 mg/d PO **Caution:** [C (1st tri), D (2nd & 3rd tri); ?]; Avoid w/ CrCl <30 mL/min; ketoconazole and other CYP3A4 inhib may ↑ aliskiren levels **CI:** Anuria, sulfur sensitivity **Disp:** Tabs 150, 300 mg **SE:** D, Abd pain, dyspepsia, GERD, cough, ↑ K^+, angioedema, ↓ BP, dizziness

Aliskiren/Hydrochlorothiazide (Tekturna HCT) BOX: May cause injury and death to a developing fetus; D/C immediately when PRG detected **Uses:** *HTN, not primary Rx* **Acts:** Renin inhib w/ diuretic **Dose:** *Monotherapy failure:* 150 mg/12.5 mg PO q day; may ↑ to 150 mg/25 mg, 300 mg/12.5 mg q day after 2–4 wk *Max:* 300 mg/25 mg **Caution:** [D, ?] Avoid w/ CrCl ≤30 mL/min; avoid w/ CYP3A4 inhib (Li, ketoconazole, etc.) may ↑ aliskiren levels; ↓ BP in salt/volume depleted pts **Disp:** Tabs (aliskiren mg/HCTZ mg) 150/12.5, 150/25, 300/12.5, 300/25 **SE:** Dizziness, influenza, D, cough, vertigo, asthenia, arthralgia, angioedema

Allopurinol (Zyloprim, Lopurin, Aloprim) **Uses:** *Gout, hyperuricemia of malignancy, uric acid urolithiasis* **Acts:** Xanthine oxidase inhib; ↓ uric acid production **Dose:** *Adults. PO:* Initial 100 mg/d; usual 300 mg/d; max 800 mg/d; ÷ dose if >300 mg/d *IV:* 200–400 mg/m²/d (max 600 mg/24 h); (after meal w/ plenty of fluid) *Peds.* Only for hyperuricemia of malignancy if <10 y: 10 mg/kg/24 h PO or 200 mg/m²/d IV ÷ q6–8h; max 600 mg/24 h; ↓ in renal impair **Caution:** [C, M] **Disp:** Tabs 100, 300 mg; Inj 500 mg/30 mL (Aloprim) **SE:** Rash, N/V, renal impair, angioedema **Notes:** Aggravates acute gout; begin after acute attack resolves; IV dose of 6 mg/mL final conc as single daily Inf or ÷ 6-, 8-, or 12-h intervals

Almotriptan (Axert) **Uses:** *Rx acute migraine* **Acts:** Vascular serotonin receptor agonist **Dose:** *Adults. PO:* 6.25–12 mg PO, repeat in 2 h PRN; 2 dose/24 h max PO dose; max 12 or 24 mg/d; w/ hepatic/renal impair 6.25 mg single dose (max 12.5 mg/d) **Caution:** [C, ?/–] **CI:** Angina, ischemic heart Dz, coronary artery vasospasm, hemiplegic or basilar migraine, uncontrolled HTN, ergot use, MAOI use w/in 14 d **Disp:** Tabs 6.25, 12.5 mg **SE:** N, somnolence, paresthesias, HA, dry mouth, weakness, numbness, coronary vasospasm, HTN

Alosetron (Lotronex) **BOX:** Serious GI SEs, some fatal, including ischemic colitis reported. Prescribed only through participation in the prescribing program **Uses:** *Severe D—predominant IBS in women who fail conventional Rx* **Acts:** Selective 5-HT$_3$ receptor antagonist **Dose:** *Adults.* 0.5 mg PO bid; ↑ to 1 mg bid max after 4 wk; D/C after 8 wk not controlled **Caution:** [B, ?/–] **CI:** Hx chronic/severe constipation, GI obst, strictures, toxic megacolon, GI perforation, adhesions, ischemic/ulcerative colitis, Crohn Dz, diverticulitis, thrombophlebitis, hypercoagulability **Disp:** Tabs 0.5, 1 mg **SE:** Constipation, Abd pain, N **Notes:** D/C immediately if constipation or Sxs of ischemic colitis develop; informed consent prior to use

Alpha-1-Protease Inhibitor (Prolastin) **Uses:** *α$_1$-Antitrypsin deficiency*; panacinar emphysema **Acts:** Replace human α$_1$-protease inhib **Dose:** 60 mg/kg IV once/wk **Caution:** [C, ?] **CI:** Selective IgA deficiencies w/ IgA antibodies **Disp:** Inj 500 mg/20 mL, 1000 mg/40 mL powder for Inj **SE:** HA, MS discomfort, fever, dizziness, flu-like Sxs, allergic Rxns, ↑ AST/ALT

Alprazolam (Xanax, Niravam) [C-IV] **Uses:** *Anxiety & panic disorders*, anxiety w/ depression **Acts:** Benzodiazepine; antianxiety agent **Dose:** *Anxiety:* Initial, 0.25–0.5 mg tid; ↑ to 4 mg/d max ÷ doses *Panic:* Initial, 0.5 mg tid; may gradually ↑ to response; ↓ in elderly, debilitated, & hepatic impair **Caution:** [D, –] **CI:** NAG, concomitant itra-/ketoconazole **Disp:** Tabs 0.25, 0.5, 1, 2 mg; Xanax XR 0.5, 1, 2, 3 mg; Niravam (ODTs) 0.25, 0.5, 1, 2 mg; soln 1 mg/mL **SE:** Drowsiness, fatigue, irritability, memory impair, sexual dysfunction, paradoxical Rxns **Notes:** Avoid abrupt D/C after prolonged use

Alprostadil [Prostaglandin E$_1$] (Prostin VR) **BOX:** Apnea in up to 12% of neonates especially <2 kg at birth **Uses:** *Conditions where ductus arteriosus flow must be maintained* (e.g., sustain pulm/systemic circulation until OR (e.g., pulm atresia/stenosis, transposition) **Acts:** Vasodilator (ductus arteriosus very sensitive), plt inhib **Dose:** 0.05 mcg/kg/min IV; ↓ to response **Caution:** [X, –] **CI:** Neonatal resp distress synd **Disp:** Inj 500 mcg/mL **SE:** Cutaneous vasodilation, Sz-like activity, jitteriness, ↑ temp, ↓ Ca^{2+}, thrombocytopenia, ↓ BP; may cause apnea **Notes:** Keep intubation kit at bedside

Alprostadil, Intracavernosal (Caverject, Edex) **Uses:** *ED* **Acts:** Relaxes smooth muscles, dilates cavernosal arteries, ↑ lacunar spaces w/ blood entrapment **Dose:** 2.5–60 mcg intracavernosal; titrate in office **Caution:** [X, –] **CI:** ↑ risk of priapism (e.g., sickle cell); penile deformities/implants; men in whom sexual activity inadvisable **Disp:** *Caverject:* 5-, 10-, 20-, 40-mcg powder for Inj vials ± diluent syringes 10-, 20-, 40-mcg amp *Caverject Impulse:* Self-contained syringe (29 gauge) 10 & 20 mcg *Edex:* 10-, 20-, 40-mcg cartridges **SE:** Local pain w/ Inj **Notes:** Counsel about priapism, penile fibrosis, & hematoma risks, titrate dose in office

Alprostadil, Urethral Suppository (Muse) **Uses:** *ED* **Acts:** Urethral absorption; vasodilator, relaxes smooth muscle of corpus cavernosa **Dose:** 125–1000-mcg system 5–10 min prior to sex; repeat × 1/24 h; titrate in office **Caution:** [X, –] **CI:** ↑

Priapism risk (especially sickle cell, myeloma, leukemia) penile deformities/implants; men in whom sex inadvisable **Disp:** 125, 250, 500, 1000 mcg w/ transurethral system **SE:** ↓ BP, dizziness, syncope, penile/testicular pain, urethral burning/bleeding, priapism **Notes:** Titrate dose in office; duration 30–60 min

Alteplase, Recombinant [tPA] (Activase)
Uses: *AMI, PE, acute ischemic stroke, & CV cath occlusion* **Acts:** Thrombolytic; binds fibrin in thrombus, initiates fibrinolysis **Dose:** *AMI:* 15 mg IV over 1–2 min, then 0.75 mg/kg (max 50 mg) over 30 min, then 0.5 mg/kg over next 60 min (max 35 mg)*(ECC 2005)* *Stroke:* w/in 3 h of onset *S&S:* 0.09 mg/kg IV over 1 min, then 0.81 mg/kg; max 90 mg/h Inf over 60 min *(ECC 2005)* *Cath occlusion:* 10–29 kg 1 mg/mL; ≥30 kg 2 mg/mL **Caution:** [C, ?] **CI:** Active internal bleeding; uncontrolled HTN (SBP >185 mm Hg, DBP >110 mm Hg); recent (w/in 3 mo) CVA, GI bleed, trauma; intracranial or intraspinal surgery or Dzs (AVM/aneurysm/subarachnoid hemorrhage/neoplasm), prolonged cardiac massage; suspected aortic dissection, w/ anticoagulants or INR >1.7, heparin w/in 48 h, plts <100,000, Sz at the time of stroke **Disp:** Powder for Inj 2, 50, 100 mg **SE:** Bleeding, bruising (e.g., venipuncture sites), ↓ BP **Notes:** Give heparin to prevent reocclusion; in AMI, doses of >150 mg associated w/ intracranial bleeding

Altretamine (Hexalen)
BOX: BM suppression, neurotox common **Uses:** *Epithelial ovarian CA* **Acts:** Unknown; cytotoxic/alkylating agent; ↓ nucleotide incorporation **Dose:** 260 mg/m²/d in 4 ÷ doses for 14–21 d of a 28-d Rx cycle; dose ↑ to 150 mg/m²/d × 14 d multiagent regimens (per protocols); after meals and hs **Caution:** [D, ?/–] **CI:** Preexisting BM depression or neurologic tox **Disp:** Gel caps 50 mg **SE:** N/V/D, cramps; neurotox (neuropathy, CNS depression); minimal myelosuppression **Notes:** ✓ CBC, routine neurologic exams

Alvimopan (Entereg)
BOX: For short-term hospital use only (max 15 doses) **Uses:** *↓ Time to GI recovery w/ bowel resection and primary anastomosis* **Action:** Opioid (μ) receptor antagonist; selectively binds GI receptors, antagonizes effects of opioids on GI motility/secretion **Dose:** 12 mg 30 min–5 h preop PO, then 12 mg bid up to 7 d; max 15 doses **Caution:** [B, ±] Not rec in complete bowel obstruction surgery, hepatic/renal impair **CI:** Therapeutic opioids > 7 consecutive days prior **Disp:** Caps 12 mg **SE:** ↓ K⁺, dyspepsia, urinary retention, anemia, back pain **Notes:** Hospitals must be registered to use.

Aluminum Hydroxide (Amphojel, AlternaGEL, Dermagran) [OTC]
Uses: *Heartburn, upset or sour stomach, or acid indigestion*; supl to Rx of ↑PO₄²⁻; *minor cuts, burns (Dermagran)* **Acts:** Neutralizes gastric acid; binds PO₄²⁻ **Dose:** *Adults.* 10–30 mL or 300–1200 mg PO q4–6h *Peds.* 5–15 mL PO q4–6h or 50–150 mg/kg/24 h PO ÷ q4–6h (hyperphosphatemia) **Caution:** [C, ?] **Disp:** Tabs 300, 600 mg; susp 320, 600 mg/5 mL; oint 0.275% (*Dermagran*) **SE:** Constipation **Notes:** OK w/ renal failure

Aluminum Hydroxide + Magnesium Carbonate (Gaviscon Extra Strength, Liquid) [OTC]
Uses: *Heartburn, acid indigestion* **Acts:** Neutralizes

gastric acid **Dose:** *Adults.* 15–30 mL PO pc & hs; 2–4 chew tabs up to qid. *Peds.* 5–15 mL PO qid or PRN; **Caution:** [C, ?] ↑ Mg^{2+}, avoid w/in renal impair **Disp:** Liq w/ AlOH 95 mg/mg carbonate 358 mg/15 mL; Extra Strength liq AlOH 254 mg/Mg carbonate 237 mg/15 mL; chew tabs AlOH 160 mg/Mg carbonate 105 mg **SE:** Constipation, D **Notes:** qid doses best pc & hs; may ↓ absorption of some drugs, take 2–3 h apart to ↓ effect

Aluminum Hydroxide + Magnesium Hydroxide (Maalox) [OTC]
Uses: *Hyperacidity* (peptic ulcer, hiatal hernia, etc) **Acts:** Neutralizes gastric acid **Dose:** *Adults.* 10–20 mL or 2–4 tabs PO qid or PRN *Peds.* 5–15 mL PO qid or PRN **Caution:** [C, ?] **Disp:** Chew tabs, susp **SE:** May ↑ Mg^{2+} w/ renal Insuff, constipation, D **Notes:** Doses qid best pc & hs

Aluminum Hydroxide + Magnesium Hydroxide & Simethicone (Mylanta, Mylanta II, Maalox Plus) [OTC]   **Uses:** *Hyperacidity w/ bloating* **Acts:** Neutralizes gastric acid & defoaming **Dose:** *Adults.* 10–20 mL or 2–4 tabs PO qid or PRN *Peds.* 5–15 mL PO qid or PRN; avoid in renal impair **Caution:** [C, ?] **Disp:** Tabs, susp, liq **SE:** ↑ Mg^{2+} in renal Insuff, D, constipation **Notes:** Mylanta II contains twice Al & Mg hydroxide of Mylanta; may affect absorption of some drugs

Aluminum Hydroxide + Magnesium Trisilicate (Gaviscon, Regular Strength) [OTC]   **Uses:** *Relief of heartburn, upset or sour stomach, or acid indigestion* **Acts:** Neutralizes gastric acid **Dose:** Chew 2–4 tabs qid; avoid in renal impair **Caution:** [C, ?] **CI:** Mg^{2+}, sensitivity **Disp:** AlOH 80 mg/Mg trisilicate 20 mg/tab **SE:** ↑ Mg^{2+} in renal Insuff, constipation, D **Notes:** May affect absorption of some drugs

Amantadine (Symmetrel)   **Uses:** *Rx/prophylaxis influenza A, parkinsonism, & drug-induced EPS* d/t **Acts:** Prevents infectious viral nucleic acid release into host cell; releases dopamine and blocks reuptake of dopamine in presynaptic nerves **Dose:** *Adults. Influenza A:* 200 mg/d PO or 100 mg PO bid w/ in 48 h of Sx *Parkinsonism:* 100 mg PO daily-bid *Peds 1–9 y:* 4.4–8.8 mg/kg/24 h to 150 mg/24 h max ÷ doses daily-bid *10–12 y:* 100–200 mg/d in 1–2 ÷ doses; ↓ in renal impair **Caution:** [C, M] **Disp:** Caps 100 mg; tabs 100 mg; soln 50 mg/5 mL **SE:** Orthostatic ↓ BP, edema, insomnia, depression, irritability, hallucinations, dream abnormalities, N/D, dry mouth **Notes:** Not for influenza use in US d/t resistance including H1N1

Ambrisentan (Letairis)   **BOX:** May cause ↑ AST/ALT to >3× ULN, LFTs monthly. CI in PRG; ✓ monthly PRG tests **Uses:** *Pulm arterial HTN* **Acts:** Endothelin receptor antagonist **Dose:** *Adults.* 5 mg PO/d, max 10 mg/d; not OK w/ hepatic impair **Caution:** [X, –] w/ Cyclosporine, strong CYP3A or 2C19 inhib, inducers of P-glycoprotein, CYPs and UGTs **CI:** PRG **Disp:** Tabs 5, 10 mg **SE:** Edema, nasal congestion, sinusitis, dyspnea, flushing, constipation, HA, palpitations, hepatotoxic **Notes:** Available only through the Letairis Education and Access Program (LEAP); D/C AST/ALT >5× ULN or bili >2× ULN or S/Sx of liver dysfunction; childbearing females must use 2 methods of contraception

Amifostine (Ethyol) Uses: *Xerostomia prophylaxis during RT (head, neck, etc) where parotid is in radiation field; ↓ renal tox w/ repeated cisplatin* **Acts:** Prodrug, dephosphorylated by alkaline phosphatase to active thiol metabolite; binds cisplatin metabolites **Dose:** 910 mg/m²/d 15-min IV Inf 30 min prechemotherapy **Caution:** [C, +/–] CV Dz **Disp:** 500-mg vials powder, reconstitute in NS **SE:** Transient ↓ BP (>60%), N/V, flushing w/ hot or cold chills, dizziness, ↓ Ca²⁺, somnolence, sneezing **Notes:** Does not ↓ effectiveness of cyclophosphamide + cisplatin chemotherapy

Amikacin (Amikin) Uses: *Serious gram(−) bacterial Infxns* & mycobacteria **Acts:** Aminoglycoside; ↓ protein synth *Spectrum:* Good gram(−) bacterial coverage: *Pseudomonas* & *Mycobacterium* sp **Dose:** *Adults & Peds. Conventional:* 5–7.5 mg/kg/dose q8h; once daily; 15–20 mg/kg q24h; ↑ interval w/ renal impair *Neonates <1200 g, 0–4 wk:* 7.5 mg/kg/dose q18h–24h *Age <7 d, 1200–2000 g:* 7.5 mg/kg/dose q12h *>2000 g:* 10 mg/kg/dose q12h *Age >7 d, 1200–2000 g:* 7 mg/kg/dose q8h *>2000 g:* 7.5–10 mg/kg/dose q8h **Caution:** [C, +/–] Avoid w/ diuretics **Disp:** Inj 50 & 250 mg/mL **SE:** Nephro-/oto-/neurotox, neuromuscular blockage, resp paralysis **Notes:** May be effective in gram(−) resistant to gentamicin & tobramycin; follow Cr; Levels: *Peak:* 30 min after Inf *Trough* <0.5 h before next dose *Therapeutic: Peak* 20–30 mcg/mL *Trough:* <8 mcg/mL *Toxic peak* >35 mcg/mL; *half-life:* 2 h

Amiloride (Midamor) Uses: *HTN, CHF, & thiazide-induced ↓ K⁺* **Acts:** K⁺-sparing diuretic; interferes w/ K⁺/Na⁺ exchange in distal tubule **Dose:** *Adults.* 5–10 mg PO daily *Peds.* 0.625 mg/kg/d; ↓ w/ renal impair **Caution:** [B, ?] **CI:** ↑ K⁺, SCr >1.5, BUN >30, diabetic neuropathy, w/ other K⁺-sparing diuretics **Disp:** Tabs 5 mg **SE:** ↑ K⁺; HA, dizziness, dehydration, impotence **Notes:** ✓ K⁺

Aminocaproic Acid (Amicar) Uses: *Excessive bleeding from systemic hyperfibrinolysis & urinary fibrinolysis* **Acts:** ↓ Fibrinolysis; inhibits TPA, inhibits conversion of plasminogen to plasmin **Dose:** *Adults.* 5 g IV or PO (1st h) then 1–1.25 g/h IV or PO × 8 h or until bleeding controlled; 30 g/d max *Peds.* 100 mg/kg IV (1st h) then 1 g/m²/h; max 18 g/m²/d; ↓ w/ renal Insuff **Caution:** [C, ?] Not for upper urinary tract bleeding **CI:** DIC **Disp:** Tabs 500, syrup 250 mg/mL; Inj 250 mg/mL **SE:** ↓ BP, ↓ HR, dizziness, HA, fatigue, rash, GI disturbance, ↓ plt Fxn **Notes:** Administer × 8 h or until bleeding controlled

Amino-Cerv pH 5.5 Cream Uses: *Mild cervicitis*, postpartum cervicitis/ cervical tears, post-cauterization/cryosurgery/conization **Acts:** Hydrating agent; removes excess keratin in hyperkeratotic conditions **Dose:** 1 Applicator-full intravag hs × 2–4 wk **Caution:** [C, ?] w/ Viral skin Infxn **Disp:** Vag cream **SE:** Stinging, local irritation **Notes:** AKA carbamide or urea; contains 8.34% urea, 0.5% sodium propionate, 0.83% methionine, 0.35% cystine, 0.83% inositol, & benzalkonium chloride

Aminoglutethimide (Cytadren) Uses: *Cushing synd*, adrenocortical carcinoma, breast CA & PCa **Acts:** ↓ Adrenal steroidogenesis & conversion of androgens to estrogens; 1st gen aromatase inhib **Dose:** Initial 250 mg PO 4 × d, titrate q1–2wk max 2 g/d; w/ hydrocortisone 20–40 mg/d; ↓ w/ renal Insuff **Caution:** [D, ?] **Disp:** Tabs 250 mg **SE:** Adrenal Insuff ("medical adrenalectomy"), hypothyroidism, masculinization; ↓ BP, N/V, rare hepatotox, rash, myalgia, fever, drowsiness, lethargy, anorexia **Notes:** Give q6h to ↓ N

Aminophylline (Generic) **Uses:** *Asthma, COPD* & bronchospasm **Acts:** Relaxes smooth muscle (bronchi, pulm vessels); stimulates diaphragm **Dose:** *Adults. Acute asthma:* Load 6 mg/kg IV, then 0.4–0.9 mg/kg/h IV cont Inf, not > than 25 mg/min *Chronic asthma:* 24 mg/kg/24 h PO ÷ q6h *Peds.* Load 6 mg/kg IV, then 6 wk-6 mo 0.5 mg/kg/h, 6 mo-1 y 0.6–0.7 mg/kg/h, 1–9 y 1 mg/kg/h IV Inf; ↓ w/ hepatic Insuff & w/ some drugs (macrolide & quinolone antibiotics, cimetidine, propranolol) **Caution:** [C, +] Uncontrolled arrhythmias, HTN, Sz disorder, hyperthyroidism, peptic ulcers **Disp:** Tabs 100, 200 mg; PR tabs 100, 200 mg, soln 105 mg/5 mL, Inj 25 mg/mL **SE:** N/V, irritability, tachycardia, ventricular arrhythmias, Szs **Notes:** Individualize dosage *Level:* 10 to 20 mcg/mL, toxic >20 mcg/mL; aminophylline 85% theophylline; erratic rectal absorption

Amiodarone (Cordarone, Nexterone, Pacerone) **BOX:** Liver tox, exacerbation of arrhythmias and lung damage reported **Uses:** *Recurrent VF or unstable VT*, supraventricular arrhythmias, AF **Acts:** Class III antiarrhythmic (Table 9 p 279) **Dose:** *Adults. Ventricular arrhythmias:* IV: 15 mg/min × 10 min, then 1 mg/min × 6 h, maint 0.5-mg/min cont Inf or PO: Load: 800–1600 mg PO × 1–3 wk Maint: 600–800 mg/d PO for 1 mo, then 200–400 mg/d *Supraventricular arrhythmias:* IV: 300 mg IV over 1 h, then 20 mg/kg for 24 h, then 600 mg PO daily for 1 wk, maint 100–400 mg daily *or PO:* Load 600–800 mg/d PO for 1–4 wk *Maint:* Slow ↓ to 100–400 mg daily *(ECC 2005) Cardiac arrest:* 300 mg IV push; 150 mg IV push 3–5 min PRN *Refractory pulseless VT, VF:* 5 mg/kg rapid IV bolus *Perfusing arrhythmias:* Load: 5 mg/kg IV/IO over 20–60 min; repeat PRN, max 15 mg/kg/d *Peds.* 10–15 mg/kg/24 h ÷ q12h PO for 7–10 d, then 5 mg/kg/24 h ÷ q12h or daily (infants require ↑ loading); ↓ w/ liver Insuff **Caution:** [D, –] May require ↓ digoxin/warfarin dose, many drug interactions **CI:** Sinus node dysfunction, 2nd-/3rd-degree AV block, sinus brady (w/o pacemaker), iodine sensitivity **Disp:** Tabs 100, 200, 400 mg; Inj 50 mg/mL **SE:** Pulm fibrosis, exacerbation of arrhythmias, ↑ QT interval; CHF, hypo-/hyperthyroidism, ↑ LFTs, liver failure, corneal microdeposits, optic neuropathy/neuritis, peripheral neuropathy, photosens **Notes:** IV conc >2.0 mg/mL central line only Levels: *Trough:* just before next dose *Therapeutic:* 1–2.5 mcg/mL *Toxic:* >2.5 mcg/mL *1/2-life:* 30–100 h

Amitriptyline (Elavil) **BOX:** Antidepressants may ↑ suicide risk; consider risks/benefits of use. Monitor pts closely **Uses:** *Depression (not bipolar depression)* peripheral neuropathy, chronic pain, tension HAs **Acts:** TCA; ↓ reuptake of serotonin & norepinephrine by presynaptic neurons **Dose:** *Adults. Initial:* 30–50 mg PO hs; may ↑ to 300 mg hs. *Peds.* Not OK <12 y unless for chronic pain *Initial:* 0.1 mg/kg PO hs, ↑ over 2–3 wk to 0.5–2 mg/kg PO hs; taper to D/C

Caution: CV Dz, Szs [D,+/−] NAG, hepatic impair **CI:** w/ MAOIs or w/in 14 d of use, during acute MI recovery **Disp:** Tabs 10, 25, 50, 75, 100, 150 mg; Inj 10 mg/mL **SE:** Strong anticholinergic SEs; OD may be fatal; urine retention, sedation, ECG changes, photosens **Notes:** Levels: *Therapeutic:* 120 to 150 ng/mL *Toxic:* >500 mg/mL; levels may not correlate w/ effectiveness

Amlodipine (Norvasc) **Uses:** *HTN, stable or unstable angina* **Acts:** CCB; relaxes coronary vascular smooth muscle **Dose:** 2.5–10 mg/d PO; ↓ w/ hepatic impair **Caution:** [C, ?] **Disp:** Tabs 2.5, 5, 10 mg **SE:** Edema, HA, palpitations, flushing, dizziness **Notes:** Take w/o regard to meals

Amlodipine/Atorvastatin (Caduet) **Uses:** *HTN, chronic stable/ vasospastic angina, control cholesterol & triglycerides* **Acts:** CCB & HMG-CoA reductase inhib **Dose:** Amlodipine 2.5–10 mg w/ atorvastatin 10–80 mg PO daily **Caution:** [X, −] **CI:** Active liver Dz, ↑ LFTs **Disp:** Tabs amlodipine/atorvastatin: 2.5/10, 2.5/20, 2.5/40, 5/10, 5/20, 5/40, 5/80, 10/10, 10/20, 10/40, 10/80 mg **SE:** Edema, HA, palpitations, flushing, myopathy, arthralgia, myalgia, GI upset, liver failure **Notes:** ✓ LFTs; instruct pt to report muscle pain/weakness

Amlodipine/Olmesartan (Azor) **BOX:** Use of renin-angiotensin agents in PRG can cause injury and death to fetus, D/C immediately when PRG detected **Uses:** *Hypertension* **Acts:** CCB w/ angiotensin II receptor blocker **Dose:** *Adults.* Initial 2 mg/20 mg, max 10 mg/40 mg q day **Caution:** [C 1st tri, D 2nd, 3rd tri, −] w/ K+ supl or K+-sparing diuretics, renal impair, RAS, severe CAD, AS **CI:** PRG **Disp:** Tabs amlodipine/olmesartan 5mg/20mg, 10/20, 5/40, 10/40 **SE:** Edema, vertigo, dizziness, ↓ BP

Amlodipine/Valsartan (Exforge) **BOX:** Use of renin-angiotensin agents in PRG can cause fetal injury and death, D/C immediately when PRG detected **Uses:** * ↑ BP not controlled on single med* **Acts:** CCB w/ angiotensin II receptor blocker **Dose:** *Adults.* Initial 5 mg/160 mg, may ↑ after 1–2 wk, max 10 mg/ 320 mg q day, start elderly at 1/2 initial dose **Caution:** [C 1st tri, D 2nd, 3rd tri, −] w/ K+ supl or K+-sparing diuretics, renal impair, RAS, severe CAD **CI:** PRG, **Disp:** Tabs amlodipine/valsartan 5/160, 10/160, 5/320,10mg/320 mg **SE:** Edema, vertigo, nasopharyngitis, URI, dizziness, ↓ BP

Amlodipine/Valsartan/HCTZ (Exforge HCT) **BOX:** Use of reninangiotensin agents in PRG can cause fetal injury and death, D/C immediately when PRG detected **Uses:** *Hypertension* **Acts:** CCB, angiotensin II receptor blocker, & thiazide diuretic **Dose:** 1 tab 1 × daily, may ↑ dose after 2 wk; max dose 10/320/25 mg **Caution:** [D, −] w/ Severe hepatic or renal impair **CI:** Anuria, sulfonamide allergy **Disp:** Tabs amlodipine/valsartan/HCTZ: 5/160/12.5, 10/160/12.5, 5/160/25, 10/160/25, 10/320/25 mg **SE:** edema, dizziness, headache, fatigue, nasopharyngitis, dyspepsia, N, back pain, muscle spasm, ↓ BP

Ammonium Aluminum Sulfate [Alum] [OTC] **Uses:** *Hemorrhagic cystitis when saline bladder irrigation fails* **Acts:** Astringent **Dose:** 1–2% soln w/ constant NS bladder irrigation **Caution:** [+/−] **Disp:** Powder for recons **SE:**

Encephalopathy possible; ✓ aluminum levels, especially w/ renal Insuff; can precipitate & occlude catheters **Notes:** Safe w/o anesthesia & w/ vesicoureteral reflux

Amoxicillin (Amoxil, Polymox) **Uses:** *Ear, nose, & throat, lower resp, skin, urinary tract Infxns from susceptible gram(+) bacteria* endocarditis prophylaxis, *H. pylori* eradication w/ other agents (gastric ulcers) **Acts:** β-Lactam antibiotic; ↓ cell wall synth **Spectrum:** Gram(+) (*Streptococcus* sp, *Enterococcus* sp); some gram(−) (*H. influenzae, E. coli, N. gonorrhoeae, H. pylori,* & *P. mirabilis*) **Dose:** *Adults.* 250–500 mg PO tid or 500–875 mg bid **Peds.** 25–100 mg/kg/24 h PO ÷ q8h, 200–400 mg PO bid (equivalent to 125–250 mg tid); ↓ in renal impair **Caution:** [B, +] **Disp:** Caps 250, 500 mg; chew tabs 125, 200, 250, 400 mg; susp 50 mg/mL, 125, 200, 250, & 400 mg/5 mL; tabs 500, 875 mg **SE:** D; rash **Notes:** Cross hypersens w/ PCN; many *E. coli* strains resistant; chew tabs contain phenylalanine

Amoxicillin & Clavulanic Acid (Augmentin, Augmentin 600 ES, Augmentin XR) **Uses:** *Ear, lower resp, sinus, urinary tract, skin Infxns caused by β-lactamase–producing H. influenzae, S. aureus,* & *E. coli** **Acts:** β-Lactam antibiotic w/ β-lactamase inhib **Spectrum:** Gram(+) same as amoxicillin alone, MSSA; gram(−) as w/ amoxicillin alone, β-lactamase–producing *H. influenzae, Klebsiella* sp, *M. catarrhalis* **Dose:** *Adults.* 250–500 mg PO q8h or 875 mg q12h; XR 2000 mg PO q12h **Peds.** 20–40 mg/Kg/d as amoxicillin PO ÷ q8h or 45 mg/kg/d ÷ q12h; ↓ in renal impair; take w/ food **Caution:** [B, enters breast milk] **Disp:** Supplied (as amoxicillin/clavulanic): Tabs 250/125, 500/125, 875/125 mg; chew tabs 125/31.25, 200/28.5, 250/62.5, 400/57 mg; susp 125/31.25, 250/62.5, 200/28.5, 400/57 mg/5 mL; susp ES 600/42.9 mg/5 mL; XR tab 1000/62.5 mg **SE:** Abd discomfort, N/V/D, allergic Rxn, vaginitis **Notes:** Do not substitute two 250-mg tabs for one 500-mg tab (OD of clavulanic acid); max clavulanic acid 125 mg/dose

Amphotericin B (Amphocin, Fungizone) **Uses:** *Severe, systemic fungal Infxns; oral & cutaneous candidiasis* **Acts:** Binds ergosterol in the fungal membrane to alter permeability **Dose:** *Adults & Peds.* Test dose: 1 mg IV adults or 0.1 mg/kg to 1 mg IV in children; then 0.25–1.5 mg/kg/24 h IV over 2–6 h (25–50 mg/d or q other day). Total varies w/ indication *PO:* 1 mL qid **Caution:** [B, ?] **Disp:** Powder (Inj) 50 mg/vial **SE:** ↓ K$^+$/Mg^{2+} from renal wasting; anaphylaxis, HA, fever, chills, nephrotox, ↓ BP, anemia, rigors **Notes:** ✓ Cr/LFTs/K/Mg; ↓ in renal impair; pretreatment w/ APAP & antihistamines (Benadryl) ↓ SE

Amphotericin B Cholesteryl (Amphotec) **Uses:** *Aspergillosis if intolerant/refractory to conventional amphotericin B*, systemic candidiasis* **Acts:** Binds ergosterol in fungal membrane, alters permeability **Dose:** *Adults & Peds.* Test dose: 1.6–8.3 mg, over 15–20 min, then 3–4 mg/kg/d; 1 mg/kg/h Inf, 7.5 mg/kg/d max; ↓ w/ renal Insuff **Caution:** [B, ?] **Disp:** Powder for Inj 50, 100 mg/vial **SE:** Anaphylaxis; fever, chills, HA, ↓ K$^+$, ↓ Mg^{2+}, nephrotox, ↓ BP, anemia **Notes:** Do not use in-line filter; ✓ LFTs/lytes

Amphotericin B Lipid Complex (Abelcet) Uses: *Refractory invasive fungal Infxn in pts intolerant to conventional amphotericin B* Acts: Binds ergosterol in fungal membrane, alters permeability Dose: *Adults & Peds.* 5 mg/kg/d IV × 1 daily Caution: [B, ?] Disp: Inj 5 mg/mL SE: Anaphylaxis; fever, chills, HA, ↓ K⁺, ↓ Mg²⁺, nephrotox, ↓ BP, anemia Notes: Filter w/ 5-micron needle; do not mix in electrolyte containing solns; if Inf >2 h, manually mix bag

Amphotericin B Liposomal (AmBisome) Uses: *Refractory invasive fungal Infxn w/ intolerance to conventional amphotericin B; cryptococcal meningitis in HIV; empiric for febrile neutropenia; visceral leishmaniasis* Acts: Binds ergosterol in fungal membrane, alters membrane permeability Dose: *Adults & Peds.* 3–6 mg/kg/d, Inf 60–120 min; varies by indication; ↓ in renal Insuff Caution: [B, ?] Disp: Powder Inj 50 mg SE: Anaphylaxis, fever, chills, HA, ↓ K⁺, ↓ Mg²⁺ nephrotox, ↓ BP, anemia Notes: Do not use < 1-micron filter

Ampicillin (Amcill, Omnipen) Uses: *Resp, GU, or GI tract Infxns, meningitis d/t gram(−) & (+) bacteria; SBE prophylaxis* Acts: β-Lactam antibiotic; ↓ cell wall synth Spectrum: Gram(+) (*Streptococcus* sp, *Staphylococcus* sp, *Listeria*); gram(−) (*Klebsiella* sp, *E. coli, H. influenzae, P. mirabilis, Shigella* sp, *Salmonella* sp) Dose: *Adults.* 500 mg–2 g IM or IV q6h or 250–500 mg PO q6h; varies by indication *Peds Neonates <7 d:* 50–100 mg/kg/24 h IV ÷ q8h *Term infants:* 75–150 mg/kg/24 h ÷ q6–8h IV or PO *Children >1 mo:* 100–200 mg/kg/24 h ÷ q4–6h IM or IV; 50–100 mg/kg/24 h ÷ q6h PO up to 250 mg/dose *Meningitis:* 200–400 mg/kg/24 h ÷ q4–6h IV; ↓ w/ renal impair; take on empty stomach Caution: [B, M] Cross-hypersens w/ PCN Disp: Caps 250, 500 mg; susp 100 mg/mL (reconstituted drops), 125 mg/5 mL, 250 mg/5 mL; powder (Inj) 125, 250, 500 mg, 1, 2, 10 g/vial SE: D, rash, allergic Rxn Notes: Many *E. coli* resistant

Ampicillin-Sulbactam (Unasyn) Uses: *Gynecologic, intra-Abd, skin Infxns d/t β-lactamase–producing S. aureus, Enterococcus, H. influenzae, P. mirabilis, & Bacteroides* sp* Acts: β-Lactam antibiotic & β-lactamase inhib Spectrum: Gram(+) & (−) as for amp alone; also *Enterobacter, Acinetobacter, Bacteroides* Dose: *Adults.* 1.5–3 g IM or IV q6h *Peds.* 100–400 mg ampicillin/kg/d (150–300 mg Unasyn) q6h; ↓ w/ renal Insuff Caution: [B, M] Disp: Powder for Inj 1.5, 3 g/vial, 15 g bulk package SE: Allergic Rxns, rash, D, Inj site pain Notes: A 2:1 ratio ampicillin:sulbactam

Anakinra (Kineret) BOX: Associated w/ ↑ incidence of serious Infxn; D/C w/ serious Infxn Uses: *Reduce S/Sxs of mod/severe active RA, failed 1 or more DMARD* Acts: Human IL-1 receptor antagonist Dose: 100 mg SQ daily; w/ CrCl <30 mL/min, q other day Caution: [B, ?] CI: *E. coli*-derived protein allergy, active Infxn, <18 y Disp: 100-mg prefilled syringes; 100 mg (0.67 mL/vial) SE: ↓ WBC especially w/ TNF-blockers, Inj site Rxn (may last up to 28 d), Infxn, N/D, Abd pain, flu-like sx, HA

Anastrozole (Arimidex) Uses: *Breast CA: postmenopausal w/ metastatic breast CA, adjuvant Rx postmenopausal early hormone-receptor(+) breast CA*

Acts: Selective nonsteroidal aromatase inhib, ↓ circulatory estradiol **Dose:** 1 mg/d **Caution:** [D, ?] **CI:** PRG **Disp:** Tabs 1 mg **SE:** May ↑ cholesterol; N/V/D, HTN, flushing, ↑ bone/tumor pain, HA, somnolence, mood disturbance, depression, rash **Notes:** No effect on adrenal steroids or aldosterone

Anidulafungin (Eraxis) **Uses:** *Candidemia, esophageal candidiasis, other *Candida* Infxn (peritonitis, intra-Abd abscess)* **Acts:** Echinocandin; ↓ cell wall synth *Spectrum: C. albicans, C. glabrata, C. parapsilosis, C. tropicalis* **Dose:** Candidemia, others: 200 mg IV × 1, then 100 mg IV daily [Tx ≥14 d after last (+)culture]; Esophageal candidiasis: 100 mg IV × 1, then 50 mg IV daily (Tx >14 d and 7 d after resolution of Sx); 1.1 mg/min max Inf rate **Caution:** [C, ?/−] **CI:** Echinocandin hypersens **Disp:** Powder 50, 100 mg/vial **SE:** Histamine-mediated Inf Rxns (urticaria, flushing, ↓ BP, dyspnea, etc), fever, N/V/D, ↓ K⁺, HA, ↑ LFTs, hep, worsening hepatic failure **Notes:** ↓ Inf rate to <1.1 mg/min w/ Inf Rxns

Anistreplase (Eminase) **Uses:** *AMI* **Acts:** Thrombolytic; activates conversion of plasminogen to plasmin, ↑ thrombolysis **Dose:** 30 units IV over 2–5 min *(ECC 2005)* **Caution:** [C, ?] **CI:** Active internal bleeding, Hx CVA, recent (<2 mo) intracranial or intraspinal surgery/trauma/neoplasm, AVM, aneurysm, bleeding diathesis, severe HTN **Disp:** 30 units/vial **SE:** Bleeding, ↓ BP, hematoma **Notes:** Ineffective if readministered >5 d after the previous dose of anistreplase or streptokinase, or streptococcal Infxn (production of antistreptokinase Ab)

Anthralin (Anthra-Derm) **Uses:** *Psoriasis* **Acts:** Keratolytic **Dose:** Apply daily **Caution:** [C, ?] **CI:** Acutely inflamed psoriatic eruptions, erythroderma **Disp:** Cream, oint 0.1, 0.25, 0.4, 0.5, 1% **SE:** Irritation; hair/fingernails/skin discoloration

Antihemophilic Factor [AHF, Factor VIII] (Monoclate) **Uses:** *Classic hemophilia A, von Willebrand Dz* **Acts:** Provides factor VIII needed to convert prothrombin to thrombin **Dose:** *Adults & Peds.* 1 AHF unit/kg ↑ factor VIII level by 2 Int Unit/dL; units required = (wgt in kg) (desired factor VIII ↑ as % nl) × (0.5); prevent spontaneous hemorrhage = 5% nl; hemostasis after trauma/surgery = 30% nl; head injuries, major surgery, or bleeding = 80–100% nl **Caution:** [C, ?] **Disp:** ✓ each vial for units contained, powder for recons **SE:** Rash, fever, HA, chills, N/V **Notes:** Determine % nl factor VIII before dosing

Antihemophilic Factor (Recombinant) (Xyntha) **Uses:** *Control/prevent bleeding & surgical prophylaxis in hemophilia A* **Acts:** ↑ Levels of factor VIII **Dose:** *Adults.* Required units = body wgt (kg) × desired factor VIII rise (Int Units/dL or % of nl) × 0.5 (Int Units/kg per Int Units/dL); frequency/duration determined by type of bleed (see PI) **Caution:** [C, ?/−] Severe hypersens Rxn possible **CI:** None **Disp:** Inj powder: 250, 500, 1000, 2000 Int Units **SE:** HA, fever, N/V/D, weakness, allergic Rxn **Notes:** Monitor for the development of factor VIII neutralizing antibodies

Antithrombin, recombinant (Atryn) **Uses:** * Prevent peri-op/peri-partum thromboembolic events w/ hereditary antithrombin (AT) deficiency* **Acts:** Inhibits thrombin and Factor Xa **Dose: *Adults.*** Based on pre-Rx AT level, BW (kg) and drug monitoring; see package. Goal AT levels 0.8 - 1.2 IU/mL **Caution:** [C, +/-] Hypersensitivity rxns; ↑ effect of heparin/LMWH **CI:** Hypersens to goat/goat milk proteins **Disp:** Powder 1750 IU/vial **SE:** Bleeding, infusion site rxn **Notes:** ✓aPTT and anti-Factor Xa; monitor for bleeding or thrombosis

Antithymocyte Globulin (See Lymphocyte Immune Globulin, page 162)

Apomorphine (Apokyn) **BOX:** Do not administer IV **Uses:** *Acute, intermittent hypomobility ("off") episodes of Parkinson Dz* **Acts:** Dopamine agonist **Dose: *Adults.*** 0.2 mL SQ supervised test dose; if BP OK, initial 0.2 mL (2 mg) SQ during "off" periods; only 1 dose per "off" period; titrate dose; 0.6 mL (6 mg) max single doses; use w/ antiemetic; ↓ in renal impair **Caution:** [C, +/−] Avoid EtOH; antihypertensives, vasodilators, cardio-/cerebrovascular Dz, hepatic impair **CI:** 5-HT₃ antagonists, sulfite allergy **Disp:** Inj 10 mg/mL, 3-mL pen cartridges; 2-mL amp **SE:** Emesis, syncope, ↑ QT, orthostatic ↓ BP, somnolence, ischemia, Inj site Rxn, abuse potential, dyskinesia, fibrotic conditions, priapism, chest pain/angina, yawning, rhinorrhea **Notes:** Daytime somnolence may limit activities; trimethobenzamide 300 mg tid PO or other non–5-HT₃ antagonist antiemetic given 3 d prior to & up to 2 mo following initiation

Apraclonidine (Iopidine) **Uses:** *Glaucoma, intraocular HTN* **Acts:** α₂-Adrenergic agonist **Dose:** 1–2 gtt of 0.5% tid; 1 gtt of 1% before and after surgical procedure **Caution:** [C, ?] **CI:** w/in 14 d of or w/ MAOI **Disp:** 0.5, 1% soln **SE:** Ocular irritation, lethargy, xerostomia

Aprepitant (Emend, Oral) **Uses:** *Prevents N/V associated w/ emetogenic CA chemotherapy (e.g., cisplatin) (use in combo w/ other antiemetics)*, postop N/V **Acts:** Substance P/neurokinin 1(NK₁) receptor antagonist **Dose:** 125 mg PO day 1, 1 h before chemotherapy, then 80 mg PO qam days 2 & 3; postop N/V: 40 mg w/in 3 h of induction **Caution:** [B, ?/−]; substrate & mod CYP3A4 inhib; CYP2C9 inducer (Table 10 p 280); ↓ Effect OCP and warfarin **CI:** Use w/ pimozide **Disp:** Caps 40, 80, 125 mg **SE:** Fatigue, asthenia, hiccups **Notes:** See also fosaprepitant (Emend, Injection)

Apriso (Salix) **Uses:** *Maintenance of UC remission* **Acts:** Locally acting aminosalicylate **Dose:** 1.5 g (0.375 g caps × 4) PO daily in am; not w/ antacids **Caution:** [B, ±] May cause renal impair, exacerbation of colitis **CI:** Hypersens to salicylates/aminosalicylates **Disp:** Caps ER 0.375 g **SE:** HA, N/D, Abd pain, nasopharyngitis, influenza, sinusitis, acute intolerance synd **Notes:** for PKU patients, product contains aspartame; monitor CBC, SCr

Arformoterol (Brovana) **BOX:** Long-acting β₂-adrenergic agonists may increase the risk of asthma-related death. Use only for pts not adequately controlled on other asthma-controller meds **Uses:** *Maint in COPD* **Acts:** Selective LA β₂-adrenergic agonist **Dose: *Adults.*** 15 mcg bid nebulization **Caution:** [C, ?] **CI:** Hypersens **Disp:** Soln 15 mcg/2 mL **SE:** Pain, back pain, CP, D, sinusitis, nervousness, palpitations, allergic Rxn **Notes:** Not for acute bronchospasm. Refrigerate, use immediately after opening

Argatroban (Acova) **Uses:** *Prevent/Tx thrombosis in HIT, PCI in pts w/ HIT risk* **Acts:** Anticoagulant, direct thrombin inhib **Dose:** 2 mcg/kg/min IV; adjust until aPTT 1.5–3 × baseline not to exceed 100 s; 10 mcg/kg/min max; ↓ w/ hepatic impair **Caution:** [B, ?] Avoid PO anticoagulants, ↑ bleeding risk; avoid use w/ thrombolytics **CI:** Overt major bleed **Disp:** Inj 100 mg/mL **SE:** AF, cardiac arrest, cerebrovascular disorder, ↓ BP, VT, N/V/D, sepsis, cough, renal tox, ↓ Hgb **Note:** Steady state in 1–3 h; ✓ aPTT w/ Inf start and after each dose change

Aripiprazole (Abilify, Abilify Discmelt) **BOX:** Increased mortality in elderly w/ dementia-related psychosis; ↑ suicidal thinking in children, adolescents, and young adults w/ MDD **Uses:** *Schizophrenia adults and peds 13–17 y, mania or mixed episodes associated w/ bipolar disorder, MDD in adults, agitation w/ schizophrenia* **Acts:** Dopamine & serotonin antagonist **Dose:** *Adults. Schizophrenia:* 10–15 mg PO/d *Acute agitation:* 9.75 mg/1.3 mL IM *Bipolar:* 15 mg/d; *MDD adjunct* w/ other antidepressants initial 2 mg/d, 10 mg/d OK **Peds.** *Schizophrenia:* **13–17y:** Start 2 mg/d, usual 10 mg/d; max 30 mg/d for all adult and peds uses; ↓ dose w/ CYP3A4/CYP2D6 inhib (Table 10 p 280); ↑ dose w/ CYP3A4 inducer **Caution:** [C, −] w/ Low WBC **Disp:** Tabs 2, 5, 10, 15, 20, 30 mg; Discmelt (disintegrating tabs 10, 15, 20, 30 mg), soln 1 mg/mL, Inj 7.5 mg/mL **SE:** Neuroleptic malignant synd, tardive dyskinesia, orthostatic ↓ BP, cognitive & motor impair, ↑ glucose, leukopenia, neutropenia, and agranulocytosis **Notes:** Discmelt contains phenylalanine; monitor CBC

Artemether & Lumefantrine (Coartem) **Uses:** *Acute, uncomplicated malaria (P. falciparum)* **Action:** Antiprotozoal/Antimalarial **Dose:** *Adults >16 y:* 25-<35 kg: 3 tabs hour 0 & 8 day 1, then 3 tabs bid day 2 & 3 (18 tabs/course) ≥35 kg: 4 tabs hour 0 & 8 day 1, then 4 tabs bid day 2 & 3 (24 tabs/course) **Peds.** *2 mo to <16 y:* 5-<15 kg: 1 tab at hour 0 & 8 day 1, then 1 tab bid day 2 & 3 (6 tabs/course) 15-<25 kg: 2 tabs hour 0 & 8 day 1, then 2 tabs bid day 2 & 3 (12 tabs/course) 25-<35 kg: 3 tabs at hour 0 & 8 day 1, then 3 tabs bid on day 2 & 3 (18 tabs/course) ≥35 kg: See Adult dose **Caution:** [C, ?] ↑ QT, hepatic/renal impair, CYP3A4 inhib **CI:** Component hypersens **Disp:** Tabs artemether 20 mg/ lumefantrine 120 mg **SE:** Palp, HA, dizziness, chills, sleep disturb, fatigue, anorexia, N/V/D, Abd pain, weakness, arthralgia, myalgia, cough, splenomegaly, hepatomegaly, ↑ AST, ↑ QT **Notes:** Not rec w/ other agents that ↑ QT

Artificial Tears (Tears Naturale) [OTC] **Uses:** *Dry eyes* **Acts:** Ocular lubricant **Dose:** 1–2 gtt tid-qid **Disp:** OTC soln **SE:** mild stinging, temp blurred vision

Armodafinil (Nuvigil) **Uses:** *Narcolepsy, shift work sleep disorder SWSD, and OSAHS* **Acts:** ?; binds dopamine receptor, ↓ dopamine reuptake **Dose:** *Adults. OSAHS/narcolepsy:* 150 or 250 mg PO daily in AM *SWSD:* 150 mg PO q day 1 h prior to start of shift; ↓ w/ hepatic impair; adjust w/ substrates for CYP3A4/5, CYP2C19 **Caution:** [C, ?] **CI:** Hypersens to modafinil/armodafinil

Disp: Tabs 50, 150, 200 mg **SE:** HA, N, dizziness, insomnia, xerostomia, rash including SJS, angioedema, anaphylactoid Rxns, multiorgan hypersens Rxns

L-Asparaginase (Elspar, Oncaspar) **Uses:** *ALL* (in combo w/ other agents) **Acts:** Protein synth inhib **Dose:** 500–20,000 Int Units/m²/d for 1–14 d (per protocols) **Caution:** [C, ?] **CI:** Active/Hx pancreatitis; Hx of allergic Rxn, thrombosis or hemorrhagic event w/ prior Rx w/ asparaginase **Disp:** Powder (Inj) 10,000 units/vial **SE:** Allergy 20–35% (urticaria to anaphylaxis); fever, chills, N/V, anorexia, Abd cramps, depression, agitation, Sz, pancreatitis, ↑ glucose or LFTs, coagulopathy **Notes:** Test dose OK, ✓ glucose, coagulation studies, LFTs

Asenapine maleate (Saphris) **BOX:** ↑Mortality in elderly w/ dementia-related psychosis **Uses:** *Schizophrenia; manic/mixed bipolar disorder* **Acts:** Dopamine/serotonin antagonist **Dose:** *Adults. Schizophrenia:* 5mg twice daily; *Bipolar disorder:* 10mg twice daily **Caution:** [C, ?/–] **Disp:** SL Tabs 5, 10mg **SE:** Dizziness, somnolence, akathisia, oral hypoesthesia, EPS, ↑ weight, ↓ glucose, ↓ BP, ↑QT interval, hyperprolactinemia,↓ WBC, neuroleptic malignant syndrome **Notes:** Do not swallow/crush/chew tab; avoid eating/drinking 10 min after dose

Aspirin (Bayer, Ecotrin, St. Joseph's) [OTC] **Uses:** *Angina, CABG, PTCA, carotid endarterectomy, ischemic stroke, TIA, MI, arthritis, pain*, HA, *fever*, inflammation, Kawasaki Dz **Acts:** Prostaglandin inhib by COX-2 inhib **Dose:** *Adults. Pain, fever:* 325–650 mg q4–6h PO or PR (4 g/d max) *RA:* 3–6 g/d PO in ÷ doses; *Plt inhib:* 81–325 mg PO daily; *Prevent MI:* 81 (preferred)–325 mg PO daily; *Acute coronary synd:* 160–325 mg PO ASAP, chewing preferred at onset *(ECC 2005) Peds. Antipyretic:* 10–15 mg/kg/dose PO or PR q4–6h up to 80 mg/kg/24 h RA: 60–100 mg/kg/24 h PO ÷ q4–6h (levels 15–30 mg/dL); *Kawasaki Dz:* 80–100 mg/kg/d ÷ q6h, 3–5 mg/kg/d after fever resolves; for all uses 4 g/d max; avoid w/ CrCl <10 mL/min, severe liver Dz **Caution:** [C, M] Linked to Reye synd; avoid w/ viral illness in peds <18 y **CI:** Allergy to ASA, chickenpox/flu Sxs, synd of nasal polyps, angioedema, & bronchospasm to NSAIDs **Disp:** Tabs 325, 500 mg; chew tabs 81 mg; EC tabs 81, 162, 325, 500, 650, 975 mg; SR tabs 650, 800 mg; effervescent tabs 325, 500 mg; supp 125, 200, 300, 600 mg **SE:** GI upset, erosion, & bleeding **Notes:** D/C 1 wk preop; avoid/limit EtOH; Salicylate levels: *Therapeutic:* 100 to 250 mcg/mL *Toxic:* >300 mcg/mL

Aspirin & Butalbital Compound (Fiorinal) [C-III] **Uses:** *Tension HA*, pain **Acts:** Barbiturate w/ analgesic **Dose:** 1–2 PO q4h PRN, max 6 tabs/d; avoid w/ CrCl <10 mL/min or severe liver Dz **Caution:** [C (D w/ prolonged use or high doses at term), ?] **CI:** ASA allergy, GI ulceration, bleeding disorder, porphyria, synd of nasal polyps, angioedema, & bronchospasm to NSAIDs **Disp:** Caps *(Fiorgen PF, Lanorinal)*, Tabs *(Lanorinal)* ASA 325 mg/butalbital 50 mg/caffeine 40 mg **SE:** Drowsiness, dizziness, GI upset, ulceration, bleeding **Notes:** Butalbital habit-forming; D/C 1 wk prior to surgery, avoid or limit EtOH

Aspirin + Butalbital, Caffeine, & Codeine (Fiorinal + Codeine) [C-III] **Uses:** Mild *pain*, HA, especially tension HA w/ stress **Acts:** Sedative and narcotic analgesic **Dose:** 1–2 tabs/caps PO q4–6h PRN max 6/d **Caution:** [C, ?] **CI:** Allergy to ASA and codeine; synd of nasal polyps, angioedema, & bronchospasm to NSAIDs, bleeding diathesis, peptic ulcer or sig GI lesions, porphyria **Disp:** Caps/tabs contains 325 mg ASA, 40 mg caffeine, 50 mg butalbital, 30 mg codeine **SE:** Drowsiness, dizziness, GI upset, ulceration, bleeding **Notes:** D/C 1 wk prior to surgery, avoid/limit EtOH

Aspirin + Codeine (Empirin No. 3, 4) [C-III] **Uses:** Mild–*mod pain*, symptomatic nonproductive cough **Acts:** Combined effects of ASA & codeine **Dose:** *Adults.* 1–2 tabs PO q4–6h PRN **Peds.** ASA 10 mg/kg/dose; codeine 0.5–1 mg/kg/dose q4h **Caution:** [D, M] **CI:** Allergy to ASA/codeine, PUD, bleeding, anticoagulant Rx, children w/ chickenpox or flu Sxs, synd of nasal polyps, angioedema, & bronchospasm to NSAIDs **Disp:** Tabs 325 mg of ASA & codeine (codeine in No. 3 = 30 mg, No. 4 = 60 mg) **SE:** Drowsiness, dizziness, GI upset, ulceration, bleeding **Notes:** D/C 1 wk prior to surgery; avoid/limit EtOH

Atazanavir (Reyataz) **BOX:** Hyperbilirubinemia may require drug D/C **Uses:** *HIV-1 Infxn* **Acts:** Protease inhib **Dose:** Antiretroviral naïve 400 mg PO daily w/ food; experienced pts 300 mg w/ ritonavir 100 mg; when given w/ efavirenz 600 mg, administer atazanavir 300 mg + ritonavir 100 mg once/d; separate doses from didanosine; ↓ w/ hepatic impair **Caution:** CDC rec: HIV-infected mothers not breast-feed [B, –]; ↑ levels of statins (avoid use) sildenafil, antiarrhythmics, warfarin, cyclosporine, TCAs; ↓ w/ St. John's wort, H_2-receptor antagonists; do not use w/salmeterol, colchicine (w/renal/hepatic failure); adjust dose w/ bosentan, tadalafil for PAH **CI:** w/ Midazolam, triazolam, ergots, pimozide, alpha 1-adrenoreceptor antagonist (alfuzosin), PDE5 Inhibitor sildenafil **Disp:** Caps 100, 150, 200, 300 mg **SE:** HA, N/V/D, rash, Abd pain, DM, photosens, ↑ PR interval **Notes:** May have less-adverse effect on cholesterol; if given w/ H_2 blocker, give together or at least 10 h after H_2; if given w/ proton pump inhib, separate by 12 h; concurrent use not OK in experienced pts

Atenolol (Tenormin) **Uses:** *HTN, angina, MI* **Acts:** selective β-adrenergic receptor blocker **Dose:** *HTN & angina:* 50–100 mg/d PO *AMI:* 5 mg IV slowly over 5 min, may repeat in 10 min then 50 mg PO bid if tolerated; *(ECC 2005);* ↓ in renal impair **Caution:** [D, M] DM, bronchospasm; abrupt D/C can exacerbate angina & ↑ MI risk **CI:** ↓ HR, cardiogenic shock, cardiac failure, 2nd-/3rd-degree AV block, sinus node dysfunction, pulm edema **Disp:** Tabs 25, 50, 100 mg; Inj 5 mg/10 mL **SE:** ↓ HR, ↓ BP, 2nd-/3rd-degree AV block, dizziness, fatigue

Atenolol & Chlorthalidone (Tenoretic) **Uses:** *HTN* **Acts:** β-Adrenergic blockade w/ diuretic **Dose:** 50–100 mg/d PO based on atenolol; ↓ dose w/ CrCl <35 mL/min **Caution:** [D, M] DM, bronchospasm **CI:** See Atenolol; anuria, sulfonamide cross-sensitivity **Disp:** *Tenoretic 50:* Atenolol 50 mg/chlorthalidone 25 mg *Tenoretic 100:* Atenolol 100 mg/chlorthalidone 25 mg **SE:** ↓ HR, ↓ BP, 2nd-/3rd-degree AV block, dizziness, fatigue, ↓ K^+, photosens

Atomoxetine (Strattera) **BOX:** Severe liver injury may rarely occur; DC w/ jaundice or ↑ LFTs, ↑ frequency of suicidal thinking; monitor closely **Uses:** *ADHD* **Acts:** Selective norepinephrine reuptake inhib **Dose:** *Adults & children >70 kg:* 40 mg PO/d, after 3 d minimum, ↑ to 80–100 mg ÷ daily-bid *Peds <70 kg:* 0.5 mg/kg × 3 d, then ↑ 1.2 mg/kg daily or bid (max 1.4 mg/kg or 100 mg); ↓ dose w/ hepatic Insuff or in combo w/ CYP2D6 inhib (Table 10 p 280) [C, ?/–] **Caution:** w/ Known structural cardiac anomalies, cardiac Hx **CI:** NAG, w/ or w/in 2 wk of D/C an MAOI **Disp:** Caps 5, 10, 18, 25, 40, 60, 80, 100 mg **SE:** HA, insomnia, dry mouth, Abd pain, N/V, anorexia ↑ BP, tachycardia, wgt loss, sexual dysfunction, jaundice, ↑ LFTs **Notes:** AHA rec: All children receiving stimulants for ADHD receive CV assessment before Rx initiated; D/C immediately w/ jaundice

Atorvastatin (Lipitor) **Uses:** *↑ Cholesterol & triglycerides* **Acts:** HMG-CoA reductase inhib **Dose:** Initial 10 mg/d, may ↑ to 80 mg/d **Caution:** [X, –] **CI:** Active liver Dz, unexplained ↑ LFTs **Disp:** Tabs 10, 20, 40, 80 mg **SE:** Myopathy, HA, arthralgia, myalgia, GI upset, chest pain, edema, insomnia dizziness, liver failure **Notes:** Monitor LFTs, instruct pt to report unusual muscle pain or weakness

Atovaquone (Mepron) **Uses:** *Rx & prevention PCP and Toxoplasma gondii encephalitis* **Acts:** ↓ Nucleic acid & ATP synth **Dose:** *Rx:* 750 mg PO bid for 21 d *Prevention:* 1500 mg PO once/d (w/ meals) **Caution:** [C, ?] **Disp:** Susp 750 mg/5 mL **SE:** Fever, HA, anxiety, insomnia, rash, N/V, cough

Atovaquone/Proguanil (Malarone) **Uses:** *Prevention or Rx P. falciparum malaria* **Acts:** Antimalarial **Dose:** *Adults. Prevention:* 1 tab PO 2 d before, during, & 7 d after leaving endemic region *Rx:* 4 tabs PO single dose daily × 3 d *Peds.* See PI **Caution:** [C, ?] **CI:** prophylactic use when CrCl <30 mL/min **Disp:** Tabs atovaquone 250 mg/proguanil 100 mg; peds 62.5/25 mg **SE:** HA, fever, myalgia, N/V, ↑ LFTs

Atracurium (Tracrium) **Uses:** *Anesthesia adjunct to facilitate ET intubation* **Acts:** Nondepolarizing neuromuscular blocker **Dose:** *Adults & Peds >2 y.* 0.4–0.5 mg/kg IV bolus, then 0.08–0.1 mg/kg q20–45min PRN **Caution:** [C, ?] **Disp:** Inj 10 mg/mL **SE:** Flushing **Notes:** Pt must be intubated & on controlled ventilation; use adequate amounts of sedation & analgesia

Atropine, Systemic (AtroPen Auto-injector) **BOX:** Primary protection against exposure to chemical nerve agent and insecticide poisoning is the wearing of specially designed protective garments **Uses:** *Preanesthetic; symptomatic ↓ HR & asystole, AV block, organophosphate (insecticide) and acetylcholinesterase (nerve gas) inhib antidote; cycloplegic* **Acts:** Antimuscarinic; blocks acetylcholine at parasympathetic sites, cycloplegic **Dose:** *Adults. (2005 ECC):* Asystole or PEA: 1 mg IV/IO push. Repeat PRN q3–5min to 0.03–0.04 mg/kg max *Bradycardia:* 0.5–1.0 mg IV q3–5min as needed; max 0.03–0.04 mg/kg; ET 2–3 mg in 10 mL NS *Preanesthetic:* 0.3–0.6 mg IM *Poisoning:* 1–2 mg IV bolus, repeat q3–5min PRN to reverse effects *Peds. (ECC 2005):* 0.01–0.03 mg/kg IV q2–5min, max 1 mg, min dose 0.1 mg *Preanesthetic:* 0.01 mg/kg/dose SQ/IV (max 0.4 mg)

Poisoning: 0.05 mg/kg IV, repeat q3–5min PRN to reverse effects **Caution:** [C, +] **CI:** NAG, adhesions between iris and lens, tachycardia, GI obst, ileus, severe ulcerative colitis, obstructive uropathy, Mobitz II block **Disp:** Inj 0.05, 0.1, 0.3, 0.4, 0.5, 0.8, 1 mg/mL AtroPen Auto-injector: 0.25, 0.5, 1, 2 mg/dose; tabs 0.4 mg, MDI 0.36 mg/Inh **SE:** Flushing, mydriasis, tachycardia, dry mouth & nose, blurred vision, urinary retention, constipation, psychosis **Notes:** SLUDGE are Sx of organophosphate poisoning; Auto-injector limited distribution; see ophthal forms below

Atropine, Benzoic Acid, Hyoscyamine Sulfate, Methenamine, Methylene Blue, Phenyl Salicylate (Urised)

Uses: *Lower urinary tract discomfort* **Acts:** Methenamine in acid urine releases formaldehyde (antiseptic), methylene blue/benzoic acid mild antiseptic, phenyl salicylate mild analgesic, hyoscyamine, and atropine parasympatholytic ↓ muscle spasm **Dose:** *Adults.* 2 tabs PO qid *Peds >6 y:* Individualize **Caution:** [C, ?/–] avoid w/ sulfonamides **CI:** NAG, pyloric/duodenal obst, BOO, coronary artery spasm **Disp:** Tabs: Atropine 0.03 mg/benzoic acid 4.5 mg/hyoscyamine 0.03 mg/methenamine 40.8 mg/methylene blue 5.4 mg/phenyl salicylate 18.1 mg **SE:** Rash, dry mouth, flushing, ↑ pulse, dizziness, blurred vision, urine/feces discoloration, voiding difficulty **Notes:** Take w/ plenty of fluid, can cause crystalluria

Atropine, Ophthalmic (Isopto Atropine, Generic)

Uses: *Cycloplegic refraction, uveitis, amblyopia* **Acts:** Antimuscarinic; cycloplegic, dilates pupils **Dose:** *Adults. Refraction:* 1–2 gtt 1 h before *Uveitis:* 1–2 gtt daily-qid *Peds.* 1 gtt in nonamblyopic eye daily **Caution:** [C, +] **CI:** NAG, adhesions between iris and lens **Disp:** 2.5- & 15-mL bottle 1% ophthal soln, 1% oint 3.5 g **SE:** Local irritation, burning, blurred vision, light sensitivity **Notes:** Compress lacrimal sac 2–3 min after instillation; effects can last 1–2 wk

Atropine/Pralidoxime (DuoDote)

BOX: For use by personnel w/ appropriate training; wear protective garments; do not rely solely on medication: evacuation and decontamination ASAP **Uses:** *Nerve agent (tabun, sarin, others), insecticide poisoning* **Acts:** Atropine blocks effects of excess acetylcholine; pralidoxime reactivates acetylcholinesterase inactivated by poisoning **Dose:** 1 Inj mid-lateral thigh; 10–15 min for effect; w/ severe Sx, give 2 additional Inj; if alert/oriented no more doses **Caution:** [C, ?] **Disp:** Auto-injector 2.1 mg atropine/600 mg pralidoxime **SE:** Dry mouth, blurred vision, dry eyes, photophobia, confusion, HA, tachycardia, ↑ BP, flushing, urinary retention, constipation, Abd pain N, V, emesis **Notes:** See "SLUDGE" in Atropine, Systemic; limited distribution

Azathioprine (Imuran)

BOX: May ↑ neoplasia w/ chronic use; mutagenic and hematologic tox possible **Uses:** *Adjunct to prevent renal transplant rejection, RA*, SLE, Crohn Dz, ulcerative colitis **Acts:** Immunosuppressive; antagonizes purine metabolism **Dose:** *Adults. Crohn and ulcerative colitis:* Start 50 mg/d, ↑ 25 mg/d q1–2wk, target dose 2–3 mg/kg/d *Adults & Peds. Renal transplant:* 3–5 mg/kg/d IV/PO single daily dose, taper by 0.5 mg/kg q4wk to lowest effective dose *RA:* 1 mg/kg/d once daily or ÷ bid × 6–8 wk, ↑ 0.5 mg/kg/d q4wk to 2.5 mg/kg/d; ↓ w/ renal Insuff **Caution:** [D, ?] **CI:** PRG **Disp:** Tabs 50, 75, 100 mg; powder for Inj 100 mg **SE:** GI intolerance, fever, chills, leukopenia, thrombocytopenia **Notes:** Handle Inj w/ cytotoxic precautions; interaction w/ allopurinol; do not administer live vaccines on drug; ✓ CBC and LFTs; dose per local transplant protocol, usually start 1–3 d pretransplant

Azelastine (Astelin, Astepro, Optivar) **Uses:** *Allergic rhinitis (rhinorrhea, sneezing, nasal pruritus), vasomotor rhinitis; allergic conjunctivitis* **Acts:** Histamine H$_1$-receptor antagonist **Dose:** *Adults & Peds > 12 y.* Nasal: 1-2 sprays/nostril bid *Ophth:* 1 gtt in each affected eye bid *Peds 5-11 y:* 1 spray/nostril 1× d **Caution:** [C, ?/–] **CI:** Component sensitivity **Disp:** Nasal 137 mcg/spray; ophthal soln 0.05% **SE:** Somnolence, bitter taste, HA, colds Sx (rhinitis, cough)

Azithromycin (Zithromax) **Uses:** *Community-acquired pneumonia, pharyngitis, otitis media, skin Infxns, nongonococcal (chlamydial) urethritis, chancroid & PID; Rx & prevention of MAC in HIV* **Acts:** Macrolide antibiotic; bacteriostatic; ↓ protein synth *Spectrum: Chlamydia, H. ducreyi, H. influenzae, Legionella, M. catarrhalis, M. pneumoniae, M. hominis, N. gonorrhoeae, S. aureus, S. agalactiae, S. pneumoniae, S. pyogenes* **Dose:** *Adults.* Resp tract Infxns: PO: Caps 500 mg day 1, then 250 mg/d PO × 4 d *Sinusitis:* 500 mg/d PO × 3 d *IV:* 500 mg × 2 d, then 500 mg PO × 7–10 d or 500 mg IV daily × 2 d, then 500 mg PO × 7–10 d *Nongonococcal urethritis:* 1 g PO × 1 *Gonorrhea, uncomplicated:* 2 g PO × 1 *Prevent MAC:* 1200 mg PO once/wk *Peds. Otitis media:* 10 mg/kg PO day 1, then 5 mg/kg/d days 2–5 *Pharyngitis:* 12 mg/kg/d PO × 5 d; take susp on empty stomach; tabs OK w/ or w/o food; ↓ w/ CrCl <10 mL/min **Caution:** [B, +] **Disp:** Tabs 250, 500, 600 mg; Z-Pack (5-d, 250 mg); Tri-Pack (500-mg tabs × 3); susp 1 g; single-dose packet (ZMAX) ER susp (2 g); susp 100, 200 mg/5 mL; Inj powder 500 mg; 2.5 mL ophthal soln 1% **SE:** GI upset, metallic taste

Azithromycin Ophthalmic 1% (AzaSite) **Uses:** *Bacterial conjunctivitis* **Acts:** Bacteriostatic **Dose:** *Adults.* 1 gtt bid, q8–12 h × 2 d, then 1 gtt q day × 5 d *Peds ≥1 y:* 1 gtt bid, q8–12h × 2 d, then 1 gtt q day × 5 d **Caution:** [B, +/–] **CI:** None **Disp:** 1% in 2.5-mL bottle **SE:** Irritation, burning, stinging, contact dermatitis, corneal erosion, dry eye, dysgeusia, nasal congestion, sinusitis, ocular discharge, keratitis

Aztreonam (Azactam) **Uses:** *Aerobic gram(−) UTIs, lower resp, intra-Abd, skin, gynecologic Infxns & septicemia* **Acts:** Monobactam; ↓ Cell wall synth *Spectrum:* Gram(−) *(Pseudomonas, E. coli, Klebsiella, H. influenzae, Serratia, Proteus, Enterobacter, Citrobacter)* **Dose:** *Adults.* 1–2 g IV/IM q6–12h *UTI:* 500–1 g IV q8–12h *Meningitis:* 2 g IV q6–8h *Peds. Premature:* 30 mg/kg/dose IV q12h *Term & children:* 30 mg/kg/dose q6–8h; ↓ in renal impair **Caution:** [B, +] **Disp:** Inj (soln), 1 g, 2 g/50 mL Inj powder for recons 500 mg 1 g, 2 g **SE:** N/V/D, rash, pain at Inj site **Notes:** No gram(+) or anaerobic activity; OK in PCN-allergic pts

Bacitracin, Ophthalmic (AK-Tracin Ophthalmic); Bacitracin & Polymyxin B, Ophthalmic (AK-Poly-Bac Ophthalmic, Polysporin Ophthalmic); Bacitracin, Neomycin, & Polymyxin B, Ophthalmic (AK-Spore Ophthalmic, Neosporin Ophthalmic); Bacitracin, Neomycin, Polymyxin B, & Hydrocortisone, Ophthalmic (AK-Spore HC Ophthalmic, Cortisporin Ophthalmic) Uses: *Steroid-responsive inflammatory ocular conditions* Acts: Topical antibiotic w/ anti-inflammatory Dose: Apply q3–4h into conjunctival sac Caution: [C, ?] CI: Viral, mycobacterial, fungal eye Infxn Disp: See Bacitracin, Topical equivalents, next listing

Bacitracin, Topical (Baciguent); Bacitracin & Polymyxin B, Topical (Polysporin); Bacitracin, Neomycin, & Polymyxin B, Topical (Neosporin); Bacitracin, Neomycin, Polymyxin B, & Hydrocortisone, Topical (Cortisporin); Bacitracin, Neomycin, Polymyxin B, & Lidocaine, Topical (Clomycin) Uses: Prevent/Rx of *minor skin Infxns* Acts: Topical antibiotic w/ added components (anti-inflammatory & analgesic) Dose: Apply sparingly bid–qid Caution: [C, ?] Not for deep wounds, puncture, or animal bites Disp: Bacitracin 500 units/g oint; bacitracin 500 units/polymyxin B sulfate 10,000 units/g oint & powder; bacitracin 400 units/neomycin 3.5 mg/polymyxin B 5000 units/g oint; bacitracin 400 units/ neomycin 3.5 mg/polymyxin B 5000 units/hydrocortisone 10 mg/g oint; Bacitracin 500 units/neomycin 3.5 mg/polymyxin B 5000 units/lidocaine 40 mg/g oint Notes: Ophthal, systemic, & irrigation forms available, not generally used d/t potential tox

Baclofen (Lioresal Intrathecal, Generic) BOX: IT abrupt discontinuation can lead to organ failure, rhabdomyolysis, and death Uses: *Spasticity d/t severe chronic disorders (e.g., MS, amyotrophic lateral sclerosis, or spinal cord lesions)*, trigeminal neuralgia, intractable hiccups Acts: Centrally acting skeletal muscle relaxant; ↓ transmission of monosynaptic & polysynaptic cord reflexes Dose: *Adults.* Initial, 5 mg PO tid; ↑ q3d to effect; max 80 mg/d *IT:* Via implantable pump (see PI) *Peds 2–7 y:* 10–15 mg/d ÷ q8h; titrate, max 40 mg/d *>8 y:* Max 60 mg/d *IT:* Via implantable pump (see PI); ↓ in renal impair; take w/ food or milk Caution: [C, +] Epilepsy, neuropsychological disturbances; Disp: Tabs 10, 20 mg; IT Inj 50 mcg/mL, 10 mg/20 mL, 10 mg/5 mL SE: Dizziness, drowsiness, insomnia, ataxia, weakness, ↓ BP

Balsalazide (Colazal) Uses: *Ulcerative colitis* Acts: 5-ASA derivative, anti-inflammatory, ↓ leukotriene synth Dose: 2.25 g (3 caps) tid × 8–12 wk Caution: [B, ?] Severe renal failure CI: Mesalamine or salicylate hypersens Disp: Caps 750 mg SE: Dizziness, HA, N, Abd pain, agranulocytosis, renal impair, allergic Rxns Notes: Daily dose of 6.75 g = 2.4 g mesalamine

Basiliximab (Simulect) BOX: Use only under the supervision of a physician experienced in immunosuppression Rx in an appropriate facility Uses: *Prevent acute transplant rejection* Acts: IL-2 receptor antagonists Dose: *Adults & Peds >35 kg:* 20 mg IV 2 h before transplant, then 20 mg IV 4 d posttransplant.

Peds <35 kg: 10 mg 2 h prior to transplant; same dose IV 4 d posttransplant **Caution:** [B, ?/–] **CI:** Hypersens to murine proteins **Disp:** Inj powder 10, 20 mg **SE:** Edema, HTN, HA, dizziness, fever, pain, Infxn, GI effects, electrolyte disturbances **Notes:** A murine/human MoAb

BCG [Bacillus Calmette-Guérin] (TheraCys, Tice BCG) **BOX:** Contains live, attenuated mycobacteria; transmission risk; handle as biohazard; nosocomial Infxns reported in immunosuppressed; fatal Rxns reported **Uses:** *Bladder CA (superficial)*, TB prophylaxis: Routine US adult BCG immunization not recommended. Children who are PPD(–) and continually exposed to untreated/ineffectively treated adults or whose TB strain is INH/rifampin resistant. Healthcare workers in high-risk environments **Acts:** Attenuated live BCG culture, immunomodulator **Dose:** Bladder CA, 1 vial prepared & instilled in bladder for 2 h. Repeat once/wk × 6 wk; then 1 Tx at 3, 6, 12, 18, & 24 mo after **Caution:** [C, ?] Asthma **CI:** Immunosuppression, PRG, steroid use, febrile illness, UTI, gross hematuria, w/ traumatic catheterization **Disp:** Powder 81 mg (10.5 ± 8.7 × 10^8 CFU/vial) (TheraCys), 50 mg (1–8 × 10^8 CFU/vial) (Tice BCG) **SE:** Intravesical: Hematuria, urinary frequency, dysuria, bacterial UTI, rare BCG sepsis **Notes:** PPD is not CI in BCG vaccinated persons; intravesical use, dispose/void in toilet w/ chlorine bleach

Becaplermin (Regranex Gel) **BOX:** Increased mortality d/t malignancy reported; use w/ caution in known malignancy **Uses:** Local wound care adjunct w/ *diabetic foot ulcers* **Acts:** Recombinant PDGF, enhances granulation tissue **Dose:** *Adults. Based on lesion:* Calculate the length of gel, measure the greatest length of ulcer by the greatest width; tube size and measured result determine the formula used in the calculation. Recalculate q1-2wk based on change in lesion size. *15-g tube:* [length × width] × 0.6 = length of gel (in inches) or for *2-g tube:* [length × width] × 1.3 = length of gel (in inches); rinse after 12 h; do not reapply w/in 24 h; repeat in 12 h *Peds.* See PI **Caution:** [C, ?] **CI:** Neoplasmatic site **Disp:** 0.01% gel in 2-, 15-g tubes **SE:** Rash **Notes:** Use w/ good wound care; wound must be vascularized; reassess after 10 wk if ulcer not ↓ by 30% or not healed by 20 wk

Beclomethasone Nasal (Beconase AQ) **Uses:** *Allergic rhinitis* refractory to antihistamines & decongestants; *nasal polyps* **Acts:** Inhaled steroid **Dose:** *Adults & Peds. Aqueous inhaler:* 1–2 sprays/nostril bid **Caution:** [C, ?] **Disp:** Nasal metered-dose inhaler 42 mcg/spray **SE:** Local irritation, burning, epistaxis **Notes:** Effect in days to 2 wk

Beclomethasone (QVAR) **Uses:** Chronic *asthma* **Acts:** Inhaled corticosteroid **Dose:** *Adults & Peds 5–11 y:* 40–160 mcg 1–4 Inhs bid; initial 40–80 mcg Inh bid if on bronchodilators alone; 40–160 mcg w/ other inhaled steroids; 320 mcg bid max; taper to lowest effective dose bid; rinse mouth/throat after **Caution:** [C, ?] **CI:** Acute asthma **Disp:** PO metered-dose inhaler; 40, 80 mcg/Inh **SE:** HA, cough, hoarseness, oral candidiasis **Notes:** Not effective for acute asthma; effect in 1-2 days or as long as 2 wks

Belladonna & Opium Suppositories (B&O Supprettes) [C-II] Uses: *Bladder spasms; mod/severe pain* Acts: Antispasmodic, analgesic Dose: 1 supp PR q6h PRN; Caution: [C, ?] CI: Glaucoma, resp depression Disp: 15A = 30 mg opium/16.2 mg belladonna extract; 16A = 60 mg opium/16.2 mg belladonna extract SE: Anticholinergic (e.g., sedation, urinary retention, constipation)

Benazepril (Lotensin) Uses: *HTN*, DN, CHF Acts: ACE inhib Dose: 10–80 mg/d PO Caution: [C (1st tri), D (2nd & 3rd tri), +] CI: Angioedema, Hx edema, bilateral RAS Disp: Tabs 5, 10, 20, 40 mg SE: Symptomatic ↓ BP w/ diuretics; dizziness, HA, ↑ K+, nonproductive cough

Bendamustine (Treanda) Uses: *CLL* Acts: Mechlorethamine derivative; alkylating agent Dose: *Adults.* 100 mg/m² IV over 30 min days 1 & 2 of 28-d cycle, up to 6 cycles (w/ tox see PI for dose changes); do not use w/ CrCl <40 mL/min, severe hepatic impair) Caution: [D, ?/–] do not use w/ CrCl <40 mL/min, severe hepatic impair CI: Hypersens to bendamustine or mannitol Disp: Inj powder 100 mg SE: Pyrexia, N/V, dry mouth, fatigue, cough, stomatitis, rash, myelosuppression, Infxn, Inf Rxns & anaphylaxis, tumor lysis synd, skin Rxns Notes: Consider use of allopurinol to prevent tumor lysis synd

Benzocaine (Americaine, Hurricane Lanacane, Various [OTC]) Uses: *topical anesthetic, lubricant on ET tubes, catheters, etc; pain relief in external otitis, cerumen removal, skin conditions, sunburn, insect bites, mouth and gum irritation, hemorrhoids* Acts: topical local anesthetic Dose: *Adults & Peds> 1 year: Anesthetic lubricant:* apply evenly to tube/instrument; *Cerumen removal:* Instill 3 X d for 2-3 days; *Otic drops:* 4-5 gtt in external canal, insert cotton plug, repeat q1-2h PRN; other uses per manufacturer instructions Caution: [C, –] do not use on broken skin; see provider if condition does not respond; avoid in infants and those w/ pulmonary Dzs Disp: Many site-specific OTC forms creams, gels, liquids, sprays, 2–20% SE: itching, irritation, burning, edema, erythema, pruritus, rash, stinging, tenderness, urticaria; methemoglobinemia (infants or in COPD) Notes: Use minimum amount to obtain effect; methemoglobinemia S&Sxs: HA, lightheadedness, SOB, anxiety, fatigue, pale, gray or blue colored skin, and tachycardia; treat w/ IV methylene blue

Benzocaine & Antipyrine (Auralgan) Uses: *Analgesia in severe otitis media* Acts: Anesthetic w/ local decongestant Dose: Fill ear, & insert a moist cotton plug; repeat 1–2 h PRN Caution: [C, ?] CI: w/ Perforated eardrum Disp: Soln 5.4% antipyrine, 1.4% benzocaine SE: Local irritation

Benzonatate (Tessalon Perles) Uses: Symptomatic relief of *cough* Acts: Anesthetizes the stretch receptors in the resp passages Dose: *Adults & Peds >10 y:* 100 mg PO tid (max 600 mg/d) Caution: [C, ?] Disp: Caps 100, 200 mg SE: Sedation, dizziness, GI upset Notes: Do not chew or puncture the caps

Benztropine (Cogentin) Uses: *Parkinsonism & drug-induced extrapyramidal disorders* Acts: Partially blocks striatal cholinergic receptors Dose: *Adults. Parkinsonism:* initial 0.5–1 mg PO/IM/IV qhs, ↑ q 5–6 d PRN by 0.5 mg, usual dose 1–2 mg, 6 mg/d max. *Extrapyramidal:* 1–4 mg PO/IV/IM q day-bid. *Acute Dystonia:* 1–2 mg IM/IV, then 1–2 mg PO bid. **Peds >3 y:** 0.02–0.05 mg/kg/dose 1–2/d **Caution:** [C, ?] w/ Urinary Sxs, NAG, hot environments, CNS or mental disorders, other phenothiazines or TCA **CI:** <3 y **Disp:** Tabs 0.5, 1, 2 mg; Inj 1 mg/mL **SE:** Anticholinergic (tachycardia, ileus, N/V, etc), anhidrosis, heat stroke **Notes:** Physostigmine 1–2 mg SQ/IV to reverse severe Sxs

Benzyl Alcohol (Ulesfia) Uses: *Head lice* **Action:** Topical antiparasitic, pediculicide **Dose:** Apply volume for hair length to dry hair; saturate the scalp; leave on 10 min; rinse w/ water; repeat in 7 days; *Hair length 0-2 in:* 4-6 oz; *2-4 in:* 6-8 oz; *4-8 in:* 8-12 oz; *8-16 in:* 12-24 oz; *16-22 in:* 24-32 oz; *>22 inches:* 32-48 oz **Caution:** [B, ?] Avoid eyes **CI:** none **Disp:** Lotion 5%, 240 mL **SE:** Pruritus, erythema, irritation (local, eyes) **Notes:** Use fine-tooth/nit comb to remove nits and dead lice.

Bepotastine besilate (Bepreve) Uses: *Allergic conjunctivitis * **Acts:** H_1 receptor antagonist **Dose:** *Adults.* 1 gtt into affected eye(s) twice daily **Caution:** [C, ?/–] Do not use while wearing contacts **Disp:** Soln 1.5% **SE:** Mild taste, eye irritation, HA, nasopharyngitis

Beractant (Survanta) Uses: *Prevention & Rx RDS in premature infants* **Acts:** Replaces pulm surfactant **Dose:** 100 mg/kg via ET tube; repeat 3 × q6h PRN; max 4 doses/48 h **Disp:** Susp 25 mg of phospholipid/mL **SE:** Transient ↓ HR, desaturation, apnea **Notes:** Administer via 4-quadrant method

Besifloxacin (Besivance) Uses: *Bacterial conjunctivitis* **Action:** Inhibits DNA gyrase & topoisomerase IV. **Dose:** *Adults & Peds > 1 yo.* 1 gtt into eye(s) TID 4-12 hrs apart × 7 d **Caution:** [C, ?] Remove contacts during Tx **CI:** None **Disp:** 0.6% susp **SE:** HA, redness, blurred vision, irritation

Betaxolol (Kerlone) Uses: *HTN* **Acts:** Competitively blocks β-adrenergic receptors, β_1 **Caution:** [C (1st tri), D (2nd or 3rd tri), +/–] Sinus ↓ HR, AV conduction abnormalities, uncompensated cardiac failure **Dose:** 5–20 mg/d **Disp:** Tabs 10, 20 mg **SE:** Dizziness, HA, ↓ HR, edema, CHF

Betaxolol, Ophthalmic (Betoptic) Uses: Open-angle glaucoma **Acts:** Competitively blocks β_1-adrenergic receptors, **Dose:** 1–2 gtt bid **Caution:** [C (1st tri), D (2nd or 3rd tri), ?/–] **Disp:** Soln 0.5%; susp 0.25% **SE:** Local irritation, photophobia

Bethanechol (Duvoid, Urecholine, Others) Uses: *Acute post-op/ postpartum nonobstructive urinary retention; neurogenic bladder w/ retention* **Acts:** Stimulates cholinergic smooth muscle in bladder & GI tract **Dose:** *Adults.* Initial 5–10 mg PO, then repeat qh until response or 50 mg, typical 10–50 mg tid-qid, 200 mg/d max tid-qid; 2.5–5 mg SQ tid-qid & PRN. *Peds.* 0.3–0.6 mg/kg/24 h PO ÷ tid-qid or 0.15–2 mg/kg/d SQ ÷ 3–4 doses; take on empty stomach **Caution:** [C, –] **CI:** BOO, PUD, epilepsy, hyperthyroidism, ↓ HR, COPD, AV conduction defects, Parkinsonism, ↓ BP, vasomotor instability **Disp:** Tabs 5, 10, 25, 50 mg; Inj 5 mg/mL **SE:** Abd cramps, D, salivation, ↓ BP **Notes:** Do not use IM/IV

Bevacizumab (Avastin) BOX: Associated w/ GI perforation, wound dehiscence, & fatal hemoptysis Uses: *Met colorectal CA w/5-FU, NSCLC w/ paclitaxel and carboplatin; metastatic RCC w/ IFN- alpha* Acts: Vascular endothelial GF inhibitor Dose: *Adults. Colon:* 5 mg/kg or 10 mg/kg IV q14d; *NSCLC:* 15 mg/kg q21d; 1st dose over 90 min; 2nd over 60 min, 3rd over 30 min if tolerated; *RCC:* 10 mg/kg IV q2 wks w/ IFN-α alfa Caution: [C, –] Do not use w/in 28 d of surgery if time for separation of drug & anticipated surgical procedures is unknown; D/C w/ serious adverse effects CI: serious hemorrhage or hemoptysis Disp: 100 mg/4 mL, 400 mg/16 mL vials SE: Wound dehiscence, GI perforation, tracheoesophageal fistula, arterial thrombosis, hemoptysis, hemorrhage, HTN, proteinuria, CHF, Inf Rxns, D, leukopenia Notes: Monitor for ↑ BP & proteinuria

Bicalutamide (Casodex) Uses: *Advanced PCa w/ GnRH agonists ([e.g., leuprolide, goserelin)]*) Acts: Nonsteroidal antiandrogen Dose: 50 mg/d Caution: [X, ?] CI: Women Disp: Caps 50 mg SE: Hot flashes, ↓ loss of libido, impotence, D/N/V, gynecomastia, & ↑ LFTs elevation

Bicarbonate (See Sodium Bicarbonate, page 226)

Bisacodyl (Dulcolax) [OTC] Uses: *Constipation; pre-op bowel prep* Acts: Stimulates peristalsis Dose: *Adults.* 5–15 mg PO or 10 mg PR PRN. *Peds <2 y:* 5 mg PR PRN. *>2 y:* 5 mg PO or 10 mg PR PRN (do not chew tabs or give w/in 1 h of antacids or milk) Caution: [C, ?] CI: Acute abdomen, bowel obst, appendicitis, gastroenteritis Disp: EC tabs 5 mg; tabs 5 mg; supp 10 mg, enema soln 10 mg/30 mL SE: Abd cramps, proctitis, & inflammation w/ supps

Bismuth Subcitrate/Metronidazole/Tetracycline (Pylera) BOX: Metronidazole possibly carcinogenic (based on animal studies) Uses: *H. pylori Infxn w/ omeprazole* Acts: Eradicates H. pylori, see agents Dose: 3 caps qid w/ omeprazole 20 mg bid for × 10 d Caution: [D, –] CI: PRG, peds< 8 yrs (tetracycline during tooth development causes teeth discoloration), w/ renal/hepatic impair, component hypersens Disp: Caps w/ 140-mg bismuth subcitrate potassium, 125-mg metronidazole, & 125-mg tetracycline hydrochloride SE: Stool abnormality, D, dyspepsia, Abd pain, HA, flu-like synd, taste perversion, vaginitis, dizziness; see SE for each component

Bismuth Subsalicylate (Pepto-Bismol) [OTC] Uses: Indigestion, N, & *D*; combo for Rx of *H. pylori Infxn* Acts: Antisecretory & anti-inflammatory Dose: *Adults.* 2 tabs or 30 mL PO PRN (max 8 doses/24 h). *Peds.* (For all max 8 doses/24 h). *3–6 y:* 1/3 tab or 5 mL PO PRN. *6–9 y:* 2/3 tab or 10 mL PO PRN. *9–12 y:* 1 tab or 15 mL PO PRN Caution: [C, D (3rd tri), –] Avoid w/ renal failure; hx severe GI bleed CI: Influenza or chickenpox (↑ risk of Reye synd), ASA allergy (see aspirin) Disp: Chew tabs, caplets 262 mg; liq 262, 525 mg/15 mL; susp 262 mg/15 mL SE: May turn tongue & stools black

Bisoprolol (Zebeta) Uses: *HTN* Acts: Competitively blocks β₁-adrenergic receptors Dose: 2.5–10 mg/d (max dose 20 mg/d); ↓ w/ renal impair Caution:

[C (D 2nd & 3rd tri), +/−] **CI:** Sinus bradycardia, AV conduction abnormalities, uncompensated cardiac failure **Disp:** Tabs 5, 10 mg **SE:** Fatigue, lethargy, HA, ↓ HR, edema, CHF **Notes:** Not dialyzed

Bivalirudin (Angiomax) **Uses:** *Anticoagulant w/ ASA in unstable angina undergoing PTCA, PCI, or in pts undergoing PCI w/ or at risk of HIT/HITTS* **Acts:** Anticoagulant, thrombin inhib **Dose:** 0.75 mg/kg IV bolus, then 1.75 mg/kg/h for duration of procedure and up to 4 h postprocedure; ✓ ACT 5 min after bolus, may repeat 0.3 mg/kg bolus if necessary (give w/ aspirin ASA 300–325 mg/d; start pre-PTCA) **Caution:** [B, ?] **CI:** Major bleeding **Disp:** Powder 250 mg for Inj **SE:** Bleeding, back pain, N, HA

Bleomycin Sulfate (Blenoxane) **Uses:** *Testis CA; Hodgkin Dz & NHLs; cutaneous lymphomas; & squamous cell CA (head & neck, larynx, cervix, skin, penis); malignant pleural effusion sclerosing agent* **Acts:** Induces DNA breakage (scission) **Dose:** (per protocols); ↓ w/ renal impair **Caution:** [D, ?] **CI:** Severe pulm Dz (pulm fibrosis) **Disp:** Powder (Inj) 15, 30 units **SE:** Hyperpigmentation & allergy (rash to anaphylaxis); fever in 50%; lung tox (idiosyncratic & dose related); pneumonitis w/ fibrosis; Raynaud phenomenon, N/V **Notes:** Test dose 1 unit, especially in lymphoma pts; lung tox w/ total dose >400 units or single dose >30 units; avoid high FiO₂ in general anesthesia to ↓ tox

Bortezomib (Velcade) **BOX:** May worsen preexisting neuropathy **Uses:** *Rx multiple myeloma or mantel cell lymphoma w/ one failed previous Rx* **Acts:** Proteasome inhib **Dose:** 1.3 mg/m² bolus IV 2 ×/wk for 2 wk (days 1, 2, 8, 11), w/ 10-d rest period (=1 cycle); ↓ dose w/ hematologic tox, neuropathy **Caution:** [D, ?/−] **Drugs** CYP450 metabolized (Table 10 p 280) **Disp:** 3.5-mg vial **SE:** Asthenia, GI upset, anorexia, dyspnea, HA, orthostatic ↓ BP, edema, insomnia, dizziness, rash, pyrexia, arthralgia, neuropathy

Botulinum Toxin Type A [OnabotulinumtoxinA] (Botox, Botox Cosmetic, Myobloc, Dysport) **BOX:** Effects may spread beyond tx area leading to swallowing and breathing difficulties (may be fatal); sxs may occur hours to wks after inj **Uses:** *Glabellar lines (cosmetic), blepharospasm, cervical dystonia, axillary hyperhidrosis, strabismus*, OAB **Acts:** Neurotoxin, ↓ acetylcholine release from nerve endings, ↓ neuro-muscular transmission; denervates sweat glands and muscles **Dose:** *Adults.* *Glabellar lines (cosmetic):* 0.1 mL IM × 5 sites q3–4mo; *Blepharospasm:* 1.25–2.5 units IM/site q3mo; max 200 units/30 d cum dose; *Cervical dystonia:* 198–300 units IM ÷ <100 units into sternocleidomastoid; *Hyperhidrosis, axillary:* 50 units intradermal/axilla divided; *Strabismus:* 1.25–2.5 units IM/site q3mo; inject extraocular muscles w/ EMG guidance **Peds.** *Blepharospasm: >12 y:* See Adults. dose *Cervical dystonia: >12 y:* 198–300 units IM ÷ among affected muscles; use <100 units in sternocleidomastoid; *Strabismus: >12 y:* 1.25–2.5 units IM/site q3mo; 25 units/site max; inject extraocular muscles w/ EMG guidance **Caution:** [C, ?] different products have different dosing units; w/ neurologic Dz; do not exceed dosing recommended; caution sedentary pt to resume activity slowly after inj; aminoglycosides and nondepolarizing muscle blockers have ↑↑ effects; risk for distant spread at the time of inj; Do not exceed dosing **CI:** Hypersens to components, infect at Inj site **Disp:** Inj powder **SE:** Anaphylaxis, erythema multiforme, dysphagia, dyspnea, syncope, HA, NAG, Inj site pain

Brimonidine (Alphagan P) Uses: *Open-angle glaucoma, ocular HTN* **Acts:** α$_2$-Adrenergic agonist **Dose:** 1 gtt in eye(s) tid (wait 15 min to insert contacts) **Caution:** [B, ?] **CI:** MAOI Rx **Disp:** 0.15, 0.1% soln **SE:** Local irritation, HA, fatigue

Brimonidine/Timolol (Combigan) Uses: *↓ IOP in glaucoma or ocular HTN* **Acts:** Selective α$_2$-adrenergic agonist and nonselective β-adrenergic antagonist **Dose:** *Adults & Peds ≥2 y:* 1 gtt bid **Caution:** [C, −] **CI:** Asthma, severe COPD, sinus brady, 2nd-/3rd-degree AV block, CHF cardiac failure, cardiogenic shock, component hypersens **Disp:** Soln: (2 mg/mL brimonidine, 5 mg/mL timolol) 5, 10, 15 mL **SE:** Allergic conjunctivitis, conjunctival folliculosis, conjunctival hyperemia, eye pruritus, ocular burning & stinging **Notes:** Instill other ophthal products 5 min apart

Brinzolamide (Azopt) Uses: *Open-angle glaucoma, ocular HTN* **Acts:** Carbonic anhydrase inhib **Dose:** 1 gtt in eye(s) tid **Caution:** [C, ?] **CI:** Sulfonamide allergy **Disp:** 1% susp **SE:** Blurred vision, dry eye, blepharitis, taste disturbance

Bromocriptine (Parlodel) Uses: *Parkinson Dz, hyperprolactinemia, acromegaly, pituitary tumors* **Acts:** Agonist to striatal dopamine receptors; ↓ prolactin secretion **Dose:** Initial, 1.25 mg PO bid; titrate to effect, w/ food **Caution:** [B, ?] **CI:** Severe ischemic heart Dz or PVD **Disp:** Tabs 2.5 mg; caps 5 mg **SE:** ↓ BP, Raynaud phenomenon, dizziness, N, GI upset, hallucinations

Bromocriptine mesylate (Cycloset) Uses: *Improve glycemic control in adults w/ Type 2 DM* **Acts:** Dopamine receptor agonist; ?? DM mechanism **Dose:** *Initial:* 0.8 mg PO daily, ↑ ↑weekly by 1 tab; usual dose 1.6–4.8 mg 1×X day; w/in 2 hrs after waking w/ food **Caution:** [B, −] may cause orthostatic ↓ BP, psychotic disorders, w/ strong inducers/inhib of CYP3A4, avoid w/ dopamine antagonists/receptor agonists **CI:** hypersens to ergots drugs, w/ syncopal migraine, nursing mothers **Disp:** Tabs 0.8 mg **SE:** N/V, fatigue, HA, dizziness, somnolence

Budesonide (Rhinocort Aqua, Pulmicort) Uses: *Allergic & nonallergic rhinitis, asthma* **Acts:** Steroid **Dose:** *Adults. Rhinocort Aqua:* 1–4 sprays/nostril/d; *Turbohaler:* 1–4 Inh bid; *Pulmicort Flexhaler:* 1–2 Inh bid *Peds. Rhinocort Aqua intranasal:* 1–2 sprays/nostril/d; *Pulmicort Turbuhaler:* 1–2 Inh bid; *Respules:* 0.25–0.5 mg daily or bid (rinse mouth after PO use) **Caution:** [B, ?/−] **CI:** w/ Acute asthma **Disp:** Metered-dose *Turbuhaler:* 200 mcg/Inh; *Flexhaler:* 90, 180 mcg/Inh; *Respules:* 0.25, 0.5,1 mg/2 mL; *Rhinocort Aqua:* 32 mcg/spray **SE:** HA, N, cough, hoarseness, *Candida* Infxn, epistaxis

Budesonide, oral (Entocort EC) Uses: *Mild-mod Crohn Dz* Acts: Steroid, anti-inflammatory Dose: *Adults.* initial:, 9 mg PO q A.M. to 8 wk max: maint 6 mg PO q A.M. taper by 3 mo; avoid grapefruit juice CI: Active TB and fungal Infxn Caution: [C, ?/–] DM, glaucoma, cataracts, HTN, CHF Disp: Caps 3 mg ER SE: HA, N, ↑ wgt, mood change, *Candida* Infxn, epistaxis Notes: Do not cut/crush/chew; taper on D/C

Budesonide/Formoterol (Symbicort) BOX: Long-acting β₂-adrenergic agonists may ↑ risk of asthma-related death. Use only for pts not adequately controlled on other meds Uses: *Rx of asthma, main in COPD (chronic bronchitis and emphysema)* Acts: Steroid w/ LA β₂-adrenergic agonist Dose: *Adults & Peds >12 y:* 2 inh bid (use lowest effective dose), 640/18 mcg/d max Caution: [C, ?/–] CI: Status asthmaticus/acute asthma Disp: Inh (budesonide/formoterol): 80/4.5 mcg, 160/4.5 mcg SE: HA, GI discomfort, nasopharyngitis, palpitations, tremor, nervousness, URI, paradoxical bronchospasm, hypokalemia, cataracts, glaucoma Notes: Not for acute bronchospasm; not for transferring pt from chronic systemic steroids; rinse & spit w/ water after each dose

Bumetanide (Bumex) Uses: *Edema from CHF, hepatic cirrhosis, & renal Dz* Acts: Loop diuretic; ↓ reabsorption of Na⁺ & Cl⁻, in ascending loop of Henle & the distal tubule Dose: *Adults.* 0.5–2 mg/d PO; 0.5–1 mg IV/IM q8–24h (max 10 mg/d). *Peds.* 0.015–0.1 mg/kg PO q6h-24h (max 10 mg/d) Caution: [D,?] CI: Anuria, hepatic coma, severe electrolyte depletion Disp: Tabs 0.5, 1, 2 mg; Inj 0.25 mg/mL SE: ↓ K⁺, ↓ Na⁺, ↑ Cr, ↑ uric acid, dizziness, ototox Notes: Monitor fluid & lytes

Bupivacaine (Marcaine) BOX: Administration only by clinicians experienced in local anesthesia d/t potential tox; avoid 0.75% for OB anesthesia d/t reports of cardiac arrest and death Uses: *Local, regional, & spinal anesthesia, local & regional analgesia* Acts: Local anesthetic Dose: *Adults & Peds.* Dose dependent on procedure (tissue vascularity, depth of anesthesia, etc) (Table 1 p 264) Caution: [C, ?] CI: Severe bleeding, ↓ BP, shock & arrhythmias, local Infxns at site, septicemia Disp: Inj 0.25, 0.5, 0.75% SE: ↓ BP, ↓ HR, dizziness, anxiety

Buprenorphine (Buprenex) [C-III] Uses: *Mod/severe pain* Acts: Opiate agonist-antagonist Dose: 0.3–0.6 mg IM or slow IV push q6h PRN Caution: [C, ?/–] Disp: 0.3 mg/mL SE: Sedation, ↓ BP, resp depression Notes: Withdrawal if opioid-dependent

Bupropion (Aplenzin) BOX: ↑ suicide risk in pts <24 y w/ major depressive/other psychiatric disorders; not for peds use Uses: *Depression* Acts: Aminoketone, ? action Dose: *Adults.* 174 mg PO, q day q A.M., ↑ PRN to 348 mg q day on day 4 if tolerated, max 522 mg/d; see PI if switching from Wellbutrin; mild–mod hepatic/renal impair ↓ frequency/dose; severe hepatic impair 174 mg max q other day Caution: [C, –] w/ Drugs that ↓ Sz threshold, ↑ w/ stimulants, CYP2D6-metabolized meds (Table 10 p 280) CI: Sz disorder, bulimia, anorexia nervosa, w/ in 14 d of MAOIs, other forms of bupropion, abrupt D/C of EtOH, or sedatives

Disp: ER tab 174, 348, 522 mg **SE:** Dry mouth, N, Abd pain, insomnia, dizziness, pharyngitis, agitation, anxiety, tremor, palpitation, tremor, sweating, tinnitus, myalgia, anorexia, urinary frequency, rash **Notes:** Do not cut/crush/chew, avoid EtOH

Bupropion (Wellbutrin, Wellbutrin SR, Wellbutrin XL, Zyban)
BOX: All pts being treated w/ bupropion for smoking cessation Tx should be observed for neuropsychiatric S&Sxs (hostility, agitation, depressed mood, and suicide-related events; most during/after *Zyban*; Sxs may persist following D/C;Closely monitor for worsening depression or emergence of suicidality, increased suicidal behavior in young adults **Uses:** *Depression, smoking cessation adjunct*, ADHD **Acts:** Weak inhib of neuronal uptake of serotonin & norepinephrine; ↓ neuronal dopamine reuptake **Dose:** *Depression:* 100–450 mg/d ÷ bid-tid; SR 150–200 mg bid; XL 150–450 mg daily. *Smoking cessation (Zyban, Wellbutrin XR):* 150 mg/d × 3 d, then 150 mg bid × 8–12 wks, last dose before 6 P.M.; ↓ dose w/ renal/hepatic impair **Caution:** [C, ?/–] **CI:** Sz disorder, Hx anorexia nervosa or bulimia, MAOI w/ or w/in 14 d; abrupt D/C of EtOH or sedatives; inhibitors/inducers of CYP2B6 (Table 10 p 280); w/ritonavir and lopinavir/ritonavir **Disp:** Tabs 75, 100 mg; SR tabs 100, 150, 200 mg; XL tabs 150, 300 mg; Zyban 150 mg tabs **SE:** Szs, agitation, insomnia, HA, tachycardia, ↓ wgt **Notes:** Avoid EtOH & other CNS depressants, SR & XR do not cut/chew/crush, may ↑ adverse events including Szs

Buspirone (BuSpar) BOX: Closely monitor for worsening depression or emergence of suicidality **Uses:** *Short-term relief of *anxiety* **Acts:** Anti-anxiety; antagonizes CNS serotonin and dopamine receptors **Dose:** Initial: 7.5 mg PO bid; ↑ by 5 mg q2–3d to effect; usual 20–30 mg/d; max 60 mg/d **CI:** w/ MAOI **Caution:** [B, ?/–] Avoid w/ severe hepatic/renal Insuff **Disp:** Tabs ÷ dose 5, 10, 15, 30 mg **SE:** Drowsiness, dizziness, HA, N, EPS, serotonin synd, hostility, depression **Notes:** No abuse potential or physical/psychological dependence

Busulfan (Myleran, Busulfex) BOX: Can cause severe bone marrow suppression **Uses:** *CML*, preparative regimens for allogeneic & ABMT in high doses **Acts:** Alkylating agent **Dose:** (per protocol) **Caution:** [D, ?] **Disp:** Tabs 2 mg, Inj 60 mg/10 mL **SE:** Bone marrow suppression, ↑ BP, pulm fibrosis, N (w/ high dose), gynecomastia, adrenal Insuff, skin hyperpigmentation

Butabarbital, Hyoscyamine Hydrobromide, Phenazopyridine (Pyridium Plus) Uses: *Relieve urinary tract pain w/ UTI, procedures, trauma* **Acts:** Phenazopyridine (topical anesthetic), hyoscyamine (parasympatholytic, ↓ spasm) & butabarbital (sedative) **Dose:** 1 PO qid, pc & hs; w/ antibiotic for UTI, 2 d max **Caution:** [C, ?] **Disp:** Tab butabarbital/hyoscyamine/phenazopyridine, 15 mg/0.3 mg/150 mg **SE:** HA, rash, itching, GI distress, methemoglobinemia, hemolytic anemia, anaphylactoid-like Rxns, dry mouth, dizziness, drowsiness, blurred vision **Notes:** Colors urine orange, may tint skin, sclera; stains clothing/contacts

Butorphanol (Stadol) [C-IV] Uses: *Anesthesia adjunct, pain* & migraine HA **Acts:** Opiate agonist-antagonist w/ central analgesic actions **Dose:** 1–4 mg IM or IV q3–4h PRN. *Migraine:* 1 spray in 1 nostril, repeat × 1 60–90 min, then q3–4h;. ↓ in renal impair **Caution:** [C (D if high dose or prolonged use at term), +] **Disp:** Inj 1, 2 mg/mL; nasal 1 mg/spray (10 mg/mL) **SE:** Drowsiness, dizziness, nasal congestion **Notes:** May induce withdrawal in opioid dependency

C1 Esterase Inhibitor, Human (Berinert) Uses: *Acute abdominal or facial attacks of hereditary angioedema (HAE) * Acts: ↓ contact system by ↓ Factor XIIa and kallikrein activation Dose: *Adults & Adolescents.* 20units/kg IV × 1 Caution: [C, ?/–] Hypersens rxns, monitor for thrombotic events, may contain infectious agents CI: Hypersens rxns to C1 esterase inhibitor preparations Disp: Lyophilized 500 units/vial SE: HA, abd pain, N/V/D, muscle spasms, pain, subsequent HAE attack, anaphylaxis, thromboembolism

Calcipotriene (Dovonex) Uses: *Plaque psoriasis* Acts: Keratolytic Dose: Apply bid Caution: [C, ?] CI: ↑ Ca^{2+}; vit D tox; do not apply to face Disp: Cream; oint; soln 0.005% SE: Skin irritation, dermatitis

Calcitonin (Fortical, Miacalcin) Uses: *Miacalcin:* *Paget Dz, emergent Rx hypercalcemia, postmenopausal osteoporosis*; *Fortical:* *postmenopausal osteoporosis*; osteogenesis imperfecta Acts: Polypeptide hormone (salmon derived), inhibits osteoclasts Dose: *Paget Dz:* 100 units/d IM/SQ initial, 50 units/d or 50–100 units q1–3d maint. *Hypercalcemia:* 4 units/kg IM/SQ q12h; ↑ to 8 units/kg q12h, max q6h. *Osteoporosis:* 100 units/q other day IM/SQ; intranasal 200 units = 1 nasal spray/d Caution: [C, ?] Disp: *Fortical, Miacalcin* nasal spray 200 Int Units/activation; Inj, *Miacalcin* 200 units/mL (2 mL) SE: Facial flushing, N, Inj site edema, nasal irritation, polyuria, may ↑ granular casts in urine Notes: For nasal spray alternate nostrils daily; insure adequate calcium and vit D intake; *Fortical* is rDNA derived from salmon

Calcitriol (Rocaltrol, Calcijex) Uses: *Predialysis reduction of ↑ PTH levels to treat bone Dz; ↑ Ca^{2+} on dialysis* Acts: 1,25-Dihydroxycholecalciferol (vit D analog); ↑ Ca^{2+} and phosphorus absorption; ↑ bone mineralization Dose: *Adults.* Renal failure: 0.25 mcg/d PO, ↑ 0.25 mcg/d q4–6wk PRN; 0.5 mcg 3 ×/wk IV, ↑ PRN *Hypoparathyroidism:* 0.5–2 mcg/d. *Peds.* Renal failure: 15 ng/kg/d, ↑ PRN; maint 30–60 ng/kg/d. *Hypoparathyroidism:* <5 *y:* 0.25–0.75 mcg/d. >6 *y:* 0.5–2 mcg/d Caution: [C, ?] ↑ Mg^{2+} possible w/ antacids ↑: ↑ Ca^{2+}; vit D tox Disp: Inj 1 mcg/mL (in 1 mL); caps 0.25, 0.5 mcg; soln 1 mcg/mL SE: ↑ Ca^{2+} possible Notes:✓ to keep Ca^{2+} WNL; Use non–aluminum phosphate binders and low-phosphate diet to control serum phosphate

Calcitriol, ointment (Vectical) Uses: *mild/moderate plaque psoriasis * Acts: Vitamin D_3 analog Dose: *Adults.* Apply to area BID; max 200g /wk Caution: [C, ?/–] avoid excess sunlight CI: None Disp: Oint 3 mcg/g (5-, 100 -g tube) SE: Hypercalcemia, hypercalciuria, nephrolithiasis, worsening psoriasis, pruritus, skin discomfort

Calcium Acetate (PhosLo) Uses: *ESRD-associated hyperphosphatemia* Acts: Ca^{2+} supl w/o aluminum to ↓ PO_4^{2-} absorption Dose: 2–4 tabs PO w/ meals

Caution: [C, ?] **CI:** $\uparrow$ Ca^{2+} **Disp:** Gel-Cap 667 mg **SE:** Can $\uparrow$ Ca^{2+}, hypophosphatemia, constipation **Notes:** Monitor Ca^{2+}

Calcium Carbonate (Tums, Alka-Mints) [OTC] **Uses:** *Hyperacidity-associated w/ peptic ulcer Dz, hiatal hernia, etc* **Acts:** Neutralizes gastric acid **Dose:** 500 mg–2 g PO PRN, 7 g/d max; $\downarrow$ w/ renal impair **Caution:** [C, ?] **Disp:** Chew tabs 350, 420, 500, 550, 750, 850 mg; susp **SE:** $\uparrow$ Ca^{2+}, $\downarrow$ PO_4^{-}, constipation

Calcium Glubionate (Neo-Calglucon) [OTC] **Uses:** *Rx & prevent calcium deficiency* **Acts:** Ca^{2+} supl **Dose:** *Adults.* 6–18 g/d ÷ doses. *Peds.* 600–2000 mg/kg/d ÷ qid (9 g/d max); $\downarrow$ in renal impair **Caution:** [C, ?] **CI:** $\uparrow$ Ca^{2+} **Disp:** OTC syrup 1.8 g/5 mL = elemental Ca 115 mg/5 mL **SE:** $\uparrow$ Ca^{2+}, $\downarrow$ PO_4^{-}, constipation

Calcium Salts (Chloride, Gluconate, Gluceptate) **Uses:** *Ca^{2+} replacement*, VF, Ca^{2+} blocker tox (CCB), Mg^{2+} intoxication, tetany, *hyperphosphatemia in ESRD* **Acts:** Ca^{2+} supl/replacement **Dose:** *Adults.* Replacement: 1–2 g/d PO. *Tetany:* 1 g CaCl over 10–30 min; repeat in 6 h PRN; *Hyperkalemia/ CCB OD:* 8–16 mg/kg (usually 5–10 mL) IV; 2–4 mg/kg (usually 2 mL) IV before IV calcium blockers *(ECC 2005)* *Peds.* Replacement: 200–500 mg/kg/24 h PO or IV ÷ qid. *Cardiac emergency:* 100 mg/kg/dose IV gluconate salt q10min. *Tetany:* 10 mg/kg CaCl over 5–10 min; repeat in 6 h or use Inf (200 mg/kg/d max). *Adults & Peds.* $\downarrow$ Ca^{2+} d/t citrated blood Inf: 0.45 mEq Ca/100 mL citrated blood Inf ($\downarrow$ in renal impair) **Caution:** [C, ?] **CI:** $\uparrow$ Ca^{2+} **Disp:** CaCl Inj 10% = 100 mg/mL = Ca 27.2 mg/mL = 10-mL amp; Ca gluconate Inj 10% = 100 mg/mL = Ca 9 mg/mL; tabs 500 mg = 45-mg Ca, 650 mg = 58.5-mg Ca, 975 mg = 87.75-mg Ca, 1 g = 90-mg Ca; Ca gluceptate Inj 220 mg/mL = 18-mg/mL Ca **SE:** $\downarrow$ HR, cardiac arrhythmias, $\uparrow$ Ca^{2+}, constipation **Notes:** CaCl 270 mg (13.6 mEq) elemental Ca/g, & calcium gluconate 90 mg (4.5 mEq) Ca/g. RDA for Ca intake: *Peds <6 mo:* 210 mg/d; *6 mo–1 y:* 270 mg/d; *1–3 y:* 500 mg/d; *4–9 y:* 800 mg/d; *10–18 y:* 1200 mg/d. *Adults.* 1000 mg/d; *>50 y:* 1200 mg/d

Calfactant (Infasurf) **Uses:** *Prevention & Rx of RSD in infants* **Acts:** Exogenous pulm surfactant **Dose:** 3 mL/kg instilled into lungs. Can repeat 3 total doses given 12 h apart **Caution:** [?, ?] **Disp:** Intratracheal susp 35 mg/mL **SE:** Monitor for cyanosis, airway obst, $\downarrow$ HR during administration

Candesartan (Atacand) **Uses:** *HTN*, DN, CHF **Acts:** Angiotensin II receptor antagonist **Dose:** 4–32 mg/d (usual 16 mg/d) **Caution:** [C (1st tri, D) (2nd & 3rd tri), –] **CI:** Primary hyperaldosteronism; bilateral RAS **Disp:** Tabs 4, 8, 16, 32 mg **SE:** Dizziness, HA, flushing, angioedema

Capsaicin (Capsin, Zostrix, others) [OTC] **Uses:** Pain d/t *postherpetic neuralgia*, chronic neuralgia, *arthritis*, diabetic neuropathy*, post-op pain, psoriasis, intractable pruritus **Acts:** Topical analgesic **Dose:** Apply tid-qid **Caution:** [C, ?] **Disp:** OTC creams; gel; lotions; roll-ons **SE:** Local irritation, neurotox, cough **Note:** Wk to onset of action

Captopril (Capoten, others) Uses: *HTN, CHF, MI*, LVD, DN **Acts:** ACE inhib **Dose:** *Adults. HTN:* Initial, 25 mg PO bid-tid; ↑ to maint q1–2wk by 25-mg increments/dose (max 450 mg/d) to effect. *CHF:* Initial, 6.25–12.5 mg PO tid; titrate PRN *LVD:* 50 mg PO tid. *DN:* 25 mg PO tid. **Peds** *Infants <2 mo:* 0.05–0.5 mg/kg/dose PO q8–24h. *Children:* Initial, 0.3–0.5 mg/kg/dose PO; ↑ to 6 mg/kg/d max in 2–4 ÷ doses; 1 h ac **Caution:** [C (1st tri); D (2nd & 3rd tri) +]; unknown effects in renal impair **CI:** Hx angioedema, bilateral RAS **Disp:** Tabs 12.5, 25, 50, 100 mg **SE:** Rash, proteinuria, cough, ↑ K+

Carbamazepine (Tegretol XR, Carbatrol, Epitol, Equetro) BOX: Aplastic anemia & agranulocytosis have been reported w/ carbamazepine; pts w/ Asian ancestry should be tested to determine potential for skin Rxns Uses: *Epilepsy, trigeminal neuralgia, acute mania w/ bipolar disorder (Equetro)* EtOH withdrawal **Acts:** Anticonvulsant **Dose:** *Adults. Initial:* 200 mg PO bid or 100 mg 4 ×times/d as susp; ↑ by 200 mg/d; usual 800–1200 mg/d ÷ doses. *Acute Mania (Equetro):* 400 mg/d, ÷ bid, adjust by 200 mg/d to response 1600 mg/d max. **Peds** *<6 y:* 5 mg/kg/d, ↑ to 10–20 mg/kg/d ÷ in 2–4 doses. *6–12 y:* Initial: 100 mg PO bid or 10 mg/kg/24 h PO ÷ daily-bid; ↑ to maint 20–30 mg/kg/24 h ÷ tid-qid; ↓ in renal impair; take w/ food **Caution:** [D, +] **CI:** MAOI use, Hx BM suppression **Disp:** Tabs 100, 200, 300, 400 mg; chew tabs 100 mg, 200 mg; XR tabs 100, 200, 400 mg; *Equetro* Caps ER 100, 200, 300 mg; susp 100 mg/5 mL **SE:** Drowsiness, dizziness, blurred vision, N/V, rash, SJS/toxic epidermal necrolysis (TEN), ↓ Na+, leukopenia, agranulocytosis **Notes:** Monitor CBC & levels; *Trough:* Just before next dose; *Therapeutic: Peak:* 8–12 mcg/mL (monotherapy), 4–8 mcg/ml (polytherapy); *Toxic Trough:* >15 mcg/mL; *1/2-life:* 15–20 h; generic products not interchangeable, many drug interactions, administer susp in 3–4 ÷ doses daily; skin tox (SJS/TEN) ↑ w/ HLA-B*1502 allele

Cabazitaxel (Jevtana) BOX: Neutropenic deaths reported; check frequent CBC; do not give if neutrophil ≤1,500 cells/mm³ ; severe hypersensitivity possible Uses: *Combo w/prednisone in CRPC that has failed docetaxel* **Acts:** Microtubule inhib **Dose:** 25 mg/m² IV over 1 hr every 3 wks w/10 mg PO prednisone daily throughout treatment. **Caution:** [D, +/–] w/meds that induce or inhibit CYP3A (Table 10 p 280); avoid w/hepatic impair **CI:** Component hypersens or to polysorbate (see Box) **Disp:** Inj 60 mg/1.5 mL; two dilutions prior to admin; infuse 10 mg/mL **SE:** pancytopenia (↓ WBC, HBG, plt) fatigue, constipation, asthenia, abd/back pain, hematuria, anorexia, N/V/D, flatulence, peripheral neuropathy, pyrexia, dyspnea, dysgeusia, cough, arthralgia **Notes:** Suggested premed reg IV 30 min before: Antihistamine (diphenhydramine 25 mg); corticosteroid (dexamethasone 8 mg);H₂ antagonist (ranitidine 50 mg); Antiemetic prophylaxis; ✓CBC, LFT, Cr

Carbidopa/Levodopa (Sinemet, Parcopa) Uses: *Parkinson Dz* **Acts:** ↑ CNS dopamine levels **Dose:** 25/100 mg bid-qid; ↑ as needed (max 200/2000 mg/d) **Caution:** [C, ?] **CI:** NAG, suspicious skin lesion (may activate melanoma), melanoma, MAOI use **Disp:** Tabs (mg carbidopa/mg levodopa) 10/100, 25/100, 25/250; tabs SR (mg carbidopa/mg levodopa) 25/100, 50/200; ODT 10/100, 25/100, 25/250 **SE:** Psych disturbances, orthostatic ↓ BP, dyskinesias, cardiac arrhythmias

Carboplatin (Paraplatin) **BOX:** Administration only by physician experienced in cancer CA chemotherapy; BM suppression possible; anaphylaxis may occur **Uses:** *Ovarian*, lung, head & neck, testicular, urothelial, & brain *CA, NHL* & allogeneic & ABMT in high doses **Acts:** DNA cross-linker; forms DNA-platinum adducts **Dose:** 360 mg/m² (ovarian carcinoma); AUC dosing 4–8 mg/mL (Culvert formula: mg = AUC × [25 + calculated GFR]); adjust based on plt count, CrCl, & BSA (Egorin formula); up to 1500 mg/m² used in ABMT setting (per protocols) **Caution:** [D, ?] **CI:** Severe BM suppression, excessive bleeding **Disp:** Inj 50-, 150-, 450 -mg vial (10 mg/mL) **SE:** Anaphylaxis, ↓ BM, N/V/D, nephrotox, hematuria, neurotox, ↑ LFTs **Notes:** Physiologic dosing based on Culvert or Egorin formula allows ↑ doses w/ ↓ tox

Carisoprodol (Soma) **Uses:** *Adjunct to sleep & physical therapy to relieve painful musculoskeletal conditions* **Acts:** Centrally acting muscle relaxant **Dose:** 250–350 mg PO tid-qid **Caution:** [C, M] Tolerance may result; w/ renal/hepatic impair **CI:** Allergy to meprobamate; acute intermittent porphyria **Disp:** Tabs 250, 350 mg **SE:** CNS depression, drowsiness, dizziness, HA, tachycardia **Notes:** Avoid EtOH use; available in combo w/ ASA or codeine.

Carmustine [BCNU] (BiCNU, Gliadel) **BOX:** BM suppression, dose-related pulm tox possible; administer under direct supervision of experienced physician **Uses:** *Primary or adjunct brain tumors, multiple myeloma, Hodgkin and non-Hodgkin lymphomas*, multiple myeloma, induction for allogeneic & ABMT (high dose)* surgery & RT adjunct high-grade glioma and recurrent glioblastoma *(Gliadel implant)* **Acts:** Alkylating agent; nitrosourea forms DNA cross-links to inhibit DNA synth **Dose:** 150–200 mg/m² q6–8wk single or ÷ dose daily Inj over 2 d; 20–65 mg/m² q4–6wk; 300–900 mg/m² in BMT (per protocols); up to 8 implants in CNS op site; ↓ w/ hepatic & renal impair **Caution:** [D, ?] ↓ WBC, RBC, plt counts, renal/hepatic impair **CI:** ↓ BM, PRG **Disp:** Inj 100 mg/vial; *Gliadel* wafer 7.7 mg **SE:** ↓ BP, N/V, ↓ WBC & plt, phlebitis, facial flushing, hepatic/renal dysfunction, pulm fibrosis (may occur years after), optic neuroretinitis; heme tox may persist 4–6 wk after dose **Notes:** Do not give course more frequently than q6wk (cumulative tox); ✓ baseline PFTs, monitor pulm status

Carteolol (Ocupress, Carteolol Ophthalmic) **Uses:** *HTN, ↑ IOP pressure, chronic open-angle glaucoma* **Acts:** Blocks β-adrenergic receptors (β₁, β₂), mild ISA **Dose:** Ophthal 1 gtt in eye(s) bid **Caution:** [C, ?/–] Cardiac failure, asthma **CI:** Sinus bradycardia; heart block >1st degree; bronchospasm **Disp:** Ophthal soln 1% **SE:** conjunctival hyperemia, anisocoria, keratitis, eye pain **Notes:** Oral forms no longer available in US

Carvedilol (Coreg, Coreg CR) **Uses:** *HTN, Mild to severe CHF, LVD post-MI* **Acts:** Blocks adrenergic receptors, β₁, β₂, α₁ **Dose:** *HTN:* 6.25–12.5 mg bid or CR 20–80 mg PO daily. *CHF:* 3.125–25 mg bid; w/ food to minimize ↓ BP **Caution:** [C (1st tri); D (2nd & 3rd tri); ?/–] asthma, DM **CI:** Decompensated CHF, 2nd-/3rd-degree heart block, SSS, severe ↓ HR w/o pacemaker, asthma, severe hepatic impair **Disp:** Tabs 3.125, 6.25, 12.5, 25 mg; CR Tabs 10, 20, 40, 80 mg **SE:** Dizziness, fatigue, hyperglycemia, may mask/potentiate hypoglycemia, ↓ HR, edema, hypercholesterolemia **Notes:** Do not D/C abruptly; ↑ digoxin levels

Caspofungin (Cancidas) Uses: *Invasive aspergillosis refractory/intolerant to standard Rx, esophageal candidiasis* **Acts:** Echinocandin; ↓ fungal cell wall synth; highest activity in regions of active cell growth **Dose:** 70 mg IV load day 1, 50 mg/d IV; slow Inf; ↓ in hepatic impair **Caution:** [C, ?/–] Do not use w/ cyclosporine; not studied as initial Rx **CI:** Allergy to any component **Disp:** Inj 50, 70 mg powder for recons **SE:** Fever, HA, N/V, thrombophlebitis at site, ↑ LFTs **Notes:** Monitor during Inf; limited experience beyond 2 wk of Rx

Cefaclor (Ceclor, Raniclor) Uses: *Bacterial Infxns of the upper & lower resp tract, skin, bone, urinary tract, Abd* **Acts:** 2nd-gen cephalosporin; ↓ cell wall synth. *Spectrum:* More gram(–) activity than 1st-gen cephalosporins; effective against gram(+) (*Streptococcus* sp, *S. aureus*); good gram(–) against *H. influenzae, E. coli, Klebsiella, Proteus* **Dose:** *Adults.* 250–500 mg PO tid; ER 375–500 mg bid. *Peds.* 20–40 mg/kg/d PO ÷ 8–12 h; ↓ renal impair **Caution:** [B, +] antacids ↓ absorption **CI:** Cephalosporin/PCN allergy **Disp:** Caps 250, 500 mg; Tabs ER 375, 500 mg; chew tabs (*Raniclor*) 250, 375 mg; susp 125, 187, 250, 375 mg/5 mL **SE:** N/D, rash, eosinophilia, ↑ LFTs, HA, rhinitis, vaginitis

Cefadroxil (Duricef) Uses: *Infxns skin, bone, upper & lower resp tract, urinary tract* **Acts:** 1st-gen cephalosporin; ↓ cell wall synth. *Spectrum:* Good gram(+) (group A β-hemolytic *Streptococcus* & *Staphylococcus*); gram(–) (*E. coli, Proteus, Klebsiella*) **Dose:** *Adults.* 1–2 g/d PO, 2 ÷ doses *Peds.* 30 mg/kg/d ÷ bid; ↓ in renal impair **Caution:** [B, +] Cephalosporin/PCN allergy **Disp:** Caps 500 mg; tabs 1 g; susp, 250, 500 mg/5 mL **SE:** N/V/D, rash, eosinophilia, ↑ LFTs

Cefazolin (Ancef, Kefzol) Uses: *Infxns of skin, bone, upper & lower resp tract, urinary tract* **Acts:** 1st-gen cephalosporin; β-lactam ↓ cell wall synth. *Spectrum:* Good gram(+) bacilli & cocci, (*Streptococcus, Staphylococcus* [except *Enterococcus*]); some gram(–) (*E. coli, Proteus, Klebsiella*) **Dose:** *Adults.* 1–2 g IV q8h *Peds.* 25–100 mg/kg/d IV ÷ q6–8h; ↓ in renal impair **Caution:** [B, +] **CI:** Cephalosporin/PCN allergy **Disp:** Inj: 500 mg, 1, 10, 20 g **SE:** D, rash, eosinophilia, ↑ LFTs, Inj site pain **Notes:** Widely used for surgical prophylaxis

Cefdinir (Omnicef) Uses: * Infxns of the resp tract, skin, bone, & urinary tract* **Acts:** 3rd-gen cephalosporin; ↓ cell wall synth *Spectrum:* Many gram (+) & (–) organisms; more active than cefaclor & cephalexin against *Streptococcus, Staphylococcus;* some anaerobes **Dose:** *Adults.* 300 mg PO bid or 600 mg/d PO. *Peds.* 7 mg/kg PO bid or 14 mg/kg/d PO; ↓ in renal impair **Caution:** [B, +] w/ PCN-sensitive pts, serum sickness-like Rxns reported **CI:** Hypersens to cephalosporins **Disp:** Caps 300 mg; susp 125, 250 mg/5 mL **SE:** Anaphylaxis, D, rare pseudomembranous colitis

Cefditoren (Spectracef) **Uses:** *Acute exacerbations of chronic bronchitis, pharyngitis, tonsillitis; skin Infxns* **Acts:** 3rd-gen cephalosporin; ↓ cell wall synth. *Spectrum:* Good gram(+) (*Streptococcus & Staphylococcus*); gram (–) (*H. influenzae* & *M. catarrhalis*) **Dose:** *Adults & Peds >12 y:* *Skin:* 200 mg PO bid × 10 d. *Chronic bronchitis, pharyngitis, tonsillitis:* 400 mg PO bid × 10 d; avoid antacids w/ in 2 h; take w/ meals; ↓ in renal impair **Caution:** [B, ?] Renal/hepatic impair **CI:** Cephalosporin/PCN allergy, milk protein, or carnitine deficiency **Disp:** 200 mg tabs **SE:** HA, N/V/D, colitis, nephrotox, hepatic dysfunction, SJS, toxic epidermal necrolysis, allergic Rxns **Notes:** Causes renal excretion of carnitine; tabs contain milk protein

Cefepime (Maxipime) **Uses:** *Comp/uncomp UTI, pneumonia, empiric febrile neutropenia, skin/soft-tissue Infxns, comp intra-Abd Infxns* **Acts:** 4th-gen cephalosporin; ↓ cell wall synth. *Spectrum:* Gram(+) *S. pneumoniae, S. aureus*, gram(–) *K. pneumoniae, E. coli, P. aeruginosa, & Enterobacter* sp **Dose:** *Adults.* 1–2 g IV q8–12h. *Peds.* 50 mg/kg q8h for febrile neutropenia; 50 mg/kg bid for skin/soft-tissue Infxns; ↓ in renal impair **Caution:** [B, +] **CI:** Cephalosporin/PCN allergy **Disp:** Inj 500 mg, 1, 2 g **SE:** Rash, pruritus, N/V/D, fever, HA, (+) Coombs test w/o hemolysis **Notes:** Can give IM or IV; concern over ↑ death rates not confirmed by FDA

Cefixime (Suprax) **Uses:** *Resp tract, skin, bone, & urinary tract Infxns* **Acts:** 3rd-gen cephalosporin; ↓ cell wall synth. *Spectrum:* *S. pneumoniae, S. pyogenes, H. influenzae, & enterobacteria* **Dose:** *Adults.* 400 mg PO ÷ daily-bid. *Peds.* 8–20 mg/kg/d PO ÷ daily-bid; ↓ w/ renal impair **Caution:** [B, +] **CI:** Cephalosporin/PCN allergy **Disp:** Susp 100, 200 mg/5 mL **SE:** N/V/D, flatulence, & Abd pain **Notes:** ✓renal & hepatic Fxn; use susp for otitis media

Cefoperazone (Cefobid) **Uses:** *Rx Infxns of the resp, skin, urinary tract, sepsis* **Acts:** 3rd-gen cephalosporin; ↓ bacterial cell wall synth. *Spectrum:* gram(–) (e.g., *E. coli, Klebsiella*), *P. aeruginosa* but < ceftazidime; gram(+) variable against *Streptococcus & Staphylococcus* sp **Dose:** *Adults.* 2–4 g/d IM/IV ÷ q 8–12h (16 g/d max). *Peds.* (Not approved) 100–150 mg/kg/d IM/IV ÷ bid-tid (12 g/d max); ↓ in renal/hepatic impair **Caution:** [B, +] May ↑ bleeding risk **CI:** Cephalosporin/PCN allergy **Disp:** Powder for Inj 1, 2, 10 g **SE:** D, rash, eosinophilia, ↑ LFTs, hypoprothrombinemia, & bleeding (d/t MTT side chain) **Notes:** May interfere w/ warfarin; disulfiram-like Rxn

Cefotaxime (Claforan) **Uses:** *infxns of lower resp tract, skin, bone & joint, urinary tract, meningitis, sepsis, PID, GC* **Acts:** 3rd-gen cephalosporin; ↓ cell wall synth. *Spectrum:* Most gram(–) (not *Pseudomonas*), some gram(+) cocci *S. pneumoniae, S. aureus* (penicillinase/nonpenicillinase producing), *H. influenzae* (including ampicillin-resistant), not *Enterococcus*; many PCN-resistant pneumococci **Dose:** *Adults.* *Uncomplicated Infxn:* 2 g IV/IM q12h; *Mod–severe Infxn:* 1–2 g IV/IM q 8–12 h; *Severe/septicemia:* 2 g IV/IM q4–8h; *GC urethritis, cervicitis, rectal in female:* 0.5 g IM × 1; *rectal GC men* 1 g IM × 1; *Peds.* 50–200 mg/kg/d

IV ÷ q6–8h; ↓ w/ renal/hepatic impair **Caution:** [B, +] Arrhythmia w/ rapid Inj; w/ colitis **CI:** Cephalosporin/PCN allergy **Disp:** Powder for Inj 500 mg, 1, 2, 10, 20 g, premixed Inf 20 mg/mL, 40 mg/mL **SE:** D, rash, pruritus, colitis, eosinophilia, ↑ transaminases

Cefotetan (Cefotan) Uses: *Infxns of the upper & lower resp tract, skin, bone, urinary tract, abd, & gynecologic system* **Acts:** 2nd-gen cephalosporin; ↓ cell wall synth **Spectrum:** Less active against gram(+) anaerobes including *B. fragilis*; gram(−), including *E. coli, Klebsiella, & Proteus* **Dose:** *Adults.* 1–3 g IV q12h. *Peds.* 20–40 mg/kg/d IV ÷ q12h (6 g/d max) ↓ w/ renal impair **Caution:** [B, +] May ↑ bleeding risk; w/ Hx of PCN allergies, w/ other nephrotoxic drugs **CI:** Cephalosporin/PCN allergy **Disp:** Powder for Inj 1, 2, 10 g **SE:** D, rash, eosinophilia, ↑ transaminases, hypoprothrombinemia, & bleeding (d/t MTT side chain) **Notes:** May interfere w/ warfarin

Cefoxitin (Mefoxin) Uses: *infxns of the upper & lower resp tract, skin, bone, urinary tract, abd, & gynecologic system* **Acts:** 2nd-gen cephalosporin; ↓ cell wall synth. **Spectrum:** Good gram(−) against enteric bacilli (i.e., *E. coli, Klebsiella, & Proteus*); anaerobic *B. fragilis* **Dose:** *Adults.* 1–2 g IV q6–8h. *Peds.* 80–160 mg/kg/d ÷ q4–6h (12 g/d max); ↓ w/ renal impair **Caution:** [B, +] **CI:** Cephalosporin/PCN allergy **Disp:** Powder for Inj 1, 2, 10 g **SE:** D, rash, eosinophilia, ↑ transaminases

Cefpodoxime (Vantin) Uses: *Rx resp, skin, & urinary tract infxns* **Acts:** 3rd-gen cephalosporin; ↓ cell wall synth. **Spectrum:** *S. pneumoniae* or non-β-lactamase-producing *H. influenzae*; acute uncomplicated *N. gonorrhoeae*; some uncomplicated gram(−) (*E. coli, Klebsiella, Proteus*) **Dose:** *Adults.* 100–400 mg PO q12h. *Peds.* 10 mg/kg/d PO ÷ bid; ↓ in renal impair, w/ food **Caution:** [B, +] **CI:** Cephalosporin/PCN allergy **Disp:** Tabs 100, 200 mg; susp 50, 100 mg/5 mL **SE:** D, rash, HA, eosinophilia, ↑ transaminases **Notes:** Drug interactions w/ agents that ↑ gastric pH

Cefprozil (Cefzil) Uses: *Rx resp tract, skin, & urinary tract infxns* **Acts:** 2nd-gen cephalosporin; ↓ cell wall synth. **Spectrum:** Active against MSSA, *Streptococcus*, & gram(−) bacilli (*E. coli, Klebsiella, P. mirabilis, H. influenzae, Moraxella*) **Dose:** *Adults.* 250–500 mg PO daily-bid. *Peds.* 7.5–15 mg/kg/d PO ÷ bid; ↓ in renal impair **Caution:** [B, +] **CI:** Cephalosporin/PCN allergy **Disp:** Tabs 250, 500 mg; susp 125, 250 mg/5 mL **SE:** D, dizziness, rash, eosinophilia, ↑ transaminases **Notes:** Use higher doses for otitis & pneumonia

Ceftazidime (Fortaz, Tazicef) Uses: *Rx resp, skin, bone, urinary tract Infxns, meningitis, & septicemia* **Acts:** 3rd-gen cephalosporin; ↓ cell wall synth. **Spectrum:** *P. aeruginosa* sp, good gram(−) activity **Dose:** *Adults.* 500–2 g IV/IM q8–12h. *Peds.* 30–50 mg/kg/dose IV q8h; ↓ in renal impair **Caution:** [B, +] PCN sensitivity **CI:** Cephalosporin/PCN allergy **Disp:** Powder for Inj 500 mg, 1, 2, 6 g **SE:** D, rash, eosinophilia, ↑ transaminases **Notes:** Use only for proven or strongly suspected Infxn to ↓ development of drug resistance

Ceftibuten (Cedax) **Uses:** *Rx resp tract, skin, urinary tract infxns & otitis media* **Acts:** 3rd-gen cephalosporin; ↓ cell wall synth. *Spectrum: H. influenzae & M. catarrhalis*; weak against *S. pneumoniae* **Dose:** *Adults.* 400 mg/d PO. *Peds.* 9 mg/kg/d PO; ↓ in renal impair; take on empty stomach (susp) **Caution:** [B, +] **CI:** Cephalosporin/PCN allergy **Disp:** Caps 400 mg; susp 90 mg/5 mL **SE:** D, rash, eosinophilia, ↑ transaminases

Ceftizoxime (Cefizox) **Uses:** *Rx resp tract, skin, bone, & urinary tract infxns, meningitis, septicemia* **Acts:** 3rd-gen cephalosporin; ↓ cell wall synth. *Spectrum:* Good gram(–) bacilli (not *Pseudomonas*), some gram(+) cocci (not *Enterococcus*), & some anaerobes **Dose:** *Adults.* 1–4 g IV q8–12h. *Peds.* 150–200 mg/kg/d IV ÷ q6–8h; ↓ in renal impair **Caution:** [B, +] **CI:** Cephalosporin/PCN allergy **Disp:** Inj 1, 2, 10 g **SE:** D, fever, rash, eosinophilia, thrombocytosis, ↑ transaminases

Ceftriaxone (Rocephin) **BOX:** Avoid in hyperbilirubinemic neonates or co-infusion w/ calcium-containing products **Uses:** *Resp tract (pneumonia), skin, bone, abd & urinary tract infxns, meningitis, & septicemia* **Acts:** 3rd-gen cephalosporin; ↓ cell wall synth. *Spectrum:* Mod gram(+); excellent β-lactamase producers **Dose:** *Adults.* 1–2 g IV/IM q12–24h. *Peds.* 50–100 mg/kg/d IV/IM ÷ q12–24h; ↓ w/ renal impair **Caution:** [B, +] **CI:** Cephalosporin allergy; hyperbilirubinemic neonates **Disp:** Powder for Inj 250 mg, 500 mg, 1, 2, 10 g; premixed 20, 40 mg/mL **SE:** D, rash, leukopenia, thrombocytosis, eosinophilia, ↑ LFTs

Cefuroxime (Ceftin [PO], Zinacef [Parenteral]) **Uses:** *Upper & lower resp tract, skin, bone, urinary tract, abd, gynecologic infxns* **Acts:** 2nd-gen cephalosporin; ↓ cell wall synth *Spectrum:* Staphylococci, group B streptococci, *H. influenzae, E. coli, Enterobacter, Salmonella, & Klebsiella* **Dose:** *Adults.* 750 mg–1.5 g IV q6h or 250–500 mg PO bid *Peds.* 75–150 mg/kg/d IV ÷ q8h or 20–30 mg/kg/d PO ÷ bid; ↓ w/ renal impair; take PO w/ food **Caution:** [B, +] **CI:** Cephalosporin/PCN allergy **Disp:** Tabs 250, 500 mg; susp 125, 250 mg/5 mL; powder for Inj 750 mg, 1.5, 7.5 g **SE:** D, rash, eosinophilia, ↑ LFTs **Notes:** Cefuroxime film-coated tabs & susp not bioequivalent; do not substitute on a mg/mg basis; IV crosses blood–brain barrier

Celecoxib (Celebrex) **BOX:** ↑ Risk of serious CV thrombotic events, MI, & stroke, can be fatal; ↑ risk of serious GI adverse events including bleeding, ulceration, & perforation of the stomach or intestines; can be fatal **Uses:** *OA, RA, ankylosing spondylitis, acute pain, primary dysmenorrhea preventive in FAP* **Acts:** NSAID; ↓ COX-2 pathway **Dose:** 100–200 mg/d or bid; *FAP:* 400 mg PO bid; ↓ w/ hepatic impair; take w/ food/milk **Caution:** [C/D (3rd tri), ?] w/ Renal impair **CI:** Sulfonamide allergy, perioperative coronary artery bypass graft **Disp:** Caps 100, 200, 400 mg **SE:** See Box; GI upset, HTN, edema, renal failure, HA **Notes:** Watch for Sxs of GI bleed; no effect on plt/bleeding time; can affect drugs metabolized by P-450 pathway

Cephalexin (Keflex, Panixine DisperDose) **Uses:** *Skin, bone, upper/ lower resp tract (streptococcal pharyngitis), otitis media, uncomp cystitis infxns*

Acts: 1st-gen cephalosporin; ↓ cell wall synth. *Spectrum: Streptococcus (including β-hemolytic), Staphylococcus, E. coli, Proteus, & Klebsiella* **Dose: Adults & Peds >15 y:** 250–1000 mg PO qid; Rx cystitis 7–14 d (4 g/d max). **Peds <15 y.** 25–100 mg/kg/d PO ÷ bid-qid; ↓ in renal impair; on empty stomach **Caution:** [B, +] **CI:** Cephalosporin/PCN allergy **Disp:** Caps 250, 500 mg; *(Panixine Disper-Dose)* tabs for oral susp 100, 125, 250 mg; susp 125, 250 mg/5 mL **SE:** D, rash, eosinophilia, gastritis, dyspepsia, ↑ LFTs, *C. difficile* colitis, vaginitis

Cephradine (Velosef) **Uses:** *Resp, GU, GI, skin, soft-tissue, bone, & joint infxns* **Acts:** 1st-gen cephalosporin; ↓ cell wall synth. *Spectrum:* Gram(+) bacilli & cocci (not *Enterococcus*); some gram(–) (*E. coli, Proteus, & Klebsiella*) **Dose: Adults.** 250–500 mg q6–12h (8 g/d max) **Peds >9 mo:** 25–100 mg/kg/d ÷ bid-qid (4 g/d max); ↓ in renal impair **Caution:** [B, +] **CI:** Cephalosporin/PCN allergy **Disp:** Caps: 250, 500 mg; powder for susp 125, 250 mg/5 mL **SE:** Rash, eosinophilia, ↑ LFTs, N/V/D

Certolizumab Pegol (Cimzia) **BOX:** Serious Infxns (bacterial, fungal, TB, opportunistic) possible. D/C w/ severe Infxn/sepsis, test and monitor for TB w/ Tx; lymphoma/other CA possible in children/adolescents **Uses:** *Crohn Dz w/inadequate response to conventional tx; moderate/severe RA* **Action:** TNF –α blocker **Dose:** *Crohn:* Initial: 400 mg SQ, repeat 2 & 4 wk after; *Maint:* 400 mg SQ q 4 wk. *RA:* Initial: 400 mg SQ, repeat 2 & 4 wk after; *Maint:* 200 mg SQ q other wk or 400 mg SQ q 4 wk. **Caution:** [B, ?] Infection, TB, autoimmune dz, demyelinating CNS Dz, hepatitis B reactivation **CI:** None **Disp:** Inj, powder for reconstitution 200 mg; Inj, soln: 200 mg/mL (1 mL) **SE:** HA, N, upper respiratory Infxns, serious Infxns, TB, opportunistic Infxns, malignancies, demyelinating Dz, CHF, pancytopenia, lupus-like synd, new onset psoriasis **Notes:** 400 mg dose is 2 inj of 200 mg each. Monitor for Infxn. Do not give live/attenuated vaccines during Rx; avoid use w/ anakinra

Cetirizine (Zyrtec, Zyrtec D) [OTC] **Uses:** *Allergic rhinitis & other allergic Sxs including urticaria* **Acts:** Nonsedating antihistamine; *Zyrtec D* contains decongestant **Dose: Adults & Children >6 y:** 5–10 mg/d;. *Zyrtec D* 5/120 mg PO bid whole **Peds 6–11 mo:** 2.5 mg daily. *12 mo-5 y:* 2.5 mg daily-bid; ↓ to q day in renal/hepatic impair **Caution:** [C, ?/–] w/ HTN, BPH, rare CNS stimulation, DM, heart Dz **CI:** Allergy to cetirizine, hydroxyzine **Disp:** Tabs 5, 10 mg; chew tabs 5, 10 mg; syrup 1 mg/5 mL; *Zyrtec D:* Tabs 5/120 mg (cetirizine/pseudoephedrine) **SE:** HA, drowsiness, xerostomia **Notes:** Can cause sedation; swallow ER tabs whole

Cetuximab (Erbitux) **BOX:** Severe Inf Rxns including rapid onset of airway obst (bronchospasm, stridor, hoarseness), urticaria, & ↓ BP; permanent D/C required; ↑ risk sudden death and cardiopulmonary arrest **Uses:** *EGFR + metastatic colorectal CA w/ or w/o irinotecan, unresectable head/neck small cell carcinoma w/ RT; monotherapy in metastatic head/neck CA* **Acts:** Human/mouse recombinant MoAb; binds EGFR, ↓ tumor cell growth **Dose:** Per protocol; load 400 mg/m² IV over 2 h; 250 mg/m² given over 1h × 1 wk **Caution:** [C, –] **Disp:** Inj

100 mg/50 mL **SE:** Acneform rash, asthenia/malaise, N/V/D, Abd pain, alopecia, Inf Rxn, derm tox, interstitial lung Dz, fever, sepsis, dehydration, kidney failure, PE **Notes:** Assess tumor for EGFR before Rx; pretreatment w/ diphenhydramine; w/ mild SE ↓ Inf rate by 50%; limit sun exposure

Charcoal, Activated (SuperChar, Actidose, Liqui-Char) Uses: *Emergency poisoning by most drugs & chemicals (see CI)* **Acts:** Adsorbent detoxicant **Dose:** Give w/ 70% sorbitol (2 mL/kg); repeated use of sorbitol not OK **Adults.** *Acute intoxication:* 25–100 g/dose. *GI dialysis:* 20–50 g q6h for 1–2 d. **Peds 1–12 y:** *Acute intoxication:* 1–2 g/kg/dose. *GI dialysis:* 5–10 g/dose q4–8h **Caution:** [C, ?] May cause V (hazardous w/ petroleum & caustic ingestions); do not mix w/ dairy **CI:** Not effective for cyanide, mineral acids, caustic alkalis, organic solvents, iron, EtOH, methanol poisoning, Li; do not use sorbitol in pts w/ fructose intolerance, intestinal obst, non-intact GI tracts **Disp:** Powder, liq, caps **SE:** Some liq dosage forms in sorbitol base (a cathartic); V/D, black stools, constipation **Notes:** Charcoal w/ sorbitol not OK in children <1 y; monitor for ↓ K+ & Mg2+; protect airway in lethargic/comatose pts

Chloral Hydrate (Aquachloral, Supprettes) [C-IV] Uses: *Short-term nocturnal & pre-op sedation* **Acts:** Sedative hypnotic; active metabolite trichloroethanol **Dose:** **Adults.** *Hypnotic:* 500 mg–1 g PO or PR 30 min or before procedure. *Sedative:* 250 mg PO or PR tid. **Peds.** *Hypnotic:* 20–50 mg/kg/24 h PO or PR 30 min hs or before procedure. *Sedative:* 5–15 mg/kg/dose q8h; avoid w/ CrCl <50 mL/min or severe hepatic impair **Caution:** [C, +] Porphyria & in neonates, long-term care facility residents **CI:** Allergy to components; severe renal, hepatic, or cardiac Dz **Disp:** Caps 500 mg; syrup 500 mg/5 mL; supp 325, 500 mg **SE:** GI irritation, drowsiness, ataxia, dizziness, nightmares, rash **Notes:** May accumulate; tolerance may develop >2 wk; taper dose; mix syrup in H2O or fruit juice; do not crush caps; avoid EtOH & CNS depressants

Chlorambucil (Leukeran) BOX: Myelosuppressive, carcinogenic, teratogenic, associated w/ infertility **Uses:** *CLL, Hodgkin Dz*, Waldenström macroglobulinemia **Acts:** Alkylating agent (nitrogen mustard) **Dose:** (per protocol) 0.1–0.2 mg/kg/d for 3–6 wk or 0.4 mg/kg/dose q2wk; ↓ w/ renal impair **Caution:** [D, ?] Sz disorder & BM suppression; affects human fertility **CI:** Previous resistance; alkylating agent allergy; w/ live vaccines **Disp:** Tabs 2 mg **SE:** ↓ BM, CNS stimulation, N/V, drug fever, rash, secondary leukemias, alveolar dysplasia, pulm fibrosis, hepatotoxic **Notes:** Monitor LFTs, CBC, plts, serum uric acid; ↓ dose if pt has received radiation

Chlordiazepoxide (Librium, Mitran, Libritabs) [C-IV] Uses: *Anxiety, tension, EtOH withdrawal*, & pre-op apprehension **Acts:** Benzodiazepine; anti-anxiety agent **Dose:** **Adults.** *Mild anxiety:* 5–10 mg PO tid-qid or PRN. *Severe anxiety:* 25–50 mg IM, IV, or PO q6–8h or PRN **Peds >6 y:** 0.5 mg/kg/24 h PO or IM ÷ q6–8h; ↓ in renal impair, elderly **Caution:** [D, ?] Resp depression, CNS impair, Hx of drug dependence; avoid in hepatic impair **CI:** Preexisting CNS depression, NAG

Disp: Caps 5, 10, 25 mg; Inj 100 mg **SE:** Drowsiness, CP, rash, fatigue, memory impair, xerostomia, wgt gain **Notes:** Erratic IM absorption

Chlorothiazide (Diuril) Uses: *HTN, edema* **Acts:** Thiazide diuretic **Dose:** *Adults.* 500 mg–1 g PO daily-bid; 100–1000 mg/d IV (for edema only). *Peds >6 mo:* 10–20 mg/kg/24 h PO ÷ bid; 4 mg/kg/d IV; OK w/ food **Caution:** [D, +] **CI:** Sensitivity to thiazides/sulfonamides, anuria **Disp:** Tabs 250, 500 mg; susp 250 mg/5 mL; Inj 500 mg/vial **SE:** ↓ K⁺, Na⁺, dizziness, hyperglycemia, hyperuricemia, hyperlipidemia, photosens **Notes:** Do not use IM/SQ; take early in the day to avoid nocturia; use sunblock; monitor lytes

Chlorpheniramine (Chlor-Trimeton, others) [OTC] BOX: OTC meds w/ chlorpheniramine should not be used in peds <2 y Uses: *Allergic rhinitis*, common cold **Acts:** Antihistamine **Dose:** *Adults.* 4 mg PO q4–6h or 8–12 mg PO bid of SR *Peds.* 0.35 mg/kg/24 h PO ÷ q4–6h or 2 mg/kg/24 h SR **Caution:** [C, ?/−] BOO; NAG; hepatic Insuff **CI:** Allergy **Disp:** Tabs 4 mg; chew tabs 2 mg; SR tabs 8, 12 mg **SE:** Anticholinergic SE & sedation common, postural ↓ BP, QT changes, extrapyramidal Rxns, photosens **Notes:** Do not cut/crush/chew ER forms; deaths in pts <2 y; associated w/ cough and cold meds (MMWR 2007;56(01):1–4)

Chlorpromazine (Thorazine) Uses: *Psychotic disorders, N/V*, apprehension, intractable hiccups **Acts:** Phenothiazine antipsychotic; antiemetic **Dose:** *Adults. Psychosis:* 30-800 mg/day in 1–4 ÷ doses, start low dose, ↑ PRN; typical 200-600 mg/day; 1–2 g/day may be needed in some cases. *Severe Sxs:* 25 mg IM/ IV initial; may repeat in 1–4 h; then 25–50 mg PO or PR tid. *Hiccups:* 25–50 mg PO tid-qid. *Children >6 mo: Psychosis & N/V:* 0.5–1 mg/kg/dose PO q4–6h or IM/ IV q6–8h; **Caution:** [C, ?/−] Safety in children <6 mo not established; Szs, avoid w/ hepatic impair, BM suppression **CI:** Sensitivity w/ phenothiazines, NAG **Disp:** Tabs 10, 25, 50, 100, 200 mg; soln 100 mg/mL; Inj 25 mg/mL **SE:** Extrapyramidal SE & sedation; α-adrenergic blocking properties; ↓ BP; ↑ QT interval **Notes:** Do not D/C abruptly; dilute PO conc in 2–4 oz of liq

Chlorpropamide (Diabinese) Uses: *Type 2 DM* **Acts:** Sulfonylurea; ↑ pancreatic insulin release; ↑ peripheral insulin sensitivity; ↓ hepatic glucose output **Dose:** 100–500 mg/d; w/ food, ↓ hepatic impair **Caution:** [C, ?/−] CrCl < 50 mL/min; ↓ in hepatic impair **CI:** Cross-sensitivity w/ sulfonamides **Disp:** Tabs 100, 250 mg **SE:** HA, dizziness, rash, photosens, hypoglycemia, SIADH **Notes:** Avoid EtOH (disulfiram-like Rxn)

Chlorthalidone (Hygroton, others) Uses: *HTN* **Acts:** Thiazide diuretic **Dose:** *Adults.* 25–100 mg PO daily. *Peds.* (Not approved) 2 mg/kg/dose PO 3×/wk or 1–2 mg/kg/d PO; ↓ in renal impair; OK w/ food, milk **Caution:** [D, +] **CI:** Cross-sensitivity w/ thiazides or sulfonamides; anuria **Disp:** Tabs 15, 25, 50 mg **SE:** ↓ K⁺, dizziness, photosens, ↑ glucose, hyperuricemia, sexual dysfunction

Chlorzoxazone (Paraflex, Parafon Forte DSC, others) Uses: *Adjunct to rest & physical therapy Rx to relieve discomfort associated w/ acute, painful musculoskeletal conditions* **Acts:** Centrally acting skeletal muscle relaxant

Dose: *Adults.* 250–500 mg PO tid-qid. *Peds.* 20 mg/kg/d in 3–4 ÷ doses **Caution:** [C, ?] Avoid EtOH & CNS depressants **CI:** Severe liver Dz **Disp:** Tabs 250, 500 mg **SE:** Drowsiness, tachycardia, dizziness, hepatotox, angioedema

Cholecalciferol [Vitamin D₃] (Delta D) **Uses:** Dietary supl to Rx vit D deficiency **Acts:** ↑ intestinal Ca^{2+} absorption **Dose:** 400–1000 Int Units/d PO **Caution:** [A (D doses above the RDA), +] **CI:** ↑ Ca^{2+}, hypervitaminosis, allergy **Disp:** Tabs 400, 1000 Int Units **SE:** Vit D tox (renal failure, HTN, psychosis) **Notes:** 1 mg cholecalciferol = 40,000 Int Units vit D activity

Cholestyramine (Questran, Questran Light, Prevalite) **Uses:** *Hypercholesterolemia; hyperlipidemia, pruritus associated w/ partial biliary obst; D associated w/ excess fecal bile acids* pseudomembranous colitis, dig tox, hyperoxaluria **Acts:** Binds intestinal bile acids, forms insoluble complexes **Dose:** *Adults.* Titrate: 4 g/d-bid ↑ to max 24 g/d ÷ 1–6 doses/d. *Peds.* 240 mg/kg/d in 3 ÷ doses **Caution:** [C, ?] Constipation, phenylketonuria, may interfere w/other drug absorption; consider supl w/ fat-soluble vits **CI:** Complete biliary or bowel obst; w/ mycophenolate hyperlipoproteinemia types III, IV, V **Disp:** *(Questran)* 4 g cholestyramine resin/9 g powder; *(Prevalite)* w/ aspartame: 4 g resin/5.5 g powder; *(Questran Light)* 4 g resin/6.4 g powder **SE:** Constipation, Abd pain, bloating, HA, rash, vit K deficiency **Notes:** OD may cause GI obst; mix 4 g in 2–6 oz of noncarbonated beverage; take other meds 1–2 h before or 6 h after; ✓ lipids

Ciclesonide, Inhalation (Alvesco) **Uses:** *Asthma maint* **Acts:** Inhaled steroid **Dose:** *Adults & Peds >12 y: On bronchodilators alone:* 80 mcg bid (320 mcg/d max). *Inhaled corticosteroids:* 80 mcg bid (640 mcg/d max). *On oral corticosteroids:* 320 mcg bid, 640 mcg/d max **Caution:** [C, ?] **CI:** Status asthmaticus or other acute episodes of asthma, hypersens **Disp:** Inh 80, 160 mcg/actuation **SE:** HA, nasopharyngitis, sinusitis, pharyngolaryngeal pain, URI, arthralgia, nasal congestion **Notes:** Oral *Candida* risk, rinse mouth and spit after, taper systemic steroids slowly when transferring to ciclesonide, monitor growth in pediatric pts, counsel on use of device, clean mouthpiece weekly

Ciclesonide, nasal (Omnaris) **Uses:** Allergic rhinitis **Acts:** Nasal corticosteroid **Dose:** *Adults & Peds >12 y.* 2 sprays each nostril 1×/d **Caution:** [C, ?/–] w/ Ketoconazole; monitor peds for growth reduction **CI:** Component allergy **Disp:** Intranasal spray susp, 50 mcg/spray, 120 doses **SE:** Adrenal suppression, delayed nasal wound healing, URI, HA, ear pain, epistaxis ↑ risk viral Dz (e.g., chickenpox), delayed growth in children

Ciclopirox (Loprox, Penlac) **Uses:** *Tinea pedis, tinea cruris, tinea corporis, cutaneous candidiasis, tinea versicolor, tinea rubrum* **Acts:** Antifungal antibiotic; cellular depletion of essential substrates &/or ions **Dose:** *Adults & Peds >10 y:* Massage into affected area bid. *Onychomycosis:* apply to nails daily, w/ removal q7d **Caution:** [B, ?] **CI:** Component sensitivity **Disp:** Cream 0.77%, gel 0.77%, topical susp 0.77%, shampoo 1%, nail lacquer 8% **SE:** Pruritus, local irritation, burning **Notes:** D/C w/ irritation; avoid dressings; gel best for athlete's foot

Cidofovir (Vistide) BOX: Renal impair is the major tox. Follow administration instructions; possible carcinogenic, teratogenic Uses: *CMV retinitis w/ HIV* Acts: Selective inhibition of viral DNA synth Dose: *Rx*: 5 mg/kg IV over 1 h once/wk for 2 wk w/ probenecid. *Maint*: 5 mg/kg IV once/2 wk w/ probenecid (2 g PO 3 h prior to cidofovir, then 1 g PO at 2 h & 8 h after cidofovir); ↓ in renal impair Caution: [C, −] SCr >1.5 mg/dL or CrCl <55 mL/min or urine protein >100 mg/dL; w/ other nephrotoxic drugs CI: Probenecid or sulfa allergy Disp: Inj 75 mg/mL SE: Renal tox, chills, fever, HA, N/V/D, thrombocytopenia, neutropenia Notes: Hydrate w/ NS prior to each Inf

Cilostazol (Pletal) Uses: *Reduce Sxs of intermittent claudication* Acts: Phosphodiesterase III inhib; ↑ s cAMP in plts & blood vessels, vasodilation & inhibit plt aggregation Dose: 100 mg PO bid, 1/2 h before or 2 h after breakfast & dinner Caution: [C, +/−] ↓ dose w/ drugs that inhibit CYP3A4 & CYP2C19 (Table 10 p 280) CI: CHF, hemostatic disorders, active pathologic bleeding Disp: Tabs 50, 100 mg SE: HA, palpitation, D

Cimetidine (Tagamet, Tagamet HB 200 [OTC]) Uses: *Duodenal ulcer; ulcer prophylaxis in hypersecretory states (e.g., trauma, burns); GERD* Acts: H₂-receptor antagonist Dose: *Adults*. *Active ulcer*: 2400 mg/d IV cont Inf or 300 mg IV q6h; 400 mg PO bid or 800 mg hs. *Maint*: 400 mg PO hs. *GERD*: 300–600 mg PO q6h; maint 800 mg PO hs. *Peds*. *Infants*: 10–20 mg/kg/24 h PO or IV ÷ q6–12h. *Children*: 20–40 mg/kg/24 h PO or IV ÷ q6h; ↓ w/ renal Insuff & in elderly Caution: [B, +] Many drug interactions (P-450 system); do not use w/ clopidogrel (↓ effect) CI: Component sensitivity Disp: Tabs 200 (OTC), 300, 400, 800 mg; liq 300 mg/5 mL; Inj 300 mg/2 mL SE: Dizziness, HA, agitation, ↓ plt, gynecomastia Notes: 1 h before or 2 h after antacids; avoid EtOH

Cinacalcet (Sensipar) Uses: *Secondary hyperparathyroidism in CRF; ↑ Ca²⁺ in parathyroid carcinoma* Acts: ↓ PTH by ↑ calcium-sensing receptor sensitivity Dose: *Secondary hyperparathyroidism*: 30 mg PO daily. *Parathyroid carcinoma*: 30 mg PO bid; titrate q2–4wk based on calcium & PTH levels; swallow whole; take w/ food Caution: [C, ?/−] w/ Szs, adjust w/ CYP3A4 inhib (Table 10 p 280) SE: N/V/D, myalgia, dizziness, ↓ Ca²⁺ Notes: Monitor Ca²⁺, PO₄²⁻, PTH

Ciprofloxacin (Cipro, Cipro XR, Proquin XR) BOX: ↑ risk of tendonitis and tendon rupture Uses: *Rx lower resp tract, sinuses, skin & skin structure, bone/joints, & UT infxns, including prostatitis* Acts: Quinolone antibiotic; ↓ DNA gyrase. *Spectrum*: Broad gram(+) & (−) aerobics; little *Streptococcus*; good *Pseudomonas, E. coli, B. fragilis, P. mirabilis, K. pneumoniae, C. jejuni,* or *Shigella* Dose: *Adults*. 250–750 mg PO q12h; XR 500–1000 mg PO q24h; or 200–400 mg IV q12h; ↓ in renal impair Caution: [C, ?/−] Children <18 y CI: Component sensitivity Disp: Tabs 100, 250, 500, 750 mg; Tabs XR 500, 1000 mg; susp 5 g/100 mL, 10 g/100 mL; Inj 200, 400 mg; premixed piggyback 200, 400 mg/100 mL SE: Restlessness, N/V/D, rash, ruptured tendons, ↑ LFTs Notes: Avoid antacids; reduce/

restrict caffeine intake; interactions w/ theophylline, caffeine, sucralfate, warfarin, antacids, most tendon problems in Achilles, rare shoulder and hand

Ciprofloxacin, ophthalmic (Ciloxan) Uses: *Rx & prevention of ocular infxns (conjunctivitis, blepharitis, corneal abrasions)* Acts: Quinolone antibiotic; ↓ DNA gyrase Dose: 1–2 gtt in eye(s) q2h while awake for 2 d, then 1–2 gtt q4h while awake for 5 d, oint 1/2-inch ribbon in eye tid × 2 d, then bid × 5 d Caution: [C, ?/–] CI: Component sensitivity Disp: Soln 3.5 mg/mL; oint 0.3%, 35 g SE: Local irritation

Ciprofloxacin, otic (Cetraxal) Uses: *Otitis externa* Acts: Quinolone antibiotic; ↓ DNA gyrase. Spectrum: *P aeruginosa, S. aureus* Dose: Adults & Peds *> 1 yr.* 0.25 mL in ear(s) q 12 h × 7 d Caution: [C, ?/–] CI: Component sensitivity Disp: Sol 0.2% SE: hypersens rxn, ear pruritus/pain, HA, fungal superinfection

Ciprofloxacin & Dexamethasone, otic (Ciprodex Otic) Uses: *Otitis externa, otitis media peds* Acts: Quinolone antibiotic; ↓ DNA gyrase; w/ steroid Dose: Adults. 4 gtt in ear(s) bid × 7 d. Peds *>6 mo:* 4 gtt in ear(s) bid for 7 d Caution: [C, ?/–] CI: Viral ear infxns Disp: Susp ciprofloxacin 0.3% & dexamethasone 1% SE: Ear discomfort Notes: OK w/ tympanostomy tubes

Ciprofloxacin & Hydrocortisone, otic (Cipro HC Otic) Uses: *Otitis externa* Acts: Quinolone antibiotic; ↓ DNA gyrase; w/ steroid Dose: Adults & Peds *>1 mo.* 1–2 gtt in ear(s) bid × 7 d Caution: [C, ?/–] CI: Perforated tympanic membrane, viral infxns of the external canal Disp: Susp ciprofloxacin 0.2% & hydrocortisone 1% SE: HA, pruritus

Cisplatin (Platinol, Platinol AQ) BOX: Anaphylactic-like Rxn, ototox, cumulative renal tox; doses >100 mg/m² q3–4wk rarely used, do not confuse w/ carboplatin Uses: *Testicular, bladder, ovarian*, SCLC, NSCLC, breast, head & neck, & penile CAs; osteosarcoma; peds brain tumors Acts: DNA-binding; denatures double helix; intrastrand cross-linking Dose: 10–20 mg/m²/d for 5 d q3wk; 50–120 mg/m² q3–4wk (per protocols); ↓ w/ renal impair Caution: [D, –] Cumulative renal tox may be severe; ↓ BM, hearing impair, preexisting renal Insuff CI: w/ Anthrax or live vaccines, platinum-containing compound allergy; w/ cidofovir Disp: Inj 1 mg/mL SE: Allergic Rxns, N/V, nephrotox (↑ w/ administration of other nephrotoxic drugs; minimize by NS Inf & mannitol diuresis), high-frequency hearing loss in 30%, peripheral "stocking glove"-type neuropathy, cardiotox (ST, T-wave changes), ↓ Mg²⁺, mild ↓ BM, hepatotox; renal impair dose-related & cumulative Notes: Give taxanes before platinum derivatives; ✓ Mg²⁺, lytes before & w/in 48 h after cisplatin

Citalopram (Celexa) BOX: Closely monitor for worsening depression or emergence of suicidality, particularly in pts <24 y Uses: *Depression* Acts: SSRI Dose: Initial 20 mg/d, may ↑ to 40 mg/d; ↓ in elderly & hepatic/ renal Insuff Caution: [C, +/–] Hx of mania, Szs & pts at risk for suicide CI: MAOI or w/in 14 d of MAOI use Disp: Tabs 10, 20, 40 mg; soln 10 mg/5 mL SE: Somnolence, insomnia, anxiety, xerostomia, N, diaphoresis, sexual dysfunction Notes: May cause ↓ Na⁺/SIADH

Cladribine (Leustatin) BOX: Dose-dependent reversible myelosuppression; neurotox, nephrotox, administer by physician with w/ experience in chemotherapy regimens Uses: *HCL, CLL, NHLs, progressive MS* Acts: Induces DNA strand breakage; interferes w/ DNA repair/synth; purine nucleoside analog Dose: 0.09–0.1 mg/kg/d cont IV Inf for 1–7 d (per protocols); ↓ w/ renal impair Caution: [D, ?/–] Causes neutropenia & Infxn CI: Component sensitivity Disp: Inj 1 mg/mL SE: ↓ BM, T -lymphocyte ↓ may be prolonged (26–34 wk), fever in 46%, tumor lysis synd, Infxns (especially lung & IV sites), rash (50%), HA, fatigue, N/V Notes: Consider prophylactic allopurinol; monitor CBC

Clarithromycin (Biaxin, Biaxin XL) Uses: *Upper/lower resp tract, skin/skin structure infxns, H. pylori infxns, & infxns caused by non-tuberculosis (atypical) Mycobacterium; prevention of MAC infxns in HIV-Infxn* Acts: Macrolide antibiotic, ↓ protein synth. Spectrum: H. influenzae, M. catarrhalis, S. pneumoniae, M. pneumoniae, & H. pylori Dose: Adults. 250–500 mg PO bid or 1000 mg (2 × 500 mg XL tab)/d. Mycobacterium: 500 mg PO bid. Peds >6 mo: 7.5 mg/kg/dose PO bid; ↓ w/ renal impair Caution: [C, ?] Antibiotic-associated colitis; rare QT prolongation & ventricular arrhythmias, including torsades de pointes CI: Macrolide allergy; w/ ranitidine in pts w/ Hx of porphyria or CrCl <25 mL/min Disp: Tabs 250, 500 mg; susp 125, 250 mg/5 mL; 500 mg XL tab SE: ↑ QT interval, causes metallic taste, N/D, Abd pain, HA, rash Notes: Multiple drug interactions, ↑ theophylline & carbamazepine levels; do not refrigerate susp

Clemastine Fumarate (Tavist, Dayhist, Antihist-1) [OTC] Uses: *Allergic rhinitis & Sxs of urticaria* Acts: Antihistamine Dose: Adults & Peds >12 y: 1.34 mg bid-2.68 mg tid; max 8.04 mg/d. 6–12 y: 0.67–1.34 mg bid (max 4.02 /d). <6 y: 0.335–0.67 mg/d ÷ into 2–3 doses (max 1.34 mg/d), Caution: [B, M] BOO: Do not take w/ MAOI CI: NAG Disp: Tabs 1.34, 2.68 mg; syrup 0.67 mg/5 mL SE: Drowsiness, dyscoordination, epigastric distress, urinary retention Notes: Avoid EtOH

Clevidipine (Cleviprex) Uses: *HTN when PO not available/desirable* Action: Dihydropyridine CCB, potent arterial vasodilator Dose: 1-2 mg/h IV then maint 4-6 mg/h; 21 mg/h MAX Caution: [C, ?] ↓ BP, syncope, rebound HTN, reflex tachycardia, CHF CI: Hypersens: component or formulation (soy, egg products); impaired lipid metabolism; severe aortic stenosis Disp: Inj 0.5 mg/mL (50 mL, 100 mL) SE: AF, fever, insomnia, N/V, HA, renal impair

Clindamycin (Cleocin, Cleocin-T, others) BOX: Pseudomembranous colitis may range from mild to life-threatening uses: *Rx aerobic & anaerobic Infxns; topical for severe acne & vag Infxns* Acts: Bacteriostatic; interferes w/ protein synth. Spectrum: Streptococci, pneumococci, staphylococci, & gram(+) & (–) anaerobes; no activity against gram(–) aerobes Dose: Adults. PO: 150–450 mg PO q6–8h. IV: 300–600 mg IV q6h or 900 mg IV q8h. Vaginal: 1 applicator hs for 7 d. Topical: Apply 1% gel, lotion, or soln bid. Peds Neonates: (Avoid use; contains benzyl alcohol) 10–15 mg/kg/24 h ÷ q8–12h. Children >1 mo: 10–30 mg/kg/24 h ÷ q6–8h, to a max of 1.8 g/d PO or 4.8 g/d IV. *Topical:* Apply 1%, gel, lotion, or soln bid; ↓ in severe hepatic impair **Caution:** [B, +] Can cause fatal colitis **CI:** Hx pseudomembranous colitis **Disp:** Caps 75, 150, 300 mg; susp 75 mg/5 mL; Inj 300 mg/2 mL; vag cream 2%, topical soln 1%, gel 1%, lotion 1%, vag supp 100 mg **SE:** D may be *C. difficile* pseudomembranous colitis, rash, ↑ LFTs **Notes:** D/C drug w/ D, evaluate for *C. difficile*

Clofarabine (Clolar) **Uses:** Rx relapsed/refractory ALL after at least 2 regimens in children 1–21 y **Acts:** Antimetabolite; ↓ ribonucleotide reductase w/ false nucleotide base-inhibiting DNA synth **Dose:** 52 mg/m² IV over 2 h daily × 5 d (repeat q2–6wk); per protocol **Caution:** [D, –] **Disp:** Inj 20 mg/20 mL **SE:** N/V/D, anemia, leukopenia, thrombocytopenia, neutropenia, Infxn, ↑ AST/ALT **Notes:** Monitor for tumor lysis synd & systemic inflammatory response synd (SIRS)/capillary leak synd; hydrate well

Clonazepam (Klonopin) [C-IV] **Uses:** *Lennox-Gastaut synd, akinetic & myoclonic Szs, absence Szs, panic attacks*, restless legs synd, neuralgia, parkinsonian dysarthria, bipolar disorder **Acts:** Benzodiazepine; anticonvulsant **Dose:** *Adults.* 1.5 mg/d PO in 3 ÷ doses; ↑ by 0.5–1 mg/d q3d PRN up to 20 mg/d. *Peds.* 0.01–0.03 mg/kg/24 h PO ÷ tid; ↑ to 0.1–0.2 mg/kg/24 h ÷ tid; avoid abrupt D/C **Caution:** [D, M] Elderly pts, resp Dz, CNS depression, severe hepatic impair, NAG **CI:** Severe liver Dz, acute NAG **Disp:** Tabs 0.5, 1, 2 mg, oral disintegrating tabs 0.125, 0.25, 0.5, 1, 2 mg **SE:** CNS (drowsiness, dizziness, ataxia, memory impair) **Notes:** Can cause retrograde amnesia; a CYP3A4 substrate

Clonidine, oral (Catapres) **Uses:** *HTN*, opioid, EtOH, & tobacco withdrawal, ADHD **Acts:** Centrally acting α-adrenergic stimulant **Dose:** *Adults.* 0.1 mg PO bid, adjust daily by 0.1–0.2-mg increments (max 2.4 mg/d). *Peds.* 5–10 mcg/kg/d ÷ q8–12h (max 0.9 mg/d); ↓ in renal impair **Caution:** [C, +/–] Avoid w/ β-blocker, elderly, severe CV Dz, renal impair; use w/agents that affect sinus node may cause severe ↓ HR **CI:** Component sensitivity **Disp:** Tabs 0.1, 0.2, 0.3 mg **SE:** drowsiness, orthostatic ↓ BP, xerostomia, constipation, ↓ HR, dizziness **Notes:** More effective for HTN if combined w/ diuretics; withdraw slowly, rebound HTN w/ abrupt D/C of doses >0.2 mg bid; ADHD use in peds needs CV assessment before starting epidural clonidine (Duraclon) used for chronic CA pain

Clonidine, transdermal (Catapres TTS) **Uses:** *HTN* **Acts:** Centrally acting α-adrenergic stimulant **Dose:** 1 patch q7d to hairless area (upper arm/torso); titrate to effect; ↓ w/ severe renal impair; **Caution:** [C, +/–] Avoid w/ β-blocker, withdraw slowly, in elderly, severe CV Dz and w/ renal impair; use w/agents that affect sinus node may cause severe ↓ HR **CI:** Component sensitivity **Disp:** TTS-1, TTS-2, TTS-3 (delivers 0.1, 0.2, 0.3 mg, respectively, of clonidine/d for 1 wk) **SE:** Drowsiness, orthostatic ↓ BP, xerostomia, constipation, ↓ HR **Notes:** Do not D/C abruptly (rebound HTN) Doses >2 TTS-3 usually not associated w/ ↑ efficacy; steady state in 2–3 d

Clopidogrel (Plavix) Uses: *Reduce atherosclerotic events*, administer ASAP in ECC setting w/ high-risk ST depression or T-wave inversion Acts: ↓ Plt aggregation Dose: 75 mg/d; 300–600 mg PO × 1 dose can be used to load pts; 300 mg PO, then 75 mg/d 1–9 mo *(ECC 2005)* Caution: [B, ?] Active bleeding; risk of bleeding from trauma & other; TTP; liver Dz; do not use w/ PPI (e.g., omeprazole, cimetidine)or other CYP2C19 (e.g., fluconazole); OK with ranitidne, famotidine CI: Coagulation disorders, active/ intracranial bleeding; CABG planned w/in 5–7 d Disp: Tabs 75, 300 mg SE: ↑ bleeding time, GI intolerance, HA, dizziness, rash, thrombocytopenia, ↓ WBC Notes: Plt aggregation to baseline ~ 5 d after D/C, plt transfusion to reverse acutely; clinical response highly variable

Clorazepate (Tranxene) [C-IV] Uses: *Acute anxiety disorders, acute EtOH withdrawal Sxs, adjunctive therapy Rx in partial Szs* Acts: Benzodiazepine; antianxiety agent Dose: *Adults.* 15–60 mg/d PO single or ÷ doses. *Elderly & debilitated pts:* Initial 7.5–15 mg/d in ÷ doses. *EtOH withdrawal:* Day 1: Initial 30 mg; then 30–60 mg ÷ doses; Day 2: 45–90 mg ÷ doses; Day 3: 22.5–45 mg ÷ doses; Day 4: 15–30 mg ÷ doses. *Peds.* 3.75–7.5 mg/dose bid to 60 mg/d max ÷ bid-tid Caution: [D, ?/–] Elderly; Hx depression CI: NAG; Not OK <9 y of age Disp: Tabs 3.75, 7.5, 15 mg; Tabs-SD (daily) 11.25, 22.5 mg SE: CNS depressant effects (drowsiness, dizziness, ataxia, memory impair), ↓ BP Notes: Monitor pts w/ renal/hepatic impair (drug may accumulate); avoid abrupt D/C; may cause dependence

Clotrimazole (Lotrimin, Mycelex, others) [OTC] Uses: *Candidiasis & tinea Infxns* Acts: Antifungal; alters cell wall permeability. *Spectrum:* Oropharyngeal candidiasis, dermatophytoses, superficial mycoses, cutaneous candidiasis, & vulvovaginal candidiasis Dose: *PO: Prophylaxis:* 1 troche dissolved in mouth tid *Rx:* 1 troche dissolved in mouth 5×/d for 14 d. *Vaginal 1% Cream:* 1 applicatorfull hs for 7 d. *2% Cream:* 1 applicator-full hs for 3 d *Tabs:* 100 mg vaginally hs for 7 d or 200 mg (2 tabs) vaginally hs for 3 d or 500-mg tabs vaginally hs once. *Topical:* Apply bid 10–14 d Caution: [B (C if PO), ?] Not for systemic fungal Infxn; safety in children <3 y not established CI: Component allergy Disp: 1% cream; soln; lotion; troche 10 mg; vag tabs 100, 200, 500 mg; vag cream 1%, 2% SE: *Topical:* Local irritation; *PO:* N/V, ↑ LFTs Notes: PO prophylaxis immunosuppressed pts

Clotrimazole & Betamethasone (Lotrisone) Uses: *Fungal skin Infxns* Acts: Imidazole antifungal & anti-inflammatory. *Spectrum:* Tinea pedis, cruris, & corporis Dose: ≥*17 y.* Apply & massage into area bid for 2–4 wk Caution: [C, ?] Varicella Infxn CI: Children <12 y Disp: Cream 1/0.05% 15, 45 g; lotion 1/0.05% 30 mL SE: Local irritation, rash Notes: Not for diaper dermatitis or under occlusive dressings

Clozapine (Clozaril & FazaClo) BOX: Myocarditis, agranulocytosis, Szs, & orthostatic ↓ BP associated w/ clozapine; ↑ mortality in elderly w/ dementia-related psychosis Uses: *Refractory severe schizophrenia*; childhood psychosis;

obsessive-compulsive disorder (OCD), bipolar disorder **Acts:** "Atypical" TCA **Dose:** 25 mg daily-bid initial; ↑ to 300–450 mg/d over 2 wk; maintain lowest dose possible; do not D/C abruptly **Caution:** [B, +/−] Monitor for psychosis & cholinergic rebound **CI:** Uncontrolled epilepsy; comatose state; WBC <3500 cells/mm³ and ANC <2000 cells/mm³ before Rx or <3000 cells/mm³ during Rx **Disp:** Orally disintegrating tabs (ODTs) 12.5, 25, 100 mg; tabs 25, 100 mg **SE:** Sialorrhea, tachycardia, drowsiness, ↑ wgt, constipation, incontinence, rash, Szs, CNS stimulation, hyperglycemia **Notes:** Avoid activities where sudden loss of consciousness could cause harm; benign temperature ↑ may occur during the 1st 3 wk of Rx, weekly CBC mandatory 1st 6 mo, then q other wk

Cocaine [C-II] **Uses:** *Topical anesthetic for mucous membranes* **Acts:** Narcotic analgesic, local vasoconstrictor **Dose:** Lowest topical amount that provides relief; 1 mg/kg max **Caution:** [C, ?] **CI:** PRG, ocular anesthesia **Disp:** Topical soln & viscous preparations 4–10%; powder **SE:** CNS stimulation, nervousness, loss of taste/smell, chronic rhinitis, CV tox, abuse potential **Notes:** Use only on PO, laryngeal, & nasal mucosa; do not use on extensive areas of broken skin

Codeine [C-II] **Uses:** *Mild-mod pain; symptomatic relief of cough* **Acts:** Narcotic analgesic; ↓ cough reflex **Dose:** *Adults. Analgesic:* 15–20 mg PO or IM qid PRN. *Antitussive:* 10–20 mg PO q4h PRN; max 120 mg/d. *Peds. Analgesic:* 0.5–1 mg/kg/dose PO q4–6h PRN. *Antitussive:* 1–1.5 mg/kg/24 h PO ÷ q4h; max 30 mg/24 h; ↓ in renal/hepatic impair **Caution:** [C (D if prolonged use or high dose at term), +] CNS depression, Hx drug abuse, severe hepatic impair **CI:** Component sensitivity **Disp:** Tabs 15, 30, 60 mg; soln 15 mg/5 mL; Inj 15, 30 mg/mL **SE:** Drowsiness, constipation, ↓ BP **Notes:** Usually combined w/ APAP for pain or w/ agents (e.g., terpin hydrate) as an antitussive; 120 mg IM = 10 mg IM morphine

Colchicine (Colcrys) **Uses:** *Acute gouty arthritis & prevention of recurrences; familial Mediterranean fever*; primary biliary cirrhosis **Acts:** ↓ migration of leukocytes; ↓ leukocyte lactic acid production **Dose:** *Initial:* 0.6–1.2 mg PO, then 0.6 mg q1–2h until relief or GI SE develop (max 8 mg/d); do not repeat for 3 d. *Prophylaxis:* PO: 0.6 mg/d or 3–4 d/wk; ↓ renal impair **Caution:** [D, +] w/ P-glycoprotein or CYP3A4 inhib in pt w/renal or hepatic impair, ↓ dose or avoid in elderly or w/indinavir **CI:** Serious renal, GI, hepatic, or cardiac disorders; blood dyscrasias **Disp:** Tabs 0.6 mg **SE:** N/V/D, Abd pain, BM suppression, hepatotox; local Rxn w/ SQ/IM **Notes:** IV no longer available

Colesevelam (Welchol) **Uses:** *Reduction of LDL & total cholesterol alone or in combo w/ an HMG-CoA reductase inhib* **Acts:** Bile acid sequestrant **Dose:** 3 tabs PO bid or 6 tabs daily w/ meals **Caution:** [B, ?] Severe GI motility disorders; in pts w/ triglycerides >300 mg/dL (may ↑ levels); use not established in peds **CI:** Bowel obst, serum triglycerides >500; hx hypertriglyceridemia-pancreatitis **Disp:** Tabs 625 mg **SE:** Constipation, dyspepsia, myalgia, weakness **Notes:** May ↓ absorption of fat-soluble vits

Colestipol (Colestid) Uses: *Adjunct to ↓ serum cholesterol in primary hypercholesterolemia, relieve pruritus associated w/ ↑ bile acids* Acts: Binds intestinal bile acids to form insoluble complex Dose: *Granules:* 5–30 g/d ÷ 2–4 doses; tabs: 2–16 g/d ÷ daily-bid Caution: [C, ?] Avoid w/ high triglycerides, GI dysfunction CI: Bowel obst Disp: Tabs 1 g; granules 5 g/pack or scoop SE: Constipation, Abd pain, bloating, HA, GI irritation & bleeding Notes: Do not use dry powder; mix w/ beverages, cereals, etc; may ↓ absorption of other meds and fat-soluble vits

Conivaptan HCL (Vaprisol) Uses: Euvolemic & hypervolemic hyponatremia Acts: Dual arginine vasopressin V_{1A}/V_2 receptor antagonist Dose: 20 mg IV × 1 over 30 min, then 20 mg cont IV Inf over 24 h; 20 mg/d cont IV Inf for 1–3 more d; may ↑ to 40 mg/d if Na^+ not responding; 4 d max use; use large vein, change site q24h Caution: [C, ?/–] Rapid ↑ Na^+ (>12 mEq/L/24 h) may cause osmotic demyelination synd; impaired renal/hepatic Fxn; may ↑ digoxin levels; CYP3A4 inhib (Table 10 p 280) CI: Hypovolemic hyponatremia; w/ CYP3A4 inhib; anuria Disp: Amp 20 mg/4 mL SE: Inf site Rxns, HA, N/V/D, constipation, ↓ K^+, orthostatic ↓ BP, thirst, dry mouth, pyrexia, pollakiuria, polyuria, Infxn Notes: Monitor Na^+, vol and neurologic status; D/C w/ very rapid ↑ Na^+; mix only w/ 5% dextrose

Copper IUD Contraceptive (ParaGard T 380A) Uses: *Contraception, long-term (up to 10 y)* Acts: ?, interfere w/ sperm survival/transport Dose: Insert any time during menstrual cycle; replace at 10 y max Caution: [C, ?] Remove w/ intrauterine PRG, increased risk of comps w/ PRG and device in place CI: Acute PID or in high-risk behavior, postpartum endometritis, cervicitis Disp: 52 mg IUD SE: PRG, ectopic PRG, pelvic Infxn w/ or w/o immunocompromised, embedment, perforation, expulsion, Wilson Dz, fainting w/ insert, vag bleeding, expulsion Notes: Counsel pt does not protect against STD/HIV; see PI for detailed instructions; 99% effective

Cortisone, Systemic and Topical See Steroids (page 229) and Tables 2 p 265 & 3 p 266

Cromolyn Sodium (Intal, NasalCrom, Opticrom, others) Uses: *Adjunct to the Rx of asthma; prevent exercise-induced asthma; allergic rhinitis; ophthal allergic manifestations*; food allergy, systemic mastocytosis, IBD Acts: Antiasthmatic; mast cell stabilizer Dose: *Adults & Children >12 y:* Inh: 20 mg (as powder in caps) inhaled qid or metered-dose inhaler 2 puffs qid. *PO:* 200 mg qid 15–20 min ac, up to 400 mg qid. *Nasal instillation:* Spray once in each nostril 2–6 ×/d. *Ophthal:* 1–2 gtt in each eye 4–6 × d. *Peds. Inh:* 2 puffs qid of metered-dose inhaler. *PO: Infants <2 y:* (not OK) 20 mg/kg/d in 4 ÷ doses. *2–12 y:* 100 mg qid ac Caution: [B, ?] w/ Renal/hepatic impair CI: Acute asthmatic attacks Disp: PO conc 100 mg/5 mL; soln for nebulizer 20 mg/2 mL; metered-dose inhaler (contains ozone-depleting CFCs; will be gradually removed from US market); nasal soln 40 mg/mL; ophthal soln 4% SE: Unpleasant taste, hoarseness, coughing

Notes: No benefit in acute Rx; 2–4 wk for maximal effect in perennial allergic disorders

Cyanocobalamin [Vitamin B₁₂] (Nascobal) Uses: *Pernicious anemia & other vit B₁₂ deficiency states; ↑ requirements d/t PRG; thyrotoxicosis; liver or kidney Dz* **Acts:** Dietary vit B₁₂ supl **Dose:** *Adults.* 30 mcg/d × 5–10 d; 100 mcg IM or SQ daily; intranasal: 500 mcg once/wk for pts in remission, for 5–10 d, then 100 mcg IM 2 ×/wk for 1 mo, then 100 mcg IM monthly. *Peds.* Use 0.2 mcg/kg × 2 d test dose; if OK 30–50 mcg/d for 2 or more wk (total 1000 mcg) then maint: 100 mg/mo. **Caution:** [A (C if dose exceeds RDA), +] **CI:** Allergy to cobalt; hereditary optic nerve atrophy; Leber Dz **Disp:** Tabs 50, 100, 250, 500, 1000, 2500, 5000 mcg; Inj 100, 1000 mcg/mL; intranasal (Nascobal) gel 500 mcg/0.1 mL **SE:** Itching, D, HA, anxiety **Notes:** PO absorption erratic and not; ok for use w/ hyperalimentation

Cyclobenzaprine (Flexeril) Uses: *Relief of muscle spasm* **Acts:** Centrally acting skeletal muscle relaxant; reduces tonic somatic motor activity **Dose:** 5–10 mg PO bid-qid (2–3 wk max) **Caution:** [B, ?] Shares the toxic potential of the TCAs; urinary hesitancy, NAG **CI:** Do not use concomitantly or w/in 14 d of MAOIs; hyperthyroidism; heart failure; arrhythmias **Disp:** Tabs 5, 10 mg **SE:** Sedation & anticholinergic effects **Notes:** May inhibit mental alertness or physical coordination

Cyclobenzaprine, extended release (Amrix) Uses: *Muscle spasm* **Acts:** ? Centrally acting long-term muscle relaxant **Dose:** 15–30 mg PO daily 2–3 wk; 30 mg/d max **Caution:** [B, ?/–] w/ Urinary retention, NAG, w/ EtOH/CNS depressant **CI:** MAOI w/in 14 d, elderly, arrhythmias, heart block, CHF, MI recovery phase, ↑ thyroid **Disp:** Caps 15, 30 ER **SE:** Dry mouth, drowsiness, dizziness, HA, N, blurred vision, dysgeusia **Notes:** Avoid abrupt D/C w/ long-term use

Cyclopentolate, ophthalmic (Cyclogyl, Cylate) Uses: *Cycloplegia, mydriasis* **Acts:** Cycloplegic mydriatic, anticholinergic inhibits iris sphincter and ciliary body **Dose:** *Adults.* 1 gtt in eye 40–50 min preprocedure, may repeat × 1 in 5–10 min *Peds.* As adult, children 0.5%; infants use 0.5% **Caution:** [C (may cause late-term fetal anoxia/↓ HR), +/–], w/premature infants, HTN, Down synd, elderly, **CI:** NAG **Disp:** Ophthal soln 0.5, 1, 2% **SE:** Tearing, HA, irritation, eye pain, photophobia, arrhythmia, tremor, ↑ IOP, confusion **Notes:** Compress lacrimal sac for several min after dose; heavily pigmented irises may require ↑ strength; peak 25–75 min, cycloplegia 6–24 h; mydriasis up to 24 h; 2% soln may result in psychotic Rxns and behavioral disturbances in peds

Cyclopentolate with w/ Phenylephrine (Cyclomydril) Uses: *Mydriasis greater than cyclopentolate alone* **Acts:** Cycloplegic mydriatic, α-adrenergic agonist w/ anticholinergic to inhibit iris sphincter **Dose:** 1 gtt in eye q 5–10 min (max 3 doses) 40–50 min preprocedure **Caution:** [(C ([may cause late-term fetal anoxia/↓ HR), +/–] HTN, w/ elderly w/ CAD **CI:** NAG **Disp:** Ophthal soln cyclopentolate 0.2%/phenylephrine 1% (2, 5 mL) **SE:** Tearing, HA, irritation, eye pain, photophobia, arrhythmia, tremor **Notes:** Compress lacrimal sac for several min after dose; heavily pigmented irises may require ↑ strength; peak 25–75 min, cycloplegia 6–24 h, mydriasis up to 24 h

Cyclophosphamide (Cytoxan, Neosar) **Uses:** *Hodgkin Dz & NHLs; multiple myeloma; small cell lung, breast, & ovarian CAs; mycosis fungoides; neuroblastoma, retinoblastoma; acute leukemias; allogeneic & ABMT in high doses; severe rheumatologic disorders (SLE, JRA)* **Acts:** Alkylating agent **Dose:** *Adults.* (per protocol) 500–1500 mg/m²; single dose at 2- to 4-wk intervals; 1.8 g/m² to 160 mg/kg (or at 12 g/m² in 75-kg individual) in the BMT setting (per protocols). **Peds.** *SLE:* 500–750 mg/m² q mo. *JRA:* 10 mg/kg q 2 wk; ↓ w/ renal impair **Caution:** [D, ?] w/ BM suppression, hepatic Insuff **CI:** Component sensitivity **Disp:** Tabs 25, 50 mg; Inj 500 mg, 1 g, 2 g **SE:** ↓ BM; hemorrhagic cystitis, SIADH, alopecia, anorexia; N/V; hepatotox; rare interstitial pneumonitis; irreversible testicular atrophy possible; cardiotox rare; 2nd malignancies (bladder, ALL), risk 3.5% at 8 y, 10.7% at 12 y **Notes:** Hemorrhagic cystitis prophylaxis: cont bladder irrigation & MESNA uroprotection; encourage hydration, long-term bladder Ca screening

Cyclosporine (Sandimmune, Neoral, Gengraf) **BOX:** ↑ risk neoplasm, ↑ risk skin malignancies, ↑ risk HTN and nephrotox **Uses:** *Organ rejection in kidney, liver, heart, & BMT w/ steroids; RA; psoriasis* **Acts:** Immunosuppressant; reversible inhibition of immunocompetent lymphocytes **Dose:** *Adults & Peds. PO:* 15 mg/kg/d12h pretransplant; after 2 wk, taper by 5 mg/wk to 5–10 mg/kg/d. *IV:* If NPO, give 1/3 PO dose IV; ↓ in renal/hepatic impair **Caution:** [C, ?] Dose-related risk of nephrotox/hepatotox/serious fatal infections; live, attenuated vaccines may be less effective; may induce fatal malignancy; many drug interactions; ↑ risk of infections after D/C **CI:** Renal impair; uncontrolled HTN **Disp:** Caps 25, 100 mg; PO soln 100 mg/mL; Inj 50 mg/mL **SE:** May ↑ BUN & Cr & mimic transplant rejection; HTN; HA; hirsutism **Notes:** Administer in glass container; *Neoral & Sandimmune* not interchangeable; monitor BP, Cr, CBC, LFTs, interaction w/ St. John's wort; Levels: *Trough:* Just before next dose: *Therapeutic:* Variable 150–300 ng/mL RIA

Cyclosporine, ophthalmic (Restasis) **Uses:** *↑ Tear production suppressed d/t ocular inflammation* **Acts:** Immune modulator, anti-inflammatory **Dose:** 1 gtt bid each eye 12 h apart; OK w/ artificial tears, allow 15 min between **Caution:** [C, –] **CI:** Ocular Infxn, component allergy **Disp:** Single-use vial 0.05% **SE:** Ocular burning/hyperemia **Notes:** Mix vial well

Cyproheptadine (Periactin) **Uses:** *Allergic Rxns; itching* **Acts:** Phenothiazine antihistamine; serotonin antagonist **Dose:** *Adults.* 4–20 mg PO ÷ q8h; max 0.5 mg/kg/d. *Peds 2–6 y:* 2 mg bid-tid (max 12 mg/24 h). *7–14 y:* 4 mg bid-tid; ↓ in hepatic impair **Caution:** [B, ?] Elderly, CV Dz, Asthma, thyroid Dz, BPH **CI:** Neonates or <2 y; NAG; BOO; acute asthma; GI obst; w/ MAOI **Disp:** Tabs 4 mg; syrup 2 mg/5 mL **SE:** Anticholinergic, drowsiness **Notes:** May stimulate appetite

Cytarabine [ARA-C] (Cytosar-U) BOX: Administration by experienced physician in properly equipped facility; potent myelosuppressive agent Uses: *Acute leukemias, CML, NHL; IT for leukemic meningitis or prophylaxis* Acts: Antimetabolite; interferes w/ DNA synth Dose: 100–150 mg/m²/d for 5–10 d (low dose); 3 g/m² q12h for 6–12 doses (high dose); 1 mg/kg 1–2/wk (SQ maint); 5–70 mg/m² up to 3/wk IT (per protocols); ↓ in renal/hepatic impair Caution: [D, ?] in elderly, w/ marked BM suppression, ↓ dosage by ↓ the number of days of administration CI: Component sensitivity Disp: Inj 100, 500 mg, 1, 2 g, also 20, 100 mg/mL SE: ↓ BM, N/V/D, stomatitis, flu-like synd, rash on palms/soles, hepatic/cerebellar dysfunction w/ high doses, noncardiogenic pulm edema, neuropathy, fever Notes: Little use in solid tumors; high-dose tox limited by corticosteroid ophthal soln

Cytarabine Liposome (DepoCyt) BOX: Can cause chemical arachnoiditis (N/V/HA, fever) ↓ severity w/ dexamethasone. Administer by experienced physician in properly equipped facility Uses: *Lymphomatous meningitis* Acts: Antimetabolite; interferes w/ DNA synth Dose: 50 mg IT q14d for 5 doses, then 50 mg IT q28d × 4 doses; use dexamethasone prophylaxis Caution: [D, ?] May cause neurotox; blockage to CSF flow may ↑ the risk of neurotox; use in peds not established CI: Active meningeal Infxn Disp: IT Inj 50 mg/5 mL SE: Neck pain/rigidity, HA, confusion, somnolence, fever, back pain, N/V, edema, neutropenia, ↓ plt, anemia Notes: Cytarabine liposomes are similar in microscopic appearance to WBCs; caution in interpreting CSF studies

Cytomegalovirus Immune Globulin [CMV-IG IV] (CytoGam) Uses: *Prophylaxis/attenuation CMV Dz w/ transplantation* Acts: IgG antibodies to CMV Dose: 150 mg/kg/dose w/in 72 hrs of transplant and, wks 2, 4, 6, 8, and 100 mg/kg/dose wks 12, 16 post-transplant.; see PI Caution: [C, ?] Anaphylactic Rxns; renal dysfunction CI: Allergy to immunoglobulins; IgA deficiency Disp: Inj 50 mg/mL SE: Flushing, N/V, muscle cramps, wheezing, HA, fever, non-cardiogenic pulm edema, renal insuff, aseptic meningitis Notes: IV only in separate line; do not shake

Dacarbazine (DTIC) BOX: Causes hematopoietic depression, hepatic necrosis, may be carcinogenic, teratogenic Uses: *Melanoma, Hodgkin Dz, sarcoma* Acts: Alkylating agent; antimetabolite as a purine precursor; ↓ protein synth, RNA, & especially DNA Dose: 2–4.5 mg/kg/d for 10 consecutive d or 250 mg/m²/d for 5 d (per protocols); ↓ in renal impair Caution: [C, ?] In BM suppression; renal/hepatic impair CI: Component sensitivity Disp: Inj 100, 200 mg SE: ↓ BM, N/V, hepatotox, flu-like synd, ↓ BP, photosens, alopecia, facial flushing, facial paresthesias, urticaria, phlebitis at Inj site Notes: Avoid extrav, ✓ CBC, plt

Daclizumab (Zenapax) BOX: Administer under skilled supervision in equipped facility Uses: *Prevent acute organ rejection* Acts: IL-2 receptor antagonist Dose: 1 mg/kg/dose IV; 1st dose pretransplant, then 1 mg/kg q 14d × 4 doses Caution: [C, ?] CI: Component sensitivity Disp: Inj 5 mg/mL SE: Hyperglycemia, edema, HTN, ↓ BP, constipation, HA, dizziness, anxiety, nephrotox, pulm edema, pain, anaphylaxis/hypersens Notes: Administer w/in 4 h of prep

Dactinomycin (Cosmegen) **BOX:** Administer under skilled supervision in equipped facility; powder and soln toxic, corrosive, mutagenic, carcinogenic, and teratogenic; avoid exposure and use precautions **Uses:** *Choriocarcinoma, Wilms tumor, Kaposi and Ewing sarcomas, rhabdomyosarcoma, uterine and testicular CA* **Acts:** DNA-intercalating agent **Dose:** *Adults.* 0.5 mg/d for 5 d; 2 mg/wk for 3 consecutive wk; 15 mcg/kg or 0.45 mg/m^2/d (max 0.5 mg) for 5 d q3–8wk *Peds.* Sarcoma (per protocols); ↓ in renal impair **Caution:** [C, ?] **CI:** Concurrent/recent chickenpox or herpes zoster; infants <6 mo **Disp:** Inj 0.5 mg **SE:** Myelo-/immuno-suppression, severe N/V/D, alopecia, acne, hyperpigmentation, radiation recall phenomenon, tissue damage w/ extrav, hepatotox **Notes:** Classified as antibiotic but not used as antimicrobial

Dalteparin (Fragmin) **BOX:** ↑ Risk of spinal/epidural hematoma w/LP **Uses:** *Unstable angina, non–Q-wave MI, prevent & Rx DVT following surgery (hip, Abd), pt w/ restricted mobility, extended therapy Rx for PE DVT in CA pt* **Acts:** LMW heparin **Dose:** *Angina/MI:* 120 units/kg (max 10,000 units) SQ q12h w/ ASA. *DVT prophylaxis:* 2500–5000 units SQ 1–2 h pre-op, then daily for 5–10 d. *Systemic anticoagulation:* 200 units/kg/d SQ or 100 units/kg bid SQ. *CA:* 200 Int Units/kg (max 18,000 Int Units) SQ q24h × 30 d, mo 2–6 150 Int Units/kg SQ q24h (max 18,000 Int Units) **Caution:** [B, ?] In renal/hepatic impair, active hemorrhage, cerebrovascular Dz, cerebral aneurysm, severe HTN **CI:** HIT; pork product allergy; w/ mifepristone **Disp:** Inj 2500 units (16 mg/0.2 mL), 5000 units (32 mg/0.2 mL), 7500 units (48 mg/0.3 mL), 10,000 units (64 mg/mL), 25,000 units/mL (3.8 mL); prefilled vials 10,000 units/mL (9.5 mL) **SE:** Bleeding, pain at site, ↓ plt **Notes:** Predictable effects eliminates lab monitoring; not for IM/IV use

Dantrolene (Dantrium) **BOX:** Hepatotox reported; D/C after 45 d if no benefit observed **Uses:** *Rx spasticity d/t upper motor neuron disorders (e.g., spinal cord injuries, stroke, CP, MS); malignant hyperthermia* **Acts:** Skeletal muscle relaxant **Dose:** *Adults.* Spasticity: 25 mg PO daily; ↑ 25 mg to effect to 100 mg max PO qid PRN. *Peds.* 0.5 mg/kg/dose bid; ↑ by 0.5 mg/kg to effect, to 3 mg/kg/dose max qid PRN. *Adults & Peds.* Malignant hyperthermia: *Rx:* Cont rapid IV, start 1 mg/kg until Sxs subside or 10 mg/kg is reached. *Post-crisis follow-up:* 4–8 mg/kg/d in 3–4 ÷ doses for 1–3 d to prevent recurrence **Caution:** [C, ?] Impaired cardiac/pulm/hepatic Fxn **CI:** Active hepatic Dz; where spasticity needed to maintain posture or balance **Disp:** Caps 25, 50, 100 mg; powder for Inj 20 mg/vial **SE:** Hepatotox, ↑ LFTs, drowsiness, dizziness, rash, muscle weakness, D/N/V, pleural effusion w/ pericarditis, D, blurred vision, hep, photosens **Notes:** Monitor LFTs; avoid sunlight/EtOH/CNS depressants

Dapsone, oral **Uses:** *Rx & prevent PCP; toxoplasmosis prophylaxis; leprosy* **Acts:** Unknown; bactericidal **Dose:** *Adults.* PCP prophylaxis 50–100 mg/d PO; Rx PCP 100 mg/d PO w/ TMP 15–20 mg/kg/d for 21 d. *Peds. PCP prophylaxis alternated dose:* (>1 mo) 4 mg/kg/dose once/wk (max 200 mg); prophylaxis of PCP 1–2 mg/kg/24 h PO daily; max 100 mg/d **Caution:** [C, +] G6PD deficiency;

severe anemia **CI:** Component sensitivity **Disp:** Tabs 25, 100 mg **SE:** Hemolysis, methemoglobinemia, agranulocytosis, rash, cholestatic jaundice **Notes:** Absorption ↑ by an acidic environment; for leprosy, combine w/ rifampin & other agents

Dapsone, topical (Aczone) **Uses:** *Topical for acne vulgaris* **Acts:** Unknown; bactericidal **Dose:** Apply pea-size amount and rub into areas bid; wash hands after **Caution:** [C, +] G6PD deficiency; severe anemia **CI:** Component sensitivity **Disp:** 5% gel **SE:** Skin oiliness/peeling, dryness erythema **Notes:** Not for oral, ophthal, or intravag use; check G6PD levels before use; follow CBC if G6PD deficient

Daptomycin (Cubicin) **Uses:** *Complicated skin/skin structure Infxns d/t gram(+) organisms* S. aureus, bacteremia, MRSA endocarditis **Acts:** Cyclic lipopeptide; rapid membrane depolarization & bacterial death. *Spectrum:* S. aureus (including MRSA), S. pyogenes, S. agalactiae, S. dysgalactiae subsp Equisimilis, & E. faecalis (vancomycin-susceptible strains only) **Dose:** *Skin:* 4 mg/kg IV daily × 7–14 d (over 30 min); *Bacteremia & Endocarditis:* 6 mg/kg q48h; ↓ w/ CrCl <30 mL/min or dialysis: q48h **Caution:** [B, ?] w/ HMG-CoA inhib **Disp:** Inj 250, 500 mg/10 mL **SE:** Anemia, constipation, N/V/D, HA, rash, site Rxn, muscle pain/ weakness, edema, cellulitis, hypo-/hyperglycemia, ↑ alkaline phosphatase, cough, back pain, Abd pain, ↓ K⁺, anxiety, chest pain, sore throat, cardiac failure, confusion, *Candida* Infxns **Notes:** ✓ CPK baseline & weekly; consider D/C HMG-CoA reductase inhib to ↓ myopathy risk; not for Rx PNA

Darbepoetin Alfa (Aranesp) **BOX:** Associated w/ ↑ CV, thromboembolic events and/or mortality; D/C if Hgb >12 g/dL; may increase tumor progression and death in cancer CA pts **Uses:** *Anemia associated w/ CRF*, anemia in nonmyeloid malignancy w/ concurrent chemotherapy **Acts:** ↑ Erythropoiesis, recombinant erythropoietin variant **Dose:** 0.45 mcg/kg single IV or SQ q wk; titrate, do not exceed target Hgb of 12 g/dL; use lowest doses possible, see PI to convert from *Epogen* **Caution:** [C, ?] May ↑ risk of CV &/or neurologic SE in renal failure; HTN; w/ Hx Szs **CI:** Uncontrolled HTN, component allergy **Disp:** 25, 40, 60, 100, 200, 300 mcg/ mL, 150 mcg/0.075 mL in polysorbate or albumin excipient **SE:** May ↑ cardiac risk, CP, hypo-/hypertension, N/V/D, myalgia, arthralgia, dizziness, edema, fatigue, fever, ↑ risk Infxn **Notes:** Longer 1/2-life than *Epogen*; weekly CBC until stable

Darifenacin (Enablex) **Uses:** *OAB* Urinary antispasmodic **Acts:** Muscarinic receptor antagonist **Dose:** 7.5 mg/d PO; 15 mg/d max (7.5 mg/d w/ mod hepatic impair or w/ CYP3A4 inhib); w/ drugs metabolized by CYP2D (Table 10 p 280); swallow whole **Caution:** [C, ?/–] w/ Hepatic impair **CI:** Urinary/gastric retention, uncontrolled NAG, paralytic ileus **Disp:** Tabs ER 7.5, 15 mg **SE:** Xerostomia/eyes, constipation, dyspepsia, Abd pain, retention, abnormal vision, dizziness, asthenia

Darunavir (Prezista) **Uses:** *Rx HIV w/ resistance to multiple protease inhib* **Acts:** HIV-1 protease inhib **Dose:** 600 mg PO bid, administer w/ ritonavir 100 mg bid; w/ food **Caution:** [B, ?/–] Hx Sulfa allergy, CYP3A4 substrate, changes levels of many meds (↑ amiodarone, ↑ dihydropyridine, ↑ HMG-CoA reductase inhib [statins], ↓ SSRIs, ↓ rifampin, ↓ methadone); do not use w/salmeterol, colchicine (w/renal/hepatic failure); adjust dose w/ bosentan, tadalafil for PAH **CI:** w/ Astemizole, terfenadine, dihydroergotamine, ergonovine, ergotamine, methylergonovine, pimozide, midazolam, triazolam, alpha 1-adrenoreceptor antagonist (alfuzosin), PDE5 Inhibitor sildenafil **Supplied:** Tabs 300 mg **SE:** ↑ glucose, cholesterol, triglycerides, central redistribution of fat (metabolic synd), N, ↓ neutrophils & ↑ amylase

Dasatinib (Sprycel) Uses: CML, Ph + ALL Acts: Multi-TKI Dose: 100–140 mg PO day; adjust w/ CYP3A4 inhib/inducers (Table 10 p 280) **Caution:** [D, ?/–] **CI:** None **Disp:** Tabs 20, 50, 70, 100 mg **SE:** ↓ BM, edema, fluid retention, pleural effusions, N/V/D, Abd pain, bleeding, fever, ↑ QT **Notes:** Replace K, Mg before Rx

Daunorubicin (Daunomycin, Cerubidine) **BOX:** Cardiac Fxn should be monitored d/t potential risk for cardiac tox & CHF, renal/hepatic dysfunction Uses: *Acute leukemias* Acts: DNA-intercalating agent; ↓ topoisomerase II; generates oxygen free radicals **Dose:** 45–60 mg/m²/d for 3 consecutive d; 25 mg/m²/wk (per protocols); ↓ w/renal/hepatic impair **Caution:** [D, ?] **CI:** Component sens **Disp:** Inj 20, 50 mg **SE:** ↓ BM, mucositis, N/V, orange urine, alopecia, radiation recall phenomenon, hepatotox (↑ bili), tissue necrosis w/ extrav, cardiotox (1–2% CHF w/ 550 mg/m² cumulative dose) **Notes:** Prevent cardiotox w/ dexrazoxane (w/>300 mg/m² daunorubicin cum dose);IV use only; allopurinol prior to ↓ hyperuricemia

Decitabine (Dacogen) Uses: *MDS* Acts: Inhibits DNA methyltransferase **Dose:** 15 mg/m² cont Inf over 3 h; repeat q8h × 3 d; repeat cycle q6wk, min 4 cycles; delay Tx and ↓ dose if inadequate hematologic recovery at 6 wk (see PI); delay Tx w/ Cr >2 mg/dL or bili >2× ULN **Caution:** [D, ?/–]; avoid PRG; males should not father a child during or 2 mo after; renal/hepatic impair **Disp:** Powder 50 mg/vial **SE:** ↓ WBC, ↓ HgB, ↓ plt, febrile neutropenia, edema, petechiae, N/V/D, constipation, stomatitis, dyspepsia, cough, fever, fatigue, ↑ LFTs/bili, hyperglycemia, Infxn, HA **Notes:** ✓ CBC & plt before cycle and prn; premedicate w/ antiemetic

Deferasirox (Exjade) Uses: *Chronic iron overload d/t transfusion in pts >2 y* Acts: Oral iron chelator **Dose:** 20 mg/kg PO/d; adjust by 5–10 mg/kg q3–6mo based on monthly ferritin; 30 mg/kg/d max; on empty stomach 30 min ac; hold dose w/ferritin <500 mcg/L; dissolve in water/, orange/apple juice (<1 g/3.5 oz; >1 g in 7 oz) drink immediately; resuspend residue and swallow; do not chew, swallow whole tabs or take w/ Al-containing antacids **Caution:** [B, ?/–] elderly, renal impair, heme disorders; ↑ MDS in pt 60 yrs **Disp:** Tabs for oral susp 125, 250, 500 mg **SE:** N/V/D, Abd pain, skin rash, HA, fever, cough, ↑ Cr & LFTs, Infxn, hearing loss, dizziness, cataracts, retinal disorders, ↑ IOP **Notes:** ARF, cytopenias possible; ✓ Cr weekly 1st mo then q mo, ✓ CBC, urine protein, LFTs; do not use w/ other iron-chelator therapies; dose to nearest whole tab; initial auditory/ophthal testing and q12mo

Degarelix (Firmagon) Uses:* Advanced PCa* Action: Reversible LHRH antagonist, ↓ LH and testosterone w/o flare seen w/ LHRH agonists (transient ↑ in testosterone Dose: Initial 240 mg SQ in two 120 mg doses (40 mg/mL); maint 80 mg SQ (20 mg/mL) Q28d Caution: [not for women] CI: Women Supplied: Inj vial 120 mg (initial); 80 mg (maint)SE: inj site Rxns, hot flashes, ↑ wgt, ↑ serum GGT Notes: Requires 2 inj initial (volume); 44% testosterone castrate (< 50 ng/dL) at day 1, 96% day 3

Delavirdine (Rescriptor) Uses: *HIV Infxn* Acts: Nonnucleoside RT inhib Dose: 400 mg PO tid Caution: [C, ?] CDC rec: HIV-infected others not breast-feed (transmission risk); w/ renal/hepatic impair CI: w/ drugs dependent on CYP3A (Table 10 p 280) Disp: Tabs 100, 200 mg SE: Fat redistribution, immune reconstitution synd, HA, fatigue, rash, ↑ transaminases, N/V/D Notes: Avoid antacids; ↓ cytochrome P-450 enzymes; numerous drug interactions; monitor LFTs

Demeclocycline (Declomycin) Uses: *SIADH* Acts: Antibiotic, antagonizes ADH action on renal tubules Dose: 300–600 mg PO q12h on empty stomach; ↓ in renal failure; avoid antacids Caution: [D, +] Avoid in hepatic/renal impair & children CI: Tetracycline allergy Disp: Tabs 150, 300 mg SE: D, Abd cramps, photosens, DI Notes: Avoid sunlight; numerous drug interactions; not for peds <8 y

Desipramine (Norpramin) BOX: Closely monitor for worsening depression or emergence of suicidality Uses: *Endogenous depression*, chronic pain, peripheral neuropathy Acts: TCA; ↑ synaptic serotonin or norepinephrine in CNS Dose: *Adults.* 100–200 mg/d single or ÷ dose; usually single hs dose (max 300 mg/d) *Peds 6–12 y:* 1–3 mg/kg/d ÷ dose, 5 mg/kg/d max; ↓ dose in elderly Caution: [C, ?/–] CV Dz, Sz disorder, hypothyroidism, elderly, liver impair CI: MAOIs w/in 14 d; during AMI recovery phase Disp: Tabs 10, 25, 50, 75, 100, 150 mg; caps 25, 50 mg SE: Anticholinergic (blurred vision, urinary retention, xerostomia); orthostatic ↓ BP; ↑ QT, arrhythmias Notes: Numerous drug interactions; blue-green urine; avoid sunlight

Desloratadine (Clarinex) Uses: *Seasonal & perennial allergic rhinitis; chronic idiopathic urticaria* Acts: Active metabolite of Claritin, H₁-antihistamine, blocks inflammatory mediators Dose: *Adults & Peds >12 y:* 5 mg PO daily; 5 mg PO q other day w/ hepatic/renal impair Caution: [C, ?/–] RediTabs contain phenylalanine Disp: Tabs & RediTabs (rapid dissolving) 5 mg, syrup 0.5 mg/mL SE: Allergy, anaphylaxis, somnolence, HA, dizziness, fatigue, pharyngitis, xerostomia, N, dyspepsia, myalgia

Desmopressin (DDAVP, Stimate) BOX: Not for hemophilia B or w/ factor VIII antibody; not for hemophilia A w/ factor VIII levels <5% Uses: *DI (intranasal & parenteral); bleeding d/t uremia, hemophilia A & type I von Willebrand Dz (parenteral); nocturnal enuresis* Acts: Synthetic analog of vasopressin (human ADH); ↑ factor VIII Dose: *DI: Intranasal: Adults.* 0.1–0.4 mL (10–40 mcg/d in 1–3 ÷ doses). *Peds 3 mo–12 y:* 0.05–0.3 mL/d in 1 or 2 doses. *Parenteral: Adults.* 0.5–1 mL (2–4 mcg/d in 2 ÷ doses); converting from nasal to parenteral, use 1/10 nasal dose. *PO: Adults.* 0.05 mg bid; ↑ to max of 1.2 mg. *Hemophilia A & von Willebrand Dz (type I): Adults & Peds >10 kg:* 0.3 mcg/kg in 50 mL NS, Inf over 15–30 min. *Peds <10 kg:* As above w/ dilution to 10 mL w/ NS. *Nocturnal enuresis: Peds >6 y:* 20 mcg intranasally hs **Caution:** [B, M] Avoid overhydration **CI:** Hemophilia B; CrCl <50 mL/min, severe classic von Willebrand Dz; pts w/ factor VIII antibodies; hyponatremia **Disp:** Tabs 0.1, 0.2 mg; Inj 4, 15 mcg/mL; nasal soln 0.1, 1.5 mg/mL **SE:** Facial flushing, HA, dizziness, vulval pain, nasal congestion, pain at Inj site, ↓ Na⁺, H₂O intoxication **Notes:** In very young & old pts, ↓ fluid intake to avoid H₂O intoxication & ↓ Na⁺

Desvenlafaxine (Pristiq) **BOX:** Monitor for worsening or emergence of suicidality, particularly in peds, adolescent, and young adult pts **Uses:** *Major depressive disorder* **Acts:** Selective serotonin and norepinephrine reuptake inhib **Dose:** 50 mg PO daily, ↓ w/ renal impair **Caution:** [C, ±/M] **CI:** Hypersens, MAOI w/ or w/in 14 d of stopping MAOI **Disp:** Tabs 50, 100 mg **SE:** N, dizziness, insomnia, hyperhidrosis, constipation, somnolence, decreased appetite, anxiety, and specific male sexual Fxn disorders **Notes:** Tabs should be taken whole, allow 7 d after stopping before starting an MAOI

Dexamethasone, nasal (Dexacort Phosphate Turbinaire) **Uses:** *Chronic nasal inflammation or allergic rhinitis* **Acts:** Anti-inflammatory corticosteroid **Dose:** *Adults & Peds >12 y:* 2 sprays/nostril bid–tid, max 12 sprays/d. *Peds 6–12 y:* 1–2 sprays/nostril bid, max 8 sprays/d **Caution:** [C, ?] **CI:** Untreated Infxn **Disp:** Aerosol, 84 mcg/activation **SE:** Local irritation

Dexamethasone, Ophthalmic (AK-Dex Ophthalmic, Decadron Ophthalmic) **Uses:** *Inflammatory or allergic conjunctivitis* **Acts:** Anti-inflammatory corticosteroid **Dose:** Instill 1–2 gtt tid–qid **Caution:** [C, ?/–] **CI:** Active untreated bacterial, viral, & fungal eye infxns **Disp:** Susp & soln 0.1%; oint 0.05% **SE:** Long-term use associated w/ cataracts

Dexamethasone, Systemic, Topical (Decadron) See Steroids, Systemic, page 229, & Tables 2 p 265 & 3 p 266.

Dexlansoprazole (Dexilant, Kapidex) **Uses:** *Heal and maint of erosive esophagitis (EE), GERD* **Acts:** Proton pump inhib, delayed release **Dose:** EE: 60 mg QD up to 8 wks; maint healed EE: 30 mg QD up to 6 mos; GERD 30 mg/ QD × 4 wks; ↓ w/ hepatic impair **Caution:** [B, +/–] do not use w/ atazanavir or drugs w/pH based absorption (e.g., ampicillin, iron salts, ketoconazole); may alter warfarin and tacrolimus levels **CI:** Component hypersensitivity **Disp:** Caps 30,60 mg **SE:** N/V/D, flatulence, abd pain, URI **Notes:** w or w/o food; take whole or sprinkle on tsp applesauce; clinical response does not r/o gastric malignancy; see also lansoprazole; ? ↑ risk of fractures w/ all PPI

Dexpanthenol (Ilopan-Choline, oral, Ilopan) **Uses:** *Minimize paralytic ileus, Rx post-op distention* **Acts:** Cholinergic agent **Dose:** *Adults. Relief of gas:* 2–3 tabs PO tid. *Prevent post-op ileus:* 250–500 mg IM stat, repeat in 2 h, then q6h PRN. *Ileus:* 500 mg IM stat, repeat in 2 h, then q6h, PRN **Caution:** [C, ?]

CI: Hemophilia, mechanical bowel obst **Disp:** Inj 250 mg/mL; tabs 50 mg; cream 2% **SE:** GI cramps

Dexrazoxane (Zinecard, Totect) **Uses:** *Prevent anthracycline-induced (e.g., doxorubicin) cardiomyopathy (Zinecard), extrav of anthracycline chemotherapy (Totect)* **Acts:** Chelates heavy metals; binds intracellular iron & prevents anthracycline-induced free radicals **Dose:** *Systemic(cardiomyopathy, Zinecard):* 10:1 ratio dexrazoxane: doxorubicin 30 min before each dose, 5:1 ratio w/ CrCl <40 mL/min. *Extrav (Totect):* IV Inf over 1–2 h q day × 3 d, w/in 6 h of extrav. *Day 1:* 1000 mg/m² (max 2000 mg); *Day 2:* 1000 mg/m² (max 2000 mg); *Day 3:* 500 mg/m² (max: 1000 mg); w/ CrCl <40 mL/min, ↓ dose by 50% **Caution:** [D, –] **CI:** Component sensitivity **Disp:** Inj powder 250, 500 mg (10 mg/mL) **SE:** ↓ BM, fever, Infxn, stomatitis, alopecia, N/V/D; ↑ LFTs, Inj site pain

Dextran 40 (Gentran 40, Rheomacrodex) **Uses:** *Shock, prophylaxis of DVT & thromboembolism, adjunct in peripheral vascular surgery* **Acts:** Expands plasma vol; ↓ blood viscosity **Dose:** *Shock:* 10 mL/kg Inf rapidly; 20 mL/kg max 1st 24 h; beyond 24 h 10 mL/kg max; D/C after 5 d. *Prophylaxis of DVT & thromboembolism:* 10 mL/kg IV day of surgery, then 500 mL/d IV for 2–3 d, then 500 mL IV q2–3d based on risk for up to 2 wk **Caution:** [C, ?] Inf Rxns; w/ corticosteroids **CI:** Major hemostatic defects; cardiac decompensation; renal Dz w/ severe oliguria/anuria **Disp:** 10% dextran 40 in 0.9% NaCl or 5% dextrose **SE:** Allergy/anaphylactoid Rxn (observe during 1st min of Inf), arthralgia, cutaneous Rxns, ↓ BP, fever **Notes:** Monitor Cr & lytes; keep well hydrated

Dextromethorphan (Benylin DM, Delsym, Mediquell, PediaCare 1, others) [OTC] **Uses:** *Control nonproductive cough* **Acts:** Suppresses medullary cough center **Dose:** *Adults.* 10–30 mg PO q4h PRN (max 120 mg/24 h). *Peds 2–6 y:* 2.5–7.5 mg q4–8h (max 30 mg/24 h). *7–12 y:* 5–10 mg q4–8h (max 60 mg/24 h) **Caution:** [C, ?/–] Not for persistent or chronic cough **CI:** <2 y **Disp:** Caps 30 mg; lozenges 2.5, 5, 7.5, 15 mg; syrup 15 mg/15 mL, 10 mg/5 mL; liq 10 mg/15 mL, 3.5, 7.5, 15 mg/5 mL; sustained-action liq 30 mg/5 mL **SE:** GI disturbances **Notes:** Found in combo OTC products w/ guaifenesin; deaths reported in pts <2 y; abuse potential; efficacy in children debated; do not use w/in 14 d of D/C MAOI

Diazepam (Valium, Diastat) [C-IV] **Uses:** *Anxiety, EtOH withdrawal, muscle spasm, status epilepticus, panic disorders, amnesia, pre-op sedation* **Acts:** Benzodiazepine **Dose:** *Status epilepticus:* 5–10 mg q10–20min to 30 mg max in 8-h period. *Anxiety, muscle spasm:* 2–10 mg PO bid-qid or IM/IV q3–4h PRN. *Pre-op:* 5–10 mg PO or IM 20–30 min or IV just prior to procedure. *EtOH withdrawal:* Initial 2–5 mg IV, then 5–10 mg q5–10min, 100 mg in 1 h max. May require up to 1000 mg/24 h for severe withdrawal; titrate to agitation; avoid excessive sedation; may lead to aspiration or resp arrest. *Peds. Status epilepticus:* **<5 y:** 0.05–0.3 mg/kg/dose IV q15–30min up to a max of 5 mg. *>5 y:* to max of 10 mg. *Sedation, muscle relaxation:* 0.04–0.3 mg/kg/dose q2–4h IM or IV to max of 0.6 mg/kg in 8 h, or 0.12–0.8 mg/kg/24 h PO ÷ tid-qid; ↓ w/ hepatic impair

Caution: [D, ?/–] **CI:** Coma, CNS depression, resp depression, NAG, severe uncontrolled pain, PRG **Disp:** Tabs 2, 5, 10 mg; soln 1, 5 mg/mL; Inj 5 mg/mL; rectal gel 2.5, 5, 10, 20 mg/mL **SE:** Sedation, amnesia, ↓ HR, ↓ BP, rash, ↓ resp rate **Notes:** 5 mg/min IV max in adults or 1–2 mg/min in peds (resp arrest possible); IM absorption erratic; avoid abrupt D/C

Diazoxide (Proglycem) **Uses:** *Hypoglycemia d/t hyperinsulinism (Proglycem); hypertensive crisis (Hyperstat)* **Acts:** ↓ Pancreatic insulin release; antihypertensive **Dose:** Repeat in 5–15 min until BP controlled; repeat q4–24h; monitor BP closely. *Hypoglycemia: Adults & Peds.* 3–8 mg/kg/24 h PO ÷ q8–12h. *Neonates.* 8–15 mg/kg/24 h ÷ in 3 equal doses; maint 8–10 mg/kg/24 h PO in 2–3 equal doses **Caution:** [C, ?] ↓ Effect w/ phenytoin; ↑ effect w/ diuretics, warfarin **CI:** Allergy to thiazides or other sulfonamide-containing products; HTN associated w/ aortic coarctation, AV shunt, or pheochromocytoma **Disp:** Caps 50 mg; PO susp 50 mg/mL; IV 15 mg/mL **SE:** Hyperglycemia, ↓ BP, dizziness, Na$^+$ & H$_2$O retention, N/V, weakness **Notes:** Can give false(–)-negative insulin response to glucagons; Rx extrav w/ warm compress

Dibucaine (Nupercainal) **Uses:** *Hemorrhoids & minor skin conditions* **Acts:** Topical anesthetic **Dose:** Insert PR w/ applicator bid & after each bowel movement; apply sparingly to skin **Caution:** [C, ?] topical use only **CI:** Component sensitivity **Disp:** 1% oint w/ rectal applicator; 0.5% cream **SE:** Local irritation, rash

Diclofenac (Arthrotec, Cataflam, Flector, Flector Patch, Voltaren, Voltaren XR, Voltaren gel) **BOX:** May ↑ risk of CV events & GI bleeding; CI in post-op CABG **Uses:** *Arthritis & pain, oral and topical, actinic keratosis* **Acts:** NSAID **Dose:** 50–75 mg PO bid; w/ food or milk; 1 patch to painful area bid. Topical gel upper extremity 2 g qid (max 8 g/d); lower extremity 4 g qid (max 16 g/d) **Caution:** [C, ?] CHF, HTN, renal/hepatic dysfunction, & Hx PUD, asthma **CI:** NSAID/aspirin ASA allergy; porphyria; following CABG **Disp:** Tabs 50 mg; tabs DR 25, 50, 75, 100 mg; XR tabs 100 mg; *Flector Patch: 1.3%* 10 × 14 cm, gel 1% **SE:** *Oral:* Abd cramps, heartburn, GI ulceration, rash, interstitial nephritis; *patch/gel:* pruritus, dermatitis, burning, N, HA **Notes:** Do not crush tabs; watch for GI bleed; do not apply patch/gel to damaged skin or while bathing; ✓ CBC, LFTs periodically

Diclofenac, ophthalmic (Voltaren ophthalmic) **Uses:** *Inflammation postcataract or pain/photophobia post corneal refractive surgery* * **Acts:** NSAID **Dose:** *Post-op cataract:* 1 gtt qid, start 24 h post-op× 2 wk. *Post-op refractive:* 1–2 gtt w/in 1 h preop- and w/in 15 min post-op then qid up to 3 d **Caution:** [C, ?] May ↑ bleed risk in ocular tissues **CI:** NSAID/ASA allergy **Disp:** ophthal soln 0.1% 2.5-, 5 -mL bottle **SE:** Burning/stinging/itching, keratitis, ↑ IOP, lacrimation, abnormal vision, conjunctivitis, lid swelling, discharge, iritis

Dicloxacillin (Dynapen, Dycill) **Uses:** *Rx of pneumonia, skin, & soft-tissue infxns, & osteomyelitis caused by penicillinase-producing staphylococci* **Acts:** Bactericidal; ↓ cell wall synth. *Spectrum: S. aureus & Streptococcus* **Dose:**

Adults. 150–500 mg qid (2 g/d max) *Peds <40 kg:* 12.5–100 mg/kg/d ÷ qid; take on empty stomach **Caution:** [B, ?] **CI:** Component or PCN sensitivity **Disp:** Caps 125, 250, 500 mg; soln 62.5 mg/5 mL **SE:** N/D, Abd pain **Notes:** Monitor PTT if pt on warfarin

Dicyclomine (Bentyl) Uses: *Functional IBS* **Acts:** Smooth-muscle relaxant **Dose:** *Adults.* 20 mg PO qid; ↑ to 160 mg/d max or 20 mg IM q6h, 80 mg/d ÷ qid then ↑ to 160 mg/d, max 2 wk *Peds Infants >6 mo:* 5 mg/dose tid-qid. *Children:* 10 mg/dose tid-qid **Caution:** [B, −] **CI:** Infants <6 mo, NAG, MyG, severe UC, BOO, GI obst, reflux esophagitis **Disp:** Caps 10, 20 mg; tabs 20 mg; syrup 10 mg/5 mL; Inj 10 mg/mL **SE:** Anticholinergic SEs may limit dose **Notes:** Take 30–60 min ac; avoid EtOH, do not administer IV

Didanosine [ddl] (Videx) **BOX:** Allergy manifested as fever, rash, fatigue, GI/resp Sxs reported; stop drug immediately & do not rechallenge; lactic acidosis & hepatomegaly/steatosis reported Uses: *HIV Infxn* in zidovudine-intolerant pts* **Acts:** NRTI **Dose:** *Adults. >60 kg:* 400 mg/d PO or 200 mg PO bid. *<60 kg:* 250 mg/d PO or 125 mg PO bid; adults should take 2 tabs/administration. *Peds 2 wk–8 mo:* 100 mg/m². *>8 mo:* 120 mg/m² PO bid; on empty stomach; ↓ w/ renal impair **Caution:** [B, −] CDC rec: HIV-infected mothers not breast-feed **CI:** Component sensitivity **Disp:** Chew tabs 25, 50, 100, 150, 200 mg; powder packets 100, 167, 250, 375 mg; powder for soln 2, 4 g **SE:** Pancreatitis, peripheral neuropathy, D, HA **Notes:** Do not take w/ meals; thoroughly chew tabs, do not mix w/ fruit juice or acidic beverages; reconstitute powder w/ H₂O, many drug interactions

Diflunisal (Dolobid) **BOX:** May ↑ risk of CV events & GI bleeding; CI in post-op CABG Uses: *Mild–mod pain;* OA* **Acts:** NSAID **Dose:** *Pain:* 500 mg PO bid. *OA:* 500–1500 mg PO in 2–3 ÷ doses; ↓ in renal impair, take w/ food/milk **Caution:** [C (D 3rd tri or near delivery), ?] CHF, HTN, renal/hepatic dysfunction, & Hx PUD **CI:** Allergy to NSAIDs or ASA, active GI bleed, post-CABG **Disp:** Tabs 250, 500 mg **SE:** May ↑ bleeding time; HA, Abd cramps, heartburn, GI ulceration, rash, interstitial nephritis, fluid retention

Digoxin (Lanoxin, Lanoxicaps, Digitek) Uses: *CHF, AF & A flutter, & PAT* **Acts:** Positive inotrope; ↑ AV node refractory period **Dose:** *Adults. PO digitalization:* 0.5–0.75 mg PO, then 0.25 mg PO q6–8h to total 1–1.5 mg. *IV or IM digitalization:* 0.25–0.5 mg IM or IV, then 0.25 mg q4–6h to total 0.125–0.5 mg/d PO, IM, or IV (average daily dose 0.125–0.25 mg). *Peds. Preterm infants: Digitalization:* 30 mcg/kg PO or 25 mcg/kg IV; give 1/2 of dose initial, then 1/4 of dose at 8–12-h intervals for 2 doses. *Maint:* 5–7.5 mcg/kg/24 h PO or 4–6 mcg/kg/24 h IV ÷ q12h. *Term infants: Digitalization:* 25–35 mcg/kg PO or 20–30 mcg/kg IV; give 1/2 the initial dose, then 1/3 of dose at 8–12 h. *Maint:* 6–10 mcg/kg/24 h PO or 5–8 mcg/kg/24 h ÷ q12h. *1 mo–2 y: Digitalization:* 35–60 mcg/kg PO or 30–50 mcg/kg IV; give 1/2 the initial dose, then 1/3 dose at 8–12-h intervals for 2 doses. *Maint:* 10–15 mcg/kg/24 h PO or 7.5–15 mcg/kg/24 h IV ÷ q12h. *2–10 y: Digitalization:* 30–40 mcg/kg PO or 25 mcg/kg IV; give 1/2 initial dose, then 1/3 of the dose at 8–12-h intervals for 2 doses. *Maint:* 8–10 mcg/kg/24 h PO or 6–8 mcg/kg/24 h IV ÷ q12h. *7–10 y:* Same as for adults; ↓ in renal impair **Caution:** [C, +] w/ ↓ K^+, Mg^{2+}, renal failure **CI:** AV block; idiopathic hypertrophic subaortic stenosis; constrictive pericarditis; cardiac arrhythmias **Disp:** Caps 0.05, 0.1, 0.2 mg; tabs 0.125, 0.25, 0.5 mg; elixir 0.05 mg/mL; Inj 0.1, 0.25 mg/mL **SE:** Can cause heart block; ↓ K^+ potentiates tox; N/V, HA, fatigue, visual disturbances (yellow-green halos around lights); cardiac arrhythmias **Notes:** Multiple drug interactions; IM Inj painful, has erratic absorption & should not be used. *Levels: Trough:* Just before next dose: *Therapeutic:* 0.8–2 ng/mL; *Toxic:* >2 ng/mL; *1/2Half-life:* 36 h

Digoxin Immune Fab (Digibind, DigiFab) Uses: *Life-threatening digoxin intoxication* **Acts:** Antigen-binding fragments bind & inactivate digoxin **Dose:** *Adults & Peds.* Based on serum level & pt's wgt; see charts provided w/ drug **Caution:** [C, ?] **CI:** Sheep product allergy **Disp:** Inj 38 mg/vial **SE:** Worsening of cardiac output or CHF, ↓ K^+, facial swelling, & redness **Notes:** Each vial binds ~ 0.6 mg of digoxin; renal failure may require redosing in several days

Diltiazem (Cardizem, Cardizem CD, Cardizem LA, Cardizem SR, Cartia XT, Dilacor XR, Diltia XT, Taztia XT, Tiamate, Tiazac) Uses: *Angina, prevention of reinfarction, HTN, AF or A flutter, & PAT* **Acts:** CCB **Dose:** *Stable angina PO:* Initial, 30 mg PO qid; ↑ to 180–360 mg/d in 3–4 ÷ doses PRN; XR 120 mg/d (540 mg/d max), *LA:* 180–360 mg/d. *HTN:* SR: 60–120 mg PO bid; ↑ to 360 mg/d max. *CD or XR:* 120–360 mg/d (max 540 mg/d) or LA 180–360 mg/d. *IV:* 0.25 mg/kg IV bolus over 2 min; may repeat in 15 min at 0.35 mg/kg; begin Inf of 5–15 mg/h. *Acute rate control:* 15–20 mg (0.25 mg/kg) IV over 2 min, repeat in 15 min at 20–25 mg (0.35 mg/kg) over 2 min (*ECC 2005*) **Caution:** [C, +] ↑ effect w/ amiodarone, cimetidine, fentanyl, Li, cyclosporine, digoxin, β-blockers, theophylline **CI:** SSS, AV block, ↓ BP, AMI, pulm congestion **Disp:** *Cardizem CD:* Caps 120, 180, 240, 300, 360 mg; *Cardizem LA:* Tabs 120, 180, 240, 300, 360, 420 mg; *Cardizem SR:* caps 60, 90, 120 mg; *Cardizem:* Tabs 30, 60, 90, 120 mg; *Cartia XT:* Caps 120, 180, 240, 300 mg; *Dilacor XR:* Caps 180, 240 mg; *Diltia XT:* Caps 120, 180, 240 mg; *Tiazac:* Caps 120, 180, 240, 300, 360, 420 mg; *Tiamate (XR):* Tabs 120, 180, 240 mg; Inj 5 mg/mL; *Taztia XT:* 120, 180, 240, 300, 360 mg **SE:** Gingival hyperplasia, ↓ HR, AV block, ECG abnormalities, peripheral edema, dizziness, HA **Notes:** Cardizem CD, Dilacor XR, & Tiazac not interchangeable

Dimenhydrinate (Dramamine, others) Uses: *Prevention & Rx of N/V, dizziness, or vertigo of motion sickness* **Acts:** Antiemetic, action unknown **Dose:** *Adults.* 50–100 mg PO q4–6h, max 400 mg/d; 50 mg IM/IV PRN. *Peds 2–6 y:* 12.5–25 mg q6–8h max 75 mg/d. *6–12 y:* 25–50 mg q6–8h max 150 mg/d **Caution:** [B, ?] **CI:** Component sensitivity **Disp:** Tabs 50 mg; chew tabs 50 mg; liq 12.5 mg/4 mL, 12.5 mg/5 mL, 15.62 mg/5 mL **SE:** Anticholinergic SE **Notes:** Take 30 min before travel for motion sickness

Dimethyl Sulfoxide [DMSO] (Rimso-50) Uses: *Interstitial cystitis* **Acts:** Unknown **Dose:** Intravesical, 50 mL, retain for 15 min; repeat q2wk until relief **Caution:** [C, ?] **CI:** Component sensitivity **Disp:** 50% & 100% soln **SE:** Cystitis, eosinophilia, GI, & taste disturbance

Dinoprostone (Cervidil Vaginal Insert, Prepidil Vaginal Gel, Prostin E2) BOX: Should only be used by trained personnel in an appropriate hospital setting **Uses:** *Induce labor; terminate PRG (12–20 wk); evacuate uterus in missed abortion or fetal death* **Acts:** Prostaglandin, changes consistency, dilatation, & effacement of the cervix; induces uterine contraction **Dose:** *Gel:* 0.5 mg; if no cervical/uterine response, repeat 0.5 mg q6h (max 24-h dose 1.5 mg). *Vaginal insert:* 1 insert (10 mg = 0.3 mg dinoprostone/h over 12 h); remove w/ onset of labor or 12 h after insertion. *Vaginal supp:* 20 mg repeated q3–5h; adjust PRN supp: 1 high in vagina, repeat at 3–5-h intervals until abortion (240 mg max) **Caution:** [X, ?] **CI:** Ruptured membranes, allergy to prostaglandins, placenta previa or AUB, when oxytocic drugs CI or if prolonged uterine contractions are inappropriate (Hx C-section, cephalopelvic disproportion, etc) **Disp:** *Endocervical gel:* 0.5 mg in 3-g syringes (w/ 10- & 20-mm shielded catheter). *Vaginal gel:* 0.5 mg/3 g *Vaginal supp:* 20 mg. *Vaginal insert, CR:* 10 mg **SE:** N/V/D, dizziness, flushing, HA, fever, abnormal uterine contractions

Diphenhydramine (Benadryl) [OTC] **Uses:** *Rx & prevent allergic Rxns, motion sickness, potentiate narcotics, sedation, cough suppression, & Rx of extrapyramidal Rxns* **Acts:** Antihistamine, antiemetic **Dose:** *Adults.* 25–50 mg PO, IV, or IM bid–tid. *Peds >2 y:* 5 mg/kg/24 h PO or IM ÷ q6h (max 300 mg/d); ↑ dosing interval w/ mod–severe renal Insuff **Caution:** [B, −] elderly, NAG, BPH, w/ MAOI **CI:** acute asthma **Disp:** Tabs & caps 25, 50 mg; chew tabs 12.5 mg; elixir 12.5 mg/5 mL; syrup 12.5 mg/5 mL; liq 6.25 mg/5 mL, 12.5 mg/5 mL; Inj 50 mg/mL, cream 2% **SE:** Anticholinergic (xerostomia, urinary retention, sedation)

Diphenoxylate + Atropine (Lomotil, Lonox) [C-V] **Uses:** *D* **Acts:** Constipating meperidine congener, ↓ GI motility **Dose:** *Adults.* Initial, 5 mg PO tid-qid until controlled, then 2.5–5 mg PO bid; 20 mg/d max *Peds >2 y:* 0.3–0.4 mg/kg/24 h (of diphenoxylate) bid-qid, 10 mg/d max **Caution:** [C, +] elderly, w/ renal impair **CI:** Obstructive jaundice, D d/t bacterial Infxn; children <2 y **Disp:** Tabs 2.5 mg diphenoxylate/0.025 mg atropine; liq 2.5 mg diphenoxylate/0.025 mg atropine/5 mL **SE:** Drowsiness, dizziness, xerostomia, blurred vision, urinary retention, constipation

Diphtheria & Tetanus Toxoids (Td) (Decavac—for > 7 y) **Uses:** *primary immunization, booster (peds 7-9 y; peds 11-12 y if 5 yrs since last shot then q 10 yrs); tetanus protection after wound.* **Acts:** Active immunization **Dose:** 0.5 mL IM × 1; **Caution:** [C, ?/−] **CI:** Component sensitivity **Disp:** Single-dose syringes 0.5 mL **SE:** Inj site pain, redness, swelling; fever, fatigue, HA, malaise, neuro disorders rare **Notes:** If IM, use only preservative-free Inj; Use DTaP (Adacel) rather than TT or Td all adults 19-64 y who have not previously received one dose of DTaP (protection adult pertussis) and Tdap for ages 10-18 y (Boostrix); do not confuse Td (for adults) w/ DT (for children < 7 y)

Diphtheria & Tetanus Toxoids (DT)(Generic only for < 7 y) Uses: primary immunization ages <7 y (DTaP is recommended vaccine) **Acts:** Active immunization **Dose:** 0.5 mL IM ×X1 **Caution:** [C, N/A] **CI:** Component sensitivity **Disp:** Single-dose syringes 0.5 mL **SE:** Inj site pain, redness, swelling; fever, fatigue, myalgias/arthralgias, N/V, seizures, other neurological disorders rare **Notes:** If IM, use only preservative-free Inj. Do not confuse DT (for children < 7 y) w Td (for adults); DTaP is recommended for primary immunization

Diphtheria, Tetanus Toxoids, & Acellular pertussis adsorbed (Tdap) (Ages > 10-11 y) (Boosters: Adacel, Boostrix); **Acts:** active immunization, ages >10-11 y **Uses:** "Catch-up" vaccination if 1 or more of the 5 childhood doses of DTP or DTaP missed; all adults 19–64 y who have **not** received one dose previously (adult pertussis protection) or if around infants < 12 mo; booster q10 yrs; tetanus protection after fresh wound. **Actions:** Active immunization **Dose:** 0.5 mL IM X1; **Caution:** [C, ?/–] **CI:** Component sensitivity; if previous pertussis vaccine caused progressive neurologic disorder/encephalopathy w/in 7 d of shot **Disp:** Single-dose vials 0.5 mL **SE:** Inj site pain, redness, swelling; abd pain, arthralgias/myalgias, fatigue, fever, headache, N/V/D, rash, tiredness **Notes:** If IM, use only preservative-free Inj; ACIP rec: Tdap for ages 10-18 y (*Boostrix*) or 11-64 y (*Adacel*); Td should be used in children 7-9 y

Diphtheria, Tetanus Toxoids, & Acellular Pertussis Adsorbed (DTaP) (Ages < 7 y) (Daptacel, Infanrix, Tripedia) Uses: primary vaccination; 5 Inj at 2, 4, 6, 15–18 mo and 4–6 y **Acts:** Active immunization **Dose:** 0.5 mL IM X1 as in previous above; **Caution:** [C, N/A] **CI:** Component sensitivity; if previous pertussis vaccine caused progressive neurologic disorder/encephalopathy w/in 7 d of shot **Disp:** Single-dose vials 0.5 mL **SE:** Inj site nodule/pain/swelling/redness; drowsiness, fatigue, fever, fussiness, irritability, lethargy, V, prolonged crying; rare ITP and neurologic disorders **Notes:** If IM, use only preservative-free Inj; DTaP recommended for primary immunization age <7 y, if age 7–9 y use Td, ages >10–11 y use Tdap; if encephalopathy or other neurologic disorder w/in 7 d of previous dose **DO NOT USE** DTaP use DT or Td depending on age

Diphtheria, Tetanus Toxoids, & Acellular Pertussis Adsorbed, Hep B (Recombinant), & Inactivated Poliovirus Vaccine [IPV] combined (Pediarix) Uses: *Vaccine against diphtheria, tetanus, pertussis, HBV, polio (types 1, 2, 3) as a 3-dose primary series in infants & children <7 y, born to HBsAg(–) mothers* **Acts:** Active immunization **Dose:** *Infants:* Three 0.5-mL doses IM, at 6–8-wk intervals, start at 2 mo; child given 1 dose of hep B vaccine, same; previously vaccinated w/ one1 or more doses inactivated poliovirus vaccine, use to complete series **Caution:** [C, N/A] w/ bleeding disorders **CI:** HBsAg(+) mother, adults, children >7 y, immunosuppressed, component sensitivity or allergy to yeast/neomycin/polymyxin B; encephalopathy, or progressive neurologic disorders **Disp:** Single-dose vials 0.5 mL **SE:** Drowsiness, restlessness, fever, fussiness, ↓ appetite, Inj site pain/swelling/nodule/redness **Notes:** If IM, use only preservative-free Inj

Dipivefrin (Propine) **Uses:** *Open-angle glaucoma* **Acts:** α-Adrenergic agonist **Dose:** 1 gtt in eye q12h **Caution:** [B, ?] **CI:** NAG **Disp:** 0.1% soln **SE:** HA, local irritation, blurred vision, photophobia, HTN

Dipyridamole (Persantine) **Uses:** *Prevent post-op thromboembolic disorders, often in combo w/ ASA or warfarin (e.g., CABG, vascular graft); w/ warfarin after artificial heart valve; chronic angina; w/ ASA to prevent coronary artery thrombosis; dipyridamole IV used in place of exercise stress test for CAD* **Acts:** Anti-plt activity; coronary vasodilator **Dose:** *Adults.* 75–100 mg PO tid-qid; stress test 0.14 mg/kg/min (max 60 mg over 4 min). *Peds >12 y;* : 3–6 mg/kg/d ÷ tid (safety/efficacy not established) **Caution:** [B, ?/–] w/ Other drugs that affect coagulation **CI:** Component sensitivity **Disp:** Tabs 25, 50, 75 mg; Inj 5 mg/mL **SE:** HA, ↓ BP, N, Abd distress, flushing rash, dizziness, dyspnea **Notes:** IV use can worsen angina

Dipyridamole & Aspirin (Aggrenox) **Uses:** *↓ Reinfarction after MI; prevent occlusion after CABG; ↓ risk of stroke* **Acts:** ↓ Plt aggregation (both agents) **Dose:** 1 cap PO bid **Caution:** [C, ?] **CI:** Ulcers, bleeding diathesis **Disp:** Dipyridamole (XR) 200 mg/ ASA 25 mg **SE:** ASA component: allergic Rxns, skin Rxns, ulcers/GI bleed, bronchospasm; dipyridamole component: dizziness, HA, rash **Notes:** Swallow caps whole

Disopyramide (Norpace, Norpace CR, NAPAmide, Rythmodan) **BOX:** Excessive mortality or nonfatal cardiac arrest rate w/ use in asymptomatic non–life-threatening ventricular arrhythmias w/ MI 6 d to 2 y prior. Restrict use to life-threatening arrhythmias only **Uses:** *Suppression & prevention of VT* **Acts:** Class IA antiarrhythmic; stabilizes membranes, ↓depresses action potential **Dose:** *Adults.* Immediate <50 kg 200 mg, >50 kg 300 mg, maint 400–800 mg/d ÷ q6h or q12h for CR, max 1600 mg/d **Peds** *<1 y:* 10–30 mg/kg/24 h PO (÷ qid). *1–4 y:* 10–20 mg/kg/24 h PO (÷ qid). *4–12 y:* 10–15 mg/kg/24 h PO (÷ qid). *12–18 y:* 6–15 mg/kg/24 h PO (÷ qid); ↓ in renal/hepatic impair **Caution:** [C, +] Elderly, w/ abnormal ECG, lytes, liver/renal impair, NAG **CI:** AV block, cardiogenic shock, ↓ BP, CHF **Disp:** Caps 100, 150 mg; CR caps 100, 150 mg **SE:** Anticholinergic SEs; negative inotrope, may induce CHF **Notes:** Levels: *Trough:* just before next dose; *Therapeutic:* 2–5 mcg/mL; *Toxic* >5 mcg/mL; half-life: 4–10 h

Dobutamine (Dobutrex) **Uses:** *Short-term in cardiac decompensation secondary to ↓ contractility* **Acts:** Positive inotrope **Dose:** *Adults & Peds.* Cont IV Inf of 2.5–15 mcg/kg/min; rarely, 40 mcg/kg/min required; titrate; 2–20 mcg/kg/min; titrate to HR not >10% of baseline *(ECC 2005)* **Caution:** [C, ?] w/ Arrhythmia, MI, severe CAD, ↓ vol **CI:** Sensitivity to sulfites, IHSS **Disp:** Inj 250 mg/20 mL, 12.5/mL **SE:** Chest pain, HTN, dyspnea **Notes:** Monitor PWP & cardiac output if possible; ✓ ECG for ↑ HR, ectopic activity; follow BP

Docetaxel (Taxotere) BOX: Do not administer if neutrophil count <1500 cell/mm³; severe Rxns possible in hepatic dysfunction Uses: *Breast (anthracycline-resistant), ovarian, lung, & prostate CA* Acts: Antimitotic agent; promotes microtubular aggregation; semisynthetic taxoid Dose: 100 mg/m² over 1 h IV q3wk (per protocols); dexamethasone 8 mg bid prior & continue for 3–4 d; ↓ dose w/ ↑ bili levels Caution: [D, –] CI: Sensitivity to meds w/ polysorbate 80, component sensitivity **Disp:** Inj 20 mg/0.5 mL, 80 mg/2 mL SE: ↓ BM, neuropathy, N/V, alopecia, fluid retention synd; cumulative doses of 300–400 mg/m² w/o steroid prep & post-treatment & 600–800 mg/m² w/ steroid prep; allergy possible (rare w/ steroid prep) Notes: ✓ Bili/SGOT/SGPT prior to each cycle; frequent CBC during Rx

Docusate Calcium (Surfak)/Docusate Potassium (Dialose)/ Docusate Sodium (DOSS, Colace) Uses: *Constipation; adjunct to painful anorectal conditions (hemorrhoids)* Acts: Stool softener Dose: *Adults.* 50–500 mg PO ÷ daily–qid. *Peds Infants–3 y:* 10–40 mg/24 h ÷ daily–qid. *3–6 y:* 20–60 mg/24 h ÷ daily–qid. *6–12 y:* 40–120 mg/24 h ÷ daily–qid Caution: [C, ?] CI: Use w/ mineral oil; intestinal obst, acute Abd pain, N/V Disp: *Ca:* Caps 50, 240 mg. *K:* Caps 100, 240 mg. *Na:* Caps 50, 100 mg; syrup 50, 60 mg/15 mL; liq 150 mg/15 mL; soln 50 mg/mL SE: Rare Abd cramping, D Notes: Take w/ full glass of H₂O; no laxative action; do not use >1 wk

Dofetilide (Tikosyn) BOX: To minimize the risk of induced arrhythmia, hospitalize for minimum of 3 d to provide calculations of CrCl, cont ECG monitoring, & cardiac resuscitation Uses: *Maintain nl sinus rhythm in AF/A flutter after conversion* Acts: Class III antiarrhythmic, prolongs action potential Dose: Based on CrCl & QTc; CrCl >60 mL/min 500 mcg PO q12h, QTc 2–3 h after, if QTc >15% over baseline or >500 msec, ↓ to 250 mcg q 12h, ✓ after each dose; if CrCl <60 mL/min, see PI; D/C if QTc >500 msec after dosing adjustments Caution: [C, –] w/ AV block, renal Dz, electrolyte imbalance CI: Baseline QTc >440 msec, CrCl <20 mL/min; w/ verapamil, cimetidine, trimethoprim, ketoconazole, quinolones, ACE inhib/HCTZ combo Disp: Caps 125, 250, 500 mcg SE: Ventricular arrhythmias, QT ↑, torsades de pointes, rash, HA, CP, dizziness Notes: Avoid w/ other drugs that ↑ QT interval; hold Class I/III antiarrhythmics for 3 1/2-lives prior to dosing; amiodarone level should be <0.3 mg/L before use, do not initiate if HR <60 BPM; restricted to participating prescribers; correct K⁺ and Mg²⁺ before use.

Dolasetron (Anzemet) Uses: *Prevent chemotherapy and post–op–associated N/V* Acts: 5-HT₃ receptor antagonist Dose: *Adults & Peds. IV:* 1.8 mg/kg IV as single dose 30 min prior to chemotherapy *Adults. PO:* 100 mg PO as a single dose 1 h prior to chemotherapy. *Post-op:* 12.5 mg IV, or 100 mg PO 2 h pre-op *Peds 2–16 y:* 1.8 mg/kg PO (max 100 mg) as single dose. *Post-op:* 0.35 mg/kg IV or 1.2 mg/kg PO Caution: [B, ?] w/ Cardiac conduction problems CI: Component sensitivity Disp: Tabs 50, 100 mg; Inj 20 mg/mL SE: ↑ QT interval, D, HTN, HA, Abd pain, urinary retention, transient ↑ LFTs

Donepezil (Aricept) Uses: *Severe Alzheimer dementia* ADHD; behavioral synds in dementia; dementia w/ Parkinson Dz; Lewy-body dementia Acts: ACH inhib Dose: *Adults.* 5 mg qhs, ↑ to 10 mg PO qhs after 4–6 wk Peds. ADHD: 5 mg/d Caution: [C, ?] risk for ↓ HR w/ preexisting conduction abnormalities, may exaggerate succinylcholine-type muscle relaxation w/ anesthesia, ↑ gastric acid secretion CI: Hypersens Disp: Tabs 5, 10 mg; ODT tab 5, 10 mg SE: N/V/D, insomnia, Infxn, muscle cramp, fatigue, anorexia Notes: N/V/D dose-related & resolves in 1–3 wk

Dopamine (Intropin) BOX: Vesicant, give phentolamine w/ extrav Uses: *Short-term use in cardiac decompensation secondary to ↓ contractility; ↑ organ perfusion (at low dose)* Acts: Positive inotropic agent w/ dose response: 1–10 mcg/kg/min β effects (↑ CO & renal perfusion); 10–20 mcg/kg/min β- effects (peripheral vasoconstriction, pressor); >20 mcg/kg/min peripheral & renal vasoconstriction Dose: *Adults & Peds.* 5 mcg/kg/min by cont Inf, ↑ by 5 mcg/kg/min to 50 mcg/kg/min max to effect *(ECC 2005)* Caution: [C, ?] ↓ Dose w/ MAOI CI: Pheochromocytoma, VF, sulfite sensitivity Disp: Inj 40, 80, 160 mg/mL, premixed 0.8, 1.6, 3.2 mg/mL SE: Tachycardia, vasoconstriction, ↓ BP, HA, N/V, dyspnea Notes: >10 mcg/kg/min ↓ renal perfusion; monitor urinary output & ECG for ↑ HR, BP, ectopy; monitor PCWP & cardiac output if possible, phentolamine used for extrav 10 to 15 mL NS w/5 to 10 mg of phentolamine

Doripenem (Doribax) Uses: *Complicated intra-Abd infection and UTI including pyelo* Acts: Carbapenem, ↓ cell wall synth, a β-lactam Spectrum: Excellent gram(+) (except MRSA and Enterococcus sp.), excellent gram(−) coverage including β-lactamase producers, good anaerobic Dose: 500 mg IV q8h, ↓ w/ renal impair Caution: [B, ?] CI: carbapenem β-lactams hypersens Disp: 500 mg single-use vial SE: HA, N/D, rash, phlebitis Notes: May ↓ valproic acid levels; overuse may ↑ bacterial resistance; monitor for *C. difficile*-associated D

Dornase Alfa (Pulmozyme, DNase) Uses: *↓ Frequency of resp infxns in CF* Acts: Enzyme cleaves extracellular DNA, ↓ mucous viscosity Dose: *Adults.* Inh 2.5 mg/bid dosing w/ FVC >85% w/ recommended nebulizer Peds >5 y: Inh 2.5 mg/daily-bid if forced vital capacity >85% Caution: [B, ?] CI: Chinese hamster product allergy Disp: Soln for Inh 1 mg/mL SE: Pharyngitis, voice alteration, CP, rash

Dorzolamide (Trusopt) Uses: *Open-angle glaucoma, ocular hypertension* Acts: Carbonic anhydrase inhib Dose: 1 gtt in eye(s) tid Caution: [C, ?] w/ NAG, CrCl <30 mL/min CI: Component sensitivity Disp: 2% soln SE: irritation, bitter taste, punctate keratitis, ocular allergic Rxn

Dorzolamide & Timolol (Cosopt) Uses: *Open-angle glaucoma, ocular hypertension* Acts: Carbonic anhydrase inhib w/ β-adrenergic blocker Dose: 1 gtt in eye(s) bid Caution: [C, ?] CrCl <30 mL/min CI: Component sensitivity, asthma, severe COPD, sinus bradycardia, AV block Disp: Soln dorzolamide 2% & timolol 0.5% SE: Irritation, bitter taste, superficial keratitis, ocular allergic Rxn

Doxazosin (Cardura, Cardura XL) Uses: *HTN & symptomatic BPH* Acts: α_1-Adrenergic blocker; relaxes bladder neck smooth muscle Dose: *HTN:* Initial 1 mg/d PO; may be ↑ to 16 mg/d PO. *BPH:* Initial 1 mg/d PO, may ↑ to 8 mg/d; XL 2–8 mg q A.M. Caution: [B, ?] w/ Liver impair CI: Component sensitivity; use w/ PDE-5 inhib (e.g., sildenafil) can cause ↓ BP Disp: Tabs 1, 2, 4, 8 mg; XL 4, 8 mg SE: Dizziness, HA, drowsiness, fatigue, malaise, sexual dysfunction, doses >4 mg ↑ postural ↓ BP risk; intraoperative floppy iris synd Notes: 1st dose hs; syncope may occur w/in 90 min of initial dose

Doxepin (Adapin) BOX: Closely monitor for worsening depression or emergence of suicidality Uses: *Depression, anxiety, chronic pain* Acts: TCA; ↑ synaptic CNS serotonin or norepinephrine Dose: 25–150 mg/d PO, usually hs but can ÷ doses; up to 300 mg/d for depression ↓ in hepatic impair Caution: [C, ?/–] w/ EtOH abuse, elderly, w/ MAOI CI: NAG, urinary retention, MAOI use w/in 14 d, in recovery phase of MI Disp: Caps 10, 25, 50, 75, 100, 150 mg; PO conc 10 mg/mL SE: Anticholinergic SEs, ↓ BP, tachycardia, drowsiness, photosens

Doxepin, Topical (Zonalon, Prudoxin) Uses: *Short-term Rx pruritus (atopic dermatitis or lichen simplex chronicus)* Acts: Antipruritic; H_1- & H_2-receptor antagonism Dose: Apply thin coating qid, 8 d max Caution: [C, ?/–] CI: Component sensitivity Disp: 5% cream SE: ↓ BP, tachycardia, drowsiness, photosens Notes: Limit application area to avoid systemic tox

Doxorubicin (Adriamycin, Rubex) Uses: *Acute leukemias; Hodgkin Dz & NHLs; soft tissue, osteo- & Ewing sarcoma; Wilms tumor; neuroblastoma; bladder, breast, ovarian, gastric, thyroid, & lung CAs* Acts: Intercalates DNA; ↓ DNA topoisomerase I & II Dose: 60–75 mg/m² q3wk; ↓ w/ hepatic impair; IV use only ↓ cardiotox w/ weekly (20 mg/m²/wk) or cont Inf (60–90 mg/m² over 96 h); (per protocols) Caution: [D, ?] CI: Severe CHF, cardiomyopathy, preexisting ↓ BM, previous Rx w/ total cumulative doses of doxorubicin, idarubicin, daunorubicin Disp: Inj 10, 20, 50, 75, 150, 200 mg/mL SE: ↓ BM, venous streaking & phlebitis, N/V/D, mucositis, radiation recall phenomenon, cardiomyopathy rare (dose-related) Notes: Limit of 550 mg/m² cumulative dose (400 mg/m² w/ prior mediastinal irradiation); dexrazoxane may limit cardiac tox; tissue damage w/ extrav; red/orange urine; vesicant w/ extrav, Rx w/ dexrazoxane

Doxycycline (Adoxa, Periostat, Oracea, Vibramycin, Vibra-Tabs) Uses: *Broad-spectrum antibiotic* acne vulgaris, uncomplicated GC, chlamydia, PID, Lyme Dz, skin infxns, anthrax, malaria prophylaxis Acts: Tetracycline; bacteriostatic; ↓ protein synth. *Spectrum:* Limited gram(+) and (–), *Rickettsia* sp, *Chlamydia, M. pneumoniae, B. anthracis* Dose: *Adults.* 100 mg PO q12h on 1st d, then 100 mg PO daily–bid or 100 mg IV q12h; acne q day, chlamydia ×7d, Lyme ×21 d, PID ×14 d *Peds >8 y:* 5 mg/kg/24 h PO, 200 mg/d max ÷ daily–bid Caution: [D, +] hepatic impair CI: Children <8 y, severe hepatic dysfunction Disp: Tabs 20, 50, 75, 100, 150 mg; caps 50, 100 mg; Oracea 40 mg caps (30 mg timed release, 10 mg DR); syrup 50 mg/5 mL; susp 25 mg/5 mL; Inj 100, 200 mg/vial SE: D, GI disturbance, photosens **Notes:** ↓ effect w/ antacids; tetracycline of choice w/in renal impair; for inhalational anthrax use w/ 1–2 additional antibiotics, not for CNS anthrax

Dronabinol (Marinol) [C-II] **Uses:** *N/V associated w/ CA chemotherapy; appetite stimulation* **Acts:** Antiemetic; ↓ V center in the medulla **Dose:** *Adults & Peds.* Antiemetic: 5–15 mg/m²/dose q4–6h PRN. *Adults. Appetite stimulant:* 2.5 mg PO before lunch & dinner; max 20 mg/d **Caution:** [C, ?] elderly, Hx psychological disorder, Sz disorder, substance abuse **CI:** Hx schizophrenia, sesame oil hypersens **Disp:** Caps 2.5, 5, 10 mg **SE:** Drowsiness, dizziness, anxiety, mood change, hallucinations, depersonalization, orthostatic ↓ BP, tachycardia **Notes:** Principal psychoactive substance present in marijuana

Droperidol (Inapsine) **BOX:** Cases of QT interval prolongation and torsades de pointes (some fatal) reported **Uses:** *N/V; anesthetic premedication* **Acts:** Tranquilizer, sedation, antiemetic **Dose:** *Adults. N:* initial max 2.5 mg IV/IM, may repeat 1.25 mg based on response; *Premed:* 2.5–10 mg IV, 30–60 min pre-op. *Peds. Premed:* 0.1–0.15 mg/kg/dose **Caution:** [C, ?]w/ Hepatic/renal impair **CI:** Component sensitivity **Disp:** Inj 2.5 mg/mL **SE:** Drowsiness, ↓ BP, occasional tachycardia & extrapyramidal Rxns, ↑ QT interval, arrhythmias **Notes:** Give IV push slowly over 2–5 min

Dronedarone (Multaq) **BOX:** CI w/ NYHA Class IV HF or NYHA Class II-III HF w/ decompensation **Uses:** *A Fib/A Flutter* **Acts:** Antiarrhythmic **Dose:** 400 mg PO BID w/AM and PM meal **Caution:** [X, –] w/ other drugs (see PI) **CI:** See Box 2ⁿᵈ- /3ʳᵈ degree AV block or SSS (unless w/ pacemaker), HR <50 BPM, w/ strong CYP3A inhib, w/ drugs/herbals that ↑ QT interval, QTc interval ≥500 ms, severe hepatic impair, PRG **Disp:** Tabs 400 mg **SE:** N/V/D, Abd pain, asthenia, heart failure, ↑ K⁺, ↑ Mg²⁺, ↑ QTc, ↓ HR, ↑ SCr, rash **Notes:** Avoid grapefruit juice

Drotrecogin Alfa (Xigris) **Uses:** *↓ Mortality in adults w/ severe sepsis (w/ acute organ dysfunction) at high risk of death (e.g., determined by APACHE II score [www.ncemi.org])* **Acts:** Recombinant human-activated protein C; antithrombotic and anti-inflammatory, unclear mechanism **Dose:** 24 mcg/kg/h, total of 96 h **Caution:** [C, ?] w/ Anticoagulation, INR >3, plt <30,000 cells/mm³, GI bleed w/in 6 wk **CI:** Active bleeding, recent stroke/CNS surgery, head trauma/CNS lesion w/ herniation risk, trauma w/ ↑ bleeding risk, epidural catheter, mifepristone **Disp:** 5-, 20-mg vials **SE:** Bleeding **Notes:** Single-organ dysfunction & recent surgery may not be at high risk of death irrespective of APACHE II score & therefore not indicated. *Percutaneous procedures:* Stop Inf 2 h before & resume 1 h after; major surgery: stop Inf 2 h before & resume 12 h after in absence of bleeding

Duloxetine (Cymbalta) **BOX:** Antidepressants may ↑ risk of suicidality; consider risks/benefits of use. Closely monitor for clinical worsening, suicidality, or behavior changes **Uses:** *Depression; DM peripheral neuropathic pain, generalized anxiety disorder (GAD)* **Acts:** Selective serotonin & norepinephrine reuptake inhib (SSNRI) **Dose:** *Depression:* 40–60 mg/d PO ÷ bid. *DM neuropathy:* 60 mg/d PO; *GAD:* 30–60 mg/d max 120 mg/d **Caution:** [C, ?/–]; use in 3rd tri; avoid if

CrCl <30 mL/min, NAG, w/ fluvoxamine, inhib of CYP2D6 (Table 10 p 280), TCAs, phenothiazines, type class 1C antiarrhythmics (Table 9 p 279) **CI:** MAOI use w/in 14 d, w/ thioridazine, NAG, hepatic Insuff **Disp:** Caps delayed-release 20, 30, 60 mg **SE:** N, dizziness, somnolence, fatigue, sweating, xerostomia, constipation, ↓ appetite, sexual dysfunction, urinary hesitancy, ↑ LFTs, HTN **Notes:** Swallow whole; monitor BP; avoid abrupt D/C

Dutasteride (Avodart) **Uses:** *Symptomatic BPH to improve Sxs, ↓ risk of retention and BPH surgery alone or in combo w/ tamsulosin* **Acts:** 5α-Reductase inhib; ↓ intracellular dihydrotestosterone (DHT) **Dose:** *Monotherapy:* 0.5 mg PO/d. *Combo:* 0.5 mg PO q day w/ tamsulosin 0.4 mg q day **Caution:** [X, –] Hepatic impair; pregnant women should not handle pills; R/o cancer before starting **CI:** Women, peds **Disp:** Caps 0.5 mg **SE:** ↑ testosterone, ↑ TSH, impotence, ↓ libido, gynecomastia, ejaculatory disturbance, **Notes:** No blood donation until 6 mo after D/C; ↓ PSA, ✓ new baseline PSA at 6 mo (corrected PSA × 2);any PSA rise on dutasteride suspicious for cancer; under FDA review for PCa chemoprevention; now available in fixed dose combination w/tamsulosin (see *Jalyn*)

Dutasteride and tamsulosin (Jalyn) **Uses:** *Symptomatic BPH to improve Sxs * **Acts:** 5α-Reductase inhib (↓ intracellular DHT) w/ alpha blocker **Dose:** 1 capsule daily after same meal **Caution:** [X, –] w/ CYP3A4 and CYP2D6 inhib may ↑ SE's; pregnant women should not handle pills; R/o cancer before starting; IFIS (tamsulosin) discuss w/ophthalmologist before cataract surgery; rare priapism; w/warfarin **CI:** Women, peds, component sens **Disp:** Caps 0.5 mg dutasteride w/0.4 mg tamsulosin **SE:** impotence, decreased libido, ejaculation disorders, and breast disorders **Notes:** No blood donation until 6 mo after D/C; ↓ PSA,✓ new baseline PSA at 6 mo (corrected PSA × 2);any PSA rise on dutasteride suspicious for cancer (see also dutasteride and tamsulosin)

Ecallantide (Kalbitor) **BOX:** Anaphylaxis reported, administer in a setting able to manage anaphylaxis and HAE, monitor closely **Uses:** *Acute attacks of hereditary angioedema (HAE) * **Acts:** Plasma kallikrein inhibitor **Dose:** *Adult & >16yrs.* 30mg SC in three 10mg injections; if attack persists may repeat 30mg dose w/n 24 hr **Caution:** [C, ?/–] Hypersens rxns **Disp:** Inj 10mg/ml **SE:** HA, N/V/D, pyrexia, inj site rxn, nasopharyngitis, fatigue, abd pain

Echothiophate Iodine (Phospholine Ophthalmic) **Uses:** *Glaucoma* **Acts:** Cholinesterase inhib **Dose:** 1 gtt eye(s) bid w/ 1 dose hs **Caution:** [C, ?] **CI:** Active uveal inflammation, inflammatory Dz of iris/ciliary body, glaucoma iridocyclitis **Disp:** Powder, reconstitute 1.5 mg/0.03%; 3 mg/0.06%; 6.25 mg/0.125%; 12.5 mg/0.25% **SE:** Local irritation, myopia, blurred vision, ↓ BP, ↓ HR

Econazole (Spectazole) **Uses:** *Tinea, cutaneous Candida, & tinea versicolor infxns* **Acts:** Topical antifungal **Dose:** Apply to areas bid (daily for tinea versicolor) for 2–4 wk **Caution:** [C, ?] **CI:** Component sensitivity **Disp:** Topical cream 1% **SE:** Local irritation, pruritus, erythema **Notes:** Early Sx/clinical improvement; complete course to avoid recurrence

Eculizumab (Soliris) **BOX:** ↑ Risk of meningococcal infections (give meningococcal vaccine 2 wk prior to 1st dose and revaccinate per guidelines) **Uses:** *Rx paroxysmal nocturnal hemoglobinuria* **Acts:** Complement inhib **Dose:** 600 mg IV q 7 d × 4 wk, then 900 mg IV 5th dose 7 d later, then 900 mg IV q14d **Caution:** [C,; ?] **CI:** Active *N. meningitidis* Infxn; if not vaccinated against *N. meningitidis* **Disp:** 300-mg vial **SE:** Meningococcal Infxn, HA, nasopharyngitis, N, back pain, infxns, fatigue, severe hemolysis on D/C **Notes:** IV over 35 min (2-h max Inf time); monitor for 1 h for S/Sx of Inf Rxn

Edrophonium (Tensilon, Reversol) **Uses:** *Diagnosis of MyG; acute MyG crisis; curare antagonist, reverse of nondepolarizing neuromuscular blockers* **Acts:** Anticholinesterase **Dose:** *Adults.* *Test for MyG:* 2 mg IV in 1 min; if tolerated, give 8 mg IV; (+) test is brief ↑ in strength. *Peds.* *Test for MyG:* Total dose 0.2 mg/kg; 0.04 mg/kg test dose; if no Rxn, give remainder in 1 -mg increments to 10 mg max; ↓ in renal impair **Caution:** [C, ?] **CI:** GI or GU obst; allergy to sulfite **Disp:** Inj 10 mg/mL **SE:** N/V/D, excessive salivation, stomach cramps, ↑ aminotransferases **Notes:** Can cause severe cholinergic effects; keep atropine available

Efalizumab (Raptiva) Withdrawn from US market in 2009 due to progressive multifocal leukoencephalopathy (PML).

Efavirenz (Sustiva) **Uses:** *HIV infxns* **Acts:** Antiretroviral; nonnucleoside RT inhib **Dose:** *Adults.* 600 mg/d PO q hs. *Peds ≥3 y 10–<15 kg:* 200 mg PO q day; *15–<20 kg:* 250 mg PO q day; *20–<25 kg:* 300 mg PO q day; *25–<32.5 kg:* 350 mg PO q day; *32.5–<40 kg:* 400 mg PO q day ≥*40 kg:* 600 mg PO q day; on empty stomach **Caution:** [D, ?] CDC rec: HIV-infected mothers not breast-feed **CI:** w/ Astemizole, bepridil, cisapride, midazolam, pimozide, triazolam, ergot derivatives, voriconazole **Disp:** Caps 50, 100, 200; 600 mg tab **SE:** Somnolence, vivid dreams, depression, CNS Sxs, dizziness, rash, N/V/D **Notes:** ✓ LFTs (especially w/underlying liver Dz), cholesterol; not for monotherapy

Efavirenz, Emtricitabine, Tenofovir (Atripla) **BOX:** Lactic acidosis and severe hepatotoxicity w/ steatosis, including fatal cases, reported w/ nucleoside analogs alone or combo w/ other antiretrovirals **Uses:** *HIV infxns* **Acts:** Triple fixed-dose combo nonnucleoside RT inhib/nucleoside analog **Dose:** *Adults.* 1 tab q day on empty stomach; HS dose may ↓ CNS SE **Caution:** [D, ?] CDC rec: HIV-infected mothers not breast-feed, w/ obesity **CI:** <18 y, w/ astemizole, midazolam, triazolam, or ergot derivatives (CYP3A4 competition by efavirenz could cause serious/life-threatening SE) **Disp:** Tab (efavirenz 600 mg/emtricitabine 200 mg/ tenofovir 300 mg) **SE:** Somnolence, vivid dreams, HA, dizziness, rash, N/V/D, ↓ BMD **Notes:** Monitor LFTs, cholesterol; see individual agents for additional info, not for HIV/hep B coinfection

Eletriptan (Relpax) **Uses:** *Acute Rx of migraine* **Acts:** Selective serotonin receptor (5-HT$_{1B/1D}$) agonist **Dose:** 20–40 mg PO, may repeat in 2 h; 80 mg/24 h max **Caution:** [C, +] **CI:** Hx ischemic heart Dz, coronary artery spasm, stroke or TIA, peripheral vascular Dz, IBD, uncontrolled HTN, hemiplegic or basilar migraine, severe hepatic impair, w/in 24 h of another 5-HT$_1$ agonist or ergot, w/in 72 h of CYP3A4 inhib **Disp:** Tabs 20, 40 mg **SE:** Dizziness, somnolence, N, asthenia, xerostomia, paresthesias; pain, pressure, or tightness in chest, jaw, or neck; serious cardiac events

Eltrombopag (Promacta) **BOX:** May cause hepatotoxicity. ✓ baseline ALT/AST/bili, q 2 wks w/dosage adjustment, then monthly. D/C if ALT is >3× ULN w/ ↑ bili, or Sx of liver injury **Uses:** *Tx ↑ plt in idiopathic thrombocytopenia refractory to steroids, immune globulins, splenectomy* **Acts:** Thrombopoietin receptor agonist **Dose:** 50 mg PO daily, adjust to keep plt ≥50,000 cells/mm³; 75 mg/d max; start 25 mg/d if East-Asian or w/ hepatic impair; on an empty stomach; not w/in 4 hrs of product w/ polyvalent cations **Caution:** [C, ?/–] ↑ risk for BM reticulin fiber deposition, heme malignancies, rebound ↓ plt on D/C, thromboembolism **CI:** None **Disp:** Tabs 25, 50 mg **SE:** rash, bruising, menorrhagia, N/V, dyspepsia, ↓ plt, ↑ ALT/AST, limb pain, myalgia, paresthesia, cataract, conjunctival hemorrhage **Notes:** D/C if no ↑ plt count after 4 wks; restricted distribution Promacta® *Cares (1-877-9-PROMACTA)*

Emedastine (Emadine) **Uses:** *Allergic conjunctivitis* **Acts:** Antihistamine; selective H$_1$-antagonist **Dose:** 1 gtt in eye(s) up to qid **Caution:** [B, ?] **CI:** Allergy to ingredients (preservatives benzalkonium, tromethamine) **Disp:** 0.05% soln **SE:** HA, blurred vision, burning/stinging, corneal infiltrates/staining, dry eyes, foreign body sensation, hyperemia, keratitis, tearing, pruritus, rhinitis, sinusitis, asthenia, bad taste, dermatitis, discomfort **Notes:** Do not use contact lenses if eyes are red

Emtricitabine (Emtriva) **BOX:** Lactic acidosis, & severe hepatomegaly w/ steatosis reported; not for HBV Infxn **Uses:** HIV-1 Infxn **Acts:** NRTI **Dose:** 200 mg caps or 240 mg soln PO daily; ↓ w/ renal impair **Caution:** [B, –] risk of liver Dz **CI:** Component sensitivity **Disp:** Soln 10 mg/mL, caps 200 mg **SE:** HA, N/D, rash, rare hyperpigmentation of feet & hands, posttreatment exacerbation of hep **Notes:** 1st once-daily NRTI; caps/soln not equivalent; not ok as monotherapy; screen for hep B, do not use w/ HIV and HBV coinfection

Enalapril (Vasotec) **BOX:** ACE inhib used during PRG can cause fetal injury & death **Uses:** *HTN, CHF, LVD* **, DN **Acts:** ACE inhib **Dose:** *Adults.* 2.5–40 mg/d PO; 1.25 mg IV q6h. *Peds.* 0.05–0.08 mg/kg/d PO q12–24h; ↓ w/ renal impair **Caution:** [C (1st tri; D 2nd & 3rd tri), +] D/C immediately w/PRG, w/ NSAIDs, K+ supplements **CI:** Bilateral RAS, angioedema **Disp:** Tabs 2.5, 5, 10, 20 mg; IV 1.25 mg/mL (1, 2 mL) **SE:** ↓ BP w/ initial dose (especially w/ diuretics), ↑ K+, ↑ Cr nonproductive cough, angioedema **Notes:** Monitor Cr; D/C diuretic for 2–3 d prior to start

Enfuvirtide (Fuzeon) **BOX:** Rarely causes allergy; never rechallenge **Uses:** *w/ Antiretroviral agents for HIV-1 in Tx-experienced pts w/ viral replication despite ongoing Rx* **Acts:** Viral fusion inhib **Dose:** *Adults.* 90 mg (1 mL) SQ bid in upper arm, anterior thigh, or abd; rotate site *Peds.* See PI **Caution:** [B, –] **CI:** Previous allergy to drug **Disp:** 90 mg/mL recons; pt kit w/ supplies × 1 mo **SE:** Inj site Rxns;

pneumonia, D, N, fatigue, insomnia, peripheral neuropathy **Notes:** Available via restricted distribution system; use immediately on recons or refrigerate (24 h max)

Enoxaparin (Lovenox) BOX: Recent or anticipated epidural/spinal anesthesia, ↑ risk of spinal/epidural hematoma w/ subsequent paralysis **Uses:** *Prevention & Rx of DVT; Rx PE; unstable angina & non–Q-wave MI* **Acts:** LMW heparin; inhibit thrombin by complexing w/ antithrombin III **Dose:** *Adults. Prevention:* 30 mg SQ bid or 40 mg SQ q24h. *DVT/PE Rx:* 1 mg/kg SQ q12h or 1.5 mg/kg SQ q24h. *Angina:* 1 mg/kg SQ q12h; *Ancillary to AMI fibrinolysis:* 30 mg IV bolus, then 1 mg/kg SQ bid *(ECC 2005);* CrCl <30 mL/min ↓ to 1 mg/kg SQ q day *Peds. Prevention:* 0.5 mg/kg SQ q12h. *DVT/PE Rx:* 1 mg/kg SQ q12h; ↓ dose w/ CrCl <30 mL/min **Caution:** [B, ?] Not for prophylaxis in prosthetic heart valves **CI:** Active bleeding, HIT Ab **Disp:** Inj 10 mg/0.1 mL (30-, 40-, 60-, 80-, 100-, 120-, 150-mg syringes); 300-mg/mL multidose vial **SE:** Bleeding, hemorrhage, bruising, thrombocytopenia, fever, pain/hematoma at site, ↑ AST/ALT **Notes:** No effect on bleeding time, plt Fxn, PT, or aPTT; monitor plt for HIT, clinical bleeding; may monitor antifactor Xa; not for IM

Entacapone (Comtan) **Uses:** *Parkinson Dz* **Acts:** Selective & reversible carboxymethyl transferase inhib **Dose:** 200 mg w/ each levodopa/carbidopa dose; max 1600 mg/d; ↓ levodopa/carbidopa dose 25% w/ levodopa dose >800 mg **Caution:** [C, ?] Hepatic impair **CI:** Use w/ MAOI **Disp:** Tabs 200 mg **SE:** Dyskinesia, hyperkinesia, N, D, dizziness, hallucinations, orthostatic ↓ BP, brown-orange urine **Notes:** ✓ LFTs; do not D/C abruptly

Ephedrine **Uses:** *Acute bronchospasm, bronchial asthma, nasal congestion*, ↓ BP, narcolepsy, enuresis, & MyG **Acts:** Sympathomimetic; stimulates α- & β-receptors; bronchodilator **Dose:** *Adults. Congestion:* 25–50 mg PO q6h PRN; ↓ *BP:* 25–50 mg IV q5–10min, 150 mg/d max. *Peds.* 0.2–0.3 mg/kg/dose IV q4–6h PRN **Caution:** [C, ?/–] **CI:** Arrhythmias; NAG **Disp:** Nasal soln 0.48%, 0.5%; caps 25 mg; Inj 50 mg/mL; nasal spray 0.25% **SE:** CNS stimulation (nervousness, anxiety, trembling), tachycardia, arrhythmia, HTN, xerostomia, dysuria **Notes:** Protect from light; monitor BP, HR, urinary output; can cause false (+) amphetamine EMIT; take last dose 4–6 h before hs; abuse potential, OTC sales mostly banned/ restricted

Epinephrine (Adrenalin, Sus-Phrine, EpiPen, EpiPen Jr., others) **Uses:** *Cardiac arrest, anaphylactic Rxn, anaphylaxis, open-angle glaucoma* **Acts:** β-Adrenergic agonist, some α- effects **Dose:** *Adults.* 1 mg IV push, repeat q3–5min; (0.2 mg/kg max) if 1-mg dose fails. Inf: 30 mg (30 mL of 1:1000 soln) in 250 mL NS or D₅W, at 100 mL/h, titrate. ET 2–2.5 mg in 20 mL NS. *Profound bradycardia/hypotension:* 2–10 mcg/min (1 mg of 1:1000 in 500 mL NS, infuse 1–5 mL/min) *(ECC 2005). Anaphylaxis:* 0.3–0.5 mL SQ of 1:1000 dilution, repeat PRN q5–15min to max 1 mg/dose & 5 mg/d. *Asthma:* 0.1–0.5 mL SQ of 1:1000 dilution, repeat q20min to 4h, or 1 Inh (metered-dose) repeat in 1–2 min, or susp 0.1–0.3 mL SQ for extended effect. *Peds. ACLS:* 1st dose 0.1 mL/kg IV of 1:10,000 dilution, then 0.1 mL/kg IV of 1:1000 dilution q3–5min to response. *Anaphylaxis:* 0.15–0.3 mg IM depending on wgt <30 kg 0.01 mg/kg. *Asthma:* 0.01 mL/kg SQ of 1:1000 dilution q8–12h **Caution:** [C, ?/–] ↓ bronchodilator w/ β-blockers **CI:** Cardiac arrhythmias, NAG **Disp:** Inj 1:1000, 1:2000, 1:10,000, 1:100,000; susp for Inj 1:200; aerosol 220 mcg/spray; 1% Inh soln; EpiPen Autoinjector 1 dose = 0.30 mg; EpiPen Jr. 1 dose = 0.15 mg **SE:** CV (tachycardia, HTN, vasoconstriction), CNS stimulation (nervousness, anxiety, trembling), ↓ renal blood flow **Notes:** Can give via ET tube if no central line (use 2–2.5 × IV dose); EpiPen for pt self-use (www.EpiPen.com)

Epinastine (Elestat) **Uses:** Itching w/ allergic conjunctivitis **Acts:** Antihistamine **Dose:** 1 gtt bid **Caution:** [C, ?/–] **Disp:** Soln 0.05% **SE:** Burning, folliculosis, hyperemia, pruritus, URI, HA, rhinitis, sinusitis, cough, pharyngitis **Notes:** Remove contacts before, reinsert in 10 min

Epirubicin (Ellence) **BOX:** Do not give IM or SQ. Extrav causes tissue necrosis; potential cardiotox; severe myelosuppression; ↓ dose w/ hepatic impair **Uses:** *Adjuvant Rx for (+) axillary nodes after resection of primary breast CA* **Actions:** Anthracycline cytotoxic agent **Dose:** Per protocols; ↓ dose w/ hepatic impair **Caution:** [D, –] **CI:** Baseline neutrophil count <1500 cells/mm³, severe cardiac Insuff, recent MI, severe arrhythmias, severe hepatic dysfunction, previous anthracyclines Rx to max cumulative dose **Disp:** Inj 50 mg/25 mL, 200 mg/100 mL **SE:** Mucositis, N/V/D, alopecia, ↓ BM, cardiotox, secondary AML, tissue necrosis w/ extrav (see Adriamycin for Rx), lethargy **Notes:** ✓ CBC, bili, AST, Cr, cardiac Fxn before/during each cycle

Eplerenone (Inspra) **Uses:** *HTN* **Acts:** Selective aldosterone antagonist **Dose:** *Adults.* 50 mg PO daily-bid, doses >100 mg/d no benefit w/ ↑ K⁺; ↓ to 25 mg PO daily if giving w/ CYP3A4 inhib **Caution:** [B, +/–] w/ CYP3A4 inhib (Table 10 p 280); monitor K⁺ w/ ACE inhib, ARBs, NSAIDs, K⁺-sparing diuretics; grapefruit juice, St. John's wort **CI:** K⁺ >5.5 mEq/L; non–insulin-dependent diabetes mellitus (NIDDM) w/ microalbuminuria; SCr >2 mg/dL (males); >1.8 mg/dL (females); CrCl <30 mL/min; w/ K⁺ supls/K⁺-sparing diuretics, ketoconazole **Disp:** Tabs 25, 50 mg **SE:** ↑ cholesterol/triglycerides, ↑ K⁺, HA, dizziness, gynecomastia, D, orthostatic ↓ BP **Notes:** May take 4 wk for full effect

Epoetin Alfa [Erythropoietin, EPO] (Epogen, Procrit) **BOX:** ↑ Mortality, serious CV/thromboembolic events, and tumor progression. Renal failure pts experienced ↑ greater risks (death/CV events) on erythropoiesis-stimulating agents (ESAs) to target higher Hgb levels. Maintain Hgb 10–12g/dL. In cancer pts, ESAs ↓ survival/time-to progression in some cancers when dosed Hgb ≥12 g/dL. Use lowest dose needed. Use only for myelosuppressive chemo-therapy. D/C following chemotherapy. Pre-op ESA ↑ DVT. Consider DVT prophylaxis **Uses:** *CRF-associated anemia, zidovudine Rx in HIV-infected pts, CA chemotherapy; ↓ transfusions associated w/ surgery* **Acts:** Induces erythropoiesis **Dose:** *Adults & Peds.* 50–150 units/kg IV/SQ 3×/wk; adjust dose q4–6wk PRN. *Surgery:* 300 units/kg/d × 10 d before to 4 d after; ↓ dose if Hct ~ 36% or Hgb, ↑ > ≥ 12 g/dL or

Hgb ↑ >1 g/dL in 2-wk period; hold dose if Hgb >12 g/dL **Caution:** [C, +] **CI:** Uncontrolled HTN **Disp:** Inj 2000, 3000, 4000, 10,000, 20,000, 40,000 units/mL **SE:** HTN, HA, fatigue, fever, tachycardia, N/V **Notes:** Refrigerate; monitor baseline & posttreatment Hct/Hgb, BP, ferritin

Epoprostenol (Flolan) Uses: *Pulm HTN* **Acts:** Dilates pulm/systemic arterial vascular beds; ↓ plt aggregation **Dose:** Initial 2 ng/kg/min; ↑ by 2 ng/kg/min q15min until dose-limiting SE (CP, dizziness, N/V, HA, ↓ BP, flushing); IV cont Inf 4 ng/kg/min < max tolerated rate; adjust based on response; see PI **Caution:** [B, ?] ↑ tox w/ diuretics, vasodilators, acetate in dialysis fluids, anticoagulants **CI:** Chronic use in CHF 2nd degree, if pt develops pulm edema w/ dose initiation, severe LVSD **Disp:** Inj 0.5, 1.5 mg **SE:** Flushing, tachycardia, CHF, fever, chills, nervousness, HA, N/V/D, jaw pain, flu-like Sxs **Notes:** Abrupt D/C can cause rebound pulm HTN; monitor bleeding w/ other antiplatelet/anticoagulants; watch ↓ BP w/ other vasodilators/diuretics

Eprosartan (Teveten) Uses: *HTN*, DN, CHF **Acts:** ARB **Dose:** 400–800 mg/d single dose or bid **Caution:** [C (1st tri); D (2nd & 3rd tri), D/C immediately when PRG detected) w/ Li, ↑ K⁺ w/ K⁺-sparing diuretics/supls/high-dose trimethoprim **CI:** Bilateral RAS, 1st-degree aldosteronism **Disp:** Tabs 400, 600 mg **SE:** Fatigue, depression, URI, UTI, Abd pain, rhinitis/pharyngitis/cough, hypertriglyceridemia

Eptifibatide (Integrilin) Uses: *ACS, PCI* **Acts:** Glycoprotein IIb/IIIa inhib **Dose:** 180 mcg/kg IV bolus, then 2 mcg/kg/min cont Inf; ↓ in renal impair (SCr >2 mg/dL, <4 mg/dL: 135 mcg/kg bolus & 0.5 mcg/kg/min Inf); *ACS:* 180 mcg/kg IV bolus then 2 mcg/kg/min. *PCI:* 135 mcg/kg IV bolus then 0.5 mcg/kg/min; bolus again in 10 min *(ECC 2005)* **Caution:** [B, ?] Monitor bleeding w/ other anticoagulants **CI:** Other glycoprotein IIb/IIIa inhib, Hx abnormal bleeding, hemorrhagic stroke (w/in 30 d), severe HTN, major surgery (w/in 6 wk), plt count <100,000 cells/mm³, renal dialysis **Disp:** Inj 0.75, 2 mg/mL **SE:** Bleeding, ↓ BP, Inj site Rxn, thrombocytopenia **Notes:** Monitor bleeding, coagulants, plts, SCr, activated coagulation time (ACT) w/ prothrombin consumption index (keep ACT 200–300 s)

Erlotinib (Tarceva) Uses: *NSCLC after failing 1 chemotherapy; maint NSCLC who have not progressed after 4 cycles cisplatin based therapy, CA pancreas* **Acts:** HER2/EGFR TKI **Dose:** CA pancreas 100 mg, others 150 mg/d PO 1 h ac or 2 h pc; ↓ (in 50-mg decrements) w/ severe Rxn or w/ CYP3A4 inhib (Table 10 p 280); per protocols **Caution:** [D, ?/–]avoid pregnancy; w/ CYP3A4 inhib (Table 10 p 280) **Disp:** Tabs 25, 100, 150 mg **SE:** Rash, N/V/D, anorexia, Abd pain, fatigue, cough, dyspnea, edema, stomatitis, conjunctivitis, pruritus, skin/nail changes, infxn, ↑ LFTs, interstitial lung Dz **Notes:** May ↑ INR w/ warfarin, monitor INR

Ertapenem (Invanz) Uses: *Complicated intra-Abd, acute pelvic, & skin infxns, pyelonephritis, CAP* **Acts:** α carbapenem; β-lactam antibiotic, ↓ cell wall synth. *Spectrum:* Good gram(+/–) & anaerobic coverage, not *Pseudomonas,*

PCN-resistant pneumococci, MRSA, *Enterococcus*, β-lactamase (+) *H. influenzae*, *Mycoplasma*, *Chlamydia* **Dose:** *Adults.* 1 g IM/IV daily; 500 mg/d in CrCl <30 mL/min. *Peds 3 mo–12 y:* 15 mg/kg bid IM/IV, max 1 g/d **Caution:** [B, ?/–] Sz Hx, CNS disorders, β-lactam & multiple allergies, probenecid ↓ renal clearance **CI:** component hypersens or amide anesthetics **Disp:** Inj 1 g/vial **SE:** HA, N/V/D, Inj site Rxns, thrombocytosis, ↑ LFTs **Notes:** Can give IM × 7 d, IV × 14 d; 137 mg Na⁺ (6 mEq)/g ertapenem

Erythromycin (E-Mycin, E.E.S., Ery-Tab, EryPed, Ilotycin) **Uses:** *Bacterial infxns; bowel prep*; ↑ GI motility (*prokinetic*); *acne vulgaris* **Acts:** Bacteriostatic; interferes w/ protein synth. *Spectrum:* Group A streptococci (*S. pyogenes*), *S. pneumoniae*, *N. meningitidis*, *N. gonorrhoeae* (if PCN-allergic), *Legionella*, *M. pneumoniae* **Dose:** *Adults.* Base 250–500 mg PO q6–12h or ethylsuccinate 400–800 mg q6–12h; 500 mg–1 g IV q6h. *Prokinetic:* 250 mg PO tid 30 min ac. *Peds.* 30–50 mg/kg/d PO ÷ q6–8h or 20–40 mg/kg/d IV ÷ q6h, max 2 g/d **Caution:** [B, +] ↑ tox of carbamazepine, cyclosporine, digoxin, methylprednisolone, theophylline, felodipine, warfarin, simvastatin/lovastatin; ↓ sildenafil dose w/ use **CI:** Hepatic impair, preexisting liver Dz (estolate), use w/ pimozide **Disp:** *Lactobionate (Ilotycin):* Powder for Inj 500 mg, 1 g. *Base:* Tabs 250, 333, 500 mg; caps 250 mg. *Estolate (Ilosone):* Susp 125, 250 mg/5 mL. *Stearate (Erythrocin):* Tabs 250, 500 mg. *Ethylsuccinate (EES, EryPed):* Chew tabs 200 mg; tabs 400 mg; susp 200, 400 mg/5 mL **SE:** HA, Abd pain, N/V/D; [QT prolongation, torsades de pointes, ventricular arrhythmias/tachycardias (rarely)]; cholestatic jaundice (estolate) **Notes:** 400 mg ethylsuccinate = 250 mg base/estolate; w/ food minimizes GI upset; lactobionate contains benzyl alcohol (caution in neonates)

Erythromycin & Benzoyl Peroxide (Benzamycin) **Uses:** *Topical for acne vulgaris* **Acts:** Macrolide antibiotic w/ keratolytic **Dose:** Apply bid (A.M. & P.M.) **Caution:** [C, ?] **CI:** Component sensitivity **Disp:** Gel erythromycin 30 mg/benzoyl peroxide 50 mg/g **SE:** Local irritation, dryness

Erythromycin & Sulfisoxazole (Eryzole, Pediazole) **Uses:** *Upper & lower resp tract; bacterial infxns; H. influenzae otitis media in children*; infxns in PCN-allergic pts **Acts:** Macrolide antibiotic w/ sulfonamide **Dose:** *Adults.* Based on erythromycin content; 400 mg erythromycin/1200 mg sulfisoxazole PO q6h. *Peds >2 mo:* 40–50 mg/kg/d erythromycin & 150 mg/kg/d sulfisoxazole PO ÷ q6h; max 2 g/d erythromycin or 6 g/d sulfisoxazole × 10 d; ↓ in renal impair **Caution:** [C (D if near term), +] w/ PO anticoagulants, hypoglycemics, phenytoin, cyclosporine **CI:** Infants <2 mo **Disp:** Susp erythromycin ethylsuccinate 200 mg/sulfisoxazole 600 mg/5 mL (100, 150, 200 mL) **SE:** GI upset

Erythromycin, ophthalmic (Ilotycin Ophthalmic) **Uses:** *Conjunctival/corneal infxns* **Acts:** Macrolide antibiotic **Dose:** 1/2 inch 2–6×/d **Caution:** [B, +] **CI:** Erythromycin hypersens **Disp:** 0.5% oint **SE:** Local irritation

Erythromycin, topical (A/T/S, Eryderm, Erycette, T-Stat) **Uses:** *Acne vulgaris* **Acts:** Macrolide antibiotic **Dose:** Wash & dry area, apply 2%

product over area bid **Caution:** [B, +] **CI:** Component sensitivity **Disp:** Soln 1.5%, 2%; gel 2%; pads & swabs 2% **SE:** Local irritation

Escitalopram (Lexapro) **BOX:** Closely monitor for worsening depression or emergence of suicidality, particularly in peds pts **Uses:** Depression, anxiety **PCs:** SSRI **Dose:** *Adults.* 10–20 mg PO daily; 10 mg/d in elderly & hepatic impair **Caution:** [C, +/−] Serotonin synd (Table 11 p 282); use of escitalopram, w/ NSAID, ASA, or other drugs affecting coagulation associated w/ ↑ bleeding risk **CI:** w/ or w/ in 14 d of MAOI **Disp:** Tabs 5, 10, 20 mg; soln 1 mg/mL **SE:** N/V/D, sweating, insomnia, dizziness, xerostomia, sexual dysfunction **Notes:** Full effects may take 3 wk

Esmolol (Brevibloc) **Uses:** *SVT & noncompensatory sinus tachycardia, AF/A flutter* **Acts:** β_1-Adrenergic blocker; class II antiarrhythmic **Dose:** *Adults & Peds.* Initial 500 mcg/kg load over 1 min, then 50 mcg/kg/min × 4 min; if inadequate response, repeat load & maint Inf of 100 mcg/kg/min × 4 min; titrate by repeating load, then incremental ↑ in the maint dose of 50 mcg/kg/min for 4 min until desired HR reached or ↓ BP; average dose 100 mcg/kg/min; 0.5 mg/kg over 1 min, then 0.05 mg/kg/min *(ECC 2005)* **Caution:** [C (1st tri; D 2nd or 3rd tri), ?] **CI:** Sinus bradycardia, heart block, uncompensated CHF, cardiogenic shock, ↓ BP **Disp:** Inj 10, 20, 250 mg/mL; premix Inf 10 mg/mL **SE:** ↓ BP, ↑ HR, diaphoresis, dizziness, pain on Inj **Notes:** Hemodynamic effects back to baseline w/in 30 min after D/C Inf

Esomeprazole (Nexium) **Uses:** *Short-term (4–8 wk) for erosive esophagitis/GERD; H. pylori Infxn in combo w/ antibiotics* **Acts:** Proton pump inhib, ↓ gastric acid **Dose:** *Adults. GERD/erosive gastritis:* 20–40 mg/d PO × 4–8 wk; 20–40 mg IV 10–30 min Inf or >3 min IV push, 10 d max; *Maint:* 20 mg/d PO. *H. pylori Infxn:* 40 mg/d PO, plus clarithromycin 500 mg PO bid & amoxicillin 1000 mg/bid for 10 d; **Caution:** [B, ?/−] **CI:** Component sensitivity; do not use w/ clopidogrel (↓ effect) **Disp:** Caps 20, 40 mg; IV 20, 40 mg **SE:** HA, D, Abd pain **Notes:** Do not chew; may open caps & sprinkle on applesauce; ? ↑ risk of fractures w/ all PPI

Estazolam (ProSom) [C-IV] **Uses:** *Short-term management of insomnia* **Acts:** Benzodiazepine **Dose:** 1–2 mg PO qhs PRN; ↓ in hepatic impair/elderly/debilitated **Caution:** [X, −] ↑ Effects w/ CNS depressants; cross-sensitivity w/ other benzodiazepines **CI:** PRG, component hypersens, w/ itraconazole or ketoconazole **Disp:** Tabs 1, 2 mg **SE:** Somnolence, weakness, palpitations, anaphylaxis, angioedema, amnesia **Notes:** May cause psychological/physical dependence; avoid abrupt D/C after prolonged use

Esterified Estrogens (Estratab, Menest) **BOX:** ↑ Risk endometrial CA. Do not use in the prevention of CV Dz or dementia; ↑ risk of MI, stroke, breast CA, PE, DVT, in postmenopausal **Uses:** *Vasomotor Sxs or vulvar/vag atrophy w/ menopause*; female hypogonadism, PCa, prevent osteoporosis **Acts:** Estrogen supl **Dose:** *Menopausal vasomotor Sx:* 0.3–1.25 mg, cyclically 3 wk on, 1 wk off; add progestin 10–14 d w/ 28-d cycle w/ uterus intact; *Vulvovaginal atrophy:* same regimen except use 0.3–1.25 mg; *Hypogonadism:* 2.5–7.5 mg/d PO × 20 d, off

× 10 d; add progestin 10–14 d w/ 28-d cycle w/uterus intact **Caution:** [X, –] **CI:** Undiagnosed genital bleeding, breast CA, estrogen-dependent tumors, thromboembolic disorders, thrombophlebitis, recent MI, PRG, severe hepatic Dz **Disp:** Tabs 0.3, 0.625, 1.25, 2.5 mg **SE:** N, HA, bloating, breast enlargement/tenderness, edema, venous thromboembolism, hypertriglyceridemia, gallbladder Dz **Notes:** Use lowest dose for shortest time (see WHI data [www.whi.org])

Esterified Estrogens + Methyltestosterone (Estratest, Estratest HS, Syntest DS, HS) **BOX:** ↑ Risk endometrial CA. Avoid in PRG. Do not use in the prevention of CV Dz or dementia; ↑ risk of MI, stroke, breast CA, PE, DVT in postmenopausal women **Uses:** *Vasomotor Sxs*; postpartum breast engorgement **Acts:** Estrogen & androgen supl **Dose:** 1 tab/d × 3 wk, 1 wk off **Caution:** [X, –] **CI:** Genital bleeding of unknown cause, breast CA, estrogen-dependent tumors, thromboembolic disorders, thrombophlebitis, recent MI, PRG **Disp:** Tabs (estrogen/methyltestosterone) 0.625 mg/1.25 mg, 1.25 mg/2.5 mg **SE:** N, HA, bloating, breast enlargement/tenderness, edema, ↑ triglycerides, venous thromboembolism, gallbladder Dz **Notes:** Use lowest dose for shortest time; (see WHI data [www.whi.org])

Estradiol, gel (Divigel) **BOX:** ↑ Risk of endometrial CA. Do not use in the prevention of CV Dz or dementia; ↑ risk MI, stroke, breast CA, PE, and DVT in postmenopausal women (50–79 y). ↑ Dementia risk in postmenopausal women (≥65 y) **Uses:** *Vasomotor Sx in menopause* **Acts:** Estrogen **Dose:** 0.25 g q day on right or left upper thigh **Caution:** [X, +/–] may ↑ PT/PTT/plt aggregation w/ thyroid Dz **CI:** Undiagnosed genital bleeding, breast CA, estrogen-dependent tumors, thromboembolic disorders, thrombophlebitis, recent MI, PRG, severe hepatic Dz **Disp:** 0.1% gel 0.25/0.5/ 1 g single-dose foil packets w/ 0.25, 0.5, 1-mg estradiol, respectively **SE:** N, HA, bloating, breast enlargement/tenderness, edema, venous thromboembolism, ↑ BP, hypertriglyceridemia, gallbladder Dz **Notes:** If person other than pt applies, glove should be used, keep dry immediately after, rotate site; contains alcohol, caution around flames until dry, not for vag use

Estradiol, Gel (Elestrin) **BOX:** Do not use in the prevention of CV Dz or dementia; ↑ risk MI, stroke, breast CA, PE, and DVT in postmenopausal women **Uses:** *Postmenopausal vasomotor Sxs* **Acts:** Estrogen **Dose:** Apply 0.87–1.7 g to skin q day; add progestin × 10–14 d/28-d cycle w/ intact uterus; use lowest effective estrogen dose **Caution:** [X, ?] **CI:** AUB, breast CA, estrogen-dependent tumors, thromboembolic disorders, recent MI, PRG, severe hepatic Dz **Disp:** Gel 0.06% **SE:** Thromboembolic events, MI, stroke, ↑ BP, breast/ovarian/endometrial CA, site Rxns, vag spotting, breast changes, Abd bloating, cramps, HA, fluid retention **Notes:** Apply to upper arm, wait >25 min before sunscreen; avoid concomitant use for >7 d; BP, breast exams

Estradiol, Oral (Estrace, Delestrogen, Femtrace) **BOX:** ↑ Risk of endometrial CA; avoid in PRG **Uses:** *Atrophic vaginitis, menopausal vasomotor Sxs,↑ low estrogen levels, palliation breast and PCa* **Acts:** Estrogen **Dose:** *PO:* 1–2 mg/d, adjust PRN to control Sxs. *Vaginal cream:* 2–4 g/d × 2 wk, then 1 g 1–3×/wk. *Vasomotor Sx/vag Atrophy:* 10–20 mg IM q4wk, D/C or taper at 3–6-mo intervals. *Hypoestrogenism:* 10–20 mg IM q4wk. *PCa:* 30 mg IM q12wk **Caution:** [X, –] **CI:** Genital bleeding of unknown cause, breast CA, porphyria, estrogen-dependent tumors, thromboembolic disorders, thrombophlebitis; recent MI; hepatic impair **Disp** Ring 0.05, 0.1, 2 mg; gel 0.061%; tabs 0.5, 1, 2 mg; vag cream 0.1 mg/g, depot Inj (Delestrogen) 10, 20, 40 mg/mL **SE:** N, HA, bloating, breast enlargement/tenderness, edema, ↑ triglycerides, venous thromboembolism, gallbladder Dz

Estradiol, spray (Evamist) BOX: ↑ Risk of endometrial CA. Do not use in the prevention of CV Dz or dementia; ↑ risk MI, stroke, breast CA, PE, and DVT in postmenopausal women (50–79 y). ↑ Dementia risk in postmenopausal women (≥65 y) **Uses:** *Vasomotor Sx in menopause* **Acts:** Estrogen supl **Dose:** 1 spray on inner surface of forearm **Caution:** [X, +/–] May ↑ PT/PTT/plt aggregation w/ thyroid Dz **CI:** Undiagnosed genital bleeding, breast CA, estrogen-dependent tumors, thromboembolic disorders, thrombophlebitis, recent MI, PRG, severe hepatic Dz **Disp:** 1.53 mg/spray (56-sprays container) **SE:** N, HA, bloating, breast enlargement/tenderness, edema, venous thromboembolism, ↑ BP, hypertriglyceridemia, gallbladder Dz **Notes:** Contains alcohol, caution around flames until dry; not for vag use

Estradiol, Transdermal (Estraderm, Climara, Vivelle, Vivelle Dot) BOX: ↑ Risk of endometrial CA. Do not use in the prevention of CV Dz or dementia; ↑ risk MI, stroke, breast CA, PE, and DVT in postmenopausal women (50–79 y). ↑ Dementia risk in postmenopausal women (≥65 y) **Uses:** *Severe menopausal vasomotor Sxs; female hypogonadism* **Acts:** Estrogen supl **Dose:** Start 0.0375–0.05 mg/d patch 2× /wk based on product; adjust PRN to control Sxs; w/ intact uterus cycle 3 wk on 1 wk off or use cyclic progestin 10–14 d **Caution:** [X, –] See Estradiol **CI:** PRG, AUB, porphyria, breast CA, estrogen-dependent tumors, Hx thrombophlebitis, thrombosis **Disp:** Transdermal patches (mg/24 h) 0.025, 0.0375, 0.05, 0.06, 0.075, 0.1 **SE:** N, bloating, breast enlargement/tenderness, edema, HA, hypertriglyceridemia, gallbladder Dz **Notes:** Do not apply to breasts, place on trunk, rotate sites

Estradiol, vaginal (Estring, Femring, Vagifem) BOX: ↑ Risk of endometrial CA. Do not use in the prevention of CV Dz or dementia; ↑ risk MI, stroke, breast CA, PE, and DVT in postmenopausal women (50–79 y) **Uses:** *Postmenopausal vag atrophy (Estring)* *vasomotor Sxs and vulvar/vag atrophy associated w/ menopause(Femring)* *atrophic vaginitis (Vagifem)* **Acts:** Estrogen supl **Dose:** *Estring:* Insert ring into upper third of vag vault; remove and replace after 90 d; reassess 3–6 mo; *Femring:* use lowest effective dose, insert vaginally, replace q3mo; *Vagifem:* 1 tab vaginally q day × 2 wk, then maint 1 tab 2×/wk, D/C or taper at 3–6 mo **Caution:** [X, –] May ↑ PT/PTT/plt aggregation w/ thyroid Dz, toxic shock reported **CI:** Undiagnosed genital bleeding, breast CA, estrogen-dependent tumors, thromboembolic disorders, thrombophlebitis, recent MI, PRG, severe hepatic Dz **Disp:** *Estring ring:* 0.0075 mg/24 h; *Femring ring:* 0.05

and 0.1 mg/d *Vagifem tab (vag):* 25 mcg **SE:** HA, leukorrhea, back pain, candidiasis, vaginitis, vag discomfort/hemorrhage, arthralgia, insomnia, Abd pain

Estradiol/Levonorgestrel, Transdermal (Climara Pro) BOX: ↑ Risk of endometrial CA. Do not use in the prevention of CV Dz or dementia; ↑ risk MI, stroke, breast CA, PE, and DVT in postmenopausal women (50–79 y). ↑ Dementia risk in postmenopausal women (≥65 y) **Uses:** *Menopausal vasomotor Sx; prevent postmenopausal osteoporosis* **Acts:** Estrogen & progesterone **Dose:** 1 Patch 1×/wk **Caution:** [X, −] w/ ↓ Thyroid **CI:** AUB, estrogen-sensitive tumors, Hx thromboembolism, liver impair, PRG, hysterectomy **Disp:** Estradiol 0.045 mg/levonorgestrel 0.015/mg day patch **SE:** Site Rxn, vag bleed/spotting, breast changes, Abd bloating/cramps, HA, retention fluid, edema, ↑ BP **Notes:** Apply lower Abd; for osteoporosis give Ca²⁺/vit D supl; follow breast exams

Estradiol/Medroxyprogesterone (Lunelle) BOX: Cigarette smoking ↑ risk of serious CV SEs from contraceptives w/ estrogen. This risk ↑ w/ age & w/ heavy smoking (>15 cigarettes/d) & is marked in women >35 y. Women who use Lunelle should not smoke **Uses:** *Contraceptive* **Acts:** Estrogen & progestin **Dose:** 0.5 mL IM (deltoid, anterior thigh, buttock) monthly, do not exceed 33 d **Caution:** [X, M] HTN, gallbladder Dz, ↑ lipids, migraines, sudden HA, valvular heart Dz w/ comps **CI:** PRG, heavy smokers >35 y, DVT, PE, cerebro-/CV Dz, estrogen-dependent neoplasm, undiagnosed AUB, porphyria, hepatic tumors, cholestatic jaundice **Disp:** Estradiol cipionate (5 mg), medroxyprogesterone acetate (25 mg) single-dose vial or syringe (0.5 mL) **SE:** Arterial thromboembolism, HTN, cerebral hemorrhage, MI, amenorrhea, acne, breast tenderness **Notes:** Start w/in 5 d of menstruation

Estradiol/Norethindrone (FemHRT, Activella) BOX: ↑ Risk of endometrial CA. Do not use in the prevention of CV Dz or dementia; ↑ risk MI, stroke, breast CA, PE, and DVT in postmenopausal women (50–79 y). ↑ Dementia risk in postmenopausal women (≥65 y) **Uses:** *Menopause vasomotor Sxs; prevent osteoporosis* **Acts:** Estrogen/progestin; plant derived **Dose:** 1 tab/d start w/ lowest dose combo **Caution:** [X, −] w/ ↓ Ca²⁺/thyroid **CI:** PRG; Hx breast CA; estrogen-dependent tumor; abnormal genital bleeding; Hx DVT, PE, or related disorders; recent (w/in past year) arterial thromboembolic Dz (CVA, MI) **Disp:** *Femhrt:* Tabs 2.5/0.5, 5 mcg/1 mg; *Activella:* tabs 1/0.5, 0.5 mg/0.1 mg **SE:** Thrombosis, dizziness, HA, libido changes, insomnia, emotional instability, breast pain **Notes:** Use in women w/ intact uterus; caution in heavy smokers

Estramustine Phosphate (Emcyt) Uses: *Advanced PCa* **Acts:** estradiol w/ nitrogen mustard; exact mechanism unknown **Dose:** 14 mg/kg/d in 3–4 ÷ doses; on empty stomach, no dairy products **Caution:** [NA, not used in females] **CI:** Active thrombophlebitis or thromboembolic disorders **Disp:** Caps 140 mg **SE:** N/V, exacerbation of preexisting CHF, edema, hepatic disturbances, thrombophlebitis, MI, PE, gynecomastia in 20–100% **NOTE:** low-dose breast irradiation before may ↓ gynecomastia

Estrogen, Conjugated (Premarin) **BOX:** ↑ Risk of endometrial CA. Do not use in the prevention of CV Dz or dementia; ↑ risk MI, stroke, breast CA, PE, and DVT in postmenopausal women (50–79 y). ↑ Dementia risk in postmenopausal women (≥65 y) **Uses:** *Mod–severe menopausal vasomotor Sxs; atrophic vaginitis; palliative advanced CAP; prevention & Tx of estrogen deficiency osteoporosis* **Acts:** Estrogen replacement **Dose:** 0.3–1.25 mg/d PO cyclically; prostatic CA 1.25–2.5 mg PO tid; **Caution:** [X, –] **CI:** Severe hepatic impair, genital bleeding of unknown cause, breast CA, estrogen-dependent tumors, thromboembolic disorders, thrombosis, thrombophlebitis, recent MI **Disp:** Tabs 0.3, 0.45, 0.625, 0.9, 1.25, 2.5 mg; vag cream 0.625 mg/g **SE:** ↑ Risk of endometrial CA, gallbladder Dz, thromboembolism, HA, & possibly breast CA **Notes:** generic products not equivalent

Estrogen, Conjugated Synthetic (Cenestin, Enjuvia) **BOX:** ↑ Risk of endometrial CA. Do not use in the prevention of CV Dz or dementia; ↑ risk MI, stroke, breast CA, PE, and DVT in postmenopausal women (50–79 y). ↑ Dementia risk in postmenopausal women (≥65 y) **Uses:** *Vasomotor menopausal Sxs, vulvovaginal atrophy, prevent postmenopausal osteoporosis* **Acts:** Multiple estrogen replacement **Dose:** For all w/ intact uterus progestin × 10–14 d/28-d cycle; *Vasomotor:* 0.3–1.25 mg (Enjuvia) 0.625–1.25 mg (Cenestin) PO daily; *Vag atrophy:* 0.3 mg/d; *Osteoporosis:* (Cenestin) 0.625 mg/d **Caution:** [X, –] **CI:** See Estrogen, conjugated **Disp:** Tabs, Cenestin 0.3, 0.45, 0.625, 0.9 mg; Enjuvia ER 0.3, 0.45, 0.625, 1.25 mg **SE:** ↑ Risk endometrial/breast CA, gallbladder Dz, thromboembolism

Estrogen, Conjugated + Medroxyprogesterone (Prempro, Premphase) **BOX:** Should not be used for the prevention of CV Dz or dementia; ↑ risk of MI, stroke, breast CA, PE, & DVT; ↑ risk of dementia in postmenopausal women **Uses:** *Mod–severe menopausal vasomotor Sxs; atrophic vaginitis; prevent postmenopausal osteoporosis* **Acts:** Hormonal replacement **Dose:** Prempro 1 tab PO daily; Premphase 1 tab PO daily **Caution:** [X, –] **CI:** Severe hepatic impair, genital bleeding of unknown cause, breast CA, estrogen-dependent tumors, thromboembolic disorders, thrombosis, thrombophlebitis **Disp:** (As estrogen/medroxyprogesterone) *Prempro:* Tabs 0.625/2.5, 0.625/5 mg; *Premphase:* Tabs 0.625/0 (d 1–14) & 0.625/5 mg (d 15–28) **SE:** Gallbladder Dz, thromboembolism, HA, breast tenderness **Notes:** See WHI (www.whi.org)

Estrogen, Conjugated + Methyl progesterone (Premarin + Methyl progesterone) **BOX:** Do not use in the prevention of CV Dz or dementia; ↑ risk of endometrial CA **Uses:** *Menopausal vasomotor Sxs; osteoporosis* **Acts:** Estrogen & androgen combo **Dose:** 1 tab/d **Caution:** [X, –] **CI:** Severe hepatic impair, AUB, breast CA, estrogen-dependent tumors, thrombosis, thrombophlebitis **Disp:** Tabs 0.625 mg estrogen, conjugated, & 2.5 or 5 mg of methyl progesterone **SE:** N, bloating, breast enlargement/tenderness, edema, HA, hypertriglyceridemia, gallbladder Dz

Estrogen, Conjugated + Methyltestosterone (Premarin + Methyltestosterone) **BOX:** Do not use in the prevention of CV Dz or dementia;

↑ risk of endometrial CA **Uses:** *Mod–severe menopausal vasomotor Sxs*; postpartum breast engorgement **Acts:** Estrogen & androgen combo **Dose:** 1 tab/d × 3 wk, then 1 wk off **Caution:** [X, –] **CI:** Severe hepatic impair, genital bleeding of unknown cause, breast CA, estrogen-dependent tumors, thromboembolic disorders, thrombophlebitis **Disp:** Tabs (estrogen/methyltestosterone) 0.625 mg/5 mg, 1.25 mg/10 mg **SE:** N, bloating, breast enlargement/tenderness, edema, HA, hypertriglyceridemia, gallbladder Dz

Eszopiclone (Lunesta) [C-IV] **Uses:** *Insomnia* **Acts:** Nonbenzodiazepine hypnotic **Dose:** 2–3 mg/d hs *Elderly:* 1–2 mg/d hs; w/ hepatic impair use w/ CYP3A4 inhib (Table 10 p 280): 1 mg/d hs **Caution:** [C, ?/–] **Disp:** Tabs 1, 2, 3 mg **SE:** HA, xerostomia, dizziness, somnolence, anaphylaxis, Infxn, unpleasant taste, anaphylaxis, angioedema **Notes:** High-fat meals ↓ absorption

Etanercept (Enbrel) **BOX:** Serious infxns (bacterial sepsis, TB, reported); D/C w/ severe Infxn. Evaluate for TB risk; test for TB before use; lymphoma/other CA possible in children/adolescents possible **Uses:** *↓ Sxs of RA in pts who fail other DMARD*, Crohn Dz **Acts:** TNF receptor blocker **Dose:** *Adults.* RA 50 mg SQ weekly or 25 mg SQ 2×/wk (separated by at least 72–96 h). *Peds 4–17 y:* 0.8 mg/kg/wk (max 50 mg/wk) or 0.4 mg/kg (max 25 mg/dose) 2×/wk 72–96 h apart **Caution:** [B, ?] w/ Predisposition to Infxn (i.e., DM); may ↑ risk of malignancy in peds and young adults **CI:** Active Infxn **Disp:** Inj 25 mg/vial, 50 mg/mL syringe **SE:** HA, rhinitis, Inj site Rxn, URI, new onset psoriasis **Notes:** Rotate Inj sites

Ethambutol (Myambutol) **Uses:** *Pulm TB* & other mycobacterial infxns, MAC **Acts:** ↓ RNA synth **Dose:** *Adults & Peds >12 y:* 15–25 mg/kg/d PO single dose; ↓ in renal impair, take w/ food, avoid antacids **Caution:** [C, +] **CI:** unconscious pts, optic neuritis **Disp:** Tabs 100, 400 mg **SE:** HA, hyperuricemia, acute gout, Abd pain, ↑ LFTs, optic neuritis, GI upset

Ethinyl Estradiol (Estinyl, Feminone) **BOX:** ↑ Risk endometrial CA. Avoid in PRG. Do not use in the prevention of CV Dz or dementia; ↑ risk of MI, stroke, breast CA, PE, DVT, in postmenopausal women **Uses:** *Menopausal vasomotor Sxs; female hypogonadism* **Acts:** Estrogen supl **Dose:** 0.02–1.5 mg/d ÷ daily–tid **Caution:** [X, –] **CI:** Severe hepatic impair; genital bleeding of unknown cause, breast CA, estrogen-dependent tumors, thromboembolic disorders, thrombophlebitis **Disp:** Tabs 0.02, 0.05, 0.5 mg **SE:** N, bloating, breast enlargement/tenderness, edema, HA, hypertriglyceridemia, gallbladder Dz

Ethinyl Estradiol & Norelgestromin (Ortho Evra) **Uses:** *Contraceptive patch* **Acts:** Estrogen & progestin **Dose:** Apply patch to abd, buttocks, upper torso (not breasts), or upper outer arm at the beginning of the menstrual cycle; new patch is applied weekly for 3 wk; wk 4 is patch-free **Caution:** [X, M] **CI:** PRG, Hx or current DVT/PE, stroke, MI, CV Dz, CAD; SBP ≥ 160 systolic mm Hg or DBP ≥ 100 diastolic mm Hg severe HTN; severe HA w/ focal neurologic Sx; breast/endometrial CA; estrogen-dependent neoplasms; hepatic dysfunction; jaundice; major surgery w/ prolonged immobilization; heavy smoking if >35 y **Disp:** 20 cm² patch (6 mg norelgestromin [active metabolite norgestimate] & 0.75 mg of ethinyl estradiol) **SE:** Breast discomfort, HA, site Rxns, N, menstrual cramps; thrombosis risks similar to OCP **Notes:** Less effective in women >90 kg; instruct pt does not protect against STD/HIV; discourage smoking

Ethosuximide (Zarontin) **Uses:** *Absence (petit mal) Szs* **Acts:** Anticonvulsant; ↑ Sz threshold **Dose:** *Adults & peds >6 y:* Initial, 500 mg PO ÷ bid; ↑ by 250 mg/d q4–7d PRN (max 1500 mg/d) usual maint 20–30 mg/kg. *Peds 3–6 y:* Initial: 15 mg/kg/d PO ÷ bid. *Maint:* 15–40 mg/kg/d ÷ bid, max 1500 mg/d **Caution:** [D, +] In renal/hepatic impair; antiepileptics may ↑ risk of suicidal behavior or ideation **CI:** Component sensitivity **Disp:** Caps 250 mg; syrup 250 mg/5 mL **SE:** Blood dyscrasias, GI upset, drowsiness, dizziness, irritability **Notes:** Levels: *Trough:* just before next dose; *Therapeutic:* *Peak:* 40–100 mcg/mL; *Toxic Trough:* >100 mcg/mL; *Half-life:* 25–60 h

Etidronate Disodium (Didronel) **Uses:** *↑Ca²⁺ of malignancy, Paget Dz, & heterotopic ossification* **Acts:** ↓ nl & abnormal bone resorption **Dose:** *Paget Dz:* 5–10 mg/kg/d PO ÷ doses (for 3–6 mo). ↑ *Ca²⁺:* 7.5 mg/kg/d IV Inf over 2 h × 3 d, then 20 mg/kg/d PO on last day of Inf ÷ 1–3 mo **Caution:** [B PO (C parenteral), ?] Bisphosphonates may cause severe musculoskeletal pain **CI:** Overt osteomalacia, SCr >5 mg/dL **Disp:** Tabs 200, 400 mg; Inj 50 mg/mL **SE:** GI intolerance (↓ by ÷ daily doses); hyperphosphatemia, hypomagnesemia, bone pain, abnormal taste, fever, convulsions, nephrotox **Notes:** Take PO on empty stomach 2 h before or 2 h pc

Etodolac **BOX:** May ↑ risk of CV events & GI bleeding; may worsen ↑ BP **Uses:** *OA & pain*, RA **Acts:** NSAID **Dose:** 200–400 mg PO bid-qid (max 1200 mg/d) **Caution:** [C (D 3rd tri), ?] ↑ Bleeding risk w/ ASA, warfarin; ↑ nephrotox w/ cyclosporine; Hx CHF, HTN, renal/hepatic impair, PUD **CI:** Active GI ulcer **Disp:** Tabs 400, 500 mg; ER tabs 400, 500, 600 mg; caps 200, 300 mg **SE:** N/V/D, gastritis, Abd cramps, dizziness, HA, depression, edema, renal impair **Notes:** Do not crush tabs

Etonogestrel/Ethinyl Estradiol vaginal insert (NuvaRing) **Uses:** *Contraceptive* **Acts:** Estrogen & progestin combo **Dose:** Rule out PRG first; insert ring vaginally for 3 wk, remove for 1 wk; insert new ring 7 d after last removed (even if bleeding) at same time of day ring removed. 1st day of menses is day 1, insert before day 5 even if bleeding. Use other contraception for 1st 7 d of starting Rx. See PI if converting from other contraceptive; after delivery or 2nd tri abortion, insert 4 wk postpartum (if not breast-feeding) **Caution:** [X, ?/–] HTN, gallbladder Dz, ↑ lipids, migraines, sudden HA **CI:** PRG, heavy smokers >35 y, DVT, PE, cerebro-/CV Dz, estrogen-dependent neoplasm, undiagnosed abnormal genital bleeding, hepatic tumors, cholestatic jaundice **Disp:** Intravag ring: ethinyl estradiol 0.015 mg/d & etonogestrel 0.12 mg/d **Notes:** If ring removed, rinse w/ cool/lukewarm H₂O (not hot) & reinsert ASAP; if not reinserted w/in 3 h, effectiveness ↓; do not use w/ diaphragm

Etonogestrel implant (Implanon) **Uses:** *Contraception* **Acts:** Transforms endometrium from proliferative to secretory **Dose:** 1 Implant subdermally q3y **Caution:** [X, +] Exclude PRG before implant **CI:** PRG, hormonally responsive tumors, breast CA, AUB, hepatic tumor, active liver Dz, Hx thromboembolic Dz **Disp:** 68-mg implant **SE:** Spotting, irregular periods, amenorrhea, dysmenorrhea, HA, tender breasts, N, wgt gain, acne, ectopic PRG, PE, ovarian cysts, stroke, ↑ BP **Notes:** 99% Effective; remove implant and replace; restricted distribution; physician must register and train; does not protect against STDs

Etoposide [VP-16] (VePesid, Toposar) **Uses:** *Testicular, NSCLC, Hodgkin Dz, & NHLs, peds ALL, & allogeneic/autologous BMT in high doses* **Acts:** Topoisomerase II inhib **Dose:** 50 mg/m²/d IV for 3–5 d; 50 mg/m²/d PO for 21 d (PO availability = 50% of IV); 2–6 g/m² or 25–70 mg/kg in BMT (per protocols); ↓ in renal/hepatic impair **Caution:** [D, –] **CI:** IT administration **Disp:** Caps 50 mg; Inj 20 mg/mL **SE:** N/V (Emesis in 10–30%), ↓ BM, alopecia, ↓ BP w/ rapid IV, anorexia, anemia, leukopenia, ↑ risk secondary leukemias

Etravirine (Intelence) **Uses:** *HIV* **Acts:** Non-NRTI **Dose:** 200 mg PO bid following a meal **Caution:** [B, ±] Many interactions: substrate/inducer (CYP3A4), substrate/inhib (CYP2C9, CYP2C19); do not use w/ tipranavir/ritonavir, fosamprenavir/ritonavir, atazanavir/ritonavir, protease inhib w/o ritonavir, and non-NRTIs **CI:** None **Disp:** Tabs 100 mg **SE:** N/V/D, rash, severe/potentially life-threatening skin Rxns, fat redistribution

Everolimus (Afinitor) **Uses:** * Advanced RCC w/ sunitinib or sorafenib failure * **Action:** mTOR inhib (mammalian rapamycin target) **Dose:** 10 mg PO daily, ↓ to 5 mg w/ SE or hepatic impair; avoid w/high fat meal **Caution:** [D, ?] Avoid live vaccines and those who received live vaccines and w/ CYP3A4 inhib **CI:** compound/ rapamycin derivative hypersens **Disp:** Tabs 5, 10 mg **SE:** Non-infectious pneumonitis, ↑ infxn risk, oral ulcers, asthenia, cough, fatigue, diarrhea, ↑ glucose/SCr/lipids; ↓ hemoglobin/WBC/plt **Notes:** Follow CBC, LFT, glucose, lipids; see also everolimus (Zortress)

Everolimus (Zortress) **Uses:** * Prevent renal transplant rejection; combo w/ basiliximab w/ ↓ dose of steroids and cyclosporine * **Action:** mTOR inhib (mammalian rapamycin target) **Dose:** 7.5 mg PO BID, adjust to trough levels 3-8 ng/mL **Caution:** [D, ?] **CI:** compound/ rapamycin derivative hypersens **Disp:** Tabs 0.25, 0.5,0.75 mg **SE:** peripheral edema, constipation, ↑ BP, n, ↓ Hct, UTI, ↑ lipids **Notes:** Follow CBC, LFT, glucose, lipids; see also everolimus (Afinitor)

Exemestane (Aromasin) **Uses:** *Advanced breast CA in postmenopausal women w/ progression after tamoxifen* **Acts:** Irreversible, steroidal aromatase inhib; ↓ estrogens **Dose:** 25 mg PO daily after a meal **Caution:** [D, ?/–] **CI:** PRG, component sensitivity **Disp:** Tabs 25 mg **SE:** Hot flashes, N, fatigue,↑ alkaline phosphate

Exenatide (Byetta) **Uses:** Type 2 DM combined w/ metformin &/or sulfonylurea **Acts:** Incretin mimetic: ↑ insulin release, ↓ glucagon secretion, ↓ gastric emptying, promotes satiety **Dose:** 5 mcg SQ bid w/in 60 min before A.M. & P.M. meals; ↑ to 10 mcg SQ bid after 1 mo PRN; do not give pc **Caution:** [C, ?/–] may

↓ absorption of other drugs (take antibiotics/contraceptives 1 h before) **CI:** CrCl <30 mL/min **Disp:** Soln 5, 10 mcg/dose in prefilled pen **SE:** Hypoglycemia, N/V/D, dizziness, HA, dyspepsia, ↓ appetite, jittery; acute pancreatitis **Notes:** Consider ↓ sulfonylurea to ↓ risk of hypoglycemia; discard pen 30 d after 1st use; monitor Cr

Ezetimibe (Zetia) **Uses:** *Hypercholesterolemia alone or w/ a HMG-CoA reductase inhib* **Acts:** ↓ cholesterol & phytosterols absorption **Dose:** *Adults & Peds >10 y:* 10 mg/d PO **Caution:** [C, +/−] Bile acid sequestrants ↓ bioavailability **CI:** Hepatic impair **Disp:** Tabs 10 mg **SE:** HA, D, Abd pain, ↑ transaminases w/ HMG-CoA reductase inhib, erythema multiforme

Ezetimibe/Simvastatin (Vytorin) **Uses:** *Hypercholesterolemia* **Acts:** ↓ Absorption of cholesterol & phytosterols w/ HMG-CoA-reductase inhib **Dose:** 10/10–10/80 mg/d PO; w/ cyclosporine/ or danazol: 10/10 mg/d max; w/ amiodarone/ or verapamil: 10/20 mg/d max; ↓ w/ severe renal Insuff; give 2 h before or 4 h after bile acid sequestrants **Caution:** [X, −]; w/ CYP3A4 inhib (Table 10 p 280), gemfibrozil, niacin >1 g/d, danazol, amiodarone, verapamil; avoid high dose w/diltiazem; w/Chinese pt on lipid modifying meds **CI:** PRG/lactation; liver Dz, ↑ LFTs **Disp:** Tabs (mg ezetimibe/mg simvastatin) 10/10, 10/20, 10/40, 10/80 **SE:** HA, GI upset, myalgia, myopathy (muscle pain, weakness, or tenderness w/ creatine kinase 10 × ULN, rhabdomyolysis), hep, Infxn **Notes:** Monitor LFTs, lipids; ezetimibe/simvastatin combo lowered LDL more than simvastatin alone in ENHANCE study, but was no difference in carotid-intima media thickness; pts to report muscle pain

Famciclovir (Famvir) **Uses:** *Acute herpes zoster (shingles) & genital herpes* **Acts:** ↓ Viral DNA synth **Dose:** *Zoster:* 500 mg PO q8h × 7 d. *Simplex:* 125–250 mg PO bid; ↓ w/ renal impair **Caution:** [B, −] **CI:** Component sensitivity **Disp:** Tabs 125, 250, 500 mg **SE:** Fatigue, dizziness, HA, pruritus, N/D **Notes:** Best w/in 72 h of initial lesion

Famotidine (Pepcid, Pepcid AC) [OTC] **Uses:** *Short-term Tx of duodenal ulcer & benign gastric ulcer; maint for duodenal ulcer, hypersecretory conditions, GERD, & heartburn* **Acts:** H_2-antagonist; ↓ gastric acid **Dose:** *Adults. Ulcer:* 20 mg IV q12h or 20–40 mg PO qhs × 4–8 wk. *Hypersecretion:* 20–160 mg PO q6h. *GERD:* 20 mg PO bid × 6 wk; maint: 20 mg PO hs. *Heartburn:* 10 mg PO PRN q12h. *Peds.* 0.5–1 mg/kg/d; ↓ in severe renal Insuff **Caution:** [B, M] **CI:** Component sensitivity **Disp:** Tabs 10, 20, 40 mg; chew tabs 10 mg; susp 40 mg/5 mL; gelatin caps 10 mg, Inj 10 mg/2 mL **SE:** Dizziness, HA, constipation, N/V/D, ↓ plt, hepatitis **Notes:** Chew tabs contain phenylalanine

Febuxostat (Uloric) **Uses:** *Hyperuricemia and gout* **Action:** Xanthine oxidase inhib (enzyme that converts hypoxanthine to xanthine to uric acid) **Dose:** 40 mg PO 1X daily, ↑ 80 mg if uric acid not <6 mg/dL after 2 wks **Caution:** [C, ?/−] **CI:** use w/azathioprine, mercaptopurine, theophylline **Supplied:** Tabs 40,80 mg **SE:** ↑ LFT's, rash, myalgia **Notes:** OK to continue w/ gouty flare or use w/ NSAIDs

Felodipine (Plendil) Uses: *HTN & CHF* Acts: CCB Dose: 2.5–10 mg PO daily; swallow whole; ↓ in hepatic impair Caution: [C, ?] ↑ effect w/ azole antifungals, erythromycin, grapefruit juice CI: Component sensitivity Disp: ER tabs 2.5, 5, 10 mg SE: Peripheral edema, flushing, tachycardia, HA, gingival hyperplasia Notes: Follow BP in elderly & w/ hepatic impair

Fenofibrate (TriCor, Antara, Lofibra, Lipofen, Triglide) Uses: *Hypertriglyceridemia, hypercholesteremia* Acts: ↓ Triglyceride synth Dose: 43–160 mg/d; ↓ w/ renal impair; take w/ meals Caution: [C, ?] CI: Hepatic/severe renal Insuff, primary biliary cirrhosis, unexplained ↑ LFTs, gallbladder Dz Disp: Caps 50, 100, 150 mg; caps (micronized): (Lofibra) 67, 134, 200 mg, tabs 54, 160 mg (Antara) 43, 130 mg; SE: GI disturbances, cholecystitis, arthralgia, myalgia, dizziness, ↑ LFTs Notes: Monitor LFTs

Fenofibric acid (Trilipix) Uses: * Adjunct to diet for ↑ triglycerides, to ↓ LDL-C, cholesterol, triglycerides, and apo B, to ↑ HDL-C in hypercholesterolemia/ mixed dyslipidemia; adjunct to diet w/ a statin to ↓ triglycerides and ↑ HDL-C w/ CHD or w/ CHD risk* Action: Agonist of peroxisome proliferator-activated receptor-alpha (PPAR-alpha),causes ↑ VLDL catabolism, fatty acid oxidation, and clearing of triglyceride-rich particles w/ ↓ VLDL, triglycerides; ↑ HDL in some Dose: Mixed dyslipidemia w/ a statin 135 mg PO X 1 daily; Hypertriglyceridemia: 45-135 mg 1× X daily; Maint based on response: Primary hypercholesterolemia/ mixed dyslipidemia: 135 mg PO 1 X daily; 135 mg/d MAX Caution: [C, /-], Multiple interactions, ↑ embolic phenomenon CI: Severe renal impair, pt on dialysis, active liver/gall bladder Dz, nursing Disp: DR Caps 45, 135 mg SE: HA, back pain, nasopharyngitis, URI, N/D, myalgia, gall stones, ↑ CPK (usually stabilizes), rare myositis/rhabdomyolysis Notes:✓CBC, lipid panel, LFT's; D/C if LFT > 3 ULN

Fenoldopam (Corlopam) Uses: *Hypertensive emergency* Acts: Rapid vasodilator Dose: Initial 0.03–0.1 mcg/kg/min IV Inf, titrate q15min by 1.6 mcg/kg/min, to max 0.05–0.1 mcg/kg/min Caution: [B, ?] ↓ BP w/ β-blockers CI: Allergy to sulfites Disp: Inj 10 mg/mL SE: ↓ BP, edema, facial flushing, N/V/D, atrial flutter/fibrillation, ↑ IOP Notes: Avoid concurrent β-blockers

Fenoprofen (Nalfon) BOX: May ↑ risk of CV events and GI bleeding Uses: *Arthritis & pain* Acts: NSAID Dose: 200–600 mg q4–8h, to 3200 mg/d max; w/ food Caution: [B (D 3rd tri), +/−] CHF, HTN, renal/hepatic impair, Hx PUD CI: NSAID sensitivity Disp: Caps 200, 300, 600 mg SE: GI disturbance, dizziness, HA, rash, edema, renal impair, hep Notes: Swallow whole

Fentanyl (Sublimaze) [C-II] Uses: *Short-acting analgesic* in anesthesia & PCA Acts: Narcotic analgesic Dose: Adults. 25–100 mcg/kg/dose IV/IM titrated; Anesthesia: 5–15 mcg/kg; Pain: 200 mcg over 15 min, titrate to effect Peds. 1–2 mcg/kg IV/IM q1–4h titrate; ↓ in renal impair Caution: [B, +] CI: Paralytic ileus ↑ ICP, resp depression, severe renal/hepatic impair Disp: Inj 0.05 mg/mL SE: Sedation, ↓ BP, ↓ HR, constipation, N, resp depression, miosis Notes: 0.1 mg fentanyl = 10 mg morphine IM

Fentanyl iontophoretic transdermal system (Ionsys) **BOX:** Use only w/ hospitalized pts, D/C on discharge; fentanyl may result in potentially life-threatening resp depression and death **Uses:** *Short-term in-hospital analgesia* **Acts:** Opioid narcotic, iontophoretic transdermal **Dose:** 40 mcg/activation by pt; dose given over 10 min; max over 24 h 3.2 mg (80 doses) **Caution:** [C, –] **CI:** See fentanyl **Disp:** Battery-operated self-contained transdermal system, 40 mcg/activation, 80 doses **SE:** See fentanyl, site Rxn **Notes:** Choose nl skin site chest or upper outer arm; titrate; to comfort, pts must have access to supplemental analgesia; instruct in device use; dispose properly at discharge

Fentanyl, transdermal (Duragesic) [C-II] **BOX:** Potential for abuse and fatal OD **Uses:** *Persistent mod–severe chronic pain in pts already tolerant to opioids* **Acts:** Narcotic **Dose:** Apply Patch to upper torso q72h; dose based on narcotic requirements in previous 24 h; start 25 mcg/h patch q72h; ↓ in renal impair **Caution:** [B, +] w/ CYP3A4 inhib (Table 10 p 280) may ↑ fentanyl effect, w/ Hx substance abuse **CI:** Not opioid tolerant, short-term pain management, post-op outpatient pain in outpatient surgery, mild pain, PRN use, ↑ ICP, resp depression, severe renal/hepatic impair, peds <2 y **Disp:** Patches 12.5, 25, 50, 75, 100 mcg/h **SE:** Resp depression (fatal), sedation, ↓ BP, ↓ HR, constipation, N, miosis **Notes:** 0.1 mg fentanyl = 10 mg morphine IM; do not cut patch; peak level in PRG 24–72 h

Fentanyl, transmucosal (Actiq, Fentora) [C-II] **BOX:** Potential for abuse and fatal OD; use only in CA pts w/ chronic pain who are opioid tolerant; buccal formulation ↑ bioavailability over transmucosal; do not substitute on a mcg-per-/mcg basis; use w/ strong CYP3A4 inhib may ↑ fentanyl levels **Uses:** *Breakthrough CA pain* **Acts:** Narcotic analgesic, transmucosal absorption **Dose:** Start 100 mcg buccal (Fentora) × 1, may repeat in 30 min, 4 tabs/dose max; titrate; start 200 mcg PO (Actiq) × 1, may repeat × 1 after 30 min; titrate **Caution:** [B, +] **CI:** ↑ ICP, resp depression, severe renal/hepatic impair, management of post-op or awake pain **Disp:** (Actiq) Lozenges on stick 200, 400, 600, 800, 1200, 1600 mcg; (Fentora) buccal tabs 100, 200, 300, 400, 600, 800 mcg **SE:** Sedation, ↓ BP, ↓ HR, constipation, N, resp depression, miosis **Notes:** 0.1 mg fentanyl = 10 mg IM morphine; for use in pts already tolerant to opioid Rx

Ferrous Gluconate (Fergon [OTC], others) **BOX:** Accidental OD of iron-containing products is a leading cause of fatal poisoning in children <6 y. Keep out of reach of children **Uses:** *Iron-deficiency anemia* & Fe supl **Acts:** Dietary supl **Dose:** *Adults.* 100–200 mg of elemental Fe/d ÷ doses. *Peds.* 4–6 mg/kg/d ÷ doses; on empty stomach (OK w/ meals if GI upset occurs); avoid antacids **Caution:** [A, ?] **CI:** Hemochromatosis, hemolytic anemia **Disp:** Tabs Fergon 240 (27 mg Fe), 246 (28 mg Fe), 300 (34 mg Fe), 325 (36 mg Fe) **SE:** GI upset, constipation, dark stools, discoloration of urine, may stain teeth **Notes:** 12% Elemental Fe; false(+) stool guaiac; keep away from children; severe tox in OD

Ferrous Gluconate Complex (Ferrlecit) **Uses:** *Iron deficiency anemia or supl to erythropoietin Rx therapy* **Acts:** Fe supl **Dose:** *Test dose:* 2 mL (25 mg

Fe) IV over 1 h, if OK, 125 mg (10 mL) IV over 1 h. *Usual cumulative dose:* 1 g Fe over 8 sessions (until favorable Hct) **Caution:** [B, ?] **CI:** non–Fe-deficiency anemia; CHF; Fe overload **Disp:** Inj 12.5 mg/mL Fe **SE:** ↓ BP, serious allergic Rxns, GI disturbance, Inj site Rxn **Notes:** Dose expressed as mg Fe; may infuse during dialysis

Ferrous Sulfate (OTC) **Uses:** *Fe-deficiency anemia & Fe supl* **Acts:** Dietary supl **Dose:** *Adults.* 100–200 mg elemental Fe/d in ÷ doses. *Peds.* 1–6 mg/kg/d ÷ daily–tid; on empty stomach (OK w/ meals if GI upset occurs); avoid antacids **Caution:** [A, ?] ↑ Absorption w/ vit C; ↓ absorption w/ tetracycline, fluoroquinolones, antacids, H_2 blockers, proton pump inhib **CI:** Hemochromatosis, hemolytic anemia **Disp:** Tabs 187 (60 mg Fe), 200 (65 mg Fe), 324 (65 mg Fe), 325 (65 mg Fe); SR caplets & tabs 160 (50 mg Fe), 200 mg (65 mg Fe); gtt 75 mg/0.6 mL (15 mg Fe/0.6 mL); elixir 220 mg/5 mL (44 mg Fe/5 mL); syrup 90 mg/5 mL (18 mg Fe/5 mL) **SE:** GI upset, constipation, dark stools, discolored urine

Ferumoxytol (Feraheme) **Uses:** *Iron deficiency anemia in chronic kidney disease* **Acts:** Fe replacement **Dose:** *Adults.* 510 mg IV × 1, then 510 mg IV × 1 3-8 days later; give 1ml/sec duration; for 30mins after dose, may alter MRI studies **Caution:** [C, ?/–] Monitor for hypersens & ↓ BP for 30mins after dose, may alter MRI studies **CI:** Iron overload; hypersens to ferumoxytol **Disp:** IV sol 30 mg/ml (510 mg elemental Fe/17ml) **SE:** N/D, constipation, dizziness, hypotension, peripheral edema, hypersens rxn **Notes:** ✓hematologic response 1 month after 2nd dose

Fesoterodine Fumarate (Toviaz) **Uses:** * OAB w/ urge urinary incontinence, urgency, frequency * **Action:** Competitive muscarinic receptor antagonist, ↓ bladder muscle contractions **Dose:** 4 mg PO q day, ↑ to 8 mg PO daily PRN **Caution:** [C, /?] Avoid > 4 mg w/ severe renal insuff or w/ CYP3A4 inhib (e.g., ketoconazole, clarithromycin); w/ BOO, ↓ GI motility/constipation, NAG, MyG **CI:** urinary/gastric retention, or uncontrolled NAG, hypersens to class **Disp:** Tabs 5, 10 mg **SE:** Dry mouth, constipation, ↓ sweating can cause heat prostration

Fexofenadine (Allegra, Allegra-D) **Uses:** *Allergic rhinitis; chronic idiopathic urticaria* **Acts:** Selective antihistamine, antagonizes H_1-receptors; Allegra D contains w/ pseudoephedrine **Dose:** *Adults & Peds >12 y:* 60 mg PO bid or 180 mg/d; 12-h ER form bid, 24-h ER form q day. *Peds 6–11 y:* 30 mg PO bid; ↓ in renal impair **Caution:** [C, ?] w/ Nevirapine **CI:** Component sensitivity **Disp:** Tabs 30, 60, 180 mg; susp 6 mg/mL; *Allegra-D* 12-h ER tab (60 mg fexofenadine/120 mg pseudoephedrine), *Allegra-D 24-h* ER (180 mg fexofenadine/240 mg pseudoephedrine) **SE:** Drowsiness (rare), HA, ischemic colitis

Fibrinogen concentrate, human (Riastap) **Uses:** *Rx acute bleeding associated w/ congenital fibrinogen deficiency* **Action:** Fibrinogen replacement **Dose:** *Adults & Peds.*70mg/kg IV, when baseline fibrinogen is known: Dose (mg/kg) = (Target fibrinogen level − actual fibrinogen level) ÷ 1.7. **Caution:** [C, ?] **Disp:** Inj 900-1300 mg (✓vial label) **SE:** Fever, HA, hypersens rxn, thromboembolism **Notes:** Target fibrinogen levels of 100 mg/dl

Filgrastim [G-CSF] (Neupogen) Uses: *↓ Incidence of Infxn in febrile neutropenic pts; Rx chronic neutropenia* Acts: Recombinant G-CSF Dose: *Adults & Peds.* 5 mcg/kg/d SQ or IV single daily dose; D/C when ANC >10,000 cells/mm^3 Caution: [C, ?] w/ Drugs that potentiate release of neutrophils (e.g., Li) CI: Allergy to *E. coli*-derived proteins or G-CSF Disp: Inj 300, 600 mcg/mL SE: Fever, alopecia, N/V/D, splenomegaly, bone pain, HA, rash Notes: ✓ CBC & plt; monitor for cardiac events; no benefit w/ ANC >10,000 cells/mm^3

Finasteride (Proscar [generic], Propecia) Uses: *BPH & androgenetic alopecia* Acts: ↓ 5α-Reductase Dose: *BPH:* 5 mg/d PO. *Alopecia:* 1 mg/d PO; food ↓ absorption Caution: [X, –] Hepatic impair CI: Pregnant women should avoid handling pills, teratogen to male fetus Disp: Tabs 1 mg (Propecia), 5 mg (Proscar) SE: ↓ Libido, vol ejaculate, ED, gynecomastia Notes: ↓ PSA by ~ 50%; reestablish PSA baseline 6 mo (double PSA for "true" reading); 3–6 mo for effect on urinary Sxs; continue to maintain new hair, not for use in women; potential chemoprevention for PCa; no role in diagnosed PCa

Flavoxate (Urispas) Uses: *Relief of Sx of dysuria, urgency, nocturia, suprapubic pain, urinary frequency, incontinence* Acts: Antispasmodic Dose: 100–200 mg PO tid-qid Caution: [B, ?] CI: GI obst, GI hemorrhage, ileus, achalasia, BPH Disp: Tabs 100 mg SE: Drowsiness, blurred vision, xerostomia

Flecainide (Tambocor) BOX: ↑ Mortality in pts w/ ventricular arrhythmias and recent MI; pulm effects reported; ventricular proarrhythmic effects in AF/A flutter, not ok for chronic AF Uses: Prevent AF/A flutter & PSVT, *prevent/suppress life-threatening ventricular arrhythmias* Acts: Class 1C antiarrhythmic Dose: *Adults.* 100 mg PO q12h; ↑ by 50 mg q12h q4d, to max 4400 mg/d MAX *Peds.* 3–6 mg/kg/d in 3 ÷ doses; ↓ w/ renal impair, Caution: [C, +] Monitor w/ hepatic impair, ↑ conc w/ amiodarone, digoxin, quinidine, ritonavir/amprenavir, β-blockers, verapamil; may worsen arrhythmias CI: 2nd-/3rd-degree AV block, right BBB w/ bifascicular or trifascicular block, cardiogenic shock, CAD, ritonavir/amprenavir, alkalinizing agents Disp: Tabs 50, 100, 150 mg SE: Dizziness, visual disturbances, dyspnea, palpitations, edema, chest pain, tachycardia, CHF, HA, fatigue, rash, N Notes: Initiate Rx in hospital; dose q8h if pt is intolerant/uncontrolled at q12h; *Levels: Trough:* Just before next dose; *Therapeutic:* 0.2–1 mcg/mL; *Toxic:* >1 mcg/mL; *1/2-life:* 11–14 h

Floxuridine (FUDR) BOX: Administration by experienced physician only; pts should be hospitalized for 1st course d/t risk for severe Rxn Uses: *GI adenoma, liver, renal CAs*; colon & pancreatic CAs Acts: Converted to 5-FU; inhibits thymidylate synthase; ↓ DNA synthase (S-phase specific) Dose: 0.1–0.6 mg/kg/d for 1–6 wk (per protocols) usually intraarterial for liver mets Caution: [D, –] Interaction w/ vaccines CI: BM suppression, poor nutritional status, serious Infxn, PRG, component sensitivity Disp: Inj 500 mg SE: ↓ BM, anorexia, Abd cramps, N/V/D, mucositis, alopecia, skin rash, & hyperpigmentation; rare neurotox (blurred vision, depression, nystagmus, vertigo, & lethargy); intraarterial catheter-related problems (ischemia, thrombosis, bleeding, & Infxn) **Notes:** Need effective birth control; palliative Rx for inoperable/incurable pts

Fluconazole (Diflucan) **Uses:** *Candidiasis (esophageal, oropharyngeal, urinary tract, vag, prophylaxis); cryptococcal meningitis, prophylaxis w/ BMT* **Acts:** Antifungal; ↓ cytochrome P-450 sterol demethylation. *Spectrum:* All *Candida* sp except *C. krusei* **Dose:** *Adults.* 100–400 mg/d PO or IV. *Vaginitis:* 150 mg PO daily. *Crypto:* doses up to 800 mg/d reported; 400 mg d 1, then 200 mg × 10–12 wk after CSF (–). *Peds.* 3–6 mg/kg/d PO or IV; 12 mg/kg/d/systemic Infxn; ↓ in renal impair **Caution:** [C, –] do not use w/ clopidogrel (↓ effect) **CI:** None **Disp:** Tabs 50, 100, 150, 200 mg; susp 10, 40 mg/mL; Inj 2 mg/mL **SE:** HA, rash, GI upset, ↓ K+, ↑ LFTs **Notes:** PO (preferred) = IV levels

Fludarabine Phosphate (Flamp, Fludara) **BOX:** Administer only under supervision of qualified physician experienced in chemotherapy. Can ↓ BM and cause severe CNS effects (blindness, coma, and death). Severe/fatal autoimmune hemolytic anemia reported; monitor for hemolysis. Use w/ pentostatin not ok (fatal pulm tox) **Uses:** *Autoimmune hemolytic anemia, CLL, cold agglutinin hemolysis*, low-grade lymphoma, mycosis fungoides **Acts:** ↓ Ribonucleotide reductase; blocks DNA polymerase-induced DNA repair **Dose:** 18–30 mg/m²/d for 5 d, as a 30-min Inf (per protocols); ↓ w/ renal impair **Caution:** [D, –] Give cytarabine before fludarabine (↓ its metabolism) **CI:** w/ pentostatin, severe infxns, CrCl <30 mL/min, hemolytic anemia **Disp:** Inj 50 mg **SE:** ↓ BM, N/V/D, ↑ LFTs, edema, CHF, fever, chills, fatigue, dyspnea, nonproductive cough, pneumonitis, severe CNS tox rare in leukemia, autoimmune hemolytic anemia

Fludrocortisone Acetate (Florinef) **Uses:** *Adrenocortical Insuff, Addison Dz, salt-wasting synd* **Acts:** Mineralocorticoid **Dose:** *Adults.* 0.1–0.2 mg/d PO. *Peds.* 0.05–0.1 mg/d PO **Caution:** [C, ?] **CI:** Systemic fungal infxns; known allergy **Disp:** Tabs 0.1 mg **SE:** HTN, edema, CHF, HA, dizziness, convulsions, acne, rash, bruising, hyperglycemia, hypothalamic–pituitary–adrenal suppression, cataracts **Notes:** For adrenal Insuff, use w/ glucocorticoid; dose changes based on plasma renin activity

Flumazenil (Romazicon) **Uses:** *Reverse sedative effects of benzodiazepines & general anesthesia* **Acts:** Benzodiazepine receptor antagonist **Dose:** *Adults.* 0.2 mg IV over 15 s; repeat PRN, to 1 mg max (5 mg max in benzodiazepine OD). *Peds.* 0.01 mg/kg (0.2 mg/dose max) IV over 15 s; repeat 0.005 mg/kg at 1-min intervals to 1 mg max total; ↓ in hepatic impair **Caution:** [C, ?] **CI:** TCA OD; if pts given benzodiazepines to control life-threatening conditions (ICP/status epilepticus) **Disp:** Inj 0.1 mg/mL **SE:** N/V, palpitations, HA, anxiety, nervousness, hot flashes, tremor, blurred vision, dyspnea, hyperventilation, withdrawal synd **Notes:** Does not reverse narcotic Sx or amnesia, use associated w/ Szs

Flunisolide (AeroBid, Aerospan, Nasarel) **Uses:** *Asthma in pts requiring chronic steroid Rx; relieve seasonal/perennial allergic rhinitis* **Acts:** Topical steroid **Dose:** *Adults.* Metered-dose Inh: 2 Inh bid (max 8/d). *Nasal:* 2 sprays/nostril bid (max 8/d). *Peds >6 y:* Metered-dose Inh: 2 Inh bid (max 4/d). *Nasal:*

1–2 sprays/nostril bid (max 4/d) **Caution:** [C, ?] w/ Adrenal Insuff **CI:** Status asthmaticus, viral, TB, fungal, bacterial Infxn; **Disp:** AeroBid 0.25 mg/Inh; Nasarel 29 mcg/spray; Aerospan 80 mcg/Inh (CFC-Free) **SE:** Tachycardia, bitter taste, local effects, oral candidiasis **Notes:** Not for acute asthma

Fluorouracil [5-FU] (Adrucil) **BOX:** Administration by experienced chemotherapy physician only; pts should be hospitalized for 1st course d/t risk for severe Rxn **Uses:** *Colorectal, gastric, pancreatic, breast, basal cell*, head, neck, bladder, CAs **Acts:** Inhibits thymidylate synthetase (↓ DNA synth, S-phase specific) **Dose:** 370–1000 mg/m²/d × 1–5 d IV push to 24-h cont Inf; protracted venous Inf of 200–300 mg/m²/d (per protocol); 800 mg/d max **Caution:** [D, ?] ↑ tox w/ allopurinol; do not give live vaccine before 5-FU **CI:** Poor nutritional status, depressed BM Fxn, thrombocytopenia, major surgery w/in past mo, G6PD enzyme deficiency, PRG, serious Infxn, bili >5 mg/dL **Disp:** Inj 50 mg/mL **SE:** Stomatitis, esophago-pharyngitis, N/V/D, anorexia, ↓ BM, rash/dry skin/photosens, tingling in hands/feet w/ pain (palmar–plantar erythrodysesthesia), phlebitis/discoloration at Inj sites **Notes:** ↑ Thiamine intake; contraception OK

Fluorouracil, Topical [5-FU] (Efudex) **Uses:** *Basal cell carcinoma; actinic/solar keratosis* **Acts:** Inhibits thymidylate synthetase (↓ DNA synth, S-phase specific) **Dose:** 5% cream bid × 2–6 wk **Caution:** [D, ?] Irritant chemotherapy **CI:** Component sensitivity **Disp:** Cream 0.5, 1, 5%; soln 1, 2, 5% **SE:** Rash, dry skin, photosens **Notes:** Healing may not be evident for 1–2 mo; wash hands thoroughly; avoid occlusive dressings; do not overuse

Fluoxetine (Prozac, Sarafem) **BOX:** Closely monitor for worsening depression or emergence of suicidality, particularly in peds pts **Uses:** *Depression, OCD, panic disorder, bulimia (Prozac)* *PMDD (Sarafem)* **Acts:** SSRI **Dose:** 20 mg/d PO (max 80 mg/d ÷ dose); weekly 90 mg/wk after 1–2 wk of standard dose. *Bulimia:* 60 mg q AM. *Panic disorder:* 20 mg/d. *OCD:* 20–80 mg/d. *PMDD:* 20 mg/d or 20 mg intermittently, start 14 d prior to menses, repeat w/ each cycle; ↓ in hepatic failure **Caution:** [C, ?/–] Serotonin synd w/ MAOI, SSRI, serotonin agonists, linezolid; QT prolongation w/ phenothiazines; do not use w/ clopidogrel (↓ effect) **CI:** w/ MAOI/thioridazine (wait 5 wk after D/C before MAOI) **Disp:** *Prozac:* Caps 10, 20, 40 mg; scored tabs 10, 20 mg; SR caps 90 mg; soln 20 mg/5 mL. *Sarafem:* Caps 10, 20 mg **SE:** N, nervousness, wgt loss, HA, insomnia

Fluoxymesterone (Halotestin, Androxy)[CIII] **Uses:** Androgen-responsive metastatic *breast CA, hypogonadism* **Acts:** ↓ Secretion of LH & FSH (feedback inhibition) **Dose:** *Breast CA:* 10–40 mg/d ÷ × 1–3 mo. *Hypogonadism:* 5–20 mg/d **Caution:** [X, ?/–] ↑ Effect w/ anticoagulants, cyclosporine, insulin, Li, narcotics **CI:** Serious cardiac, liver, or kidney Dz; PRG **Disp:** Tabs 10 mg **SE:** Priapism, edema, virilization, amenorrhea & menstrual irregularities, hirsutism, alopecia, acne, N, cholestasis; suppression of factors II, V, VII, & X, & polycythemia; ↑ libido, HA, anxiety **Notes:** Radiographic exam of hand/wrist q6mo in prepubertal children; ↓ total T₄ levels

Flurazepam (Dalmane) [C-IV] Uses: *Insomnia* Acts: Benzodiazepine **Dose:** *Adults & Peds >15 y:* 15–30 mg PO qhs PRN; ↓ in elderly **Caution:** [X, ?/–] Elderly, low albumin, hepatic impair **CI:** NAG; PRG **Disp:** Caps 15, 30 mg **SE:** "Hangover" d/t accumulation of metabolites, apnea, anaphylaxis, angioedema, amnesia **Notes:** May cause dependency

Flurbiprofen (Ansaid, Ocufen) BOX: May ↑ risk of CV events and GI bleeding Uses: *Arthritis, ocular surgery* Acts: NSAID **Dose:** 50–300 mg/d w/ bid-qid, max 300 mg/d w/ food, ocular 1 gtt q 30 min × 4, beginning 2 h pre-op **Caution:** [B (D in 3rd tri), +] **CI:** PRG (3rd tri); ASA allergy **Disp:** Tabs 50, 100 mg **SE:** Dizziness, GI upset, peptic ulcer Dz, ocular irritation

Flutamide (Eulexin) BOX: Liver failure & death reported. Measure LFTs before, monthly, & periodically after; D/C immediately if ALT 2 × ULN or jaundice develops Uses: Advanced *PCa* (w/ LHRH agonists, e.g., leuprolide or goserelin); w/ radiation & GnRH for localized CAP Acts: Nonsteroidal antiandrogen **Dose:** 250 mg PO tid (750 mg total) **Caution:** [D, ?] **CI:** Severe hepatic impair **Disp:** Caps 125 mg **SE:** Hot flashes, loss of libido, impotence, N/V/D, gynecomastia, hepatic failure **Notes:** ✓ LFTs, avoid EtOH

Fluticasone Furoate, Nasal (Veramyst) Uses: *Seasonal allergic rhinitis* Acts: Topical steroid **Dose:** *Adults & Peds > 12 y:* 2 sprays/nostril/d, then 1 spray /d maint. *Peds 2–11 y:* 1–2 sprays/nostril/d **Caution:** [C, M] Avoid w/ ritonavir, other steroids, recent nasal surgery/trauma **CI:** None **Disp:** Nasal spray 27.5 mcg/actuation **SE:** HA, epistaxis, nasopharyngitis, pyrexia, pharyngolaryngeal pain, cough, nasal ulcers, back pain, anaphylaxis

Fluticasone Propionate, nasal (Flonase) Uses: *Seasonal allergic rhinitis* Acts: Topical steroid **Dose:** *Adults & Peds >12 y:* 2 sprays/nostril/d *Peds 4–11 y:* 1–2 sprays/nostril/d **Caution:** [C, M] **CI:** Primary Rx of status asthmaticus **Disp:** Nasal spray 50 mcg/actuation **SE:** HA, dysphonia, oral candidiasis

Fluticasone Propionate, inhalation (Flovent HFA, Flovent Diskus) Uses: *Chronic asthma* Acts: Topical steroid **Dose:** *Adults & Peds >12 y:* 2–4 puffs bid. *Peds 4–11 y:* 44 or 50 mcg bid **Caution:** [C, M] **CI:** Status asthmaticus **Disp:** Diskus dry powder: 50, 100, 250 mcg/action; HFA; MDI 44/110/220 mcg/Inh **SE:** HA, dysphonia, oral candidiasis **Notes:** Risk of thrush, rinse mouth after; counsel on use of devices

Fluticasone Propionate & Salmeterol Xinafoate (Advair Diskus, Advair HFA) BOX: Increased risk of worsening wheezing or asthma-related death w/ long- acting β₂-adrenergic agonists; use only if asthma not controlled on agent such as inhaled steroid Uses: *Maint Rx for asthma* Acts: Corticosteroid w/ LA bronchodilator β₂ agonist **Dose:** *Adults & Peds >12 y:* 1 Inh bid q12h; titrate to lowest effective dose (4 Inh or 920/84 mcg/d max) **Caution:** [C, M] **CI:** Acute asthma attack; conversion from PO steroids; w/ phenothiazines **Disp:** Diskus = metered-dose Inh powder (fluticasone/salmeterol in mcg) 100/50, 250/50, 500/50; HFA = aerosol 45/21, 115/21, 230/21 mg **SE:** Upper resp Infxn, pharyngitis, HA

Notes: Combo of Flovent & Serevent; do not wash mouthpiece, do not exhale into device; Advair HFA for pts not controlled on other meds (e.g., low-medium dose Inh steroids) or whose Dz severity warrants 2 maint therapies

Fluvastatin (Lescol) Uses: *Atherosclerosis, primary hypercholesterolemia, heterozygous familial hypercholesterolemia hypertriglyceridemia* **Acts:** HMG-CoA reductase inhib **Dose:** 20–40 mg bid PO or XL 80 mg/d ↓ w/ hepatic impair **Caution:** [X, –] **CI:** Active liver Dz, ↑ LFTs, PRG, breast-feeding **Disp:** Caps 20, 40 mg; XL 80 mg **SE:** HA, dyspepsia, N/D, Abd pain **Notes:** Dose no longer limited to HS ✓ LFTs

Fluvoxamine (Luvox, Luvox CR) BOX: Closely monitor for worsening depression or emergence of suicidality, particularly in peds pts Uses: *OCD, SAD* **Acts:** SSRI **Dose:** Initial 50-mg single qhs dose, ↑ to 300 mg/d in ÷ doses; *CR:* 100–300 mg PO qhs, may ↑ by 50 mg/d q wk, max 300 mg/d ↓ in elderly/hepatic impair, titrate slowly; ÷ doses >100 mg **Caution:** [C, ?/–] multiple interactions (see PI: MAOIs, phenothiazines, SSRIs, serotonin agonists, others); do not use w/ clopidogrel **CI:** MAOI w/in 14 d, w/ alosetron, tizanidine, thioridazine, pimozide **Disp:** Tabs 25, 50, 100 mg; Caps ER 100, 150 mg **SE:** HA, N/D, somnolence, insomnia, ↓ Na⁺, **Notes:** gradual taper to D/C

Folic Acid Uses: *Megaloblastic anemia; folate deficiency* **Acts:** Dietary supl **Dose:** *Adults.* Supl: 0.4 mg/d PO. *PRG:* 0.8 mg/d PO. *Folate deficiency:* 1 mg PO daily–tid. *Peds.* Supl: 0.04–0.4 mg/24 h PO, IM, IV, or SQ. *Folate deficiency:* 0.5–1 mg/24 h PO, IM, IV, or SQ **Caution:** [A, +] **CI:** Pernicious, aplastic, normocytic anemias **Disp:** Tabs 0.4, 0.8, 1 mg; Inj 5 mg/mL **SE:** Well tolerated **Notes:** OK for all women of child-bearing age; ↓ fetal neural tube defects by 50%; no effect on normocytic anemias

Fondaparinux (Arixtra) BOX: When epidural/spinal anesthesia or spinal puncture is used, pts anticoagulated or scheduled to be anticoagulated w/ LMW heparins, heparinoids, or fondaparinux are at risk for epidural or spinal hematoma, which can result in long-term or permanent paralysis Uses: *DVT prophylaxis* w/ hip fracture, hip or knee replacement, Abd surgery; w/ DVT or PE in combo w/ warfarin **Acts:** Synth inhib of activated factor X; a pentasaccharide **Dose:** *Prophylaxis* 2.5 mg SQ daily, up to 5–9 d; start >6 h post-op; Tx: 7.5 mg SQ daily (<50 kg: 5 mg SQ daily; >100 kg: 10mg SQ daily); ↓ w/ renal impair **Caution:** [B, ?] ↑ Bleeding risk w/ anticoagulants, anti-plts, drotrecogin alfa, NSAIDs **CI:** Wgt <50 kg, CrCl <30 mL/min, active bleeding, SBE ↓ plt w/ anti-plt Ab **Disp:** Prefilled syringes w/ 27-gauge needle: 2.5/0.5, 5/0.4, 7.5 /0.6, 10/0.8, mg/mL **SE:** Thrombocytopenia, anemia, fever, N **Notes:** D/C if plts <100,000 cells/mcL; only give SQ; may monitor antifactor Xa levels

Formoterol Fumarate (Foradil, Perforomist) BOX: May ↑ risk of asthma -related death Uses: *Long-term Rx of bronchoconstriction in COPD, EIB (only Foradil)* **Acts:** LA β₂-agonist **Dose:** *Adults. Perforomist:* 20-mcg Inh q12h; *Foradil:* 12-mcg Inh q12h, 24 mcg/d max; *EIB:* 12 mcg 15 min before exercise

Peds >5y: (Foradil) See Adults **Caution:** [C, M] Not for acute Sx, w/ CV Dz, w/ adrenergic meds, xanthine derivatives meds that ↑ QT; β-blockers may ↓ effect, D/C w/ ECG change **CI:** None **Disp:** Foradil caps 12 mcg for Aerolizer Inhaler (12 & 60 doses) **SE:** N/D, nasopharyngitis, dry mouth, angina, HTN, ↓ BP, tachycardia, arrhythmias, nervousness, HA, tremor, muscle cramps, palpitations, dizziness **Notes:** excess use may ↑ CV risks; not for oral use

Fosamprenavir (Lexiva) **BOX:** Do not use w/ severe liver dysfunction, reduce dose w/ mild–mod liver impair (fosamprenavir 700 mg bid w/o ritonavir) **Uses:** HIV Infxn **Acts:** Protease inhib **Dose:** 1400 mg bid w/o ritonavir; w/ritonavir, fosamprenavir 1400 mg + ritonavir 200 mg daily or fosamprenavir 700 mg + ritonavir 100 mg bid; w/ efavirenz & ritonavir: fosamprenavir 1400 mg + ritonavir 300 mg daily **Caution:** [C, ?/–] do not use w/salmeterol, colchicine (w/renal/hepatic failure); adjust dose w/ bosentan, tadalafil for PAH **CI:** w/ CYPA4 drugs (Table 10 p 280) such as w/ rifampin, lovastatin, simvastatin, delavirdine, ergot alkaloids, midazolam, triazolam, or pimozide; sulfa allergy; w/Alpha 1-adrenoreceptor antagonist (alfuzosin); w/ PDE5 Inhibitor sildenafil **Disp:** Tabs 700 mg **SE:** N/V/D, HA, fatigue, rash **Notes:** Numerous drug interactions because of hepatic metabolism; replaced amprenavir

Fosaprepitant (Emend, Injection) **Uses:** *Prevent chemotherapy-associated N/V* **Acts:** Substance P/neurokinin 1 receptor antagonist **Dose:** *Chemotherapy:* 115 mg IV 30 min before chemotherapy on d 1 (followed by aprepitant [Emend, Oral] 80 mg PO days 2 and 3) in combo w/ other antiemetics **Caution:** [B, ?/–] Potential for drug interactions, substrate and mod CYP3A4 inhib (dose-dependent); ↓ effect of OCP and warfarin **CI:** w/ Pimozide, terfenadine, astemizole, or cisapride **Disp:** Inj 115 mg **SE:** N/D, weakness, hiccups, dizziness, HA, dehydration, hot flushing, dyspepsia, Abd pain, neutropenia, ↑ LFTs, Inj site discomfort **Notes:** see also Aprepitant (Emend, Oral)

Foscarnet (Foscavir) **Uses:** *CMV retinitis*; acyclovir-resistant *herpes infxns* **Acts:** ↓ Viral DNA polymerase & RT **Dose:** *CMV retinitis: Induction:* 60 mg/kg IV q8h or 100 mg/kg q12h × 14–21 d. *Maint:* 90–120 mg/kg/d IV (Mon–Fri). *Acyclovir-resistant HSV: Induction:* 40 mg/kg IV q8–12h × 14–21 d; use central line; ↓ w/ renal impair **Caution:** [C, –] ↑ Sz potential w/ fluoroquinolones; avoid nephrotoxic Rx (cyclosporine, aminoglycosides, amphotericin B, protease inhib) **CI:** CrCl <0.4 mL/min/kg **Disp:** Inj 24 mg/mL **SE:** Nephrotox, electrolyte abnormalities **Notes:** Sodium loading (500 mL 0.9% NaCl) before & after helps minimize nephrotox; monitor-ionized Ca^{2+}

Fosfomycin (Monurol) **Uses:** *Uncomplicated UTI* **Acts:** ↓ cell wall synth *Spectrum:* gram(+)*Enterococcus,* staphylococci, pneumococci; gram(–) (*E. coli, Salmonella, Shigella, H. influenzae, Neisseria,* indole(–)-negative *Proteus, Providencia*); *B. fragilis* & anaerobic gram(–) cocci are resistant **Dose:** 3 g PO in 90–120 mL of H$_2$O single dose; ↓ in renal impair **Caution:** [B, ?] ↓ Absorption w/ antacids/Ca salts **CI:** Component sensitivity **Disp:** Granule packets 3 g **SE:** HA, GI upset **Notes:** May take 2–3 d for Sxs to improve

Fosinopril (Monopril) **Uses:** *HTN, CHF*, DN **Acts:** ACE inhib **Dose:** 10 mg/d PO initial; max 40 mg/d PO; ↓ in elderly; ↓ in renal impair **Caution:** [D, +] ↑ K+ w/ K+ supls, ARBs, K+-sparing diuretics; ↑ renal after effects w/ NSAIDs, diuretics, hypovolemia **CI:** Hereditary/idiopathic angioedema or angioedema w/ ACE inhib, bilateral RAS **Disp:** Tabs 10, 20, 40 mg **SE:** Cough, dizziness, angioedema, ↑ K+

Fosphenytoin (Cerebyx) **Uses:** *Status epilepticus* **Acts:** ↓ Sz spread in motor cortex **Dose:** As phenytoin equivalents (PE). *Load:* 15–20 mg PE/kg. *Maint:* 4–6 mg PE/kg/d; ↓ dosage, monitor levels in hepatic impair **Caution:** [D, +] May ↑ phenobarbital **CI:** Sinus bradycardia, SA block, 2nd-/3rd-degree AV block, Adams–Stokes synd, rash during Rx **Disp:** Inj 75 mg/mL **SE:** ↓ BP, dizziness, ataxia, pruritus, nystagmus **Notes:** 15 min to convert fosphenytoin to phenytoin; administer <150 mg PE/min to prevent ↓ BP; administer w/ BP monitoring

Frovatriptan (Frova) **Uses:** *Rx acute migraine* **Acts:** Vascular serotonin receptor agonist **Dose:** 2.5 mg PO repeat in 2 h PRN; max 7.5 mg/d **Caution:** [C, ?/–] **CI:** Angina, ischemic heart Dz, coronary artery vasospasm, hemiplegic or basilar migraine, uncontrolled HTN, ergot use, MAOI use w/in 14 d **Supplied:** Tabs 2.5 mg **SE:** N, V, dizziness, hot flashes, paresthesias, dyspepsia, dry mouth, hot/cold sensation, chest pain, skeletal pain, flushing, weakness, numbness, coronary vasospasm, HTN

Fulvestrant (Faslodex) **Uses:** *HR(+) metastatic breast CA in postmenopausal women w/ progression following antiestrogen Rx therapy* **Acts:** Estrogen receptor antagonist **Dose:** 250 mg IM monthly, as single 5-mL Inj or 2 concurrent 2.5-mL IM Inj in buttocks **Caution:** [X, ?/–] ↑ Effects w/ CYP3A4 inhib (Table 10 p 280); w/ hepatic impair **CI:** PRG **Disp:** Prefilled syringes 50 mg/mL (single 5 mL, dual 2.5 mL) **SE:** N/V/D, constipation, Abd pain, HA, back pain, hot flushes, pharyngitis, Inj site Rxns **Notes:** Only use IM

Furosemide (Lasix) **Uses:** *CHF, HTN, edema*, ascites **Acts:** Loop diuretic; ↓ Na & Cl reabsorption in ascending loop of Henle & distal tubule **Dose:** *Adults* 20–80 mg PO or IV bid. *Peds.* 1 mg/kg/dose IV q6–12h; 2 mg/kg/dose PO q12–24h (max 6 mg/kg/dose); ↑ doses w/ renal impair **Caution:** [C, +] ↓ K+, ↑ risk digoxin tox & ototox w/ aminoglycosides, cisplatin (especially in renal dysfunction) **CI:** Sulfonylurea allergy; anuria; hepatic coma; electrolyte depletion **Disp:** Tabs 20, 40, 80 mg; soln 10 mg/mL, 40 mg/5 mL; Inj 10 mg/mL **SE:** ↓ BP, hyperglycemia, ↓ K+ **Notes:** ✓ Lytes, renal Fxn; high doses IV may cause ototox

Gabapentin (Neurontin) **Uses:** Adjunct in *partial Szs*; postherpetic neuralgia (PHN)*; chronic pain synds **Acts:** Anticonvulsant; GABA analog **Dose:** *Adults & Peds >12 y:* *Anticonvulsant:* 300 mg PO tid, ↑ max 3600 mg/d. *PHN:* 300 mg day 1, 300 mg bid day 2, 300 mg tid day 3, titrate (1800–3600 mg/d). *Peds 3–12 y:* Start 0–15 mg/kg/d ÷ tid, ↑ over 3 d; *3–4 y:* 40 mg/kg/d given tid ≥5 y: 25–35 mg/kg/d ÷ tid, 50 mg/kg/d max; ↓ w/ renal impair **Caution:** [C, ?] Use in peds 3–12 y w/ epilepsy may ↑ CNS-related adverse events **CI:** Component sensitivity **Disp:** Caps 100, 300, 400 mg; soln 250 mg/5 mL; scored tab 600, 800 mg **SE:** Somnolence, dizziness, ataxia, fatigue **Notes:** Not necessary to monitor levels; taper ↑ or ↓ over 1 wk

Galantamine (Razadyne) **Uses:** *Mild-mod Alzheimer Dz* **Acts:** ? Acetylcholinesterase inhib **Dose:** 4 mg PO bid, ↑ to 8 mg bid after 4 wk; may ↑ to 12 mg bid in 4 wk **Caution:** [B, ?] Caution w/ heart block, ↑ effect w/ succinylcholine, bethanechol, amiodarone, diltiazem, verapamil, NSAIDs, digoxin; ↓ effect w/ anticholinergics; ↑ risk of death w/ mild impair **CI:** Severe renal/hepatic impair **Disp:** Tabs 4, 8, 12 mg; soln 4 mg/mL **SE:** GI disturbances, ↓ wgt, sleep disturbances, dizziness, HA **Notes:** Caution w/ urinary outflow obst, Parkinson Dz, severe asthma/COPD, severe heart Dz or ↓ BP

Gallium Nitrate (Ganite) **BOX:** ↑ Risk of severe renal Insuff w/ concurrent use of nephrotoxic drugs (e.g., aminoglycosides, amphotericin B). D/C if use of potentially nephrotoxic drug is indicated; hydrate several days after administration. D/C w/ SCr >2.5 mg/dL **Uses:** *↑ Ca²⁺ of malignancy*; bladder CA **Acts:** ↓ Bone resorption of Ca^{2+} **Dose:** ↑ Ca^{2+}: 100–200 mg/m² × 5 d. *CA:* 350 mg/m² cont Inf × 5 d to 700 mg/m² rapid IV Inf q2wk in antineoplastic settings (per protocols) **Caution:** [C, ?] Do not give w/ live or rotavirus vaccine **CI:** SCr >2.5 mg/dL **Disp:** Inj 25 mg/mL **SE:** Renal Insuff, ↓ Ca²⁺, hypophosphatemia, ↓ bicarb, <1% acute optic neuritis **Notes:** Bladder CA, use in combo w/ vinblastine & ifosfamide

Ganciclovir (Cytovene, Vitrasert) **Uses:** *Rx & prevent CMV retinitis, prevent CMV Dz* in transplant recipients **Acts:** ↓ viral DNA synth **Dose:** *Adults & Peds. IV:* 5 mg/kg IV q12h for 14–21 d, then maint 5 mg/kg/d IV × 7 d/wk or 6 mg/kg/d IV × 5 d/wk. *Ocular implant:* One implant q5–8mo. *Adults. PO:* Following induction, 1000 mg PO tid. *Prevention:* 1000 mg PO tid; w/ food; ↓ in renal impair **Caution:** [C, –] ↑ Effect w/ immunosuppressives, imipenem/cilastatin, zidovudine, didanosine, other nephrotoxic Rx **CI:** ANC <500 cells/mm³, plt <25,000 cells/mm³, intravitreal implant **Disp:** Caps 250, 500 mg; Inj 500 mg, ocular implant 4.5 mg **SE:** Granulocytopenia & thrombocytopenia, fever, rash, GI upset **Notes:** Not a cure for CMV; handle Inj w/ cytotoxic cautions; no systemic benefit w/ implant

Gefitinib (Iressa) **Uses:** *Rx locally advanced or metastatic NSCLC after platinum-based & docetaxel chemotherapy fails* **Acts:** selective TKI of EGFR **Dose:** 250 mg/d PO **Caution:** [D, –] **Disp:** Tabs 250 mg **SE:** D, rash, acne, dry skin, N/V, interstitial lung Dz, ↑ transaminases **Notes:** ✓ LFTs, only give to pts who have already received drug; no new pts because it has not been shown to increase survival

Gemcitabine (Gemzar) **Uses:** *Pancreatic CA (single agent),breast Ca w/ paclitaxel, NSCLC w/cisplatin, Ovarian Ca w/carboplatin*, gastric CA **Acts:** Antimetabolite; nucleoside metabolic inhibitor; ↓ ribonucleotide reductase; produces false nucleotide base-inhibiting DNA synth **Dose:** 1000–1250 mg/m² over 30 min–1 h IV Inf/wk × 3–4 wk or 6–8 wk; modify dose based on hematologic

Fxn (per protocol) **Caution:** [D, ?/–] **CI:** PRG **Disp:** Inj 200 mg, 1 g **SE:** ↓ BM, N/V/D, drug fever, skin rash **Notes:** Reconstituted soln 38 mg/mL; monitor hepatic/renal Fxn

Gemfibrozil (Lopid) **Uses:** *Hypertriglyceridemia, coronary heart Dz* **Acts:** Fibric acid **Dose:** 1200 mg/d PO ÷ bid 30 min ac A.M. & P.M. **Caution:** [C, ?] ↑ Warfarin effect, sulfonylureas; ↑ risk of myopathy w/ HMG-CoA reductase inhib; ↓ effects w/ cyclosporine **CI:** Renal/hepatic impair (SCr >2.0 mg/dL), gallbladder Dz, primary biliary cirrhosis, use w/ repaglinide (↓ glucose) **Disp:** Tabs 600 mg **SE:** Cholelithiasis, GI upset **Notes:** Avoid w/HMG-CoA reductase inhib; ✓ LFTs & serum lipids

Gemifloxacin (Factive) **Uses:** *CAP, acute exacerbation of chronic bronchitis* **Acts:** ↓ DNA gyrase & topoisomerase IV; *Spectrum:* S. pneumoniae (including multidrug-resistant strains), H. influenzae, H. parainfluenzae, M. catarrhalis, M. pneumoniae, C. pneumoniae, K. pneumoniae **Dose:** 320 mg PO daily × 5–7 d; CrCl <40 mL/min: 160 mg PO/d **Caution:** [C, ?/–]; Peds <18 y; Hx of ↑ QTc interval, electrolyte disorders, w/ class IA/III antiarrhythmics, erythromycin, TCAs, antipsychotics, ↑ INR and bleeding risk w/ warfarin **CI:** Fluoroquinolone allergy **Disp:** Tab 320 mg **SE:** Rash, N/V/D, C. difficile enterocolitis, ↑ risk of Achilles tendon rupture, tendonitis, Abd pain, dizziness, xerostomia, arthralgia, allergy/anaphylactic Rxns, peripheral neuropathy, tendon rupture **Notes:** Take 3 h before or 2 h after Al/Mg antacids, Fe 2²⁺, Zn²⁺ or other metal cations; ↑ rash risk w/ ↑ duration of Rx

Gemtuzumab Ozogamicin (Mylotarg) Withdrawn from market 2010. Fatal induction phase toxicity and lack of efficacy issues. Patients under treatment can complete course.

Gentamicin (Garamycin, G-mycitin, others) **Uses:** *Septicemia, serious bacterial Infxn of CNS, urinary tract, resp tract, GI tract, including peritonitis, skin, bone, soft tissue, including burns; severe Infxn P. aeruginosa w/ carbenicillin; group D streptococci endocarditis w/ PCN-type drug; serious staphylococcal infxns, but not the antibiotic of 1st choice; mixed Infxn w/ staphylococci and gram(–)* **Acts:** Aminoglycoside, bactericidal; ↓ protein synth *Spectrum:* gram(–) (not *Neisseria, Legionella, Acinetobacter*); weaker gram(+) but synergy w/ PCNs **Dose:** *Adults. Standard:* 1–2 mg/kg IV q8–12h or daily dosing 4–7 mg/kg q24h IV. *Gram(+) Synergy:* 1 mg/kg q8h *Peds. Infants <7 d <1200 g:* 2.5 mg/kg/dose q18–24h. *Infants >1200 g:* 2.5 mg/kg/dose q12–18h. *Infants >7 d:* 2.5 mg/kg/dose IV q8–12h. *Children:* 2.5 mg/kg/d IV q8h; ↓ w/ renal Insuff; if obese, dose based on IBW **Caution:** [C, +/–] Avoid other nephrotoxics **CI:** Aminoglycoside sensitivity **Disp:** Premixed Inf 40, 60, 70, 80, 90, 100, 120 mg; ADD-Vantage Inj vials 10 mg/mL; Inj 40 mg/mL; IT preservative-free 2 mg/mL **SE:** Nephro-/oto-/neurotox **Notes:** Follow CrCl, SCr & serum conc for dose adjustments; use IBW to dose (use adjusted if obese >30% IBW);OK to use intraperitoneal for peritoneal dialysis-related infxns *Levels: Peak:* 30 min after Inf; *Trough:* <0.5 h before next dose;

Therapeutic: Peak: 5–8 mcg/mL, *Trough:* <2 mcg/mL, if >2 mcg/mL associated w/ renal tox

Gentamicin, Ophthalmic (Garamycin, Genoptic, Gentacidin, Gentak, Others) Uses: *Conjunctival infxns* Acts: Bactericidal; ↓ protein synth Dose: *Oint:* Apply 1/2 inch bid–tid. *Soln:* 1–2 gtt q2–4h, up to 2 gtt/h for severe Infxn Caution: [C, ?] CI: Aminoglycoside sensitivity Disp: Soln & oint 0.1% and 0.3% SE: Local irritation Notes: Do not use other eye drops w/in 5–10 min; do not touch dropper to eye

Gentamicin, Topical (Garamycin, G-mycitin) Uses: *Skin infxns* caused by susceptible organisms Acts: Bactericidal; ↓ protein synth Dose: *Adults & Peds >1 y:* Apply tid-qid Caution: [C, ?] CI: Aminoglycoside sensitivity Disp: Cream & oint 0.1% SE: Irritation

Gentamicin & Prednisolone, Ophthalmic (Pred-G Ophthalmic) Uses: *Steroid-responsive ocular & conjunctival infxns* sensitive to gentamicin Acts: Bactericidal; ↓ protein synth w/ anti-inflammatory. *Spectrum: Staphylococcus, E. coli, H. influenzae, Klebsiella, Neisseria, Pseudomonas, Proteus, & Serratia* sp Dose: *Oint:* 1/2 inch in conjunctival sac daily-tid. *Susp:* 1 gtt bid-qid, up to 1 gtt/h for severe infxns CI: Aminoglycoside sensitivity Caution: [C, ?] Disp: *Oint, ophthal:* Prednisolone acetate 0.6% & gentamicin sulfate 0.3% (3.5 g). *Susp, ophthal:* Prednisolone acetate 1% & gentamicin sulfate 0.3% (2, 5, 10 mL) SE: Local irritation

Glimepiride (Amaryl) Uses: *Type 2 DM* Acts: Sulfonylurea; ↑ pancreatic insulin release; ↑ peripheral insulin sensitivity; ↓ hepatic glucose output/production Dose: 1–4 mg/d, max 8 mg Caution: [C, –] CI: DKA Disp: Tabs 1, 2, 4 mg SE: HA, N, hypoglycemia Notes: Give w/ 1st meal of day

Glimepiride/pioglitazone (Duetact) Uses: *Adjunct to exercise type 2 DM not controlled by single agent* Acts: Sulfonylurea (↓ glucose) w/ agent that ↑ insulin sensitivity & ↓ gluconeogenesis Dose: initial 30 mg/2 mg PO q AM; 45 mg pioglitazone/8 mg glimepiride/d max; w/food Caution: [C, ?/–] w/ Liver impair, elderly CI: Component hypersens, DKA Disp: Tabs 30/2, 30 mg/4 mg SE: Hct, ↑ ALT, ↓ glucose, URI, ↑ wgt, edema, HA, N/D, may ↑ CV mortality Notes: Monitor CBC, ALT, Cr, wgt

Glipizide (Glucotrol, Glucotrol XL) Uses: *Type 2 DM* Acts: Sulfonylurea; ↑ pancreatic insulin release; ↑ peripheral insulin sensitivity; ↓ hepatic glucose output/production; ↓ intestinal glucose absorption Dose: 5 mg initial, ↑ by 2.5–5 mg/d, max 40 mg/d; XL max 20 mg; 30 min ac; hold if NPO Caution: [C, ?/–] Severe liver Dz CI: DKA, type 1 DM, sulfonamide sensitivity Disp: Tabs 5, 10 mg; XL tabs 2.5, 5, 10 mg SE: HA, anorexia, N/V/D, constipation, fullness, rash, urticaria, photosens Notes: Counsel about DM management; wait several days before adjusting dose; monitor glucose

Glucagon Uses: Severe *hypoglycemic* Rxns in DM w/ sufficient liver glycogen stores; β-blocker OD Acts: Accelerates liver gluconeogenesis Dose: *Adults.*

0.5–1 mg SQ, IM, or IV; repeat in 20 min PRN. β-*blocker OD:* 3–10 mg IV; repeat in 10 min PRN; may give cont Inf 1–5 mg/h (*ECC 2005*). **Peds. Neonates:** 0.3 mg/kg/dose SQ, IM, or IV q4h PRN. *Children:* 0.025–0.1 mg/kg/dose SQ, IM, or IV; repeat in 20 min PRN **Caution:** [B, M] **CI:** Pheochromocytoma **Disp:** Inj 1 mg **SE:** N/V, ↓ BP **Notes:** Administration of dextrose IV necessary; ineffective in starvation, adrenal Insuff, or chronic hypoglycemia

Glyburide (DiaBeta, Micronase, Glynase) Uses: *Type 2 DM* Acts: Sulfonylurea; ↑ pancreatic insulin release; ↓ peripheral insulin sensitivity; ↓ hepatic glucose output/production; ↓ intestinal glucose absorption **Dose:** 1.25–10 mg daily-bid, max 20 mg/d. *Micronized:* 0.75–6 mg daily-bid, max 12 mg/d **Caution:** [C, ?] Renal impair, sulfonamide allergy **CI:** DKA, type I DM **Disp:** Tabs 1.25, 2.5, 5 mg; micronized tabs 1.5, 3, 6 mg **SE:** HA, hypoglycemia, cholestatic jaundice, and hepatitis may cause liver failure **Notes:** Not OK for CrCl <50 mL/min; hold dose if NPO; hypoglycemia may be difficult to recognize; many medications can enhance hypoglycemic effects

Glyburide/Metformin (Glucovance) Uses: *Type 2 DM* Acts: *Sulfonylurea:* ↑ Pancreatic insulin release. *Metformin:* Peripheral insulin sensitivity; ↓ hepatic glucose output/production; ↓ intestinal glucose absorption **Dose:** 1st line (naïve pts), 1.25/250 mg PO daily-bid; 2nd line, 2.5/500 mg or 5/500 mg bid (max 20/2000 mg); take w/ meals, slowly ↑ dose; hold before & 48 h after ionic contrast media **Caution:** [C, –] **CI:** SCr >1.4 mg/dL in females or >1.5 mg/dL in males; hypoxemic conditions (sepsis, recent MI); alcoholism; metabolic acidosis; liver Dz; **Disp:** Tabs 1.25/250 mg, 2.5/500 mg, 5/500 mg **SE:** HA, lactic acidosis, anorexia, N/V, rash **Notes:** Avoid EtOH; hold dose if NPO; monitor folate levels (megaloblastic anemia)

Glycerin Suppository Uses: *Constipation* Acts: Hyperosmolar laxative **Dose:** *Adults.* 1 Adult supp PR PRN. *Peds.* 1 Infant supp PR daily-bid PRN **Caution:** [C, ?] **Disp:** Supp (adult, infant); liq 4 mL/applicator-full **SE:** D

Golimumab (Simponi) BOX: Serious infxns (bacterial, fungal, TB, opportunistic) possible. D/C w/ severe infxn/sepsis, test and monitor for TB w/treatment; lymphoma/other CA possible in children/adolescents Uses: *Mod/severe RA w/ methotrexate, psoriatic arthritis w/ or w/o methotrexate, ankylosing spondylitis* Acts: TNF blocker **Dose:** 50 mg SQ 1 × mo **Caution:** [B, ?/-] do use w/active infxn; w/ malignancies, CHF, demyelinating dz; do use w/ abatacept, anakinra, live vaccines **CI:** None **Disp:** Prefilled syringe & SmartJect auto-injector 50 mg/0.5 ml **SE:** URI, nasopharyngitis, Inj site rxn, ↑ LFTs, infxn, hep B reactivation, new onset psoriasis

Gonadorelin (Factrel) Uses: *Primary hypothalamic amenorrhea* Acts: ↑ Pituitary release of LH & FSH **Dose:** 5 mcg IV over 1 min q 90 min × 21 d using pump kit **Caution:** [B, M] ↑ Levels w/ androgens, estrogens, progestins, glucocorticoids, spironolactone, levodopa; ↓ levels w/ OCP, digoxin, dopamine antagonists **CI:** Condition exacerbated by PRG or reproductive hormones, ovarian cysts, causes of anovulation other than hypothalamic, hormonally dependent tumor **Disp:** Inj 100 mcg **SE:** Multiple PRG risk; Inj site pain **Notes:** Monitor LH, FSH

Goserelin (Zoladex) **Uses:** Advanced *CA Prostate* & w/ radiation for localized high-risk Dz, *endometriosis, breast CA* **Acts:** LHRH agonist, transient ↑ then ↓ in LH, w/ ↓ testosterone **Dose:** 3.6 mg SQ (implant) q28d or 10.8 mg SQ q3mo; usually upper Abd wall **Caution:** [X, –] **CI:** PRG, breast-feeding, 10.8-mg implant not for women **Disp:** SQ implant 3.6 (1 mo), 10.8 mg (3 mo) **SE:** Hot flashes, ↓ libido, gynecomastia, & transient exacerbation of CA-related bone pain ("flare Rxn" 7–10 d after 1st dose) **Notes:** Inject SQ into fat in Abd wall; do not aspirate; females must use contraception

Granisetron (Kytril) **Uses:** *Rx and Prevention of N/V (chemo/radiation/postoperation)* **Acts:** Serotonin (5-HT₃) receptor antagonist **Dose:** *Adults & Peds. Chemotherapy:* 10 mcg/kg/dose IV 30 min prior to chemotherapy *Adults. Chemotherapy:* 2 mg PO q day 1 h before chemotherapy, then 12 h later. *Post-op N/V:* 1 mg IV over 30 s before end of case **Caution:** [B, +/–] St. John's wort ↓ levels **CI:** Liver Dz, children <2 y **Disp:** Tabs 1 mg; Inj 1 mg/mL; soln 2 mg/10 mL **SE:** HA, asthenia, somnolence, D, constipation, Abd pain, dizziness, insomnia, ↑ LFTs

Guaifenesin (Robitussin, others) **Uses:** *Relief of dry, nonproductive cough* **Acts:** Expectorant **Dose:** *Adults.* 200–400 mg (10–20 mL) PO q4h SR 600–1200 mg PO bid, (max 2.4 g/d); *Peds 2–5 y:* 50–100 mg (2.5–5 mL) PO q4h (max 600 mg/d). *6–11 y:* 100–200 mg (5–10 mL) PO q4h (max 1.2 g/d) **Caution:** [C, ?] **Disp:** Tabs 100, 200 mg; SR tabs 600, 1200 mg; caps 200 mg; SR caps 300 mg; liq 100 mg/5 mL **SE:** GI upset **Notes** Give w/ large amount of H₂O; some dosage forms contain EtOH

Guaifenesin & Codeine (Robitussin AC, Brontex, Others) [C-V] **Uses:** *Relief of dry cough* **Acts:** Antitussive w/ expectorant **Dose:** *Adults.* 5–10 mL or 1 tab PO q6–8h (max 60 mL/24 h). *Peds 2–6 y:* 1–1.5 mg/kg codeine/d ÷ dose q4–6h (max 30 mg/24 h). *6–12 y:* 5 mL q4h (max 30 mL/24 h) **Caution:** [C, +] **Disp:** Brontex tab 10 mg codeine/300 mg guaifenesin; liq 2.5 mg codeine/75 mg guaifenesin/5 mL; others 10 mg codeine/100 mg guaifenesin/5 mL **SE:** Somnolence, constipation

Guaifenesin & Dextromethorphan (Many OTC Brands) **Uses:** *Cough* d/t upper resp tract irritation **Acts:** Antitussive w/ expectorant **Dose:** *Adults & Peds >12 y:* 10 mL PO q6–8h (max 40 mL/24 h). *Peds 2–6 y:* Dextromethorphan 1–2 mg/kg/24 h ÷ 3–4 × d (max 10 mL/d). *6–12 y:* 5 mL q6–8h (max 20 mL/d) **Caution:** [C, +] **CI:** Administration w/ MAOI **Disp:** Many OTC formulations **SE:** Somnolence **Notes:** Give w/ plenty of fluids; some forms contain EtOH

Haemophilus B Conjugate Vaccine (ActHIB, HibTITER, Hiberix, PedvaxHIB, Prohibit, TriHIBit, others) **Uses:** *Immunize children against H. influenzae type B Dzs* **Acts:** Active immunization **Dose:** *Peds.* 0.5 mL (25 mg) IM (deltoid or vastus lateralis muscle) 2 doses 2 and 4 mos; booster

12–15 mo or 2, 4 and 6 mos booster at 12–15 mos depending on formulation; **Caution:** [C, +] **CI:** Component sensitivity, febrile illness, immunosuppression, thimerosal allergy **Disp:** Inj 7.5, 10, 15, 25 mcg/0.5 mL **SE:** Fever, restlessness, fussiness, anorexia, pain/redness inj site; observe for anaphylaxis; edema, ↑ risk of *Haemophilus* B Infxn the wk after vaccination **Notes:** *Prohibit* and *TriHIBit* cannot be used in children < 12 mo. *Hiberix* approved ages 15 mo-4 yrs, single dose; booster beyond 5 yrs old not required; report SAE to Vaccine Adverse Events Reporting System (VAERS: 1-800-822-7967); dosing varies, check with each product

Haloperidol (Haldol) BOX: ↑ Mortality in elderly w/ dementia-related psychosis. Risk for torsade de pointes and QT prolongation, death w/ IV administration at higher doses **Uses:** *Psychotic disorders, agitation, Tourette disorders, hyperactivity in children* **Acts:** Butyrophenone; antipsychotic, neuroleptic **Dose:** *Adults. Mod Sxs:* 0.5–2 mg PO bid–tid. *Severe Sxs/agitation:* 3–5 mg PO bid–tid or 1–5 mg IM q4h PRN (max 100 mg/d). *ICU psychosis:* 2–10 mg IV q 30 min to effect, the 25% max dose q6h *Peds 3–6 y:* 0.01–0.03 mg/kg/24 h PO daily. *6–12 y:* Initial, 0.5–1.5 mg/24 h PO; ↑ by 0.5 mg/24 h to maint of 2–4 mg/24 h (0.05–0.1 mg/kg/24 h) or 1–3 mg/dose IM q4–8h to 0.1 mg/kg/24 h max; Tourette Dz may require up to 15 mg/24 h PO; ↓ in elderly **Caution:** [C, ?] ↑ Effects w/ SSRIs, CNS depressants, TCA, indomethacin, metoclopramide; avoid levodopa (↓ antiparkinsonian effects) **CI:** NAG, severe CNS depression, coma, Parkinson Dz, ↓ BM suppression, severe cardiac/hepatic Dz **Disp:** Tabs 0.5, 1, 2, 5, 10, 20 mg; conc liq 2 mg/mL; Inj 5 mg/mL; decanoate Inj 50, 100 mg/mL **SE:** Extrapyramidal Sxs (EPS), tardive dyskinesia, neuroleptic malignant synd, ↓ BP, anxiety, dystonias, risk for torsades de pointes and QT prolongation; leukopenia, neutropenia and agranulocytosis **Notes:** Do not give decanoate IV; dilute PO conc liq w/ H2O/juice; monitor for EPS; ECG monitoring w/ off-label IV use; follow CBC if WBC counts decreased

Heparin (generic) Uses: *Rx & prevention of DVT & PE*, unstable angina, AF w/ emboli, & acute arterial occlusion **Acts:** w/ antithrombin III to inactivate thrombin & ↓ thromboplastin formation **Dose:** *Adults. Prophylaxis:* 3000–5000 units SQ q8–12h. *DVT/PE Rx:* Load 50–80 units/kg IV (max 10,000 units), then 10–20 units/kg IV qh (adjust based on PTT); bolus 60 units/kg (max 4000 units); then 12 mg/kg/h (max 1000 units/h) round to nearest 50 units; keep PTT 1.5–2.0 × control for 48 h or until angiography) *(ECC 2005) Peds Infants:* Load 50 units/kg IV bolus, then 20 units/kg/h IV by cont Inf. *Children:* Load 50 units/kg IV, then 15–25 units/kg cont Inf or 100 units/kg/dose q4h IV intermittent bolus (adjust based on PTT) **Caution:** [B, +] ↑ Risk of hemorrhage w/ anticoagulants, ASA, anti-plt, cephalosporins w/ MTT side chain **CI:** Uncontrolled bleeding, severe thrombocytopenia, suspected ICH **Disp:** Inj 10, 100, 1000, 2000, 2500, 5000, 7500, 10,000, 20,000, 40,000 units/mL **SE:** Bruising, bleeding, thrombocytopenia **Notes:** Follow PTT, thrombin time, or activated clotting time; little PT effect; therapeutic PTT 1.5–2 control for most conditions; monitor for HIT w/ plt counts; New "USP" formulation heparin is approximately 10% less effective than older formulations

Hepatitis A Vaccine (HAVRIX, VAQTA) Uses: *Prevent hep A* in high-risk individuals (e.g., travelers, certain professions, day-care workers if 1 or more children or workers are infected, high-risk behaviors, children at ↑ risk); in chronic liver Dz Acts: Active immunity Dose: *Adults.* HAVRIX 1.0-mL IM w/ 1.0-mL booster 6–12 mo later; VAQTA: 1.0 mL IM w/ 1.0 ml IM booster 6–18 mo later *Peds >12 mo.* HAVRIX 0.5-mL IM, w/ 0.5-mL booster 6–18 mo later; VAQTA 0.5 mL IM w/ booster 0.5 mL 6–18 mo later Caution: [C, +] CI: Component sensitivity; syringes contain latex Disp: *HAVRIX:* Inj 720 EL.U./0.5 mL, 1440 EL.U./1 mL; *VAQTA* 50 units/mL SE: Fever, fatigue, HA, Inj site pain Notes: Give primary at least 2 wks before anticipated exposure; do not give HAVRIX in gluteal region; report SAE to VAERS (1-800-822-7967)

Hepatitis A (Inactivated) & Hepatitis B (Recombinant) Vaccine (Twinrix) Uses: *Active immunization against hep A/B in pts >18 y* Acts: Active immunization Dose: 1 mL IM at 0, 1, & 6 mo; accelerated regimen 1 mL IM day 0, 7 and 21–20 then booster at 12 mo; 720 ELISA E.L.U. units Hep A antigen, 20 mcg/mL hep B surface antigen Caution: [C, +/–] CI: Component sensitivity Disp: Single-dose vials, syringes SE: Fever, fatigue, HA, pain/redness at site Notes: Booster OK 6–12 mo after 2nd dose; report SAE to Vaccine Adverse Events Reporting System (VAERS: 1-800-822-7967)

Hepatitis B Immune Globulin (HyperHep, HepaGam B, Nabi-HB, H-BIG) Uses: *Exposure to HBsAg(+) material (e.g., blood, accidental needlestick, mucous membrane contact, PO or sexual contact), prevent hep B in HBsAg(+) liver Tx pt* Acts: Passive immunization Dose: *Adults & Peds.* 0.06 mL/kg IM 5 mL max; w/in 24 h of exposure; w/in 14 d of sexual contact; repeat 1 mo if nonresponder or refused initial tx; liver Tx per protocols Caution: [C, ?] CI: Allergies to γ-globulin, anti-immunoglobulin Ab, or thimerosal; IgA deficiency Disp: Inj SE: Inj site pain, dizziness, HA, myalgias, arthralgias, anaphylaxis Notes: IM in gluteal or deltoid; w/ continued exposure, give hep B vaccine; not for active hep B; ineffective for chronic hep B

Hepatitis B Vaccine (Engerix-B, Recombivax HB) Uses: *Prevent hep B*: men who have sex w/ men, people who inject street drugs; chronic renal/liver Dz, healthcare workers exposed to blood, body fluids; sexually active not in monogamous relationship, people seeking evaluation for or w/ STDs, household contacts and partners of HepB infected persons, travelers to countries w/ ↑ Hep B prevalence, clients/staff working w/ people w/ developmental disabilities Acts: Active immunization; recombinant DNA Dose: *Adults.* 3 IM doses 1 mL each; 1st 2 doses 1 mo apart; the 3rd 6 mo after the 1st. *Peds.* 0.5 mL IM adult schedule Caution: [C, +] ↓ Effect w/ immunosuppressives CI: Yeast allergy, component sensitivity Disp: *Engerix-B:* Inj 20 mcg/mL; peds Inj 10 mcg/0.5 mL. *Recombivax HB:* Inj 10 & 40 mcg/mL; peds Inj 5 mcg/0.5 mL SE: Fever, HA, Inj site pain Notes: Deltoid IM Inj adults/older peds; younger peds, use anterolateral thigh

Hetastarch (Hespan) Uses: *Plasma vol expansion* adjunct in shock & leukapheresis Acts: Synthetic colloid; acts similar to albumin Dose: *Vol expansion:*

500–1000 mL (1500 mL/d max) IV (20 mL/kg/h max rate). *Leukapheresis:* 250–700 mL; ↓ in renal failure **Caution:** [C, +] **CI:** Severe bleeding disorders, CHF, oliguric/anuric renal failure **Disp:** Inj 6 g/100 mL **SE:** Bleeding (↑ PT, PTT, bleeding time) **Notes:** Not blood or plasma substitute

Human Papillomavirus Recombinant Vaccine (Cervarix [Types 16, 18], Gardasil, [Types 6, 11, 16, 18]) Uses: *Prevent cervical CA, precancerous genital lesions (*Cervarix and Gardasil*), genital warts, anal cancer and oral cancer (*Gardasil*) d/t to human papillomavirus (HPV) types 16, 18 (*Cervarix*) and types 6, 11, 16, 18 (Gardasil) in females 9-26 y*; prevent genital warts caused by types 6 and 11 in boys 9-26 y (Gardasil) * **Acts:** Recombinant vaccine, passive immunity **Dose:** 0.5 mL IM, then 1 and 6 mo (*Cervarix*), or 2 and 6 mo (*Gardasil*) (upper thigh or deltoid) **Caution:** [B, ?/-] **Disp:** Single-dose vial & prefilled syringe: 0.5 mL **SE:** Erythema, pain at inj site, fever, syncope, venous thromboembolism **Notes:** First cancer prevention vaccine, 90% effective in preventing CIN 2 or more severe dx in HPV naive populations; report adverse events to Vaccine Adverse Events Reporting System (VAERS: 1-800-822-7967); continue cervical CA screening. Hx of genital warts, abn Pap smear, or + HPV DNA test is **not** CI to vaccination

Hydralazine (Apresoline, Others) Uses: *Mod–severe HTN; CHF* (w/ Isordil) **Acts:** Peripheral vasodilator **Dose:** *Adults.* Initial 10 mg PO 3–4×/d, ↑ to 25 mg 3–4×/d, 300 mg/d max. *Peds.* 0.75–3 mg/kg/24 h PO ÷ q6–12h; ↓ in renal impair; ✓ CBC & ANA before **Caution:** [C, +] Hepatic Fxn & CAD; ↑ tox w/ MAOI, indomethacin, β-blockers **CI:** Dissecting aortic aneurysm, mitral valve/rheumatic heart Dz **Disp:** Tabs 10, 25, 50, 100 mg; Inj 20 mg/mL **SE:** SLE-like synd w/ chronic high doses; SVT following IM route;. peripheral neuropathy **Notes:** Compensatory sinus tachycardia eliminated w/ β-blocker

Hydrochlorothiazide (HydroDIURIL, Esidrix, Others) Uses: *Edema, HTN* prevent stones in hypercalciuria **Acts:** Thiazide diuretic; ↓ distal tubule Na⁺ reabsorption **Dose:** *Adults.* 25–100 mg/d PO single or ÷ doses; 200 mg/d max. *Peds <6 mo:* 2–3 mg/kg/d in 2 ÷ doses. *>6 mo:* 2 mg/kg/d in 2 ÷ doses **Caution:** [D, +] **CI:** Anuria, sulfonamide allergy, renal Insuff **Disp:** Tabs 25, 50, mg; caps 12.5 mg; PO soln 50 mg/5 mL **SE:** ↓ K⁺, hyperglycemia, hyperuricemia, ↓ Na⁺; sun sensitivity **Notes:** Follow K⁺, may need supplementation

Hydrochlorothiazide & Amiloride (Moduretic) Uses: *HTN* **Acts:** Combined thiazide & K⁺-sparing diuretic **Dose:** 1–2 tabs/d PO **Caution:** [D, ?] **CI:** Renal failure, sulfonamide allergy **Disp:** Tabs (amiloride/HCTZ) 5 mg/50 mg **SE:** ↓ BP, photosens, ↑ K⁺/↓ K⁺, hyperglycemia, ↓ Na⁺, hyperlipidemia, hyperuricemia

Hydrochlorothiazide & Spironolactone (Aldactazide) Uses: *Edema, HTN* **Acts:** Thiazide & K⁺-sparing diuretic **Dose:** 25–200 mg each component/d, ÷ doses **Caution:** [D, +] **CI:** Sulfonamide allergy **Disp:** Tabs (HCTZ/spironolactone) 25 mg/25 mg, 50 mg/50 mg **SE:** Photosens, ↓ BP, ↑ or ↓ K⁺, ↓ Na⁺, hyperglycemia, hyperlipidemia, hyperuricemia

Hydrochlorothiazide & Triamterene (Dyazide, Maxzide) Uses: *Edema & HTN* **Acts:** Combo thiazide & K+-sparing diuretic **Dose:** *Dyazide:* 1–2 caps PO daily-bid. *Maxzide:* 1 tab/d PO daily-bid. **[D, +/–] CI:** Sulfonamide allergy **Disp:** (Triamterene/HCTZ) 37.5 mg/25 mg, 75 mg/50 mg **SE:** Photosens, ↓ BP, ↑ or ↓ K+, ↓ Na+, hyperglycemia, hyperlipidemia, hyperuricemia **Notes:** HCTZ component in Maxzide more bioavailable than in Dyazide

Hydrocodone & Acetaminophen (Lorcet, Vicodin, Hycet, others) [C-III] Uses: *Mod–severe pain*; **Acts:** Narcotic analgesic w/ nonnarcotic analgesic **Dose:** *Adults.* 1–2 caps or tabs PO q4–6h PRN; soln 15 mL q4–6h **Peds.** Soln (Hycet) 0.27 mL/kg q4–6h **Caution:** [C, M] **CI:** CNS depression, severe resp depression **Disp:** Many formulations; specify hydrocodone/APAP dose; caps 5/500 mg; tabs 2.5/500, 5/325, 5/400, 5/500, 7.5/325, 7.5/400, 7.5/500, 7.5/650, 7.5/750, 10/325, 10/400, 10/500, 10/650, 10/660, 10/750 mg; soln Hycet (fruit punch) 7.5 mg hydrocodone/325 mg acetaminophen/15 mL **SE:** GI upset, sedation, fatigue **Notes:** Do not exceed >4 g APAP/d

Hydrocodone & Aspirin (Lortab ASA, others) [C-III] Uses: *Mod–severe pain* **Acts:** Narcotic analgesic w/ NSAID **Dose:** 1–2 PO q4–6h PRN, w/ food/milk **Caution:** [C, M] ↓ Renal Fxn, gastritis/PUD, **CI:** Component sensitivity; children w/chickenpox (Reye synd) **Disp:** 5 mg hydrocodone/500 mg ASA/tab **SE:** GI upset, sedation, fatigue **Notes:** Monitor for GI bleed

Hydrocodone & Guaifenesin (Hycotuss Expectorant, others) [C-III] Uses: *Nonproductive cough* associated w/ resp Infxn **Acts:** Expectorant w/ cough suppressant **Dose:** *Adults & Peds >12 y:* 5 mL q4h pc & hs. *Peds <2 y:* 0.3 mg/kg/d ÷ qid. *2–12 y:* 2.5 mL q4h pc & hs **Caution:** [C, M] **CI:** Component sensitivity **Disp:** Hydrocodone 5 mg/guaifenesin 100 mg/5 mL **SE:** GI upset, sedation, fatigue

Hydrocodone & Homatropine (Hycodan, Hydromet, others) [C-III] Uses: *Relief of cough* **Acts:** Combo antitussive (Based on hydrocodone) *Adults.* 5–10 mg q4–6h. *Peds.* 0.6 mg/kg/d ÷ tid-qid **Caution:** [C, M] **CI:** NAG, ↑ ICP, depressed ventilation **Disp:** Syrup 5 mg hydrocodone/5 mL; tabs 5 mg hydrocodone **SE:** Sedation, fatigue, GI upset **Notes:** Do not give < q4h; see individual drugs

Hydrocodone & Ibuprofen (Vicoprofen) [C-III] Uses: *Mod–severe pain (<10 d)* **Acts:** Narcotic w/ NSAID **Dose:** 1–2 tabs q4–6h PRN **Caution:** [C, M] Renal Insuff; ↓ effect w/ ACE inhib & diuretics; ↑ effect w/ CNS depressants, EtOH, MAOI, ASA, TCA, anticoagulants **CI:** Component sensitivity **Disp:** Tabs 7.5 mg hydrocodone/200 mg ibuprofen **SE:** Sedation, fatigue, GI upset

Hydrocodone & Pseudoephedrine (Detussin, Histussin-D, others) [C-III] Uses: *Cough & nasal congestion* **Acts:** Narcotic cough suppressant w/ decongestant **Dose:** 5 mL qid, PRN **Caution:** [C, M] **CI:** MAOIs **Disp:** hydrocodone/pseudoephedrine 5 mg/60 mg, 3 mg/15 mg 5 mL; tab 5 mg/60 mg **SE:** ↑ BP, GI upset, sedation, fatigue

Hydrocodone, Chlorpheniramine, Phenylephrine, Acetaminophen, & Caffeine (Hycomine Compound) [C-III] Uses: *Cough & Sxs of URI* Acts: Narcotic cough suppressant w/ decongestants & analgesic Dose: 1 tab PO q4h PRN Caution: [C, M] CI: NAG Disp: Hydrocodone 5 mg/chlorpheniramine 2 mg/phenylephrine 10 mg/APAP 250 mg/caffeine 30 mg/tab SE: ↑ BP, GI upset, sedation, fatigue

Hydrocortisone, rectal (Anusol-HC Suppository, Cortifoam Rectal, Proctocort, others) Uses: *Painful anorectal conditions*, radiation proctitis, ulcerative colitis Acts: Anti-inflammatory steroid Dose: *Adults.* Ulcerative colitis: 10–100 mg PR daily-bid for 2–3 wk Caution: [B, ?/–] CI: Component sensitivity Disp: *Hydrocortisone acetate:* Rectal aerosol 90 mg/applicator; supp 25 mg. *Hydrocortisone base:* Rectal 0.5%, 1%, 2.5%; rectal susp 100 mg/60 mL SE: Minimal systemic effect

Hydrocortisone, topical & systemic (Cortef, Solu-Cortef) See Steroids pages 228, 230 and Tables 2 p 265 & 3 p 266 Caution: [B, –] CI: Viral, fungal, or tubercular skin lesions; serious infxns (except septic shock or TB meningitis) SE: *Systemic:* ↑ Appetite, insomnia, hyperglycemia, bruising Notes: May cause hypothalamic–pituitary–adrenal axis suppression

Hydromorphone (Dilaudid, Dilaudid HP) [C-II] BOX: A potent Schedule II opioid agonist; highest potential for abuse and risk of resp depression. HP formula is highly concentrated; do not confuse w/ standard formulations, OD and death could result. Alcohol, other opioids, CNS depressants ↑ resp depressant effects Uses: *Mod/severe pain* Acts: Narcotic analgesic Dose: 1–4 mg PO, IM, IV, or PR q4–6h PRN; ↓ w/ hepatic failure Caution: [B (D if prolonged use or high doses near term), ?] ↑ Resp depression and CNS effects, CNS depressants, phenothiazines, TCA CI: CNS lesion w/ ↑ ICP, COPD, cor pulmonale, emphysema, kyphoscoliosis, status asthmaticus; HP-Inj form in OB analgesia Disp: Tabs 2, 4 mg, 8 mg scored; liq 5 mg/5 mL or 1 mg/mL; Inj 1, 2, 4 mg, *Dilaudid HP* is 10 mg/mL; supp 3 mg SE: Sedation, dizziness, GI upset Notes: Morphine 10 mg IM = hydromorphone 1.5 mg IM

Hydroxocobalamin (Cyanokit) Uses: *Cyanide poisoning* Acts: Binds cyanide to form nontoxic cyanocobalamin excreted in urine Dose: 5 g IV over 15 min, repeat PRN 5 g IV over 15 min–2 h, total dose 10 g Caution: [C, ?] CI: None known Disp: Kit 2 to 2.5 g vials w/ Inf set SE: ↑ BP (can be severe) anaphylaxis, chest tightness, edema, urticaria, rash, chromaturia, N, HA, Inj site Rxns

Hydroxyurea (Hydrea, Droxia) Uses: *CML, head & neck, ovarian & colon CA, melanoma, ALL, sickle cell anemia, polycythemia vera, HIV* Acts: ↓ Ribonucleotide reductase Dose: (per protocol) 50–75 mg/kg for WBC >100,000 cells/mL; 20–30 mg/kg in refractory CML. *HIV:* 1000–1500 mg/d in single or ÷ doses; ↓ in renal Insuff Caution: [D, –] ↑ Effects w/ zidovudine, zalcitabine, didanosine, stavudine, fluorouracil CI: Severe anemia, BM suppression, WBC <2500 cells/mL or plt <100,000 cells/mm³, PRG Disp: Caps 200, 300, 400, 500 mg, tabs 1000 mg SE: ↓ BM (mostly leukopenia), N/V, rashes, facial erythema, radiation recall Rxns, renal impair **Notes:** Empty caps into H_2O

Hydroxyzine (Atarax, Vistaril) **Uses:** *Anxiety, sedation, itching* **Acts:** Antihistamine, antianxiety **Dose:** *Adults. Anxiety/sedation:* 50–100 mg PO or IM qid or PRN (max 600 mg/d). *Itching:* 25–50 mg PO or IM tid-qid. *Peds.* 0.5–1.0 mg/kg/24 h PO or IM q6h; ↓ w/hepatic impair **Caution:** [C, +/–] ↑ Effects w/ CNS depressants, anticholinergics, EtOH **CI:** Component sensitivity **Disp:** Tabs 10, 25, 50 mg; caps 25, 50 mg; syrup 10 mg/5 mL; susp 25 mg/5 mL; Inj 25, 50 mg/mL **SE:** Drowsiness, anticholinergic effects **Notes:** Used to potentiate narcotic effects; not for IV/SQ (thrombosis & digital gangrene possible)

Hyoscyamine (Anaspaz, Cystospaz, Levsin, others) **Uses:** *Spasm w/ GI & bladder disorders* **Acts:** Anticholinergic **Dose:** *Adults.* 0.125–0.25 mg (1–2 tabs) SL/PO tid-qid, ac & hs; 1 SR caps q12h **Caution:** [C, +] ↑ Effects w/ amantadine, antihistamines, antimuscarinics, haloperidol, phenothiazines, TCA, MAOI **CI:** BOO, GI obst, NAG, MyG, paralytic ileus, ulcerative colitis, MI **Disp:** (Cystospaz-M, Levsinex) time-release caps 0.375 mg; elixir (EtOH); soln 0.125 mg/5 mL; Inj 0.5 mg/mL; tab 0.125 mg; tab (Cystospaz) 0.15 mg; XR tab (Levbid) 0.375 mg; SL (Levsin SL) 0.125 mg **SE:** Dry skin, xerostomia, constipation, anticholinergic SE, heat prostration w/ hot weather **Notes:** Administer tabs ac

Hyoscyamine, Atropine, Scopolamine, & Phenobarbital (Donnatal, Others) **Uses:** *Irritable bowel, spastic colitis, peptic ulcer, spastic bladder* **Acts:** Anticholinergic, antispasmodic **Dose:** 0.125–0.25 mg (1–2 tabs) tid-qid, 1 caps q12h (SR), 5–10 mL elixir tid-qid or q8h **Caution:** [C, ?/–] **CI:** [D, M] **Disp:** Many combos/ manufacturers. *Caps (Donnatal, others):* Hyoscyamine 0.1037 mg/atropine 0.0194 mg/ scopolamine 0.0065 mg/phenobarbital 16.2 mg. *Tabs (Donnatal, others):* Hyoscyamine 0.1037 mg/atropine 0.0194 mg/scopolamine 0.0065 mg/phenobarbital 16.2 mg. *LA (Donnatal):* Hyoscyamine 0.311 mg/atropine 0.0582 mg/scopolamine 0.0195 mg/phenobarbital 48.6 mg. *Elixirs (Donnatal, others):* Hyoscyamine 0.1037 mg/atropine 0.0194 mg/scopolamine 0.0065 mg/phenobarbital 16.2 mg/5 mL **SE:** Sedation, xerostomia, constipation

Ibandronate (Boniva) **Uses:** *Rx & prevent osteoporosis in postmenopausal women* **Acts:** Bisphosphonate, ↓ osteoclast-mediated bone-resorption **Dose:** 2.5 mg PO daily or 150 mg once/month on same day (do not lie down for 60 min after); 3 mg IV over 15–30 s q3mo **Caution:** [C, ?/–] Avoid w/ CrCl <30 mL/min **CI:** Uncorrected ↓ Ca^{2+}; inability to stand/sit upright for 60 min (PO) **Disp:** Tabs 2.5, 150 mg, Inj IV 3 mg/3 mL **SE:** Jaw osteonecrosis (avoid extensive dental procedures) N/D, HA, dizziness, asthenia, HTN, Infxn, dysphagia, esophagitis, esophageal/gastric ulcer, musculoskeletal pain **Notes:** Take 1st thing in AM. w/ H_2O (6–8 oz) >60 min before 1st food/beverage & any meds w/ multivalent cations; give adequate Ca^{2+} & vit D supls; possible association between bisphosphonates & severe muscle/bone/joint pain; may ↑ atypical subtrochanteric femur fractures

Ibuprofen, oral (Motrin, Motrin IB, Rufen, Advil, Others) [OTC]
BOX: May ↑ risk of CV events & GI bleeding **Uses:** *Arthritis, pain, fever* **Acts:** NSAID **Dose:** *Adults.* 200–800 mg PO bid-qid (max 2.4 g/d). *Peds.* 30–40 mg/kg/d in 3–4 ÷ doses (max 40 mg/kg/d); w/ food **Caution:** [B, +] May interfere w/ ASA's anti-plt effect if given <8 h before ASA **CI:** 3rd tri PRG, severe hepatic impair, allergy, use w/ other NSAIDs, upper GI bleeding, ulcers **Disp:** Tabs 100, 200, 400, 600, 800 mg; chew tabs 50, 100 mg; caps 200 mg; susp 100 mg/2.5 mL, 100 mg/5 mL, 40 mg/mL (Motrin IB & Advil OTC 200 mg are the OTC forms) **SE:** Dizziness, peptic ulcer, plt inhibition, worsening of renal insuff

Ibuprofen, parenteral (Caldolor)   **BOX:** May ↑ risk of CV events & GI bleeding **Uses:** *Mild/moderate pain, as adjunct to opioids, ↓ fever* **Acts:** NSAID **Dose:** *Pain:* 400–800 mg IV over 30 min Q 6 H PRN; *Fever:* 400 mg IV over 30 min, the 400 mg Q4-6 H or 100–200 mg Q4-6 H PRN **Caution:** [C < 30 wks, D after 30 wks, ?/-] may ↓ ACE effects; avoid w/ ASA, and < 17 yrs **CI:** Hypersens NSAID's; asthma, urticaria, or allergic Rxns w/ NSAIDs, peri-op CABG **Disp:** Vials 400 mg/4 mL, 800 mg/8 mL **SE:** N/V, HA, flatulence, hemorrhage, dizziness **Notes:** Make sure pt well hydrated

Ibutilide (Corvert) **Uses:** *Rapid conversion of AF/A flutter* **Acts:** Class III antiarrhythmic **Dose:** *Adults* >60 kg 1 mg IV over 10 min; may repeat × 1; <60 kg use 0.01 mg/kg (*ECC 2005;* DC cardioversion preferred) **Caution:** [C, –] **CI:** w/ Class I/III antiarrhythmics (Table 9 p 279); QTc >440 msec **Disp:** Inj 0.1 mg/mL **SE:** Arrhythmias, HA **Notes:** Give w/ ECG monitoring; ✓ K⁺, Mg²⁺

Idarubicin (Idamycin) **BOX:** Administer only under supervision of an MD experienced in leukemia and in an institution w/ resources to maintain a pt compromised by drug tox **Uses:** *Acute leukemias* (AML, ALL), *CML in blast crisis, breast CA* **Acts:** DNA-intercalating agent; ↓ DNA topoisomerase I & II **Dose:** (Per protocol) 10–12 mg/m²/d for 3–4 d; ↓ in renal/hepatic impair **Caution:** [D, –] **CI:** Bilirubin >5 mg/dL, PRG **Disp:** Inj 1 mg/mL (5-, 10-, 20 -mg vials) **SE:** ↓ BM, cardiotox, N/V, mucositis, alopecia, & IV site Rxns, rarely ↓ renal/hepatic Fxn **Notes:** Avoid extrav, potent vesicant; IV only

Ifosfamide (Ifex, Holoxan) **Uses:** Lung, breast, pancreatic & gastric CA, Hodgkin lymphoma/NHL, soft-tissue sarcoma **Acts:** Alkylating agent **Dose:** (Per protocol) 1.2 g/m²/d for 5 d bolus or cont Inf; 2.4 g/m²/d for 3 d; w/ MESNA uro-protection; ↓ in renal/hepatic impair **Caution:** [D, M] ↑ Effect w/ phenobarbital, carbamazepine, phenytoin; St. John's wort may ↓ levels [D-] w/ BM Fxn, PRG **Disp:** Inj 1, 3 g **SE:** Hemorrhagic cystitis, nephrotox, N/V, mild–mod leukopenia, lethargy & confusion, alopecia, ↑ hepatic enzyme **Notes:** Administer w/ mesna to prevent hemorrhagic cystitis

Iloperidone (Fanapt) **BOX:** Risk for torsades de pointes and ↑ QT. Elderly pts at ↑ risk of death, CVA **Uses:** *Acute schizophrenia* **Action:** Atypical antipsychotic **Dose:** *Initial:* 1 mg PO, ↑ daily to goal 12-24 mg/d ÷ BID **Caution:** [? /-] **CI:** component hypersens **Disp:** Tabs:1, 2, 4, 6, 8, 10, 12 mg **SE:**

Orthostatic ↓ BP, dizziness, dry mouth, ↑ wgt **Notes:** Titrate to ↓ BP risk. Monitor QT interval

Iloprost (Ventavis) **BOX:** Associated w/ syncope; may require dosage adjustment **Uses:** *NYHA class III/IV pulm arterial HTN* **Acts:** Prostaglandin analog **Dose:** Initial 2.5 mcg; if tolerated, ↑ to 5 mcg Inh 6–9×/d at least 2 h apart while awake **Caution:** [C, ?/–] Anti-plt effects, ↑ bleeding risk w/ anticoagulants; additive hypotension effects **CI:** SBP <85 mm Hg **Disp:** Inh soln 10 mcg/mL **SE:** Syncope, ↓ BP, vasodilation, cough, HA, trismus, D, dysgeusia, rash, oral irritation **Notes:** Requires *Pro-Dose AAD* or *I-neb ADD* system nebulizer; counsel on syncope risk; do not mix w/ other drugs; monitor vitals during initial Rx

Imatinib (Gleevec) **Uses:** *Rx CML Ph (+), CML blast crisis, ALL Ph(+), myelodysplastic/myeloproliferative Dz, aggressive systemic mastocytosis, chronic eosinophilic leukemia, GIST, dermatofibrosarcoma protuberans* **Acts:** ↓ BCL-ABL; TKI **Dose:** *Adults.* Typical dose 400–600 mg PO daily; w/ meal **Peds.** CML Ph (+) newly diagnosed 340 mg/m^2/d, 600 mg/d max; recurrent 260 mg/m^2/d PO ÷ daily-bid, to 340 mg/m^2/d max **Caution:** [D, ?/–] w/ CYP3A4 meds (Table 10 p 280), warfarin **CI:** Component sensitivity **Disp:** Tab 100, 400 mg **SE:** GI upset, fluid retention, muscle cramps, musculoskeletal pain, arthralgia, rash, HA, neutropenia, thrombocytopenia **Notes:** Follow CBCs & LFTs baseline & monthly; w/ large glass of H$_2$O & food to ↓ GI irritation

Imipenem–Cilastatin (Primaxin) **Uses:** *Serious infxns* d/t susceptible bacteria **Acts:** Bactericidal; ↓ cell wall synth. **Spectrum:** Gram(+) (*S. aureus,* group A & B streptococci), gram(–) (not *Legionella*), anaerobes **Dose:** *Adults.* 250–1000 mg (imipenem) IV q6–8h, 500–750 mg IM. **Peds.** 60–100 mg/kg/24 h IV ÷ q6h; ↓ if CrCl is <70 mL/min **Caution:** [C, +/–] Probenecid ↑ tox **CI:** Peds pts w/ CNS Infxn (↑ Sz risk) & <30 kg w/ renal impair **Disp:** Inj (imipenem/cilastatin) 250/250 mg, 500/500 mg **SE:** Szs if drug accumulates, GI upset, thrombocytopenia

Imipramine (Tofranil) **BOX:** Close observation for suicidal thinking or unusual changes in behavior **Uses:** *Depression, enuresis*, panic attack, chronic pain **Acts:** TCA; ↑ CNS synaptic serotonin or norepinephrine **Dose:** *Adults.* Hospitalized: Initial 100 mg/24 h PO in ÷ doses; ↑ over several wk 300 mg/d max. *Outpatient:* Maint 50–150 mg PO hs, 300 mg/24 h max. *Peds. Antidepressant:* 1.5–5 mg/kg/24 h ÷ daily-qid. *Enuresis:* >**6 y:** 10–25 mg PO qhs; ↑ by 10–25 mg at 1–2-wk intervals (max 50 mg for 6–12 y, 75 mg for >12 y); Rx for 2–3 mo, then taper **Caution:** [D, ?/–] **CI:** Use w/ MAOIs, NAG, acute recovery from MI, PRG, CHF, angina, CV Dz, arrhythmias **Disp:** Tabs 10, 25, 50 mg; caps 75, 100, 125, 150 mg **SE:** CV Sxs, dizziness, xerostomia, discolored urine **Notes:** Less sedation than amitriptyline

Imiquimod Cream, 5% (Aldara) **Uses:** *Anogenital warts, HPV, condylomata acuminata* **Acts:** Unknown; ? cytokine induction **Dose:** Apply 3×/wk, leave on 6–10 h & wash off w/ soap & water, continue 16 wk max **Caution:** [B, ?]

CI: Component sensitivity **Disp:** Single-dose packets 5% (250-mg cream) **SE:** Local skin Rxns **Notes:** Not a cure; may weaken condoms/vag diaphragms, wash hands before & after use

Immune Globulin, IV (Gamimune N, Gammaplex, Gammar IV, Sandoglobulin, others) **Uses:** *IgG deficiency Dz states, B-cell CLL, CIDP, HIV, hep A prophylaxis, ITP*, Kawasaki dx, travel to ↑ prevalence area and Hep A vaccination within 2 weeks of travel **Acts:** IgG supl **Dose:** *Adults & Peds. Immunodeficiency:* 200-(300 *Gammaplex*)-800 mg/kg/mo IV at 0.01–0.04 (0.08 *Gammaplex*) mL/kg/min; initial dose 0.01 mL/kg/min. *B-cell CLL:* 400 mg/kg/dose IV Q 3 wks, *CIDP:* 2,000 mg/kg/dose over 2–4 days then 1,000 mg/kg/day every 3 wks, *ITP:* 400 mg/kg/dose IV daily × 5 d. *BMT:* 500 mg/kg/wk; ↓ in renal Insuff **Caution:** [C, ?] Separate live vaccines by 3 mo **CI:** IgA deficiency w/ Abs to IgA, severe ↓ plt, coag disorders **Disp:** Inj **SE:** Associated mostly w/ Inf rate; GI upset, thrombotic events, hemolysis, renal failure/dysfun, TRALI **Notes:** Monitor vitals during infusion; do not give if volume depleted; Hep A prophylaxis with immunoglobulin is no better than with vaccination; advantages to using vaccination, cost similar

Immune Globulin, subcutaneous (Vivaglobin) **Uses:** *Primary immunodeficiency* **Acts:** IgG supl **Dose:** 100–200 mg/kg body wgt SQ weekly **Caution:** [C, ?] **CI:** Hx anaphylaxis to immune globulin; some IgA deficiency **Disp:** 10-, 20-mL vials w/ 160 mg/IgG/mL **SE:** Inj site Rxns, HA, GI complaint, fever, N, D, rash, sore throat **Notes:** May instruct in home administration; keep refrigerated; discard unused drug; dose >15 mL divide between sites

Inamrinone [Amrinone] (Inocor) **Uses:** *Acute CHF, ischemic cardiomyopathy* **Acts:** Inotrope w/ vasodilator **Dose:** IV bolus 0.75 mg/kg over 2–3 min; maint 5–10 mcg/kg/min, 10 mg/kg/d max; ↓ if CrCl <10 mL/min **Caution:** [C, ?] **CI:** Bisulfite allergy **Disp:** Inj 5 mg/mL **SE:** Monitor fluid, electrolyte, & renal changes **Notes:** Incompatible w/ dextrose solns, ✓ LFTs, observe for arrhythmias

Indapamide (Lozol) **Uses:** *HTN, edema, CHF* **Acts:** Thiazide diuretic; ↑ Na, Cl, & H_2O excretion in distal tubule **Dose:** 1.25–5 mg/d PO **Caution:** [D, ?] ↑ Effect w/ loop diuretics, ACE inhib, cyclosporine, digoxin, Li **CI:** Anuria, thiazide/sulfonamide allergy, renal Insuff, PRG **Disp:** Tabs 1.25, 2.5 mg **SE:** ↓ BP, dizziness, photosens **Notes:** No additional effects w/ doses >5 mg; take early to avoid nocturia; use sunscreen; OK w/ food/milk

Indinavir (Crixivan) **Uses:** *HIV Infxn* **Acts:** Protease inhib; ↓ maturation of noninfectious virions to mature infectious virus **Dose:** Typical 800 mg PO q8h in combo w/ other antiretrovirals (dose varies); on empty stomach; ↓ w/ hepatic impair **Caution:** [C, ?] Numerous drug interactions, especially CYP3A4 inhib (Table 10 p 280) **CI:** w/ Triazolam, midazolam, pimozide, ergot alkaloids, simvastatin, lovastatin, sildenafil, St. John's wort, amiodarone, salmeterol, PDE-5 inhib, Alpha 1-adrenoreceptor antagonist (alfuzosin); colchicine **Disp:** Caps 100, 200, 333, 400 mg **SE:** Nephrolithiasis, dyslipidemia, lipodystrophy, N/V, ↑ bili **Notes:** Drink six 8-oz glasses of H_2O/d

Indomethacin (Indocin) **BOX:** May ↑ risk of CV events & GI bleeding **Uses:** *Arthritis; close ductus arteriosus; ankylosing spondylitis* **Acts:** ↓ Prostaglandins **Dose:** *Adults.* 25–50 mg PO bid-tid, max 200 mg/d **Infants:** 0.2–0.25 mg/kg/dose IV; may repeat in 12–24 h up to 3 doses; w/ food **Caution:** [B, +] **CI:** ASA/NSAID sensitivity, peptic ulcer/active GI bleed, precipitation of asthma/urticaria/rhinitis by NSAIDs/ASA, premature neonates w/ NEC, ↓ renal Fxn, active bleeding, thrombocytopenia, 3rd tri PRG **Disp:** Inj 1 mg/vial; caps 25, 50 mg; SR caps 75 mg; susp 25 mg/5 mL **SE:** GI bleeding or upset, dizziness, edema **Notes:** Monitor renal Fxn

Infliximab (Remicade) **BOX:** TB, invasive fungal infxns, & other opportunistic infxns reported, some fatal; perform TB skin testing prior to use; possible association w/ rare lymphoma **Uses:** *Mod–severe Crohn Dz; fistulizing Crohn Dz; ulcerative colitis; RA (w/ MTX) psoriasis, ankylosing spondylitis* **Acts:** IgG1K neutralizes TNF-α **Dose:** *Adults. Crohn Dz: Induction:* 5 mg/kg IV Inf, w/ doses 2 & 6 wk after. *Maint:* 5 mg/kg IV Inf q8wk. *RA:* 3 mg/kg IV Inf at 0, 2, 6 wk, then q8wk. *Peds >6 y:* 5 mg/kg IV q8wk **Caution:** [B, ?/–] Active Infxn, hepatic impair, Hx or risk of TB, hep B **CI:** Murine allergy, mod–severe CHF, w/ live vaccines (e.g., smallpox) **Disp:** 100 mg Inj **SE:** Allergic Rxns; HA, fatigue, GI upset, Inf Rxns; hepatotox; reactivation hep B, pneumonia, BM suppression, systemic vasculitis, pericardial effusion, new psoriasis **Notes:** Monitor LFTs, PPD at baseline, monitor hep B carrier, skin exam for malignancy w/ psoriasis; can premedicate w/ antihistamines, APAP, and/or steroids to ↓ Inf Rxns

Influenza Vaccine, Inactivated (Afluria, Agriflu, Fluarix, FluLaval, Fluvirin, Fluzone) **Uses:** *Prevent influenza (not H1N1/swine flu)* adults >50 y, children 6–59 mo, pregnant women (2nd/3rd tri during flu season), nursing home residents, chronic dzs (asthma, CAD, DM, chronic liver or renal dx, hematologic dzs, immunosuppression), health-care workers, household contacts and caregivers of high-risk pts (children <5 yrs and adults > 50 yrs) **Acts:** Active immunization **Dose:** *Adults and Peds >9 y:* 0.5 mL/dose IM annually. *Peds 6 mo–3 y:* 0.25 mL IM annually; 0.25 mL IM × 2 doses >4 wk apart 1st vaccination; give 2 doses in 2nd vaccination year if only 1 dose given in 1st year. *3–8 y:* 0.5 mL IM annually, start 0.5 mL IM × 2 doses >4 wk apart 1st vaccination **Caution:** [C, +] **CI:** Egg hypersensitivity; neomycin, polymyxin (*Afluria*), kanamycin, neomycin (*Agriflu*), gentamicin (*Fluarix*), polymyxin, neomycin (*Fluvirin*)/thimerosal allergy (*FluLaval, Fluvirin, and multi-dose Fluzone*); infection at site, acute resp or febrile illness, Hx Guillain-Barré, immunocompromised **Disp:** Based on manufacturer, 0.25, 0.5-mL prefilled syringes **SE:** Inj site soreness, fever, chills, headache, insomnia, myalgia, malaise, rash, urticaria, anaphylactoid rxns, Guillain-Barré synd **Notes:** Not for swine flu H1N1; can be administered at same time. *Fluarix* and *Agriflu* not for peds; US Oct-Nov best, protection 1–2 wk after, lasts up to 6 mo; given yearly, vaccines based on predictions of flu season (Nov-April in US, though sporadic cases all year); whole or split virus for adults; peds <13 y split virus or purified surface antigen to ↑ febrile Rxns; see www.cdc.gov/flu; 2010–11 US trivalent vaccines will protect against 3 different flu viruses: H3N2,influenza B, H1N1

Influenza Monovalent Vaccine (H1N1), Inactivated (CSL, ID Biomedical, Novartis, Sanofi Pasteur)
The 2010–11 flu vaccines in the US/Canada will be the trivalent influenza vaccine that includes pandemic H1N1 influenza A. The monovalent vaccine against H1N1 influenza A will no longer be administered.

Influenza Virus Vaccine, Live, Intranasal [LAIV] (FluMist)
Uses: *Prevent influenza* **Acts:** Live-attenuated vaccine **Dose:** *Adults 18–49 y:* 0.1 mL each nostril × 1 annually *Peds 2–8 y:* 0.1 mL each nostril × 1 annually; initial 0.1 mL each nostril × 2 doses >6 wk apart in 1st vaccination year >*9 y:* See adults **Caution:** [C, ?/–] **CI:** Age <2 years, egg, gentamicin, gelatin, or arginine allergy, peds 2–17 y on ASA, PRG, Hx Guillain–Barré, known/suspected immune deficiency, asthma or reactive airway Dz, acute febrile illness, **Disp:** Prefilled, single-use, intranasal sprayer; shipped frozen, store 35–46°F **SE:** Runny nose, nasal congestion, HA, cough **Notes:** Do not give w/ other vaccines; avoid contact w/ immunocompromised individuals for 21 d; live influenza vaccine more effective in children than inactivated influenza vaccine; 2010–11 US trivalent vaccine will protect against 3 different flu viruses: H3N2, influenza B, H1N1.

Insulin, Injectable (see Table 4 page 269)
Uses: *Type 1 or type 2 DM refractory to diet or PO hypoglycemic agents; acute life-threatening ↑ K+* **Acts:** Insulin supl **Dose:** Based on serum glucose; usually SQ (upper arms, abd wall [most rapid absorption site], upper legs, buttocks); can give IV (only regular)/IM; type 1 typical start dose 0.5–1 units/kg/d; type 2 0.3–0.4 units/kg/d; renal failure ↓ insulin needs **Caution:** [B, +] **CI:** Hypoglycemia **Disp:** Table 4 p 269. Some can dispensed w/preloaded insulin cartridge pens w/ 29-, 30-, or 31-gauge needles and dosing adjustments. **SE:** Hypoglycemia. Highly purified insulins ↑ free insulin; monitor for several wks when changing doses/agents **Notes:** Specific agent/regimen based on patient and physician choices that maintain glycemic control. Typical type 1 regimens use a basal daily insulin w/ premeal Inj of rapidly acting insulins. Insulin pumps may achieve basal insulin levels. ↑ malignancy risk w/ glargine controversial.

Interferon Alfa (Roferon-A, Intron-A)
BOX: Can cause or aggravate fatal or life-threatening neuropsychological, autoimmune, ischemic, and infectious disorders. Monitor closely **Uses:** *Hairy cell leukemia, Kaposi sarcoma, melanoma, CML, chronic hep B & C, follicular NHL, condyloma acuminata* **Acts:** Antiproliferative; modulates host immune response; ↓ viral replication in infected cells **Dose:** Per protocols. *Adults.* Per protocols. *Hairy cell leukemia:* Alfa-2a (Roferon-A): 3 mill units/d for 16–24 wk SQ/IM then 3 mill units 3×/wk × 6–24 mo; Alfa-2b (Intron A): 2 mill units/m² IM/SQ 3×/wk for 2–6 mo. *Chronic hep B:* Alfa-2b (Intron A): 3 mill units/m² SQ 3×/wk × 1 wk, then 6 mill units/m² 3×/wk (max 10 mill units 3×/wk, total duration 16–24 wk). *Follicular NHL* (Intron A): 5 mill units SQ 3×/wk for 18 mo. *Melanoma* (Intron A): 20 mill units/m²

IV × 5 d/wk × 4 wk, then 10 mill units/m² SQ 3×/wk × 48 wk. *Kaposi sarcoma* (Intron A): 30 mill units/m² IM/SQ 3×/wk × 10–12 wk, then 36 mill units IM/SQ 3×/wk. *Chronic hep C* (Intron A): 3 mill units 3×/wk × 16 wk (continue 18–24 mo if response). *Roferon A:* 3 mill units 3×/wk for 12 mo SQ/IM. *Condyloma* (Intron A): 1 mill units/lesion (max 5 lesions) 3×/wk for 3 wk. **Peds. CML:** Alfa-2a (Roferon-A): 2.5–5 mill units/m² IM daily. **CI:** Benzyl alcohol sensitivity, decompensated liver Dz, autoimmune Dz, immunosuppressed, neonates, infants **Disp:** Inj forms (see also polyethylene glycol [PEG]-interferon) **SE:** Flu-like Sxs, fatigue, anorexia, neurotox at high doses; up to 40% neutralizing Ab w/ Rx

Interferon Alfa-2b & Ribavirin Combo (Rebetron) **BOX:** Can cause or aggravate fatal or life-threatening neuropsychological, autoimmune, ischemic, and infectious disorders. Monitor pts closely. CI in pregnant females & their male partners **Uses:** *Chronic hep C w/ compensated liver Dz who relapse after α-interferon Rx therapy* **Acts:** Combo antiviral agents (see individual agents) **Dose:** 3 mill units Intron A SQ 3× wk w/ 1000–1200 mg of Rebetron PO ÷ bid dose for 24 wk. *Pts <75 kg:* 1000 mg of Rebetron/d **Caution:** [X, ?] **CI:** PRG, males w/ PRG female partner, autoimmune hep, CrCl <50 mL/min **Disp:** *Pts <75 kg:* Combo packs: 6 vials Intron A (3 mill units/0.5 mL) w/ 6 syringes & EtOH swabs, 70 Rebetol caps; one 18-mill units multidose vial of Intron A Inj (22.8 mill units/3.8 mL; 3 mill units/0.5 mL) & 6 syringes & swabs, 70 Rebetol caps; one 18-mill units Intron A Inj multidose pen (22.5 mill units/1.5 mL; 3 mill units/0.2 mL) w/ 6 needles & swabs, 70 Rebetol caps. *Pts >75 kg:* Identical except 84 Rebetol caps/pack **SE:** See Box, flu-like synd, HA, anemia **Notes:** Monthly PRG test; instruct in self-administration of SQ Intron A

Interferon Alfacon-1 (Infergen) **BOX:** Can cause or aggravate fatal or life-threatening neuropsychological, autoimmune, ischemic, & infectious disorders. Monitor closely **Uses:** *Chronic hep C* **Acts:** Biologic response modifier **Dose:** 9 mcg SQ 3×/wk × 24 wk **Caution:** [C, M] **CI:** *E. coli* product allergy **Disp:** Inj 9, 15 mcg **SE:** Flu-like synd, depression, blood dyscrasias, colitis, pancreatitis, hepatic decompensation, ↑ SCr, eye disorders, ↓ thyroid **Notes:** Allow >48 h between Inj; monitor CBC, plt, SCr, TFT

Interferon Beta-1a (Rebif) **BOX:** Can cause or aggravate fatal or life-threatening neuropsychological, autoimmune, ischemic, & infectious disorders. Monitor closely **Uses:** *MS, relapsing* **Acts:** Biologic response modifier **Dose:** 44 mcg SQ 3×/wk; start 8.8 mcg SQ 3×/wk × 2 wk, then 22 mcg SQ 3×/wk × 2 wk **Caution:** [C, ?] w/ Hepatic impair, depression, Sz disorder, thyroid Dz **CI:** Human albumin allergy **Disp:** 0.5- mL prefilled syringes w/ 29-gauge needle *Titrate Pak* 8.8 and 22 mcg; 22 or 44 mcg **SE:** Inj site Rxn, HA, flu-like Sx, malaise, fatigue, rigors, myalgia, depression w/ suicidal ideation, hepatotox, ↓ BM **Notes:** Dose >48 h apart; ✓ CBC 1, 3, 6 mo; ✓ TFTs q6mo w/ Hx thyroid Dz

Interferon Beta-1b (Betaseron, Extavia) **Uses:** *MS, relapsing/remitting/secondary progressive* **Acts:** Biologic response modifier **Dose:** 0.0625 mg (2 MU) (0.25 mL) q other day SQ, ↑ by 0.0625 mg q2wk to target dose 0.25 mg (1 mL) q other day **Caution:** [C, ?/–] **CI:** Human albumin sensitivity **Disp:** Powder for Inj 0.3 mg (32 MU interferon [IFN]) **SE:** Flu-like synd, depression, suicide, blood dyscrasias, ↑ AST/ALT/GGT, inj site necrosis, anaphylaxis **Notes:** Teach pt self-injection, rotate sites; ✓ LFTs, CBC 1, 3, 6 mo; TFT q6mo; consider stopping w/depression

Interferon Gamma-1b (Actimmune) **Uses:** *↓ Incidence of serious in-fxns in chronic granulomatous Dz (CGD), osteoporosis* **Acts:** Biologic response modifier **Dose:** **Adults.** **CGD:** 50 mcg/m² SQ (1.5 **mill units** /m²) BSA >0.5 m²; if BSA <0.5 m², give 1.5 mcg/kg/dose; given 3× wk **Caution:** [C, ?] **CI:** Allergy to *E. coli*-derived products **Disp:** Inj 100 mcg (2 **mill units**) **SE:** Flu-like synd, depression, blood dyscrasias, dizziness, altered mental status, gait disturbance, hepatic tox **Notes:** may ↑ deaths in interstitial pulm fibrosis

Ipecac Syrup [OTC] **Uses:** *Drug OD, certain cases of poisoning* **Editorial Note: Usage is falling out of favor & is no longer recommended by some groups** **Acts:** Irritation of the GI mucosa; stimulation of the chemoreceptor trigger zone **Dose:** **Adults.** 15–30 mL PO, followed by 200–300 mL of H_2O; if no emesis in 20 min, repeat once. **Peds 6–12 mo** 5–10 mL PO, followed by 10–20 mL/kg of H_2O; if no emesis in 20 min, repeat once. **1–12 y:** 15 mL PO followed by 10–20 mL/kg of H_2O; if no emesis in 20 min, repeat once **Caution:** [C, ?] **CI:** Ingestion of petroleum distillates, strong acid, base, or other caustic agents; comatose/unconscious **Disp:** Syrup 15, 30 mL (OTC) **SE:** Lethargy, D, cardiotox, protracted V **Notes:** Caution in CNS depressant OD; activated charcoal considered more effective (www.clintox.org/PosStatements/Ipecac.html)

Ipratropium (Atrovent HFA, Atrovent nasal) **Uses:** *Bronchospasm w/ COPD, rhinitis, rhinorrhea* **Acts:** Synthetic anticholinergic similar to atropine; antagonizes acetylcholine receptors, inhibits mucous gland secretions **Dose:** **Adults & Peds >12 y:** 2–4 puffs qid, max 12 Inh/d **Nasal:** 2 sprays/nostril bid-tid; **Nebulization:** 500 mcg 3–4 ×times/d **Caution:** [B, +/–] w/ Inhaled insulin **CI:** Allergy to soya lecithin-related foods **Disp:** HFA Metered-dose inhaler 18 mcg/dose; Inh soln 0.02%; nasal spray 0.03, 0.06% **SE:** Nervousness, dizziness, HA, cough, bitter taste, nasal dryness, URI, epistaxis **Notes:** Not for acute bronchospasm

Irbesartan (Avapro) **BOX:** D/C immediately if PRG detected **Uses:** *HTN, DN*, CHF **Acts:** Angiotensin II receptor antagonist **Dose:** 150 mg/d PO, may ↑ to 300 mg/d **Caution:** [C (1st tri; D 2nd/3rd), ?/–] **CI:** PRG, component sensitivity **Disp:** Tabs 75, 150, 300 mg **SE:** Fatigue, ↓ BP ↑ K

Irinotecan (Camptosar) **BOX:** D & myelosuppression **Uses:** *Colorectal* & lung CA **Acts:** Topoisomerase I inhib; ↓ DNA synth **Dose:** Per protocol; 125–350 mg/m² q wk–q3wk (↓ hepatic dysfunction, as tolerated per tox) **Caution:** [D, –] **CI:** Allergy to component **Disp:** Inj 20 mg/mL **SE:** ↓ BM, N/V/D, Abd cramping, alopecia; D is dose limiting; Rx acute D w/ atropine; Rx subacute D w/ loperamide **Notes:** D correlated to levels of metabolite SN-38

Iron Dextran (Dexferrum, INFeD) **BOX:** Anaphylactic Rxns w/ use; use only if oral iron not possible; test dose before first dose; administer where resuscitation techniques available **Uses:** *Fe deficiency when cannot supplement PO* **Acts:** Fe supl **Dose:** *Adults. Iron deficiency anemia:* Estimate Fe deficiency, give 25–100 mg IM/IV/d until total dose; total dose (mL) = [0.0442 × (desired Hgb − observed Hgb) × lean body wgt] + (0.26 × lean body wgt); *Iron replacement, blood loss:* total dose (mg) = blood loss (mL) × Hct (as decimal fraction) max 100 mg/d; *Peds >4 mo:* As above Adults; max: 0.5 mL (wgt <5 kg), 1 mL (5–10 kg), 2 mL (>10 kg) per dose IM or direct IV **Caution:** [C, M]Anaphylaxis possible; rx w/epinephrine **CI:** Anemia w/o Fe deficiency. **Disp:** Inj 50 mg (Fe)/mL **SE:** Anaphylaxis, flushing, dizziness, Inj site & Inf Rxns, metallic taste **Notes:** Give IM w/ "Z-track" technique; IV preferred; give test dose TEST DOSE OF 0.5 mL IV >1 h before; see insert tables for requirement for hemoglobin restoration and iron stores replacement

Iron Sucrose (Venofer) **Uses:** *Fe deficiency anemia w/ chronic HD in those receiving erythropoietin* **Actions:** Fe replacement. **Dose:** 5 mL (100 mg) IV on dialysis, 1 mL (20 mg)/min max **Caution:** [C, M] **CI:** Anemia w/o Fe deficiency **Disp:** 20 mg elemental Fe/mL, 5-mL vials. **SE:** Anaphylaxis, ↓ BP, cramps, N/V/D, HA **Notes:** Most pts require cumulative doses of 1000 mg; give slowly

Isoniazid (INH) **Uses:** *Rx & prophylaxis of TB* **Acts:** Bactericidal; interferes w/ mycolic acid synth, disrupts cell wall **Dose:** *Adults. Active TB:* 5 mg/kg/24 h PO or IM (usually 300 mg/d) or *DOT:* 15 mg/kg (max 900 mg) 3×/wk. *Prophylaxis:* 300 mg/d PO for 6–12 mo or 900 mg 2×/wk. **Peds.** *Active TB:* 10–15 mg/kg/d daily-bid PO or IM 300 mg/d max. *Prophylaxis:* 10 mg/kg/24 h PO; ↓ in hepatic/renal dysfunction **Caution:** [C, +] Liver Dz, dialysis; avoid EtOH **CI:** Acute liver Dz, Hx INH hep **Disp:** Tabs 100, 300 mg; syrup 50 mg/5 mL; Inj 100 mg/mL **SE:** Hep, peripheral neuropathy, GI upset, anorexia, dizziness, skin Rxn **Notes:** Use w/ 2–3 other drugs for active TB, based on INH resistance patterns when TB acquired & sensitivity results; prophylaxis usually w/ INH alone. IM rarely used. ↓ Peripheral neuropathy w/ pyridoxine 50–100 mg/d. See CDC guidelines (*MMWR*) for current recommendations

Isoproterenol (Isuprel) **Uses:** *Shock, cardiac arrest, AV nodal block* **Acts:** β_1- & β_2-receptor stimulant **Dose:** *Adults.* 2–10 mcg/min IV Inf; titrate; 2–10 mcg/min titrate (*ECC 2005*) *Peds.* 0.2–2 mcg/kg/min IV Inf; titrate **Caution:** [C, ?] **CI:** Angina, tachyarrhythmias (digitalis-induced or others) **Disp:** 0.02 mg/mL, 0.2 mg/mL **SE:** Insomnia, arrhythmias, HA, trembling, dizziness **Notes:** Pulse >130 BPM may induce arrhythmias

Isosorbide Dinitrate (Isordil, Sorbitrate, Dilatrate-SR) **Uses:** *Rx & prevent angina*, CHF (w/ hydralazine) **Acts:** Relaxes vascular smooth muscle **Dose:** *Acute angina:* 5–10 mg PO (chew tabs) q2–3h or 2.5–10 mg SL PRN q5–10 min; do not give >3 doses in a 15–30-min period. *Angina prophylaxis:* 5–40 mg PO q6h; do not give nitrates on a chronic q6h or qid basis >7–10 d; tolerance may develop; provide 10–12-h drug-free intervals; *dose in CHF:* initial 20 mg 3–4×/d, target 120–160 mg/d **Caution:** [C, ?] **CI:** Severe anemia, NAG, postural ↓

BP, cerebral hemorrhage, head trauma (can ↑ ICP), w/ sildenafil, tadalafil, vardenafil **Disp:** Tabs 5, 10, 20, 30; SR tabs 40 mg; SL tabs 2.5, 5 mg; SR caps 40 mg **SE:** HA, ↓ BP, flushing, tachycardia, dizziness **Notes:** Higher PO dose needed for same results as SL forms

Isosorbide Mononitrate (Ismo, Imdur)
Uses: *Prevention/Rx of angina pectoris* **Acts:** Relaxes vascular smooth muscle **Dose:** 5–10 mg PO bid, w/ the 2 doses 7 h apart or XR (Imdur) 30–60 mg/d PO, max 240 mg **Caution:** [C, ?] **CI:** Head trauma/cerebral hemorrhage (can ↑ ICP), w/ sildenafil, tadalafil, vardenafil **Disp:** Tabs 10, 20 mg; XR 30, 60, 120 mg **SE:** HA, dizziness, ↓ BP

Isotretinoin [13-*cis* Retinoic Acid] (Accutane, Amnesteem, Claravis, Sotret)
BOX: Must not be used by PRG females; can induce severe birth defects; pt must be capable of complying w/ mandatory contraceptive measures; prescribed according to product-specific risk management system. Because of teratogenicity, is approved for marketing only under a special restricted distribution FDA program called iPLEDGE **Uses:** *Refractory severe acne* **Acts:** Retinoic acid derivative **Dose:** 0.5–2 mg/kg/d PO ÷ bid; ↓ in hepatic Dz, take w/ food **Caution:** [X, –] Avoid tetracyclines **CI:** Retinoid sensitivity, PRG **Disp:** Caps 10, 20, 30, 40 mg **SE:** *Rare:* Depression, psychosis, suicidal thoughts; derm sensitivity, xerostomia, photosens, ↑ LFTs, & triglycerides **Notes:** Risk management program requires 2 (–) PRG tests before Rx & use of 2 forms of contraception 1 mo before, during, & 1 mo after Rx; to prescribe isotretinoin, the prescriber must access the iPLEDGE system via the Internet (www. ipledgeprogram.com); monitor LFTs & lipids

Isradipine (DynaCirc)
Uses: *HTN* **Acts:** CCB **Dose:** *Adults.* 2.5–5 mg PO bid. **Caution:** [C, ?] **CI:** Severe heart block, sinus bradycardia, CHF, dosing w/in several hours of IV β-blockers **Disp:** Caps 2.5, 5 mg; tabs CR 5, 10 mg **SE:** HA, edema, flushing, fatigue, dizziness, palpitations

Itraconazole (Sporanox)
BOX: CI w/ cisapride, pimozide, quinidine, dofetilide, or lev acetylmethadol. Serious CV events (e.g., ↑ QT, torsades de pointes, ventricular tachycardia, cardiac arrest, and/or sudden death) reported w/ these meds and other CYP3A4 inhib. Do not use for onychomycosis w/ ventricular dysfunction **Uses:** *Fungal infxns (aspergillosis, blastomycosis, histoplasmosis, candidiasis)* **Acts:** Azole antifungal, ↓ ergosterol synth **Dose:** 200 mg PO daily-bid (caps w/ meals or cola/grapefruit juice); PO soln on empty stomach; avoid antacids **Caution:** [C, ?] Numerous interactions **CI:** See Box; PRG or considering PRG; ventricular dysfunction **Disp:** Caps 100 mg; soln 10 mg/mL **SE:** N/V, rash, hepatotoxic, ↓ K⁺, CHF, ↑ BP, neuropathy **Notes:** soln & caps not interchangeable; useful in pts who cannot take amphotericin B; follow LFTs

Ixabepilone Kit (Ixempra)
BOX: CI in combo w/ capecitabine w/ AST/ALT >2.5× ULN or bili >1× ULN d/t ↑ tox and neutropenia-related death **Uses:** *Metastatic/locally advanced breast CA after failure of an anthracycline, a taxane, and capecitabine* **Acts:** Microtubule inhib **Dose:** 40 mg/m² IV over 3 h q3wk **Caution:** [D, ?/–] **CI:** Hypersens to Cremophor EL; baseline ANC <1500 cells/mm³ or plt

<100,000 cells/mm³; AST/ or ALT >2.5× ULN, bili >1× ULN **Disp:** Inj 15, 45 mg (use supplied diluent) **SE:** neutropenia, leukopenia, anemia, thrombocytopenia, peripheral sensory neuropathy, fatigue/asthenia, myalgia/arthralgia, alopecia, N/V/D, stomatitis/ mucositis **Notes:** Substrate CYP3A4, adjust dose w/ strong CYP3A4 inhib/inducers

Japanese encephalitis vaccine, inactivated, adsorbed (Ixiaro, Je-Vax) **Uses:** *Prevent Japanese encephalitis* **Action:** Inactivated vaccine **Dose:** *Adults.*0.5 ml IM, repeat 28 days later *Peds.* Use Je-Vax, 1–3 yrs: Three 0.5 ml SQ doses day 0, 7, 30; >3 yrs: Three 1ml SQ doses on day 0, 7, 30 **Caution:** [B (Ixiaro)/C (Je-Vax), ?] **SE:** HA, fatigue, inj site pain, flu-like syndrome, hypers- ens rxns **Notes:** Abbrev admin schedules of 3 doses on day 0, 7, and 14; booster dose recommended after 2 yrs. Avoid ETOH 48 hrs after dose

Ketamine (Ketalar)[CIII] **Uses:** *Induction/maintenance of anesthesia* (in combo w/ sedatives), sedation, analgesia **Action:** dissociative anesthesia; IV onset 30 sec, duration 5–10 min **Dose:** *Adults.:* 1–4.5 mg/kg IV, typical 2 mg/kg; 3–8 mg/kg IM *Peds.:* 0.5–2 mg/kg IV; 0.5–1 mg/kg for minor procedures(also IM/ PO regimens) **Caution:** w/ CAD, ↑ BP, tachycardia, EtOH use/abuse [C, ?/–] **CI:** When ↑ BP hazardous **Disp:** Soln 10, 50, 100 mg/mL **SE:** Arrhythmia, ↑/↓ HR, ↑/↓ BP, N/V, resp depression, emergence Rxn, ↑ CSF pressure. CYP2B6 inhibs w/ ↓ metabolism **Notes:** Used in RSI protocols; street drug of abuse

Ketoconazole (Nizoral) **BOX:** (Oral use) Risk of fatal hepatotox. Concom- itant terfenadine, astemizole, and cisapride are CI d/t serious cardiovascular CV adverse events **Uses:** *Systemic fungal infxns (Candida, blastomycosis, histoplas- mosis, etc); refractory topical dermatophyte Infxn*; PCa when rapid ↓ testosterone needed or hormone refractory **Acts:** Azole, ↓ fungal cell wall synth; high dose blocks P450, to ↓ testosterone production **Dose:** *PO:* 200 mg PO daily; ↑ to 400 mg PO daily for serious Infxn. *PCa:* 400 mg PO tid w/hydrocortisone 20–40 mg ÷ bid; best on empty stomach **Caution:** [C, +/–] w/ Any agent that ↑ gastric pH (↓ absorption); may enhance anticoagulants; w/ EtOH (disulfiram-like Rxn); numerous interactions including statins, niacin; do not use w/ clopidogrel (↓ effect) **CI:** CNS fungal infxns, w/ astemizole, triazolam **Disp:** Tabs 200 mg **SE:** N, rashes, hair loss, HA, ↑ wgt gain, dizziness, disorientation, fatigue, impotence, hepatox, adrenal suppression, acquired cutaneous adherence ("sticky skin synd") **Notes:** Monitor LFTs; can rapidly ↓ testosterone levels

Ketoconazole, Topical (Extina, Kuric, Nizoral A-D Shampoo, Xolegel) [Shampoo—OTC] **Uses:** *Topical for seborrheic dermatitis, sham- poo for dandruff* local fungal infxns d/t dermatophytes & yeast **Acts:** azole, ↓ fungal cell wall synth **Dose:** *Topical:* Apply q day-bid **Caution:** [C, +/–] **CI:** Bro- ken/inflamed skin **Disp:** Tabs 200 mg; topical cream 2%; (*Xolegel*) gel 2%,(*Extina*) foam 2%, shampoo 1% & 2% **SE:** Irritation, pruritus, stinging **Notes:** Do not dispense foam in hands

Ketoprofen (Orudis, Oruvail) **BOX:** May ↑ risk of CV events & GI bleeding; CI for perioperative pain in CABG surgery **Uses:** *Arthritis (RA/OA),* pain* **Acts:** NSAID; ↓ prostaglandins **Dose:** 25–75 mg PO tid-qid, 300 mg/d/max; SR 200 mg/d; w/ food; ↓ w/ hepatic/renal impair, elderly **Caution:** [C(D 3rd tri), –] w/ ACE, diuretics; ↑ warfarin, Li, MTX **CI:** NSAID/ASA sensitivity **Disp:** Caps 50, 75 mg; caps, SR 200 mg **SE:** GI upset, peptic ulcers, dizziness, edema, rash, ↑ BP, ↑ LFTs, renal dysfunction

Ketorolac (Toradol) **BOX:** For short-term (≤5 d) Rx of mod–severe acute pain; CI w/ PUD, GI bleed, post CABG, anticipated major surgery, severe renal Insuff, bleeding diathesis, labor & delivery, nursing, and w/ ASA/NSAIDs. NSAIDs may cause ↑an increased risk of risk CV/ thrombotic events (MI, stroke). PO CI in peds <16 y **Uses:** *Pain* **Acts:** NSAID; ↓ prostaglandins **Dose:** *Adults.* 15–30 mg IV/IM q6h; 10 mg PO qid only as continuation of IM/IV; max IV/IM 120 mg/d, max PO 40 mg/d. *Peds 2–16 y:* 1 mg/kg IM × 1 dose; 30 mg max; IV: 0.5 mg/kg, 15 mg max; do not use for >5 d; ↓ if >65 y, elderly, w/ renal impair, <50 kg **Caution:** [C(D 3rd tri), –] w/ ACE inhib, diuretics, BP meds, warfarin **CI:** See Box **Disp:** Tabs 10 mg; Inj 15 mg/mL, 30 mg/mL **SE:** Bleeding, peptic ulcer Dz, ↑ Cr & LFTs, ↑ BP, edema, dizziness, allergy

Ketorolac Ophthalmic (Acular, Acular LS, Acular PF) **Uses:** *Ocular itching w/ seasonal allergies; inflammation w/ cataract extraction*; pain/photophobia w/ incisional refractive surgery (Acular PF); pain w/ corneal refractive surgery (Acular LS) **Acts:** NSAID **Dose:** 1 gtt qid **Caution:** [C, +] Possible cross-sensitivity to NSAIDs, ASA **CI:** Hypersens **Disp:** *Acular LS:* 0.4% 5 mL; *Acular:* 0.5% 3, 5, 10 mL; *Acular PF:* Soln 0.5% **SE:** Local irritation, ↑ bleeding ocular tissues, hyphemas, slow healing, keratitis **Notes:** Do not use w/ contacts

Ketotifen (Alaway, Zaditor) [OTC] **Uses:** *Allergic conjunctivitis* **Acts:** Antihistamine H₁-receptor antagonist, mast cell stabilizer **Dose:** *Adults & Peds >3 y:* 1 gtt in eye(s) q8–12h **Caution:** [C, ?/–] **Disp:** Soln 0.025%/5 & 10 mL **SE:** Local irritation, HA, rhinitis, keratitis, mydriasis **Notes:** Wait 10 min before inserting contacts

Kunecatechins [Sinecatechins] (Veregen) **Uses:** *External genital/perianal warts* **Acts:** Unknown; green tea extract **Dose:** Apply 0.5-cm ribbon to each wart 3×/d until all warts clear; not >16 wk **Caution:** [C,; ?] **Disp:** Oint 15% **SE:** Erythema, pruritus, burning, pain, erosion/ulceration, edema, induration, rash, phimosis **Notes:** Wash hands before/after use; not necessary to wipe off prior to next use; avoid on open wounds

Labetalol (Trandate) **Uses:** *HTN* & hypertensive emergencies (IV) **Acts:** α- & β-Adrenergic blocker **Dose:** *Adults.* *HTN:* Initial, 100 mg PO bid, then 200–400 mg PO bid. *Hypertensive emergency:* 20–80 mg IV bolus, then 2 mg/min IV Inf, titrate up to 300 mg; 10 mg IV over 1–2 min; repeat or double dose q10min (150 mg max); or initial bolus, then 2–8 mg/min (*ECC 2005*). **Peds.** *PO:* 1–3 mg/kg/d in ÷ doses, 1200 mg/d max. *Hypertensive emergency:* 0.4–1.5 mg/kg/h IV cont Inf **Caution:** [C (D in 2nd or 3rd tri), +] **CI:** Asthma/COPD, cardiogenic shock, uncompensated CHF, heart block, sinus brady **Disp:** Tabs 100, 200, 300 mg; Inj 5 mg/mL **SE:** Dizziness, N, ↓ BP, fatigue, CV effects

Lacosamide (Vimpat) BOX: Antiepileptics associated w/ ↑ risk of suicide ideation Uses: *Adjunct in partial-onset Szs* Action: Anticonvulsant Dose: *Initial:* 50 mg IV or PO BID, ↑ weekly; *Maint:* 200-400 mg/d; 300 mg/d max if CrCl < 30 mL/min or mild/mod hepatic Dz Caution: [C, /?] CI: None Disp: *IV:* 10 mg/mL; Tabs: 50, 100, 150, 200 mg SE: Dizziness, N/V, ataxia Notes: ✓ ECG before dosing; may ↑ PR interval

Lactic Acid & Ammonium Hydroxide [Ammonium Lactate] (Lac-Hydrin) Uses: *Severe xerosis & ichthyosis* Acts: Emollient moisturizer, humectant Dose: Apply bid Caution: [B, ?] Disp: Cream, lotion, lactic acid 12% w/ ammonium hydroxide Notes: Local irritation, photosens Notes: Shake well before use

Lactobacillus (Lactinex Granules) [OTC] Uses: *Control of D*, especially after antibiotic Rx Acts: Replaces nl intestinal flora, lactase production; *Lactobacillus acidophilus* and *Lactobacillus helveticus.* Dose: *Adults & Peds >3 y:* 1 packet, 1–2 caps, or 4 tabs q day-qid Caution: [A, +] Some products may contain whey CI: Milk/lactose allergy Disp: Tabs, caps; granules in packets (all OTC) SE: Flatulence Notes: May take granules on food

Lactulose (Constulose, Generlac, Enulose, others) Uses: *Hepatic encephalopathy; constipation* Acts: Acidifies the colon, allows ammonia to diffuse into colon; osmotic effect to ↑ peristalsis Dose: *Acute hepatic encephalopathy:* 30–45 mL PO q1h until soft stools, then tid-qid, adjust 2–3 stool/d. *Constipation:* 15–30 mL/d, ↑ to 60 mL/d 1–2 ÷ doses, adjust to 2–3 stools. *Rectally:* 200 g in 700 mL of H_2O PR, retain 30–60 min q4–6h. *Peds. Infants:* 2.5–10 mL/24 h ÷ tid-qid. *Other Peds:* 40–90 mL/24 h ÷ tid-qid. *Peds Constipation:* 5 g (7.5 mL) PO after breakfast Caution: [B, ?] CI: Galactosemia Disp: Syrup 10 g/15 mL, soln 10 g/15 mL:, 10, 20 g/packet SE: Severe D, N/V, cramping, flatulence; life-threatening electrolyte disturbances

Lamivudine (Epivir, Epivir-HBV, 3TC [Many Combo Regimens]) BOX: Lactic acidosis & severe hepatomegaly w/ steatosis reported w/ nucleoside analogs Uses: *HIV Infxn, chronic hep B* Acts: NRTI, ↓ HIV RT & hep B viral polymerase, causes viral DNA chain termination Dose: *HIV: Adults & Peds >16 y:* 150 mg PO bid or 300 mg PO daily. *Peds able to swallow pills: 14–21 kg:* 75 mg bid; *22–29 kg:* 75 mg q A.M., 150 mg q P.M.; *>30 kg:* 150 mg bid. *Neonates <30 d:* 2 mg/kg bid. *Epivir-HBV: Adults.* 100 mg/d PO. *Peds 2–17 y:* 3 mg/kg/d PO, 100 mg max; ↓ w/ CrCl <50 mL/min Caution: [C, –] w/ Interferon-α and ribavirin may cause liver failure; do not use w/ zalcitabine or w/ ganciclovir/valganciclovir Disp: Tabs 100 mg (Epivir-HBV) 150 mg, 300 mg; soln 5 mg/mL (Epivir-HBV), 10 mg/mL SE: malaise, fatigue, N/V/D, HA, pancreatitis, lactic acidosis, peripheral neuropathy, fat redistribution, rhabdomyolysis hyperglycemia, nasal Sxs Notes: Differences in formulations; do not use Epivir-HBV for hep in pt w/ unrecognized HIV d/t rapid emergence of HIV resistance

Lamotrigine (Lamictal) BOX: Serious rashes requiring hospitalization & D/C of Rx reported; rash less frequent in adults; ↑ suicidality risk for antiepileptic drug, higher for those w/ epilepsy vs. those using drug for psychological indications

Uses: *Partial Szs, tonic-clonic Szs, bipolar disorder, Lennox-Gastaut synd* Acts: Phenyltriazine antiepileptic, ↓ glutamate, stabilize neuronal membrane Dose: Adults. Szs: Initial 50 mg/d PO, then 50 mg PO bid for × 1–2 wk, maint 300–500 mg/d in 2 ÷ doses. Bipolar: Initial 25 mg/d PO × 1–2 wk, 50 mg PO daily for 2 wk, 100 mg PO daily for 1 wk, maint 200 mg/d. Peds. 0.6 mg/kg in 2 ÷ doses for wk 1 & 2, then 1.2 mg/kg for wk 3 & 4, q1–2wk to maint 5–15 mg/kg/d (max 400 mg/d) 1–2 ÷ doses; ↓ in hepatic Dz or if w/ enzyme inducers or valproic acid Caution: [C, −] Interactions w/ other antiepileptics, estrogen, rifampin Disp: Tabs 25, 100, 150, 200 mg; chew tabs 2, 5, 25 mg (color-coded for those on interacting meds) SE: Photosens, HA, GI upset, dizziness, diplopia, blurred vision, blood dyscrasias, ataxia, rash (may be much more life-threatening to peds than to adults), aseptic meningitis Notes: value of therapeutic monitoring uncertain, taper w/ D/C

Lansoprazole (Prevacid, Prevacid IV, Prevacid 24HR [OTC], aseptic meningitis) Uses: *Duodenal ulcers, prevent & Rx NSAID gastric ulcers, active gastric ulcers, H. pylori Infxn, erosive esophagitis, & hypersecretory conditions, GERD* Acts: Proton pump inhib Dose: 15–30 mg/d PO; NSAID ulcer prevention: 15 mg/d PO = 12 wk. NSAID ulcers: 30 mg/d PO × 8 wk; hypersecretory condition: 60 mg/d IV daily = 7 d change to PO for 6–8 wk; ↓ w/ severe hepatic impair Caution: [B, ?/−] may ↓ effect of Plavix Disp: Prevacid: DR Caps 15, 30 mg; Prevacid 24HR [OTC] 15 mg; Prevacid SoluTab (ODT) 15 mg (contains phenylalanine); IV 30 mg SE: N/V Abd pain HA, fatigue Notes: For IV provided inline filter must be used; do not crush/chew; granules can be given w/applesauce or apple juice (NG tube) only; ? ↑ risk of fractures w/ all PPI

Lanthanum Carbonate (Fosrenol) Uses: *Hyperphosphatemia in renal Dz* Acts: Phosphate binder Dose: 750–1500 mg PO daily ÷ doses, w/ or immediately after meal; titrate q2–3wk based on PO_4^{2-} levels Caution: [C, ?/−] No data in GI Dz; not for peds Disp: Chew tabs 250, 500, 750, 1000 mg SE: N/V, graft occlusion, HA, ↓ BP Notes: Chew tabs before swallowing; separate from meds that interact w/ antacids by 2 h

Lapatinib (Tykerb) Uses: *Advanced breast CA w/ capecitabine w/ tumors that over express HER2 and failed w/ anthracycline, taxane, & trastuzumab* Acts: TKI Dose: Per protocol, 1250 mg PO days 1–21 w/ capecitabine 2000 mg/m²/d ÷ 2 doses/d on days 1–14; ↓ w/ severe cardiac or hepatic impair Caution: [D,; ?] Avoid CYP3A4 inhib/inducers CI: w/ Phenothiazines Disp: Tabs 250 mg SE: N/V/D, anemia, ↓ plt, neutropenia, ↑ QT interval, hand-foot synd, ↑ LFTs, rash, ↓ left ventricular ejection fraction, interstitial lung Dz and pneumonitis Notes: Consider baseline LVEF & periodic ECG

Latanoprost (Xalatan) Uses: *Open-angle glaucoma, ocular HTN* Acts: Prostaglandin, ↑ outflow of aqueous humor Dose: 1 gtt eye(s) hs Caution: [C, ?] Disp: 0.005% soln SE: May darken light irides; blurred vision, ocular stinging, & itching, ↑ number & length of eyelashes Notes: Wait 15 min before using contacts; separate from other eye products by 5 min

Leflunomide (Arava) BOX: PRG must be excluded prior to start of Rx Uses: *Active RA, orphan drug for organ rejection* Acts: DMARD, ↓ pyrimidine synth Dose: Initial 100 mg/d PO for 3 d, then 10–20 mg/d Caution: [X, –] w/ Bile acid sequestrants, warfarin, rifampin, MTX CI: PRG Disp: Tabs 10, 20, 100 mg SE: D, Infxn, HTN, alopecia, rash, N, joint pain, hep, interstitial lung Dz, immunosuppression Notes: Monitor LFTs, CBC, PO⁴⁻ during initial Rx; vaccine should be up-to-date, do not give w/ live vaccines

Lenalidomide (Revlimid) BOX: Significant teratogen; pt must be enrolled in RevAssist risk-reduction program; hematologic tox, DVT & PE risk Uses: *MDS, combo w/ dexamethasone in multiple myeloma in pt failing one prior Rx* Acts: Thalidomide analog, immune modulator Dose: Adults. 10 mg PO daily; swallow whole w/ water; multiple myeloma 25 mg/d days 1–21 of 28-d cycle w/ protocol dose of dexamethasone Caution: [X, –] w/ Renal impair Disp: Caps 5, 10, 15, 25 mg SE: D, pruritus, rash, fatigue, night sweats, edema, nasopharyngitis, ↓ BM (plt, WBC), ↑ K⁺, ↑ LFTs, thromboembolism Notes: Monitor CBC and for thromboembolism, hepatotox; routine PRG tests required; Rx only in 1-mo increments; limited distribution network; males must use condom and not donate sperm; use at least 2 forms contraception > 4 wk beyond D/C

Lepirudin (Refludan) Uses: *HIT* Acts: Direct thrombin inhib Dose: Bolus: 0.4 mg/kg IV, then 0.15 mg/kg/h Inf; if >110 kg 44 mg of Inf 16.5 mg/h max; ↓ dose & Inf rate w/ if CrCl <60 mL/min or if used w/ thrombolytics Caution: [B, ?/–] Hemorrhagic event, or severe HTN CI: Active bleeding Disp: Inj 50 mg SE: Bleeding, anemia, hematoma, anaphylaxis Notes: Adjust based on aPTT ratio, maintain aPTT 1.5–2 × control

Letrozole (Femara) Uses: * • Breast Ca: Adjuvant w/postmenopausal hormone receptor positive early Dz; Adjuvant in postmenopausal women with early breast Ca w/prior adjuvant tamoxifen therapy; 1st/2nd -line in postmenopausal w/ hormone receptor positive or unknown Dx* Acts: Nonsteroidal aromatase inhib Dose: 2.5 mg/d PO; q other day w/ severe liver Dz or cirrhosis Caution: [D, ?] CI: PRG, premenopausal Disp: Tabs 2.5 mg SE: Anemia, N, hot flashes, arthralgia Notes: Monitor CBC, thyroid Fxn, lytes, LFTs, & SCr

Leucovorin (Wellcovorin) Uses: *OD of folic acid antagonist; megaloblastic anemia, augment 5-FU impaired MTX elimination; w/ 5-FU in colon CA* Acts: Reduced folate source; circumvents action of folate reductase inhib (e.g., MTX) Dose: Leucovorin rescue: 10 mg/m² PO/IM/IV q6h; start w/in 24 h after dose or 15 mg PO/IM/IV q6h, 25 mg/dose max PO; Folate antagonist OD (e.g., Pemetrexed) 100 mg/m² IM/IV × 1 then 50 mg/m² IM/IV q6h × 8 d 100 mg/m² × 1; 5-FU adjuvant tx, colon CA per protocol; low dose: 20 mg/m² IV × 5 d w/ 5-FU 425 mg/m²/d IV × 5 d, repeat q4–5wk × 6; high dose: 500 mg/m² IV q wk × 6, w/ 5-FU 500 mg/m² IV q wk × 6 wk, repeat after 2 wk off × 4; Megaloblastic anemia: 1 mg IM/IV daily Caution: [C, ?/–] CI: Pernicious anemia Disp: Tabs 5, 10, 15, 25 mg; Inj 50 mg, 100 mg, 200 mg, 350 mg, 500 mg SE: Allergic Rxn, N/V/D, fatigue, wheezing, ↑ plt **Notes:** Monitor Cr, methotrexate levels q24h w/ leucovorin rescue; do not use intrathecally/intraventricularly; w/ 5-FU CBC w/ diff, plt, LFTs, lytes

Leuprolide (Lupron, Lupron DEPOT, Lupron DEPOT-Ped, Viadur, Eligard) Uses: *Advanced PCa (all except Depot-Ped), endometriosis (Lupron), uterine fibroids (Lupron), & precocious puberty (Lupron-Ped)* Acts: LHRH agonist; paradoxically ↓ release of GnRH w/ ↓ LH from anterior pituitary; in men ↓ testosterone Dose: *Adults. PCa: Lupron DEPOT:* 7.5 mg IM q28d or 22.5 mg IM q3mo or 30 mg IM q4mo. *Eligard:* 7.5 mg SQ q28d or 22.5 mg SQ q3mo or 30 mg SQ q4mo or 45 mg SQ 6 mo. *Endometriosis (Lupron DEPOT):* 3.75 mg IM q mo × 6 or 11.25 mg IM q3mo × 2. *Fibroids:* 3.75 mg IM q mo × 3 or 11.25 mg IM × 1. *Peds. CPP (Lupron DEPOT-Ped):* 50 mcg/kg/d SQ Inj; ↑ by 10 mcg/kg/d until total downregulation achieved. *Lupron DEPOT: <25 kg:* 7.5 mg IM q4wk; *>25–37.5 kg:* 11.25 mg IM q4wk; *>37.5 kg:* 15 mg IM q4wk, ↑ by 3.75 mg q4wk until response **Caution:** [X, −] w/ Impending cord compression in PCa **CI:** AUB, implant in women/peds; PRG **Disp:** Inj 5 mg/mL; *Lupron DEPOT:* 3.75 mg (1 mo for fibroids, endometriosis); *Lupron DEPOT* for PCa: 7.5 mg (1 mo), 11.25 (3 mo), 22.5 (3 mo), 30 mg (4 mo); *Eligard depot* for PCa: 7.5 (1 mo); 22.5 (3 mo), 30 (4 mo), 45 mg (6 mo); *Viadur* 65 mg 12-mo SQ implant (unavailable to new Rx), *Lupron DEPOT-Ped:* 7.5, 11.25, 15 mg **SE:** Hot flashes, gynecomastia, N/V, alopecia, anorexia, dizziness, HA, insomnia, paresthesias, depression exacerbation, peripheral edema, & bone pain (transient "flare Rxn" at 7–14 d after the 1st dose [LH/testosterone surge before suppression]); ↓ BMD w/ >6 mo use, bone loss possible **Notes:** Nonsteroidal antiandrogen (e.g., bicalutamide) may block flare in men w/ PCa

Levalbuterol (Xopenex, Xopenex HFA) Uses: *Asthma (Rx & prevention of bronchospasm)* Acts: Sympathomimetic bronchodilator; *R*-isomer of albuterol Dose: Based on NIH Guidelines 2007 *Adults.* Acute–severe exacerbation Xopenex HFA 4–8 puffs q20min up to 4 h, the q1–4h PRN or nebulizer 1/25–2.5 mg q20min × 3, then 1.25–5 mg q1–4h PRN; *Peds <4 y:* Quick relief 0.31–1.25 mg q4–6h PRN, severe 1.25 mg q20min × 3, then 0.075–0.15 mg/kg q1–4h PRN, 5 mg max. *5–11 y:* Acute–severe exacerbation 1.25 mg q20min × 3, then 0.075–0.15 mg/kg q1–4h PRN, 5 mg max. *>11 y:* 0.63–1.25 mg nebulizer q6–8h **Caution:** [C, ?] w/ Non–K⁺-sparing diuretics, CAD, HTN, arrhythmias, ↓ K⁺ **CI:** w/ Phenothiazines & TCAs, MAOI w/in 14 d **Disp:** Multidose inhaler (Xopenex HFA) 45 mcg/puff (15 g); soln nebulizer Inh 0.31, 0.63, 1.25 mg/3 mL; concentrate 1.25 mg/0.5 mL **SE:** Paradox bronchospasm, anaphylaxis, angioedema, tachycardia, nervousness, V, ↓ K⁺ **Notes:** May ↓ CV SEs compared w/ albuterol; do not mix w/ other nebs or dilute

Levetiracetam (Keppra) Uses: *Adjunctive PO Rx in partial onset Sz (adults & peds ≥4 y), myoclonic Szs (adults & peds ≥12 y) w/ juvenile myoclonic epilepsy (JME), primary generalized tonic-clonic (PGTC) Szs (adults & peds ≥6 y)*

Levofloxacin

155

w/ idiopathic generalized epilepsy. Adjunctive Inj Rx partial-onset Szs in adults w/ epilepsy; and myoclonic Szs in adults w/ JME. Inj alternative for adults (≥16 y) when PO not possible* **Acts:** Unknown **Dose:** *Adults & Peds >16 y:* 500 mg PO bid, titrate q2wk, may ↑ 3000 mg/d max. *Peds 4–15 y:* 10–20 mg/kg/d ÷ in 2 doses, 60 mg/kg/d max (↓ in renal Insuff) **Caution:** [C, ?/–] Elderly, w/ renal impair, psychological disorders; ↑ suicidality risk for antiepileptic drugs, higher for those w/ epilepsy vs. those using drug for psychological indications; Inj not for <16 y **CI:** Component allergy **Disp:** Tabs 250, 500, 750, 1000 mg, soln 100 mg/mL; Inj 100 mg/mL **SE:** Dizziness, somnolence, HA,N/V hostility, aggression, hallucinations, myelosuppression, impaired coordination **Notes:** Do not D/C abruptly; post-market hepatic failure and pancytopenia reported

Levobunolol (A-K Beta, Betagan) **Uses:** *Open-angle glaucoma, ocular HTN* **Acts:** β-Adrenergic blocker **Dose:** 1 gtt daily-bid **Caution:** [C, ?] w/ Verapamil or systemic β-blockers **CI:** Asthma, COPD, sinus bradycardia, heart block (2nd-, 3rd-degree) CHF **Disp:** Soln 0.25, 0.5% **SE:** Ocular stinging/burning, ↓ HR, ↓ BP **Notes:** Possible systemic effects if absorbed

Levocetirizine (Xyzal) **Uses:** *Perennial/seasonal allergic rhinitis, chronic urticaria* **Acts:** Antihistamine **Dose:** *Adults.* 5 mg q day *Peds 6–11 y:* 2.5 mg q day **Caution:** [B, ?] ↓ Adult dose w/ renal impair, CrCl 50–80 mL/min 2.5 mg daily, 30–50 mL/min 2.5 mg q other day 10–30 mL/min 2.5 mg 2×/wk **CI:** Peds 6–11 y w/ renal impair, adults w/ ESRD **Disp:** Tab 5 mg, soln 0.5 mL/mL (150 mL) **SE:** CNS depression, drowsiness, fatigue, xerostomia **Notes:** Take in evening

Levofloxacin (Levaquin) **BOX:** ↑ Risk Achilles tendon rupture and tendonitis **Uses:** *Skin/skin structure Infxn(SSSI), UTI, chronic bacterial prostatitis, acute pyelo, acute bacterial sinusitis, acute bacterial exacerbation of chronic bronchitis, CAP, including multidrug-resistant S. pneumoniae, nosocomial pneumonia; Rx inhalational anthrax in adults & peds ≥6 mo* **Acts:** Quinolone, ↓ DNA gyrase. *Spectrum:* Excellent gram(+) except MRSA & E. faecium; excellent gram(–) except Stenotrophomonas maltophilia & Acinetobacter sp; poor anaerobic **Dose:** *Adults ≥18 y:* IV/PO: *Bronchitis:* 500 mg q day × 7 d. *CAP:* 500 mg q day × 7–14 d or 750 mg q day × 5 d. *Sinusitis:* 500 mg q day × 10–14 d or 750 mg q day × 5 d. *Prostatitis:* 500 mg q day × 28 d. *Uncomp SSSI:* 500 mg q day × 7–10 d. *Comp SSSI/Nosocomial Pneumonia:* 750 mg q day × 7–14 d. *Anthrax:* 500 mg q day × 60 d; *Uncomp UTI:* 250 mg q day × 3 d. *Comp UTI/Acute Pyelo:* 250 mg q day × 10 d or 750 mg q day × 5 d. CrCl 10–19 mL/min: 250 mg, then 250 mg q48h or 750 mg, then 500 mg q48h. *Hemodialysis:* 750 mg, then 500 mg q48h. *Peds ≥6 mo:* Anthrax only *>50 kg:* 500 mg q 24h × 60 d, <50 kg 8 mg/kg (250 mg/dose max) q12h for 60 d ↓ w/ renal impair avoid antacids w/ PO; oral soln 1 h before, 2 h after meals **Caution:** [C, –] w/ Cation-containing products (e.g., antacids), w/ drugs that ↑ QT interval **CI:** Quinolone sensitivity **Disp:** Tabs 250, 500, 750 mg; premixed IV 250, 500, 750 mg, Inj 25 mg/mL; Leva-Pak 750 mg × 5 d **SE:** N/D, dizziness, rash, GI upset, photosens, CNS stimulant w/ IV use, C. difficile enterocolitis; rare fatal hepatox **Notes:** Use w/ steroids ↑ tendon risk; only for anthrax in peds

Levofloxacin ophthalmic (Quixin, Iquix) Uses: *Bacterial conjunctivitis* **Acts:** See levofloxacin **Dose:** *Ophthal:* 1–2 gtt in eye(s) q2h while awake × 2 d, then q4h while awake × 5 d **Caution:** [C, –] **CI:** Quinolone sensitivity **Disp:** 25 mg/mL ophthal soln 0.5% (Quixin), 1.5% (Iquix) **SE:** Ocular burning/ pain, ↓ vision, fever, foreign body sensation, HA, pharyngitis, photophobia

Levonorgestrel (Plan B) Uses: *Emergency contraceptive ("morning-after pill")*; prevents PRG if taken <72 h after unprotected sex/contraceptive failure **Acts:** Progestin, alters tubal transport & endometrium to implantation **Dose:** *Adults & Peds (postmenarche females):* 0.75 mg q12h × 2 **Caution:** [X, +] **CI:** Known/ suspected PRG, AUB **Disp:** Tab, 0.75 mg, 2 blister pack **SE:** N/V, Abd pain, fatigue, HA, menstrual changes. **Notes:** Will not induce abortion; ↑ risk of ectopic PRG; OTC "behind the counter" if >18 y, RX if <18 y varies by state

Levonorgestrel IUD (Mirena) Uses: *Contraception, long-term* **Acts:** Progestin, alters endometrium, thicken cervical mucus, inhibits ovulation and implantation **Dose:** Up to 5 y, insert w/in 7 d menses onset or immediately after 1st tri abortion; wait 6 wk if postpartum; replace any time during menstrual cycle **Caution:** [C, ?] **CI:** PRG, w/ active hepatic Dz or tumor, uterine anomaly, breast CA, acute/Hx of PID, postpartum endometriosis, infected abortion last 3 mo, gynecological neoplasia, abnormal Pap, AUB, untreated cervicitis/vaginitis, multiple sex partners, ↑ increased susceptibility to Infxn **Disp:** 52 mg IUD **SE:** Failed insertion, ectopic PRG, sepsis, PID, infertility, PRG comps w/ IUD left in place, abortion, embedment, ovarian cysts, perforation uterus/cervix, intrauterine obst/perforation, peritonitis, N, Abd pain, ↑ BP, acne, HA **Notes:** Inform pt does not protect against STD/HIV; see PI for insertion instructions; reexamine placement after 1st menses; 80% PRG w/in 12 mo of removal

Levorphanol (Levo-Dromoran) [C-II] Uses: *Mod–severe pain; chronic pain* **Acts:** Narcotic analgesic, morphine derivative **Dose:** 2–4 mg PO PRN q6–8h; ↓ in hepatic impair **Caution:** [B/D (prolonged use/high doses at term), ?/–] w/ ↑ ICP, head trauma, adrenal Insuff **CI:** Component allergy **Disp:** Tabs 2 mg **SE:** Tachycardia, ↓ BP, drowsiness, GI upset, constipation, resp depression, pruritus

Levothyroxine (Synthroid, Levoxyl, others) BOX: Not for obesity or wgt loss; tox w/ high doses, especially when combined w/ sympathomimetic amines Uses: *Hypothyroidism, pituitary thyroid-stimulating hormone (TSH) suppression, myxedema coma* **Acts:** T_4 supl l-thyroxine **Dose:** *Adults. Hypothyroid* titrate until euthyroid >50 y w/ heart Dz or <50 w/ heart Dz 25–50 mcg/d, ↑ q6–8wk; >50 y w/ heart Dz 12.5–25 mcg/d, ↑ q6–8wk; usual 100–200 mcg/d. *Myxedema:* 200–500 mcg IV, then 100–300 mcg/d. *Peds. Hypothyroid: 0–3 mo:* 10–15 mcg/kg/24 h PO; *3–6 mo:* 8–10 mcg/kg/d PO; *6–12 mo:* 6–8 mcg/kg/d PO; *1–5 y:* 5–6 mcg/kg/d PO; *6–12 y:* 4–5 mcg/kg/d PO; *>12 y:* 2–3 mcg/kg/d PO; if growth and puberty complete 1.7 mcg/kg/d; ↓ dose by 50% if IV; titrate based on response & thyroid tests; dose can ↑ rapidly in young/middle-aged; best on empty stomach **Caution:** [A, +] **CI:** Recent MI, uncorrected adrenal Insuff; many drug interactions; in elderly w/ CV Dz **Disp:** Tabs 25, 50, 75, 88, 100, 112, 125, 137, 150, 175, 200, 300 mcg; Inj 200, 500 mcg **SE:** Insomnia, wgt loss, N/V/D, ↑ LFTs, irregular periods, ↓ BMD, alopecia, arrhythmia **Notes:** Take w/ full glass of water (prevents choking); PRG may ↑ need for higher doses; takes 6 wk to see effect on TSH; wait 6 wk before checking TSH after dose change

Lidocaine, Systemic (Xylocaine, Others) Uses: *Rx cardiac arrhythmias* **Acts:** Class IB antiarrhythmic **Dose:** *Adults. Antiarrhythmic, ET:* 5 mg/kg; follow w/ 0.5 mg/kg in 10 min if effective. *IV load:* 1 mg/kg/dose bolus over 2–3 min; repeat in 5–10 min; 200–300 mg/h max; cont Inf 20–50 mcg/kg/min or 1–4 mg/min; *Cardiac arrest from VF/VT: Initial:* 1.0–1.5 mg/kg IV. *Refractory VF:* Additional 0.5–0.75 mg/kg IV push, repeat in 5–10 min, max total 3 mg/kg. *ET:* 2–4 mg/kg. *Perfusing stable VT, wide complex tachycardia or ectopy:* 1.0–1.5 mg/kg IV push; repeat 0.5–0.75 mg/kg q 5–10 min; max total 3 mg/kg; maint 1–4 mg/min (30–50 mcg/min) (ECC 2005).* *Peds. Antiarrhythmic, ET, load:* 1 mg/kg; repeat in 10–15 min 5 mg/kg max total, then IV Inf 20–50 mcg/kg/min **Caution:** [B, +] Corn allergy **CI:** Adams-Stokes synd; heart block **Disp:** Inj IV: 1% (10 mg/mL), 2% (20 mg/mL); admixture 4, 10, 20%. *IV Inf:* 0.2, 0.4% **SE:** Dizziness, paresthesias, & convulsions associated w/ tox **Notes:** 2nd line to amiodarone in ECC; dilute ET dose 1–2 mL w/ NS; for IV forms, ↓ w/ liver Dz or CHF; *Systemic levels:* steady state 6–12 h;; *Therapeutic:* 1.2–5 mcg/mL; *Toxic:* >6 mcg/mL; *1/2half-life:* 1.5 h

Lidocaine; Lidocaine w/ Epinephrine (Anestacon Topical, Xylocaine, Xylocaine Viscous, Xylocaine MPF Others) Uses: *Local anesthetic, epidural/caudal anesthesia, regional nerve blocks, topical on mucous membranes (mouth/pharynx/urethra)* **Acts:** Anesthetic; stabilizes neuronal membranes; inhibits ionic fluxes required for initiation and conduction **Dose:** *Adults. Local Inj anesthetic:* 4.5 mg/kg max total dose or 300 mg; w/ epi 7 mg/kg max total 500 mg max dose. *Oral:* 15 mL viscous swish and spit or *pharyngeal* gargle and swallow, do not use <3-h intervals or >8 × in 24 h. *Urethra:* 10–15 mL (200–300 mg) jelly in men, 5 mL female urethra; 600 mg/24 h max. *Peds. Topical:* Apply max 3 mg/kg/dose. *Local Inj anesthetic:* Max 4.5 mg/kg (Table 1 p 264) **Caution:** [B, +] Corn allergy; epi-containing soln may interact w/ TCA or MAOI and cause severe ↑ BP **CI:** Do not use lidocaine w/ epi on digits, ears, or nose (vasoconstriction & necrosis) **Disp:** *Inj local:* 0.5, 1, 1.5, 2, 4, 10, 20%; *Inj w/ epi* 0.5%/1:200,000, 1%/1:100,000, 2%/1:100,000; (MPF) 1%/1:200,000, 1.5%/1:200,000, 2%/1:200,000; (Dental formulations) 2%/1:50,000, 2%/1:100,000; cream 2%; gel 2, 2.5%; oint 2.5, 5%; liq 2.5%; soln 2, 4%; viscous 2% **SE:** Dizziness, paresthesias, & convulsions associated w/ tox **Notes:** See Table 1

Lidocaine Powder Intradermal Injection System (Zingo) Uses: *Local anesthesia before venipuncture or IV in peds 3–18 y* **Acts:** Local amide anesthetic **Dose:** Apply 3 min before procedure **Caution:** [N/A, N/A] only on intact skin **CI:** Lidocaine allergy **Disp:** 6.5-Inch device to administer under pressure 0.5 mg lidocaine powder in 2-cm area, single use **SE:** Skin Rxn, edema, petechiae

Lidocaine/Prilocaine (EMLA, LMX) Uses: *Topical anesthetic for intact skin or genital mucous membranes*; adjunct to phlebotomy or dermal procedures

Acts: Amide local anesthetics **Dose:** *Adults. EMLA cream, anesthetic disc (1 g/10 cm^2):* Thick layer 2–2.5 g to intact skin, cover w/ occlusive dressing (e.g., Tegaderm) for at least 1 h. *Anesthetic disc:* 1 g/10 cm^2 for at least 1 h. ***Peds.*** *Max dose: <3 mo or <5 kg:* 1 g/10 cm^2 for 1 h. *3–12 mo & >5 kg:* 2 g/20 cm^2 for 4 h. *1–6 y & >10 kg:* 10 g/100 cm^2 for 4 h. *7–12 y & >20 kg:* 20 g/200 cm^2 for 4 h **Caution:** [B, +] Methemoglobinemia **CI:** Use on mucous membranes, broken skin, eyes; allergy to amide-type anesthetics **Disp:** Cream 2.5% lidocaine/2.5% prilocaine; anesthetic disc (1 g); periodontal gel 2.5/2.5% **SE:** Burning, stinging, methemoglobinemia **Notes:** Longer contact time ↑ effect

Lindane (Kwell, others) BOX: Only for pts intolerant/failed first1st-line Rx w/ safer agents. Szs and deaths reported w/ repeat/prolonged use. Caution d/t increased risk of neurotox in infants, children, elderly, w/ other skin conditions, and if <50 kg. Instruct pts on proper use and inform that itching occurs after successful killing of scabies or lice Uses: *Head lice, pubic "crab" lice, body lice, scabies* Acts: Ectoparasiticide & ovicide Dose: Adults & Peds. Cream or lotion:

Thin layer to dry skin after bathing, leave for 8–12 h, rinse; also use on laundry. *Shampoo:* Apply 30 mL to dry hair, develop a lather w/ warm water for 4 min, comb out nits **Caution:** [C, +/−] **CI:** Premature infants, uncontrolled Sz disorders open wounds **Disp:** Lotion 1%; shampoo 1% **SE:** Arrhythmias, Szs, local irritation, GI upset, ataxia, alopecia, N/V, aplastic anemia **Notes:** Caution w/ overuse (may be absorbed); may repeat Rx in 7 d; try OTC first w/ pyrethrins (Pronto, Rid, others)

Linezolid (Zyvox) Uses: *infxns caused by gram(+) bacteria (including VRE), pneumonia, skin infxns* Acts: Unique, binds ribosomal bacterial RNA; bacteriocidal for streptococci, bacteriostatic for enterococci & staphylococci. Spectrum: Excellent gram(+) including VRE & MRSA Dose: Adults. 400–600 mg IV

or PO q12h. ***Peds.*** 10 mg/kg IV or PO q8h (q12h in preterm neonates) **Caution:** [C, ?/−] w/ MAOI, avoid foods w/ tyramine & cough/cold products w/ pseudoephedrine; w/ ↓ BM **Disp:** Inj 200, 600 mg; tabs 600 mg; susp 100 mg/5 mL **SE:** Lactic acidosis, peripheral/optic neuropathy, HTN, N/D, HA, insomnia, GI upset, ↓ BM, tongue discoloration **Notes:** ✓ weekly CBC; not for gram(−) Infxn, ↑ deaths in catheter-related infxns

Liothyronine (Cytomel, Triostat, T$_3$) BOX: Not for obesity or wgt loss Uses: *Hypothyroidism, nontoxic goiter, myxedema coma, thyroid suppression Rx*

Acts: T$_3$ replacement **Dose:** *Adults.* Initial 25 mcg/24 h, titrate q1–2wk to response & TFT; maint of 25–100 mcg/d PO. *Myxedema coma:* 25–50 mcg IV. *Myxedema:* 5 mcg/d, PO ↑ 5–10 mcg/d q1–2wk; maint 50–100 mcg/d. *Nontoxic goiter:* 5 mcg/d

PO, ↑ 5–10 mcg/d q1–2wk, usual dose 75 mcg/d. *T_3 suppression test:* 75–100 mcg/d × 7d. **Peds.** Initial 5 mcg/24 h, titrate by 5-mcg/24-h increments at q3–4d intervals; maint peds 1–3 yrs: 50 mcg/d. **Infants–12 mo:** 20 mcg/d. *>3 y:* Adult dose; ↓ in elderly & CV Dz **Caution:** [A, +] **CI:** Recent MI, uncorrected adrenal Insuff, uncontrolled HTN, thyrotoxicosis, artificial rewarming **Disp:** Tabs 5, 25, 50 mcg; Inj 10 mcg/mL **SE:** Alopecia, arrhythmias, CP, HA, sweating, twitching, ↑ HR, ↑ BP, MI, CHF, fever **Notes:** Monitor TFT; separate antacids by 4 h; monitor glucose w/ DM meds; when switching from IV to PO, taper IV slowly

Lisdexamfetamine dimesylate (Vyvanse) [C-II] BOX: Amphetamines have high potential for abuse; prolonged administration may lead to dependence; misuse may cause sudden death and serious CV events **Uses:** *ADHD* **Acts:** CNS stimulant **Dose:** *Adults & Peds 6–12 y:* 30 mg daily, ↑ q wk 10–20 mg/d, 70 mg/d max **Caution:** [C, ?/–] w/ Potential for drug dependency in pt w/ psychological or Sz disorder, Tourette synd, HTN **CI:** Severe arteriosclerotic CV Dz, mod–severe ↑ BP, ↑ thyroid, sensitivity to sympathomimetic amines, NAG, agitated states, Hx drug abuse, w/ or w/in 14 d of MAOI **Disp:** Caps 30, 50, 70 mg **SE:** Headache, insomnia, decreased appetite **Notes:** AHA statement April 2008: All children diagnosed w/ ADHD who are candidates for stimulant meds should undergo CV assessment prior to use

Lisinopril (Prinivil, Zestril) BOX: ACE inhib can cause fetal injury/death in 2nd/3rd tri; D/C w/ PRG **Uses:** *HTN, CHF, prevent DN & AMI* **Acts:** ACE inhib **Dose:** 5–40 mg/24 h PO daily-bid, CHF target 40 mg/d. *AMI:* 5 mg w/in 24 h of MI, then 5 mg after 24 h, 10 mg after 48 h, then 10 mg/d; ↓ in renal insuff; use low dose, ↑ slowly in elderly **Caution:** [D, –]w/aortic stenosis/cardiomyopathy **CI:** Bilateral RAS, PRG, ACE inhib sensitivity (angioedema) **Disp:** Tabs 2.5, 5, 10, 20, 30, 40 mg **SE:** Dizziness, HA, cough, ↓ BP, angioedema, ↑ K^+, ↑ Cr, rare ↓ BM **Notes:** To prevent DN, start when urinary microalbuminuria begins; ✓ K, BUN, Cr, K^+, WBC

Lisinopril and hydrochlorothiazide (Prinzide, Zestoretic, generic) BOX: ACE inhib can cause fetal injury/death in 2nd/3rd tri; D/C w/ PRG **Uses:** *HTN* **Acts:** ACE inhib w/ diuretic (HCTZ) **Dose:** Initial 10 mg lisinopril/12.5mg HCTC, titrate upward to effect; >80 mg/d lisinopril or >50 mg/day HCTZ are not recommended; ↓ in renal insuff; use low dose, ↑ slowly in elderly **Caution:** [C 1st tri, D after, –]w/aortic stenosis/cardiomyopathy **CI:** Bilateral RAS, PRG, ACE inhib sensitivity (angioedema) **Disp:** Tabs (mg lisinopril/mg HCTZ) 10/12.5,20/12.5; Zestoretic also available as 20/25 **SE:** Anaphylactoid rxn (rare), dizziness, HA, cough, fatigue, ↓ BP, angioedema, ↑/↓ K^+, ↑ Cr, rare ↓ BM/cholestatic jaundice **Notes:** Use only when monotherapy fails; ✓ K, BUN, Cr, K^+, WBC

Lithium Carbonate (Eskalith, Lithobid, Others) BOX: Li tox related to serum levels and can be seen at close to therapeutic levels **Uses:** *Manic episodes of bipolar Dz*, augment antidepressants, aggression, posttraumatic stress disorder **Acts:** ?, Effects shift toward intraneuronal metabolism of catecholamines

Dose: *Adults. Bipolar, acute mania:* 1800 mg/d PO in 2–3 ÷ doses (target serum 1–1.5 mEq/L ✓ 2×/wk until stable). *Bipolar maint:* 900–1200 /d PO in 2–3 ÷ doses (target serum 0.6–1.2 mEq/L). *Peds ≥12 y:* See Adults; ↓ in renal Insuff, elderly **Caution:** [D, –] Many drug interactions; avoid ACE inhib or diuretics; thyroid Dz **CI:** Severe renal impair or CV Dz, lactation **Disp:** Caps 150, 300, 600 mg; tabs 300 mg; SR tabs 300 mg, CR tabs 450 mg; syrup & soln 300 mg/5 mL **SE:** Polyuria, polydipsia, nephrogenic DI, long-term may affect renal conc ability and cause fibrosis; tremor; Na retention or diuretic use may ↑ tox; arrhythmias, dizziness, alopecia, goiter ↓ thyroid, N/V/D, ataxia, nystagmus, ↓ BP **Notes:** Levels: *Trough:* just before next dose *Therapeutic:* 0.8–1.2 mEq/mL; *Toxic:* >1.5 mEq/mL *1/2-life:* 18–20h. Follow levels q1–2mo on maint

Lodoxamide (Alomide) **Uses:** *Vernal conjunctivitis/keratitis* **Acts:** Stabilizes mast cells **Dose:** *Adults & Peds >2 y:* 1–2 gtt in eye(s) qid = 3 mo **Caution:** [B, ?] **Disp:** Soln 0.1% **SE:** Ocular burning, stinging, HA **Notes:** Do not use soft contacts during use

Loperamide (Diamode, Imodium) [OTC] **Uses:** *Diarrhea* **Acts:** Slows intestinal motility **Dose:** *Adults.* Initial 4 mg PO, then 2 mg after each loose stool, up to 16 mg/d. *Peds 2–5 y, 13–20 kg:* 1 mg PO tid; *6–8 y, 20–30 kg:* 2 mg PO bid; *8–12 y, >30 kg:* 2 mg PO tid **Caution:** [C, –] Not for acute D caused by *Salmonella, Shigella,* or *C. difficile*; w/ HIV may cause toxic megacolon **CI:** Pseudomembranous colitis, bloody D, Abd pain w/ D, <2 y **Disp:** Caps 2 mg; tabs 2 mg; liq 1 mg/5 mL, 1 mg/7.5 mL (OTC) **SE:** Constipation, sedation, dizziness, Abd cramp, N

Lopinavir/Ritonavir (Kaletra) **Uses:** *HIV Infxn* **Acts:** Protease inhib **Dose:** *Adults. TX naïve:* 800/200 mg PO daily or 400/100 mg PO bid; *TX Tx-experienced pt:* 400/100 mg PO bid (↑ dose if w/ amprenavir, efavirenz, fosamprenavir, nelfinavir, nevirapine); do not use q day dosing w/ concomitant Rx. *Peds 7–15 kg:* 12/3 mg/kg PO bid. *15–40 kg:* 10/2.5 mg/kg PO bid. *>40 kg:* Adult dose; w/ food **Caution:** [C, ?/–] Numerous interactions; w/ hepatic impair; do not use w/salmeterol, colchicine (w/renal/hepatic failure); adjust dose w/ bosentan, tadalafil for PAH **CI:** w/ Drugs dependent on CYP3A/CYP2D6 (Table 10 p 280), statins, St. John's wort, fluconazole; w/Alpha 1-adrenoreceptor antagonist (alfuzosin); w/ PDE5 Inhibitor sildenafil **Disp:** (mg lopinavir/mg ritonavir) Tabs 100/25, 200/50, soln 400/100/5 mL **SE:** Avoid disulfiram (soln has EtOH), metronidazole; GI upset, asthenia, ↑ cholesterol/triglycerides, pancreatitis; protease metabolic synd

Loratadine (Claritin, Alavert) **Uses:** *Allergic rhinitis, chronic idiopathic urticaria* **Acts:** Nonsedating antihistamine **Dose:** *Adults.* 10 mg/d PO. *Peds 2–5 y:* 5 mg PO daily. *>6 y:* Adult dose; on empty stomach; ↓ in hepatic Insuff; q other day dose w/ CrCl <30 mL/min **Caution:** [B, +/–] **CI:** Component allergy **Disp:** Tabs 10 mg (OTC); rapidly disintegrating RediTabs 10 mg; chew tabs 5 mg; syrup 1 mg/mL **SE:** HA, somnolence, xerostomia, hyperkinesis in peds

Lorazepam (Ativan, Others) [C-IV] **Uses:** *Anxiety & anxiety w/ depression; sedation; control status epilepticus*; EtOH withdrawal; antiemetic **Acts:**

Benzodiazepine; antianxiety agent; works via postsynaptic GABA receptors **Dose: Adults.** Anxiety: 1–10 mg/d PO in 2–3 ÷ doses. *Pre-op:* 0.05 mg/kg to 4 mg max IM 2 h before or 0.044 mg/kg-2mg dose max IV 15–20 min before surgery. *Insomnia:* 2–4 mg PO hs. *Status epilepticus:* 4 mg/dose slow over 2–5 min IV PRN q10–15min; usual total dose 8 mg. *Antiemetic:* 0.5–2 mg IV or PO q4–6h PRN. *EtOH withdrawal:* 2–5 mg IV or 1–2 mg PO initial depending on severity; titrate. **Peds.** *Status epilepticus:* 0.05–0.1 mg/kg/dose IV over 2–5 min, repeat at 1–20-min intervals × 2 PRN. *Antiemetic, 2–15 y:* 0.05 mg/kg (to 2 mg/dose) prechemotherapy; ↓ in elderly; do not administer IV >2 mg/min or 0.05 mg/kg/min **Caution:** [D, ?/–] w/ Hepatic impair, other CNS depression, COPD; ↓ dose by 50% w/ valproic acid and probenecid **CI:** Severe pain, severe ↓ BP, sleep apnea, NAG, allergy to propylene glycol or benzyl alcohol **Disp:** Tabs 0.5, 1, 2 mg; soln, PO conc 2 mg/mL; Inj 2, 4 mg/mL **SE:** Sedation, memory impair, EPS, dizziness, ataxia, tachycardia, ↓ BP, constipation, resp depression **Notes:** ~ 10 min for effect if IV; IV Inf requires inline filter

Losartan (Cozaar) **BOX:** Can cause fatal injury and death if used in 2nd & 3rd trimesters. D/C Rx if PRG detected **Uses:** *HTN, DN, prevent CVA in HTN and LVH* **Acts:** Angiotensin II receptor antagonist **Dose: Adults.** 25–50 mg PO daily-bid, max 100 mg; ↓ in elderly/hepatic impair. **Peds ≥6 y:** *HTN:* Initial 0.7 mg/kg q day, ↑ to 50 mg PRN; 1.4 mg/kg/d or 100 mg/d max **Caution:** [C (1st tri, D 2nd & 3rd tri), ?/–] w/ NSAIDs; w/ K⁺-sparing diuretics, supl may cause ↑ K⁺; w/ RAS, hepatic impair **CI:** PRG, component sensitivity **Disp:** Tabs 25, 50, 100 mg **SE:** ↓ BP in pts on diuretics; ↑ K⁺; GI upset, facial/ angioedema, dizziness, cough, weakness, ↓ renal fxn

Lovastatin (Mevacor, Altoprev) **Uses:** *Hypercholesterolemia to ↓ risk of MI, angina* **Acts:** HMG-CoA reductase inhib **Dose: Adults.** 20 mg/d PO w/ P.M. meal; may ↑ at 4-wk intervals to 80 mg/d max or 60 mg ER tab; take w/ meals. **Peds 10–17 y (at least 1-y postmenarchal):** *Familial ↑ cholesterol:* 10 mg PO q day, ↑ q4wk PRN to 40 mg/d max (immediate release w/ P.M. meal) **Caution:** [X, –] Avoid w/ grapefruit juice, gemfibrozil; dose escalation w/ renal impair **CI:** Active liver Dz, PRG, lactation **Disp:** Tabs generic 10, 20, 40 mg; *Mevacor* 20,40 mg; *Altoprev* ER tabs 20, 40, 60 mg **SE:** HA & GI intolerance common; promptly report any unexplained muscle pain, tenderness, or weakness (myopathy) **Notes:** Maintain cholesterol-lowering diet; LFTs q12wk × 1 y, then q6mo; may alter TFT

Lubiprostone (Amitiza) **Uses:** *Chronic idiopathic constipation in adults, IBS w/ constipation in females >18 y* **Acts:** Selective Cl⁻ channel activator; ↑ intestinal motility **Dose: Adults.** *Constipation:* 24 mcg PO bid w/ food. *IBS:* 8 mcg bid; w/ food **CI:** Mechanical GI obst **Caution:** [C, ?/–] Severe D, severe renal or mod–severe hepatic impair **Disp:** Gelcaps 8, 24 mcg **SE:** N/D, HA, GI distention, Abd pain **Notes:** Not approved in males; requires (–) PRG test before; use contraception; periodically reassess drug need; not for chronic use; may experience severe dyspnea w/in 1 h of dose, usually resolves w/in 3 h

Lutropin Alfa (Luveris) Uses: *Infertility w/ profound LH deficiency* Acts: Recombinant LH Dose: 75 units SQ w/ 75–150 units FSH, 2 separate Inj max 14 d Caution: [X, ?/M] Potential for arterial thromboembolism CI: Primary ovarian failure, uncontrolled thyroid/adrenal dysfunction, intracranial lesion, AUB, hormone-dependent GU tumor, ovarian cyst, PRG Disp: Inj 75 units SE: HA, N, ovarian hyperstimulation synd, ovarian torsion, Abd pain d/t ovarian enlargement, breast pain, ovarian cysts; ↑ risk of multiple births Notes: Rotate Inj sites; do not exceed 14 d duration unless signs of imminent follicular development; monitor ovarian ultrasound and serum estradiol; specific pt information packets given

Lymphocyte Immune Globulin [Antithymocyte Globulin, ATG] (Atgam) BOX: Should only be used by physician experienced in immunosuppressive therapy or management of solid-organ and/or bone marrow transplant pts. Adequate lab and supportive resources must be readily available Uses: *Allograft rejection in renal transplant pts; aplastic anemia if not candidates for BMT *, prevent rejection of other solid-organ transplants, GVHD after BMT Acts: ↓ Circulating antigen-reactive T lymphocytes; human, & equine product Dose: *Adults. Prevent rejection:* 15 mg/kg/d IV × 14 d, then q other day × 14 d; initial w/in 24 h before/after transplant. *Rx rejection:* Same but use 10–15 mg/kg/d; max 21 doses in 28 d, Q day 1st 14 days. *Aplastic anemia:* 10–20 mg/kg/d × 8–14 d, then q other day × 7 doses for total 21 doses in 28 d. *Peds. Prevent renal allograft rejection:* 5–25 mg/kg/d IV; aplastic anemia 10–20 mg/kg/d Caution: [C, –] CI: Hx Previous Rxn or Rxn to other equine γ-globulin prep, ↓ plt and WBC Disp: Inj 50 mg/mL SE: D/C w/ severe ↓ plt and WBC; rash, fever, chills, ↓ BP, HA, CP, edema, N/V/D, lightheadedness Notes: Test dose: 0.1 mL 1:1000 dilution in NS, a systemic Rxn precludes use; give via central line; pretreat w/ antipyretic, antihistamine, and/or steroids; monitor WBC, plt;. Plt counts usually return to nl w/o D/C Rx

Lysteda (tranexamic acid) Uses: * ↓ cyclic heavy menstrual bleeding* Acts: ↓ dissolution of hemostatic fibrin by plasmin Dose: 2 tabs TID (3900 mg/d) 5 days MAX during monthly menstruation; ↓ w/ renal impair Caution: [B, +/–]↑ thrombosis risk; w/subarachnoid hemorrhage CI: Component sensitivity; Hx thrombosis; use with OCP, Factor IX or anti-inhibitor coagulant concentrates or oral tretinoin may ↑ thrombosis risk Disp: Tabs 650 mg SE: HA, sinus and nasal symptoms, abd pain, back/musculoskeletal/joint pain, muscle cramps, migraine, anemia, fatigue, retinal/ocular occlusion; allergic reactions

Magaldrate (Riopan-Plus) [OTC] Uses: *Hyperacidity associated w/ peptic ulcer, gastritis, & hiatal hernia* Acts: Low-Na^+ antacid Dose: 5–10 mL PO between meals & hs, on empty stomach Caution: [C, ?/+] CI: Ulcerative colitis, diverticulitis, appendicitis, ileostomy/colostomy, renal Insuff (d/t Mg^{2+} content) Disp: Susp magaldrate/simethicone 540/20 mg & 1080/40 mg/5 mL (OTC) SE: ↑ Mg^{2+}, ↓ PO_4, white flecked feces, constipation, N/V/D Notes: <0.3 mg Na^+/tab or tsp

Magnesium Citrate (Citroma, Others) [OTC] Uses: *Vigorous bowel prep*; constipation Acts: Cathartic laxative Dose: *Adults.* 120–300 mL PO PRN.

Peds. 0.5 mL/kg/dose, q4–6h to 200 mL PO max; w/ a beverage **Caution:** [B, +] w/ Neuromuscular Dz **CI:** Severe renal Dz, heart block, N/V, rectal bleeding intestinal obst/perforation/impaction, colostomy, ileostomy, UC, diverticulitis **Disp:** soln 290 mg/5 mL (300 mL); 100 mg tabs **SE:** Abd cramps, gas, ↓ BP, ↑ Mg²⁺, resp depression **Notes:** Only for occasional use w/ constipation

Magnesium Hydroxide (Milk of Magnesia) [OTC] **Uses:** *Constipation*, hyperacidity, Mg²⁺ replacement **Acts:** NS laxative **Dose:** *Adults.* Antacid: 5–15 mL (400 mg/5 mL) or 2-4 311 mg tabs PO PRN up to qid. *Mg²⁺ replacement:* 2–4 (500 mg) tabs PO qhs or ÷ doses. *Laxative:* 30–60 mL (400 mg/5 mL) or 15–30 mL (800 mg/5 mL) or 8 311mg tabs PO qhs or ÷ doses. *Peds.* Antacid and *Mg²⁺ replacement:* <12 y not OK. *Laxative:* <2 y not OK. *2–5 y:* 5-15 mL (400 mg/5 mL) PO qhs or ÷ doses. *6–11 y:* 15–30 mL (400 mg/5 mL) or 7.5–15 mL (800 mg/5 mL) PO qhs or ÷ doses. *3–5 y:* 2 (311-mg) tabs PO qhs or ÷ doses. *6–11 y:* 4 (311 mg) tabs PO qhs or ÷ doses **Caution:** [B, +] w/ Neuromuscular Dz or renal impair **CI:** Renal Insuff, intestinal obst, ileostomy/colostomy **Disp:** Chew tabs 311, 500 mg; liq 400, 800 mg/5 mL (OTC) **SE:** D, Abd cramps **Notes:** For occasional use in constipation

Magnesium Oxide (Mag-Ox 400, Others) [OTC] **Uses:** *Replace low Mg²⁺ levels* **Acts:** Mg²⁺ supl **Dose:** 400–800 mg/d or ÷ w/ food in full glass of H₂O; ↓ w/ renal impair **Caution:** [B, +] w/ Neuromuscular Dz & renal impair, w/ bisphosphonates, calcitriol, CCBs, neuromuscular blockers, tetracyclines, quinolones **CI:** UC, diverticulitis, ileostomy/colostomy, heart block **Disp:** Caps 140 250, 500, 600 mg; tabs 400 mg (OTC) **SE:** D, N

Magnesium Sulfate (Various) **Uses:** *Replace low Mg²⁺; preeclampsia, eclampsia, & premature labor; cardiac arrest, AMI arrhythmias, cerebral edema, barium poisoning, Szs pediatric acute nephritis*; refractory ↓ K⁺ & ↓ Ca²⁺ **Acts:** Mg²⁺ supl, bowel evacuation, ↓ acetylcholine in nerve terminals, ↓ rate of sinoatrial node firing **Dose:** *Adults.* 3 g PO q6h × 4 PRN; *Supl:* 1–2 g IM or IV; repeat PRN. *Preeclampsia/premature labor:* 4-g load then 1–4 g/h IV Inf. *Cardiac arrest:* 1–2 g IV push (2–4 mL 50% soln) in 10 mL D₅W. *AMI:* Load 1–2 g in 50–100 mL D₅W over 5–60 min IV; then 0.5–1.0 g/h IV up to 24 h *(ECC 2005).* *Peds.* 25–50 mg/kg/dose IM, IV, IO q4–6h for 3–4 doses; repeat PRN; q8–12h in neonates; max 2 g single dose; ↓ dose w/ low urinary output or renal Insuff **Caution:** [A/C (manufacturer specific), +] w/ Neuromuscular Dz; interactions see Magnesium Oxide and aminoglycosides **CI:** Heart block, renal failure **Disp:** Premix Inj: 10, 20, 40, 80 mg/mL; Inj 125, 500 mg/mL; oral/topical powder 227, 454, 480, 1810, 1920, 2721 g **SE:** CNS depression, D, flushing, heart block, ↓ BP, vasodilation **Notes:** different formulation may contain Al²⁺

Mannitol (Various) **Uses:** *Cerebral edema, ↑ IOP, renal impair, poisonings, GU irrigation* **Acts:** Osmotic diuretic **Dose:** Test dose: 0.2 g/kg/dose IV over 3–5 min; if no diuresis w/in 2 h, D/C. *Oliguria:* 50–100 g IV over 90 min ↑ IOP: 0.5–2 g/kg IV over 30 min. *Cerebral edema:* 0.25–1.5 g/kg/dose IV >30 min

Caution: [C, ?/M] w/ CHF or vol overload, w/ nephrotoxic drugs & lithium **CI:** Anuria, dehydration, heart failure, PE **Disp:** Inj 5, 10, 15, 20, 25%; GU soln 5% **SE:** May exacerbate CHF, N/V/D, ↓↑ BP, ↑ HR **Notes:** Monitor for vol depletion

Maraviroc (Selzentry) BOX: Possible drug-induced hepatotox **Uses:** *Tx of CCR5-tropic HIV Infxn* **Acts:** Antiretroviral, CCR5 coreceptor antagonist **Dose:** 300 mg bid **Caution:** [B, −] w/ Concomitant CYP3A inducers/inhib **CI:** None **Disp:** Tab 150, 300 mg **SE:** Fever, URI, cough, rash

Measles, Mumps, & Rubella Vaccine Live [MMR] (M-M-R II) **Uses:** *Vaccination against measles, mumps, & rubella 12 mo and older **Acts:** Active immunization, live attenuated viruses **Dose:** 1 (0.5 -mL) SQ Inj, 1st dose 12 mo 2nd dose 4–6 yrs, at least 3 mo between doses (28 days if > 12 yrs), adults born after 1957 unless CI, hx measles & mumps or documented immunity and childbearing age women w/ rubella immunity recommend **Caution:** [C, ?/M] Hx of cerebral injury, Szs, fam Hx Szs (febrile Rxn), ↓ plt **CI:** Component and gelatin sensitivity, Hx anaphylaxis to neomycin, blood dyscrasia, lymphoma, leukemia, malignant neoplasias affecting BM, immunosuppression, fever, PRG, hx of active untreated TB **Disp:** Inj, single dose **SE:** Fever, febrile Szs (5–12 days after vaccination), Inj site Rxn, rash, ↓ plt **Notes:** Per FDA, CDC ↑ of febrile Sz (2X) w/ MMRV vs. MMR and varicella separately; preferable to use 2 separate vaccines; allow 1 mo between Inj & any other measles vaccine or 3 mo between any other varicella vaccine; limited avail of MMRV; avoid those who have not been exposed to varicella for 6 wk post-Inj; may contain albumin or trace egg antigen; avoid salicylates for 6 wks postvaccination; avoid PRG for 3 mo following vaccination; do not give w/in 3 mo of transfusion or immune globulin

Measles, Mumps, Rubella, & Varicella Virus Vaccine Live [MMRV] (ProQuad) **Uses:** *Vaccination against measles, mumps, rubella, & varicella **Acts:** Active immunization, live attenuated viruses **Dose:** 1 (0.5- mL) vial SQ Inj 12 mo–12 y or for 2nd dose of measles, mumps & rubella (MMR)*, at least 3 mos between doses (28 days if > 12 yrs) **Caution:** [C, ?/M] Hx of cerebral injury or Szs & fam Hx Szs (febrile Rxn), ↓ plt **CI:** Component and gelatin sensitivity, Hx anaphylaxis to neomycin, blood dyscrasia, lymphoma, leukemia, malignant neoplasias affecting BM, immunosuppression, fever, active untreated TB, PRG **Disp:** Inj **SE:** Fever, febrile Szs, (5–12 days after vaccination), Inj site Rxn, rash, ↓ plt, **Notes:** Per FDA, CDC ↑ of febrile Sz (2 × risk) w/ combo vaccine (MMRV) vs. MMR and varicella separately; preferable to use 2 separate vaccines; allow 1 mo between Inj & any other measles vaccine or 3 mo between any other varicella vaccine; limited avail of MMRV; substitute MMR II and/or Varivax; avoid those who have not been exposed to varicella for 6 wk post-Inj; may contain albumin or trace egg antigen; avoid salicylates

Mecasermin (Increlex, Iplex) **Uses:** *Growth failure in severe primary IGF-1 deficiency or human growth hormone (HGH) antibodies* **Acts:** Human IGF-1(recombinant DNA origin) **Dose:** *Peds.* 0.04–0.08 mg/kg SQ bid; may ↑ by 0.04 mg/kg per dose to 0.12 mg/kg bid; take w/in 20 min of meal d/t insulin-like hypoglycemic effect **Caution:** [C,?/M] Contains benzyl alcohol **CI:** Closed epiphysis, neoplasia, not for IV **Disp:** Vial 40 mg **SE:** Tonsillar hypertrophy, ↑ AST, ↑ LDH, HA, Inj site Rxn, V, hypoglycemia; initial funduscopic exam and during Tx; consider monitoring glucose until dose stable; limited distribution; rotate Inj site

Mechlorethamine (Mustargen)

BOX: Highly toxic, handle w/ care, limit use to experienced physicians; avoid exposure during PRG; vesicant **Uses:** *Hodgkin Dz (stages III, IV), cutaneous T-cell lymphoma (mycosis fungoides), lung CA, CML, malignant pleural effusions, CLL, polycythemia vera*, psoriasis **Acts:** Alkylating agent, nitrogen analog of sulfur mustard **Dose:** Per protocol: 0.4 mg/kg single dose or 0.1 mg/kg/d for 4 d, repeat at 4–6-wk intervals; 6 mg/m² IV on days 1 & 8 of 28-d cycle; *Intracavitary:* 0.2–0.4 mg/kg × 1, may repeat PRN; *Topical:* 0.01–0.02% soln, lotion, oint **Caution:** [D, ?/–] **CI:** PRG, known infect Dz, severe myelosuppression **Disp:** Inj 10 mg; topical soln, lotion, oint **SE:** ↓ BM, thrombosis, thrombophlebitis at site; tissue damage w/ extrav (Na thiosulfate used topically to Rx); N/V/D, skin rash/allergic dermatitis w/ contact, amenorrhea, sterility (especially in men), secondary leukemia if treated for Hodgkin Dz, chromosomal alterations, hepatotox, peripheral neuropathy **Notes:** Highly volatile and emetogenic; give w/in 30–60 min of prep

Meclizine (Antivert)(Bonine, Dramamine [OTC])

Uses: *Motion sickness, vertigo* **Acts:** Antiemetic, anticholinergic, & antihistaminic properties **Dose:** *Adults & Peds >12 y: Motion Sickness:* 12.5–25 mg PO 1 h before travel, repeat PRN q12–24h. *Vertigo:* 25–100 mg/d ÷ doses **Caution:** [B, ?/–] NAG, BPH, BOO, elderly, asthma **Disp:** Tabs 12.5, 25, 50 mg; chew tabs 25 mg; caps 25, 30 mg (OTC) **SE:** Drowsiness, xerostomia, blurred vision, thickens bronchial secretions

Medroxyprogesterone (Provera, Depo Provera, Depo-Sub Q Provera)

BOX: Do not use in the prevention of CV Dz or dementia; ↑ risk MI, stroke, breast CA, PE, & DVT in postmenopausal women (50–79 y). ↑ Dementia risk in postmenopausal women (≥65 y). Risk of sig bone loss **Uses:** *Contraception; secondary amenorrhea; endometrial CA, ↓ endometrial hyperplasia* AUB caused by hormonal imbalance **Acts:** Progestin supl **Dose:** *Contraception:* 150 mg IM q3mo depo or 104 mg SQ q3mo (depo SQ). *Secondary amenorrhea:* 5–10 mg/d PO for 5–10 d. *AUB:* 5–10 mg/d PO for 5–10 d beginning on the 16th or 21st d of menstrual cycle. *Endometrial CA:* 400–1000 mg/wk IM. *Endometrial hyperplasia:* 5–10 mg/d × 12–14 d on day 1 or 16 of cycle; ↓ in hepatic Insuff **Caution:** *Provera* [X, –] *Depo Provera* [X, +] **CI:** Thrombophlebitis/embolic disorders, cerebral apoplexy, ↑ LFTs, CA breast/genital organs, undiagnosed vag bleeding, missed abortion, PRG, as a diagnostic test for PRG **Disp:** Provera tabs 2.5, 5, 10 mg; depot Inj 150, 400 mg/mL; depo SQ Inj 104 mg/10.65 mL **SE:** Breakthrough bleeding, spotting, altered menstrual flow, breast tenderness, galactorrhea, depression, insomnia, jaundice, N, wgt gain, acne, hirsutism, vision changes **Notes:** Perform breast exam & Pap smear before contraceptive Rx; obtain PRG test if last Inj >3 mo

Megestrol Acetate (Megace, Megace-ES) Uses: *Breast/endometrial CAs; appetite stimulant in cachexia (CA & HIV)* Acts: Hormone; anti-leutenizing; progesterone analog Dose: *CA:* 40–320 mg/d PO in ÷ doses. *Appetite:* 800 mg/d PO ÷ dose or Megace ES 625 mg/d Caution: [X, –] Thromboembolism; handle w/ care CI: PRG Disp: Tabs 20, 40 mg; susp 40 mg/mL, Megace ES 125 mg/mL SE: DVT, edema, menstrual bleeding, photosens, N/V/D, HA, mastodynia, ↑ CA, ↑ glucose, insomnia, rash, ↓ BM, ↑ BP, CP, palpitations, Notes: Do not D/C abruptly; Megace ES not equivalent to others mg/mg; Megace ES approved only for anorexia

Meloxicam (Mobic) BOX: May ↑ risk of cardiovascular CV events & GI bleeding; CI in post-op CABG Uses: *OA, RA, JRA* Acts: NSAID w/ ↑ COX-2 activity Dose: *Adults.* 7.5–15 mg/d PO. *Peds >2 y:* 0.125 mg/kg/d, max 7.5 mg; ↓ in renal Insuff; take w/ food Caution: [C, D (3rd tri) ?/–] w/ Severe renal Insuff, CHF, ACE inhib, diuretics, Li2+, MTX, warfarin CI: Peptic ulcer, NSAID, or ASA sensitivity, PRG, post-op coronary artery bypass graft Disp: Tabs 7.5, 15 mg; susp. 7.5 mg/5 mL SE: HA, dizziness, GI upset, GI bleeding, edema, ↑ BP, renal impair, rash (SJS), ↑ LFTs

Melphalan [L-PAM] (Alkeran) BOX: Administer under the supervision of a qualified physician experienced in the use of chemotherapy; severe BM depression, leukemogenic, & mutagenic Uses: *Multiple myeloma, ovarian CAs*, breast & testicular CA, melanoma; allogenic & ABMT (high dose), neuroblastoma, rhabdomyosarcoma Acts: Alkylating agent, nitrogen mustard Dose: *Adults. Multiple myeloma:* 16 mg/m² IV q2wk × 4 doses then at 4-wk intervals after tox resolves; w/ renal impair ↓ IV dose 50% or 6 mg PO q day × 2–3 wk, then D/C up to 4 wk, follow counts then 2 mg q day. *Ovarian CA:* 0.2 mg/kg q day × 5 d, repeat q4–5wk based on counts. *Peds. Off-label rhabdomyosarcoma:* 10–35 mg/m²/dose IV q21–28d. *w/ BMT for Neuroblastoma:* 100–220 mg/m²/dose IV × 1 or ÷ 2–5 daily doses; Inf over 60 min; ↓ in renal Insuff Caution: [D, ?/–] w/ Cisplatin, digitalis, live vaccines CI: Allergy or resistance Disp: Tabs 2 mg; Inj 50 mg SE: N/V, secondary malignancy, AF, ↓ LVEF, ↓ BM, secondary leukemia, alopecia, dermatitis, stomatitis, pulm fibrosis; rare allergic Rxns Notes: Take PO on empty stomach, false(+) direct Coombs test

Memantine (Namenda) Uses: *Mod/severe Alzheimer Dz*, mild–mod vascular dementia, mild cognitive impair Acts: *N*-methyl-D-aspartate receptor antagonist Dose: Target 20 mg/d, start 5 mg/d, ↑ 5 mg/d to 20 mg/d, wait >1 wk before ↑ dose; use ÷ doses if >5 mg/d. *Vascular dementia:* 10 mg PO bid; ↓ w/ severe renal impair Caution: [B, ?/–] Hepatic/mild–mod renal impair; Sx disorders Disp: Tabs 5, 10 mg, combo pack: 5 mg × 28 + 10 mg × 21; soln 2 mg/mL SE: Dizziness, confusion, HA, V, constipation, coughing, ↑ BP, pain, somnolence, hallucinations Notes: Renal clearance ↓ by alkaline urine (↓ 80% at pH 8)

Meningococcal Conjugate Vaccine [Quadrivalent, MCV4] (Menactra) Uses: *Immunize against Neisseria meningitidis (meningococcus) 2–55 y* high risk (college freshman, military recruits, travel to endemic areas, terminal complement deficiencies, asplenia) **Acts:** Active immunization; *N. meningitidis* A, C, Y, W-135 polysaccharide conjugated to diphtheria toxoid **Dose:** *Adults 18–55 y & Peds >2 y:* 0.5 mL IM × 1 **Caution:** [C, ?/–] w/ Immunosuppression (reduced response) and bleeding disorders (IM use only) **CI:** Allergy to class (also diphtheria toxoid/compound/latex; Hx Guillain-Barré **Disp:** Inj **SE:** Local Inj site Rxns, HA, N/V, anorexia, fatigue, irritability, arthralgia, diarrhea, Guillain-Barré **Notes:** IM only, reported accidental IV; keep epi available for Rxns; use polysaccharide vaccine (MPSV4) if >55 y; do not confuse w/ Menomune (MPSV4); ACIP rec: MCV4 for 2–55 y, can use in 2–10 yrs but ↑ local Rxn compared to Menomune (MPSV4); peds 2–10, antibody levels ↓ 3 y w/ MPSV4, need revaccination in 2-3 y, use MCV4 for revaccination

Meningococcal Polysaccharide Vaccine [MPSV4] (Menomune A/C/Y/ W-135)
Uses: *Immunize against *Neisseria meningitidis* (meningococcus)* in high risk (college freshman, military recruits, travel to endemic areas, terminal complement deficiencies, asplenia) **Acts:** Active immunization **Dose:** *Adults & Peds >2 y:* 0.5 mL SQ only ; may repeat 3–5 yrs if high risk; repeat in 2–3 yrs if first 1st dose given 2–4 yrs **Caution:** [C, ?/–] w/ Immunocompromised (↓ response) **CI:** Thimerosal/latex sensitivity; w/ pertussis or typhoid vaccine, <2 y **Disp:** Inj **SE:** SQ only; local Inj site Rxns, HA, fever **Notes:** Keep epi (1:1000) available for Rxns. Recommended 2–10 y and in >55 y, but considered alternative to MCV4 in 11–54 y if no MCV4 available (MCV4 is preferred). Active against serotypes A, C, Y, & W-135 but not group B; antibody levels ↓ 3 y, high risk revaccination q3–5y (use MCV4)

Meperidine (Demerol, Meperitab) [C–II]
Uses: *Mod–severe pain*, postoperative shivering, rigors from amphotericin B **Acts:** Narcotic analgesic **Dose:** *Adults.* 50–150 mg PO or IV/IM/SQ q3–4h PRN. *Peds.* 1–1.5 mg/kg/dose PO or IM/SQ q3–4h PRN, up to 100 mg/dose; ↓ in elderly/hepatic impair, avoid in renal impair **Caution:** [C/D (prolonged use or high dose at term), +] ↓ Sz threshold, adrenal Insuff, head injury, ↑ ICP, hepatic impair, not OK in sickle cell Dz **CI:** w/ MAOIs, renal failure, PRG **Disp:** Tabs 50, 100 mg; syrup/soln 50 mg/5 mL; Inj 10, 25, 50, 75, 100 mg/mL **SE:** Resp/CNS depression, Szs, sedation, constipation, ↓ BP, rash N/V, biliary and urethral spasms, dyspnea **Notes:** Analgesic effects potentiated w/ hydroxyzine; 75 mg IM = 10 mg morphine IM; do not best in elderly; do not use oral for acute pain; not ok for repetitive use in ICU setting

Meprobamate (Various) [C–IV]
Uses: *Short-term relief of anxiety* muscle spasm, TMJ relief **Acts:** Mild tranquilizer; antianxiety **Dose:** *Adults.* 400 mg PO tid-qid, max 2400 mg/d. *Peds 6–12 y:* 100–200 mg PO bid-tid; ↓ in renal/liver impair **Caution:** [D, +/–] Elderly, Sz Dz **CI:** NAG, porphyria, PRG **Disp:** Tabs 200, 400 mg **SE:** Drowsiness, syncope, tachycardia, edema, rash (SJS), N/V/D, ↓ WBC, agranulocytosis **Notes:** Do not abruptly D/C

Mercaptopurine [6-MP] (Purinethol)
Uses: *ALL* 2nd-line Rx for CML & NHL, maint ALL in children, immunosuppressant w/ autoimmune Dzs

(Crohn Dz, ulcerative colitis) **Acts:** Antimetabolite, mimics hypoxanthine **Dose: Adults. ALL induction:** 1.5–2.5 mg/kg/d; **maint** 80–100 mg/m²/d or 2.5–5 mg/kg/d; w/ allopurinol use 67–75% ↓ dose of 6-MP (interference w/ xanthine oxidase metabolism). **Peds. ALL induction:** 2.5–5 mg/kg/D PO or 70–100 mg/m²/d; **maint** 1.5–2.5 mg/kg/d PO or 50–75 mg/m²/d q day; ↓ w/ renal/hepatic Insuff; take on empty stomach **Caution:** [D, ?] w/ Allopurinol, immunosuppression, TMP-SMX, warfarin, salicylates **CI:** Prior resistance, severe hepatic Dz, BM suppression, PRG **Disp:** Tabs 50 mg **SE:** Mild hematotoxicity, mucositis, stomatitis, D rash, fever, eosinophilia, jaundice, hep, hyperuricemia, hyperpigmentation, alopecia **Notes:** Handle properly; limit use to experienced physicians; ensure adequate hydration; for ALL, evening dosing may ↓ risk of relapse; low emetogenicity

Meropenem (Merrem) Uses: *Intra-Abd infxns, bacterial meningitis, skin Infxn*

Acts: Carbapenem; ↓ cell wall synth. *Spectrum:* Excellent gram(+) (except MRSA, methicillin-resistant *S. epidermidis* [MRSE] & *E. faecium*); excellent gram(−) including extended-spectrum β-lactamase producers; good anaerobic **Dose: Adults.** Abd Infxn: 1 to 2 g IV q8h. Skin Infxn: 50 mg IV q8h. Meningitis: 2 g IV q8h. **Peds >3 mo, <50 kg:** Abd Infxn: 20 mg/kg IV q8h. Skin Infxn: 20 mg/kg IV q8h. Meningitis: 40 mg/kg IV q8h. **Peds >50 kg:** Use adult dose; max 2 g IV q8h; ↓ in renal Insuff (see PI) **Caution:** [B, ?] w/ Probenecid, VPA **CI:** β-Lactam sensitivity **Disp:** Inj 1 g, 500 mg **SE:** Less Sz potential than imipenem; *C. difficile* enterocolitis, D, ↓ plt **Notes:** Overuse ↑ bacterial resistance

Mesalamine (Asacol, Canasa, Lialda, Pentasa, Rowasa) Uses: *Rectal: mild–mod distal ulcerative colitis, proctosigmoiditis, proctitis; oral: treat/maint of mild-mod ulcerative colitis*

Acts: 5-ASA derivative, may inhibit prostaglandins, may ↓ leukotrienes and TNF-α **Dose:** *Rectal:* 60 mL qhs, retain 8 h (enema), 500 mg bid-tid or 1000 mg qhs (supp) *PO:* Caps: 1 g PO qid; tab: 1.6–2.4 g/d ÷ doses (tid-qid); DR 2.4–4.8 g PO daily 8 wk max, do not cut/crush/chew w/ food; ↓ initial dose in elderly **Caution:** [B, M] w/ Digitalis, PUD, pyloric stenosis, renal Insuff, elderly **CI:** Salicylate sensitivity **Disp:** Tabs ER (*Asacol*) 400, 800 mg; ER caps (*Pentasa*) 250, 500 mg; DR tab (*Lialda*) 1.2 g; supp 500, (*Canasa*) 1000 mg; (*Rowasa*) rectal susp 4 g/60 mL **SE:** Yellow-brown urine, HA, malaise, Abd pain, flatulence, rash, pancreatitis, pericarditis, dizziness, rectal pain, hair loss, intolerance synd (bloody D) **Notes:** Retain rectally 1–3 h; ✓ CBC, Cr, BUN; Sx may ↑ when starting

Mesna (Mesnex) Uses: *Prevent hemorrhagic cystitis d/t ifosfamide or cyclophosphamide*

Acts: Antidote, reacts w/ acrolein and other metabolites to form stable compounds **Dose:** Per protocol; dose as % of ifosfamide or cyclophosphamide dose. *IV bolus:* 20% (e.g., 10–12 mg/kg) IV at 0, 4, & 8 h, then 40% at 0, 1, 4, & 7 h; *IV Inf:* 20% prechemotherapy, 50–100% w/ chemotherapy, then 25–50% for 12 h following chemotherapy; *Oral:* 100% ifosfamide dose given as 20% IV at hour 0 then 40% PO at hours 4 & 8; if PO dose vomited repeat or give dose IV; mix PO w/ juice **Caution:** [B; ?/−] **CI:** Thiol sensitivity **Disp:** Inj 100 mg/mL; tabs

400 mg **SE:** ↓ BP, ↓ plt, ↑ HR, ↑ RR allergic Rxns, HA, GI upset, taste perversion **Notes:** Hydration helps ↓ hemorrhagic cystitis; higher dose for BMT; IV contains benzyl alcohol

Metaproterenol (Alupent, Metaprel) **Uses:** *Asthma & reversible bronchospasm, COPD* **Acts:** Sympathomimetic bronchodilator **Dose:** *Adults. Nebulized:* 5% 2.5 mL q4–6h or PRN. *MDI:* 1–3 Inh q3–4h, 12 Inh max/24 h; wait 2 min between Inh. *PO:* 20 mg q6–8h. *Peds ≥12 y: MDI:* 2–3 Inh q3–4h, 12 Inh/d max. *Nebulizer:* 2.5 mL (soln 0.4%, 0.6%) tid-qid, up to q4h. *Peds >9 y or >60 lbs:* 20 mg PO tid-qid; *6–9 y or <60 lbs:* 10 mg PO tid-qid; ↓ in elderly **Caution:** [C, ?/–] w/ MAOI, TCA, sympathomimetics; avoid w/ β-blockers **CI:** Tachycardia, other arrhythmias **Disp:** Aerosol 0.65 mg/Inh; soln for Inh 0.4%, 0.6%; tabs 10, 20 mg; syrup 10 mg/5 mL **SE:** Nervousness, tremor, tachycardia, HTN, ↑ glucose, ↓ K+, ↑ IOP **Notes:** Fewer β₁ effects than isoproterenol & longer acting, but not a 1st-line β-agonist. Use w/ face mask <4 y; oral ↑ ADR; contains ozone-depleting CFCs; will be gradually removed from US market

Metaxalone (Skelaxin) **Uses:** *Painful musculoskeletal conditions* **Acts:** Centrally acting skeletal muscle relaxant **Dose:** 800 mg PO tid-qid **Caution:** [C, ?/–] w/ Elderly, EtOH & CNS depression, anemia **CI:** Severe hepatic/renal impair; drug-induced, hemolytic, or other anemias **Disp:** Tabs 800 mg **SE:** N/V, HA, drowsiness, hep

Metformin (Glucophage, Glucophage XR) **BOX:** Associated w/ lactic acidosis **Uses:** *Type 2 DM*, polycystic ovary synd (PCOS) HIV lipodystrophy **Acts:** Biguanide; ↓ hepatic glucose production & intestinal absorption of glucose; ↑ insulin sensitivity **Dose:** *Adults.* Initial: 500 mg PO bid; or 850 mg daily, titrate 1–2-wk intervals may ↑ to 2550 mg/d max; take w/ A.M. & P.M. meals; can convert total daily dose to daily dose of XR. *Peds 10–16 y:* 500 mg PO bid, ↑ 500 mg/wk to 2000 mg/d max in ÷ doses; do not use XR formulation in peds **Caution:** [B, +/–] Avoid EtOH; hold dose before & 48 h after iodine imaging contrast; hepatic impair, elderly **CI:** SCr >1.4 mg/dL in females or >1.5 mg/dL in males; hypoxemic conditions (e.g., acute CHF/sepsis); metabolic acidosis **Disp:** Tabs 500, 850, 1000 mg; XR tabs 500, 750, 1000 mg; soln 100 mg/mL **SE:** Anorexia, N/V/D, flatulence, weakness, myalgia, rash

Methadone (Dolophine, Methadose) [C-II] **BOX:** Deaths reported during initiation and conversion of pain pts to methadone Rx from Rx w/ other opioids. Resp depression and QT prolongation, arrhythmias observed. Only dispensed by certified opioid treatment Tx programs for addiction. Analgesic use must outweigh risks **Uses:** *Severe pain not responsive to non-narcotics; detox w/ maint of narcotic addiction* **Acts:** Narcotic analgesic **Dose:** *Adults.* 2.5–10 mg IM/IV/ SQ q8–12h or 5–15 mg PO q8h; titrate as needed; see PI for conversion from other opioids. *Peds.* (Not FDA approved) 0.1 mg/kg q4–12h IV; ↑ slowly to avoid resp depression; ↓ in renal impair **Caution:** [C, –] Avoid w/ severe liver Dz **CI:** Resp depression, acute asthma, ileus **Disp:** Tabs 5, 10 mg; tab dispersible 40 mg; PO soln 5, 10 mg/5 mL; PO conc 10 mg/mL; Inj 10 mg/mL **SE:** Resp depression, sedation, constipation, urinary retention, ↑ QT interval, arrhythmias, ↓ HR, syncope, ↓ K⁺, ↓ Mg²⁺ **Notes:** Parenteral:oral 1:2; Equianalgesic w/ parenteral morphine; longer 1:2; resp depression occurs later and lasts longer than analgesic effect, use w/ caution to avoid iatrogenic OD

Methenamine Hippurate (Hiprex) Methenamine Mandelate (UROQUID-Acid No. 2) **Uses:** *Suppress recurrent UTI long-term. Use only after infxn cleared by antibiotics* **Acts:** Converted to formaldehyde & ammonia in acidic urine; nonspecific bactericidal action **Dose:** *Adults.* *Hippurate:* 1 g PO bid. *Mandelate:* initial 1 g qid PC pc & hs, maint 1–2 g/d. *Peds 6–12 y:* *Hippurate:* 0.5–1 g PO bid PO ÷ bid. *>2 y: Mandelate:* 50–75 mg/kg/d PO ÷ qid; take w/ food, ascorbic acid w/ hydration **Caution:** [C, +] **CI:** Renal Insuff, severe hepatic Dz, & severe dehydration **Disp:** *Methenamine hippurate* (Hiprex, Urex): Tabs 1 g. *Methenamine mandelate:* 500 mg, 1 g EC tabs **SE:** Rash, GI upset, dysuria, ↑ LFTs, superinfection w/ prolonged use, *C. difficile*-associated diarrhea. **Notes:** Use w/ sulfonamides may precipitate in urine. Hippurate not indicated in peds <6 y. Not for pts w/ indwelling catheters as dwell time in bladder required for action

Methimazole (Tapazole) **Uses:** *Hyperthyroidism, thyrotoxicosis*, prep for thyroid surgery or radiation **Acts:** Blocks T₃ & T₄ formation, but does not inactivate circulating T₃, T₄ **Dose:** *Adults.* Initial based on severity: 15–60 mg/d PO q8h. *Maint:* 5–15 mg PO daily. *Peds.* *Initial:* 0.4–0.7 mg/kg/24 h PO q8h. *Maint:* 1/3–2/3 of initial dose PO daily; take w/ food **Caution:** [D, −] w/ Other meds **CI:** Breast-feeding **Disp:** Tabs 5, 10, 20 mg **SE:** GI upset, dizziness, blood dyscrasias, dermatitis, fever, hepatic Rxns, lupus-like synd **Notes:** Follow clinically & w/ TFT, CBC w/ diff

Methocarbamol (Robaxin) **Uses:** *Relief of discomfort associated w/ painful musculoskeletal conditions* **Acts:** Centrally acting skeletal muscle relaxant **Dose:** *Adults & Peds >16 y:* 1.5 g PO qid for 2–3 d, then 1-g PO qid maint. *Tetanus:* 1–2 g IV q6h × 3 d, then use PO. *<16 y:* 15 mg/kg/dose or 500 mg/m² IV, may repeat PRN (tetanus only), max 1.8 g/m²/d × 3 d **Caution:** Sz disorders [C, +] **CI:** MyG, renal impair w/IV **Disp:** Tabs 500, 750 mg; Inj 100 mg/mL **SE:** Can discolor urine, lightheadedness, drowsiness, GI upset, ↓ HR, ↓ BP **Note:** Tabs can be crushed and added to NG, do not operate heavy machinery

Methotrexate (Rheumatrex Dose Pack, Trexall) **BOX:** Administration only by experienced physician; do not use in women of childbearing age unless absolutely necessary (teratogenic); impaired elimination w/ impaired renal Fxn, ascites, pleural effusion; severe ↓ BM w/ NSAIDs; hepatotoxic, occasionally fatal; can induce life-threatening pneumonitis; D and ulcerative stomatitis require D/C; lymphoma risk; may cause tumor lysis synd; can cause severe skin Rxn, opportunistic infxns; w/ RT can ↑ tissue necrosis risk. Preservatives make this agent unsuitable for intrathecal IT or higher dose use **Uses:** *ALL, AML, leukemic meningitis, trophoblastic tumors (choriocarcinoma, hydatidiform mole), breast, lung, head, & neck

CAs, Burkitt lymphoma, mycosis fungoides, osteosarcoma, Hodgkin Dz & NHL, psoriasis; RA, JRA, SLE*, chronic Dz **Acts:** ↓ Dihydrofolate reductase-mediated prod of tetrahydrofolate, causes ↓ DNA synth **Dose:** *Adults.* Per protocol. *RA:* 7.5 mg/wk PO 1/wk 1 or 2.5 mg q12h PO for 3 doses/wk. *Psoriasis:* 2.5–5 mg PO q12h × 3d/wk or 10–25 mg PO/IM q wk. *Chronic:* 15–25 mg IM/SQ q wk, then 15 mg/wk. *Peds.* 10 mg/m² PO/IM q wk, then 5–14 mg/m² × 1 or as 3 divided doses 12 h apart; ↓ elderly, w/ renal/hepatic impair **Caution:** [D, –] w/ renal nephro-/hepatotoxic meds, multiple interactions, w/ Sz, profound ↓ BM other than CA related **CI:** Severe renal/hepatic impair, PRG/lactation **Disp:** Dose pack 2.5 mg in 8, 12, 16, 20, or 24 doses; tabs 2.5, 5, 7.5, 10, 15 mg; Inj powder 20 mg, 1 g **SE:** ↓ BM, N/V/D, anorexia, mucositis, hepatotox (transient & reversible; may progress to atrophy, necrosis, fibrosis, cirrhosis), rashes, dizziness, malaise, blurred vision, alopecia, photosens, renal failure, pneumonitis; rare pulm fibrosis; chemical arachnoiditis & HA w/ IT delivery **Notes:** Monitor CBC, LFTs, Cr, MTX levels & CXR; "high dose" >500 mg/m² requires leucovorin rescue to ↓ tox; w/ IT, use preservative-/alcohol-free soln; systemic levels: *Therapeutic:* >0.01 micromole; *Toxic:* >10 micromoles over 24 h

Methyldopa (Aldomet) **Uses:** *HTN* **Acts:** Centrally acting antihypertensive, ↓ sympathetic outflow **Dose:** *Adults.* 250–500 mg PO bid-tid (max 2–3 g/d) or 250 mg–1 g IV q6–8h. *Peds: Neonates:* 2.5–5 mg/kg PO/IV q6–8h. *Other peds:* 10 mg/kg/24 h PO in 2–3 + doses or 5–10 mg/kg/dose IV q6–8h to max 65 mg/kg/24 h; ↓ in renal Insuff/elderly **Caution:** [B(PO), C(IV), +] **CI:** Liver Dz, w/ MAOIs, bisulfate allergy **Disp:** Tabs 250, 500 mg; Inj 50 mg/mL **SE:** Discolors urine; initial transient sedation/drowsiness, edema, hemolytic anemia, hepatic disorders, fevers, nightmares **Notes:** Tolerance may occur, false(+) Coombs test

Methylergonovine (Methergine) **Uses:** *Postpartum bleeding (atony, hemorrhage)* **Acts:** Ergotamine derivative, rapid and sustained uterotonic effect **Dose:** 0.2 mg IM after anterior shoulder delivery or puerperium, may repeat in 2–4-h intervals or 0.2–0.4 mg PO q6–12h for 2–7 d **Caution:** [C, ?] w/ Sepsis, obliterative vascular Dz, hepatic/renal impair, w/ CYP3A4 inhib (Table 10 p 280) **CI:** HTN, PRG, toxemia **Disp:** Inj 0.2 mg/mL; tabs 0.2 mg **SE:** HTN, N/V, CP, ↓ BP, Sz **Notes:** Give IV only if absolutely necessary over >1 min w/ BP monitoring

Methylnaltrexone Bromide (Relistor) **Uses:** *Opioid-induced constipation in pt w/ advanced illness such as CA* **Acts:** Peripheral opioid antagonist **Dose:** *Adults. Wgt-based <38 kg/>114 kg:* 0.15 mg/kg SQ; *38–61 kg:* 8 mg SQ; *62–114 kg:* 12 mg SQ, dose q other day PRN, max 1 dose q24h **Caution:** [B, NR] w/ CrCl <30 mL/min ↓ dose 50% **Disp:** Inj 12 mg/0.6 mL **SE:** N/D, Abd pain, dizziness **Notes:** Does not affect opioid analgesic effects or induce withdrawal

Methylphenidate, Oral (Concerta, Metadate CD, Methylin Ritalin, Ritalin LA, Ritalin SR, Others) [CII] **BOX:** w/ Hx of drug or alcohol dependence, avoid abrupt D/C; chronic use can lead to dependence or psychotic behavior; observe closely during withdrawal of drug **Uses:** *ADHD, narcolepsy*,

depression **Acts:** CNS stimulant, blocks reuptake of norepinephrine and DA **Dose:** *Adults.* Narcolepsy: 10 mg PO 2–3×/d, 60 mg/d max. *Depression:* 2.5 mg q A.M.; ↑ slowly, 20 mg/d max., ÷ bid 7 A.M. & 12 P.M.; use regular release only. **Adults and & Peds** *>6 y: ADHD: IR:* 5 mg PO bid, ↑ 5–10 mg/d to 60 mg/d max (2 mg/kg/d), *ER/SR* use total IR dose q day. *CD/LA* 20 mg PO q day, ↑ 10–20 mg q wk to 60 mg/d max. *Concerta:* 18 mg PO q A.M. Rx naïve or already on 20 mg/d, 36 mg PO q A.M. if on 40 mg/d or 54 mg/d max **Caution:** [C, +/−] w/ Hx EtOH/drug abuse, CV Dz, HTN, bipolar Dz, Sz; separate from MAOIs by 14 d **Disp:** Chew tabs 2.5, 5, 10 mg; tabs scored IR (Ritalin) 5, 10, 20 mg; *Caps ER (Ritalin LA)* 10, 20, 30, 40 mg *Caps ER (Metadate CD)* 10, 20, 30, 40, 50, 60 mg *(Methylin ER)* 10, 20 mg. Tabs SR *(Ritalin SR)* 20 mg; ER tabs *(Concerta)* 18, 27, 36, 54 mg. Oral soln 5, 10 mg/5 mL **SE:** CV/CNS stimulation, growth retard, GI upset, pancytopenia, ↑ LFTs **CI:** Marked anxiety, tension, agitation, NAG, motor tics, family Hx or diagnosis of Tourette synd, severe HTN, angina, arrhythmias, CHF, recent MI, ↑ thyroid; w/ or w/in 14 d of MAOI **Notes:** See also transdermal form; titrate dose; take 30–45 min ac; do not chew or crush; *Concerta* "ghost tablet" in stool, avoid w/ GI narrowing; Metadate contains sucrose, avoid w/ lactose/galactose problems. Do not use these meds w/ halogenated anesthetics; abuse and diversion concerns; AHA recommends: all ADHD peds need CV assessment and consideration for ECG before Rx

Methylphenidate, Transdermal (Daytrana) [CII]   **BOX:** w/ Hx of drug or alcohol dependence; chronic use can lead to dependence or psychotic behavior; observe closely during withdrawal of drug **Uses:** *ADHD in children 6–17 y* **Acts:** CNS stimulant, blocks reuptake of norepinephrine and DA **Dose:** *Adults & Peds ≥6 y:* Apply to hip in A.M. (2 h before desired effect), remove 9 h later; titrate 1st wk 10 mg/9 h, 2nd wk 15 mg/9 h, 3rd wk 20 mg/9 h, 4th wk 30 mg/9 h **Caution:** [C, +/−] See methylphenidate, oral sensitization may preclude subsequent use of oral forms; abuse and diversion concerns **CI:** significant anxiety, agitation; component allergy; glaucoma; w/ or w/in 14 d of MAOI; tics, or family hx Tourette synd **Disp:** Patches 10, 15, 20, 30 mg **SE:** Local Rxns, N/V, nasopharyngitis, ↓ wgt, ↓ appetite, lability, insomnia, tic **Notes:** Titrate dose weekly; effects last hours after removal; evaluate BP, HR at baseline and periodically; avoid heat exposure to patch, may cause OD, AHA rec: all ADHD peds need CV assessment and consideration for ECG before Rx

Methylprednisolone (Solu-Medrol) [See Steroids page 229 and Table 2 p 265]

Metoclopramide (Reglan, Clopra, Octamide)   **BOX:** Chronic use may cause tardive dyskinesia; D/C if sxs develop; avoid prolonged use (>12 wks) **Uses:** *Diabetic gastroparesis, symptomatic GERD; chemotherapy & post-op N/V, facilitate small-bowel intubation & upper GI radiologic evaluation*; stimulate gut in prolonged post-op ileus **Acts:** ↑ Upper GI motility; blocks dopamine in chemoreceptor trigger zone, sensitized tissues to ACH **Dose:** *Adults. Gastroparesis:*

10 mg PO 30 min ac & hs for 2–8 wk PRN, or same dose IM/IV for 10 d, then PO. *Reflux:* 10–15 mg PO 30 min ac & hs. *Chemotherapy Antiemetic:* 1–3 mg/kg/dose IV 30 min before chemotherapy, then q2h × 2 doses, then q3h × 3 doses. *Post-op:* 10–20 mg IV/IM q4–6h PRN. *Adults & Peds >14 y: Intestinal intubation:* 10 mg IV × 1 over 1–2 min. **Peds.** *Reflux:* 0.1 mg/kg/dose PO 30 min ac & hs, max 0.3–0.75 mg/kg/d × 2 wk-6 mo. *Chemotherapy Antiemetic:* 1–2 mg/kg/dose IV as adults. *Post-op:* 0.25 mg/kg IV q4–6h PRN. **Peds** *intestinal intubation:* **6–14 y:** 2.5–5 mg IV × 1 over 1–2 min; **<6 y:** use 0.1 mg/kg IV × 1 **Caution:** [B, –] Drugs w/ extrapyramidal ADRs, MAOIs, TCAs, sympathomimetics **CI:** EPS meds, GI bleeding, pheochromocytoma, Sz disorders, GI obst **Disp:** Tabs 5, 10 mg; syrup 5 mg/5 mL; Inj 5 mg/mL **SE:** Dystonic Rxns common w/ high doses (Rx w/IV diphenhydramine), fluid retention, restlessness, D, drowsiness

Metolazone (Zaroxolyn) Uses: *Mild–mod essential HTN & edema of renal Dz or cardiac failure* **Acts:** Thiazide-like diuretic; ↓ distal tubule Na reabsorption **Dose:** *HTN:* 2.5–5 mg PO maint 5–20 mg PO q day *Edema:* 2.5–20 mg/d PO. **Caution:** [D, +] Avoid w/ Li, gout, digitalis, SLE, many interactions **CI:** Anuria, hepatic coma or precoma. **Disp:** Tabs 2.5, 5, 10 mg **SE:** Monitor fluid/lytes; dizziness, ↓ BP, ↓ K+, ↑ HR, ↑ uric acid, CP, photosens

Metoprolol Tartrate (Lopressor) Metoprolol Succinate (Toprol XL) **BOX:** Do not acutely stop Rx as marked worsening of angina can result; taper over 1–2 wk Uses: *HTN, angina, AMI, CHF (XL form)* **Acts:** β_1-Adrenergic receptor blocker **Dose:** *Adults.* *Angina:* 50–200 mg PO bid max 400 mg/d; ER form dose q day. *HTN:* 50–200 mg PO bid max 450 mg/d, ER form dose q day. *AMI:* 5 mg IV q2min × 3 doses, then 50 mg PO q6h × 48 h, then 100 mg PO bid. *CHF: (XL form preferred)* 12.5–25 mg/d PO × 2 wk, ↑ 2-wk intervals, 200 mg/max, use low dose w/ greatest severity; 5 mg slow IV q5min, total 15 mg *(ECC 2005).* **Peds 1–17 y:** *HTN* IR form 1–2 mg/kg/d PO, max 6 mg/kg/d (200 mg/d). **≥6 y:** *HTN* ER form 1 mg/kg/d PO, initial max 50 mg/d ↑ PRN to 2 mg/kg/d max; ↓ w/ hepatic failure; take w/ meals **Caution:** [C, +] Uncompensated CHF, ↓ HR, heart block, hepatic impair, MyG, PVD, Raynaud, thyrotoxicosis **CI:** For HTN/angina SSS (unless paced), severe PVD, pheochromocytoma. For MI sinus brady <45 BPM, 1st-degree block (PR >0.24 s), 2nd-, 3rd-degree block, SBP <100 mm Hg, severe CHF, cardiogenic shock **Disp:** Tabs 25, 50, 100 mg; ER tabs 25, 50, 100, 200 mg; Inj 1 mg/mL **SE:** Drowsiness, insomnia, ED, ↓ HR, bronchospasm **Notes:** IR:ER 1:1 daily dose but ER/XL is q day. OK to split XL tab but do not crush/chew

Metronidazole (Flagyl, MetroGel) **BOX:** Carcinogenic in rats Uses: *Bone/joint, endocarditis, intra-Abd, meningitis, & skin infxns; amebiasis and amebic liver abscess; trichomoniasis in pt and partner; bacterial vaginosis; PID; giardiasis; antibiotic associated pseudomembranous colitis (C. difficile), eradicate H. pylori w/ combo Rx, rosacea, prophylactic in post-op colorectal surgery* **Acts:** Interferes w/ DNA synth. **Spectrum:** Excellent anaerobic, *C. difficile* **Dose:** *Adults.*

Anaerobic infxns: 500 mg IV q6–8h. *Amebic dysentery:* 500–750 mg/d PO q8h × 5–10 d. *Trichomonas:* 250 mg PO tid for 7 d or 2 g PO × 1 (Rx partner). *C. difficile:* 500 mg PO or IV q8h for 7–10 d (PO preferred; IV only if pt NPO), if no response, change to PO vancomycin. *Vaginosis:* 1 applicator intravag q day or bid × 5 d, or 500 mg PO bid × 7 d or 750 mg PO q day × 7 d. *Acne rosacea/skin:* Apply bid. *Giardia:* 500 mg PO bid × 5–7 d. *H. pylori:* 250–500 mg PO w/ meals & hs × 14 d, combine w/ other antibiotic & a proton pump inhib or H_2 antagonist. **Peds.** 30 mg/kg PO/IV/d ÷ q6H, 4 g/d max ÷. *Amebic dysentery:* 35–50 mg/kg/24 h PO in 3 ÷ doses for 5–10 d; Rx 7–10 d for *C. difficile.* *Trichomonas:* 15–30 mg/kg/d PO ÷ q8h × 7 d. *C. difficile:* 20 mg/kg/d PO ÷ q6h × 10 d, max 2 g/d; ↓ w/ severe hepatic/renal impair **Caution:** [B, +/–] Avoid EtOH, w/ warfarin, CYP3A4 substrates (Table 10 280), ↑ Li levels **CI:** First tri of PRG **Disp:** Tabs 250, 500 mg; XR tabs 750 mg; caps 375 mg; IV 500 mg/100 mL; lotion 0.75%; gel 0.75, 1%; intravag gel 0.75% (5 g/applicator 37.5 mg in 70-g tube); cream 0.75,1% **SE:** Disulfiram-like Rxn; dizziness, HA, GI upset, anorexia, urine discoloration, flushing, metallic taste **Notes:** For trichomoniasis, Rx pt's partner; no aerobic bacteria activity; use in combo w/ serious mixed infxns; wait 24 h after 1st dose to breast-feed or 48 h if extended Rx, take ER on empty stomach

Mexiletine (Mexitil) **BOX:** Mortality risks noted for flecainide and/or encainide (class I antiarrhythmics). Reserve for use in pts w/ life-threatening ventricular arrhythmias **Uses:** *Suppress symptomatic vent arrhythmias* **DN Acts:** Class IB antiarrhythmic (Table 9 p 279) **Dose: Adults.** 200–300 mg PO q8h. Initial 200 mg q8h, can load w/ 400 mg if needed, ↑ q2–3d, 1200 mg/d max. **Caution:** [C, +] CHF, may worsen severe arrhythmias; interacts w/ hepatic inducers & suppressors **CI:** Cardiogenic shock or 2nd/3rd-degree AV block w/o pacemaker **Disp:** Caps 150, 200, 250 mg **SE:** Light-headedness, dizziness, anxiety, incoordination, GI upset, ataxia, hepatic damage, blood dyscrasias, PVCs, N/V, tremor **Notes:** ✓ LFTs, CBC, false(+) ANA

Miconazole (Monistat 1 Combo, Monistat 3, Monistat 7) [OTC] (Monistat-Derm) **Uses:** *Candidal infxns, dermatomycoses (tinea pedis/ tinea cruris/tinea corporis/tinea versicolor/Candidiasis)* **Acts:** Azole antifungal, alters fungal membrane permeability **Dose:** *Intravag:* 100 mg supp or 2% cream intravag qhs × 7 d or 200 mg supp or 4% cream intravag qhs × 3 d. *Derm:* Apply bid, A.M./P.M. *Tinea versicolor:* Apply q day. Treat tinea pedis for 1 mo and other infxns for 2 wk. **Peds ≥12 y:** 100 mg supp or 2% cream intravag qhs × 7 d or 200 mg supp or 4% cream intravag qhs × 3 d. **Caution:** [C, ?] Azole sensitivity **Disp:** *Monistat-Derm:* (Rx) cream 2%; *Monistat 1 Combo:* 2% cream w/ 1200 mg supp, *Monistat 3:* Vag cream 4%, supp 200 mg; *Monistat 7:* cream 2%, supp 100 mg; lotion 2%; powder 2%; effervescent tab 2%; oint 2%; spray 2%; vag supp 100, 200, 1200 mg; vag cream 2%, 4%; [OTC] **SE:** Vag burning; on skin contact dermatitis, irritation, burning **Notes:** May interfere w/ condom and diaphragm, do not use w/ tampons

Miconazole/Zinc oxide/Petrolatum (Vusion) Uses: *Candidal diaper rash* Acts: Combo antifungal Dose: *Peds >4 wk:* Apply at each diaper change × 7 d Caution: [C, ?] CI: None Disp: Miconazole/zinc oxide/petrolatum oint 0.25/15/81.35%, 50-, 90- g tube SE: None Notes: Keep diaper dry, not for prevention

Midazolam (Various) [C-IV] BOX: Associated w/ resp depression and resp arrest especially when used for sedation in noncritical care settings. Reports of airway obst, desaturation, hypoxia, and apnea w/ other CNS depressants. Cont monitoring required Uses: *Pre-op sedation, conscious sedation for short procedures & mechanically ventilated pts, induction of general anesthesia* Acts: Short-acting benzodiazepine Dose: *Adults.* 1–5 mg IV or IM or 0.02–0.35 mg/kg based on indication; titrate to effect. *Peds. Pre-op: >6 mo:* 0.25–1 mg/kg PO, 20 mg max. *Conscious sedation:* 0.08 mg/kg × 1. *>6 mo:* 0.1–0.15 mg/kg IM × 1 max 10 mg. *General anesthesia:* 0.025–0.1 mg/kg IV q2min for 1–3 doses PRN to induce anesthesia (↓ in elderly, w/ narcotics or CNS depressants) Caution: [D, +/–] w/ CYP3A4 substrate (Table 9 279), multiple drug interactions CI: NAG; w/ fosamprenavir, atazanavir, nelfinavir, ritonavir Disp: Inj 1, 5 mg/mL; syrup 2 mg/mL SE: Resp depression; ↓ BP w/ conscious sedation, N Notes: Reversal w/ flumazenil; monitor for resp depression; not for epidural/intrathecal IT use

Mifepristone [RU 486] (Mifeprex) BOX: Pt counseling & information required; associated w/ fatal infxns & bleeding Uses: *Terminate intrauterine pregnancies PRGs of <49 d* Acts: Antiprogestin; ↑ prostaglandins, results in uterine contraction Dose: Administered w/ 3 office visits: Day 1: 600 mg PO × 1; day 3, unless abortion confirmed, 400 mg PO of misoprostol (*Cytotec*); about day 14, verify termination of PRG. Surgical termination if Rx fails. Caution: [X, –] w/ Infxn, sepsis CI: Ectopic PRG, undiagnosed adnexal mass, w/ IUD, adrenal failure, w/ long-term steroid Rx, hemorrhagic Dz, w/ anticoagulants, prostaglandin hypersens. Pts who do not have access to medical facilities or unable to understand treatment or comply. Disp: Tabs 200 mg SE: Abd pain & 1–2 wk of uterine bleeding, N/V/D, HA Notes: Under physician's supervision only, 9–16 d vag bleed on average after using

Miglitol (Glyset) Uses: *Type 2 DM* Acts: α-Glucosidase inhib; delays carbohydrate digestion Dose: Initial 25 mg PO tid; maint 50–100 mg tid (w/ 1st bite of each meal), titrate over 4–8 wk Caution: [B, –] w/ Digitalis & digestive enzymes CI: DKA, obstructive/inflammatory GI disorders; SCr >2 mg/dL Disp: Tabs 25, 50, 100 mg SE: Flatulence, D, Abd pain Notes: Use alone or w/ sulfonylureas

Milnacipran (Savella) BOX: Antidepressants associated w/ ↑ risk of suicide ideation in children and young adults Uses: *Fibromyalgia* Action: Antidepressant, SNRI Dose: 50 mg PO bid, max 200 mg/d; ↓ to 25 mg bid w/ CrCl < 30 mL/min Caution: [C, /?] CI: NAG, w/ recent MAOI Disp: Tabs: 12.5, 25, 50, 100 mg SE: Headache, N/V, constipation, dizziness, ↑ HR, ↑ BP Notes: Monitor HR and BP

Milrinone (Primacor) Uses: *CHF acutely decompensated*, calcium antagonist intoxication **Acts:** Phosphodiesterase inhib, (+) inotrope & vasodilator; little chronotropic activity **Dose:** 50 mcg/kg, IV over 10 min then 0.375–0.75 mcg/kg/min IV Inf; ↓ w/ renal impair **Caution:** [C, ?] Allergy to drug; w/ inamrinone **Disp:** Inj 200 mcg/mL **SE:** Arrhythmias, ↓ BP, HA **Notes:** Monitor fluids, lytes, CBC, Mg^{2+}, BP, HR; not for long-term use

Mineral Oil [OTC] Uses: *Constipation, bowel irrigation, fecal impaction* **Acts:** Lubricant laxative **Dose:** *Adults. Constipation:* 15–45 mL PO/d PRN. *Fecal impaction or after barium:* 118 mL rectally × 1. *Peds >6 y: Constipation:* 5–25 mL PO q day. *2–12 y: Fecal impaction:* 118 mL rectally × 1. **Caution:** [C, ?] w/ N/V, difficulty swallowing, bedridden pts; may ↓ absorption of vit A, D, E, K, warfarin **CI:** Colostomy/ileostomy, appendicitis, diverticulitis, ulcerative colitis **Disp:** All [OTC] liq PO 13.5 mL/15 mL, PO microemulsion 2.5 mL/5 mL, rectal enema 118 mL **SE:** Lipid pneumonia (aspiration of PO), N/V, temporary anal incontinence **Notes:** Take PO upright, do not use PO in peds <6 y

Mineral Oil-Pramoxine HCl-Zinc Oxide (Tucks Ointment, [OTC]) Uses: *Temporary relief of anorectal disorders (itching, etc)* **Acts:** Topical anesthetic **Dose:** *Adults & Peds ≥12 y:* Cleanse, rinse, & dry, apply externally or into anal canal w/ tip 5×/d × 7 d max. **Caution:** [?, ?] Do not place into rectum **CI:** None **Disp:** Oint 30-g tube **SE:** Local irritation **Notes:** D/C w/ if rectal bleeding occurs or if condition worsens or does not improve w/in 7 d

Minocycline (Dynacin, Minocin, Solodyn) Uses: *Mod–severe nonnodular acne (Solodyn), anthrax, rickettsiae, skin Infxn, URI, UTI, nongonococcal urethritis, amebic dysentery, asymptomatic meningococcal carrier, Mycobacterium marinum* **Acts:** Tetracycline, bacteriostatic; ↓ protein synth **Dose:** *Adults & Peds >12 y:* Usual: 200 mg, then 100 mg q12h or 100–200 mg, then 50 mg qid. *Gonococcal urethritis, men:* 100 mg q12h × 5 d. *Syphilis:* Usual dose × 10–15 d. *Meningococcal carrier:* 100 mg q12h × 5 d. *M. marinum:* 100 mg q12h × 6–8 wk. *Uncomp urethral, endocervical, or rectal Infxn:* 100 mg q12h × 7 d minimum. *Adults & Peds >12 y: Acne: (Solodyn)* 1 mg/kg PO q day × 12 wk. *>8 y:* 4 mg/kg initially then 2 mg/kg q12h w/ food to ↓ irritation, hydrate well, ↓ dose or extend interval w/ renal impair. **Caution:** [D, –] Associated w/ pseudomembranous colitis, w/ renal impair, may ↓ OCP, or w/ warfarin may ↑ INR **CI:** Allergy, women of childbearing potential **Disp:** Tabs 50, 75, 100 mg; tabs ER *(Solodyn)* 45, 90, 135 mg, caps *(Minocin)* 50, 100 mg, susp 50 mg/mL **SE:** D, HA, fever, rash, joint pain, fatigue, dizziness, photosens, hyperpigmentation, SLE synd, pseudotumor cerebri **Notes:** Do not cut/crush/chew; keep away from children, tooth discoloration in <8 y or w/ use last half of PRG

Minoxidil, Oral BOX: May cause pericardial effusion, occasional tamponade, and angina pectoris may be exacerbated. Only for non-responders to max doses of 2 other antihypertensives and a diuretic. Administer under supervision w/ a β-blocker and diuretic. Monitor for ↓ BP in those receiving guanethidine w/ malignant HTN **Uses:** *Severe HTN* **Acts:** Peripheral vasodilator **Dose:** *Adults & Peds >12 y:* 5 mg PO ÷ daily, titrate q3d, 10 mg/d max. *Peds.* 0.2–1 mg/kg/24 h ÷ PO q12–24h, titrate q3d, max 50 mg/d; ↓ w/ elderly, renal insuff **Caution:** [C, +] **CI:** Pheochromocytoma, component allergy, CHF, renal impair **Disp:** Tabs 2.5, 10 mg **SE:** Pericardial effusion & vol overload w/ PO use; hypertrichosis w/ chronic use, edema, ECG changes, wgt gain **Note:** Avoid for 1 mo after MI

Minoxidil, Topical (Theroxidil, Rogaine) [OTC] Uses: *Male & female pattern baldness* **Acts:** Stimulates vertex hair growth **Dose:** Apply 1 mL bid to area, D/C if no growth in 4 mo. **Caution:** [?, ?] **CI:** Component allergy **Disp:** Soln & aerosol foam 5% **SE:** Changes in hair color/texture **Note:** requires chronic use to maintain hair

Mirtazapine (Remeron, Remeron SolTab) BOX: ↑ Risk of suicidal thinking and behavior in children, adolescents, and young adults w/ major depression and other psychological disorders. Not for peds **Uses:** *Depression* **Acts:** α₂-Antagonist antidepressant, ↑ norepinephrine & 5-HT **Dose:** 15 mg PO hs, up to 45 mg/d hs **Caution:** [C, ?] Has anticholesterol effects, w/ Sz, clonidine, CNS depressant use, CYP1A2, CYP3A4 inducers/inhib **CI:** MAOIs w/in 14 d **Disp:** Tabs 15, 30, 45 mg; rapid dispersion tabs (SolTab) 15, 30, 45 mg **SE:** Somnolence, ↑ cholesterol, constipation, xerostomia, wgt gain, agranulocytosis, ↓ BP, edema, musculoskeletal pain **Notes:** Do not ↑ dose < q1–2wk; handle rapid tabs w/ dry hands, do not cut or chew

Misoprostol (Cytotec) BOX: Use in PRG can cause abortion, premature birth, or birth defects; do not use to ↓ decrease ulcer risk in women of childbearing age; must comply w/ birth control measures **Uses:** *Prevent NSAID-induced gastric ulcers; medical termination of PRG <49 d w/ mifepristone*; induce labor (cervical ripening); incomplete & therapeutic abortion **Acts:** Prostaglandin (PGE-1); antisecretory & mucosal protection; induces uterine contractions **Dose:** *Ulcer prevention:* 200 mcg PO qid w/ meals; in females, start 2nd/3rd d of next nl period. *Induction of labor (term):* 25–50 mcg intravag. *PRG termination:* 400 mcg PO on day 3 of mifepristone; take w/ food **Caution:** [X, –] **CI:** PRG, component allergy **Disp:** Tabs 100, 200 mcg **SE:** Miscarriage w/ severe bleeding; HA, D, Abd pain, constipation. **Note:** Not used for induction of labor w/ previous C-section or major uterine surgery

Mitomycin (Mutamycin) BOX: Administer only by physician experienced in chemotherapy; myelosuppressive; can induce hemolytic uremic synd w/ irreversible renal failure **Uses:** *Stomach, pancreas*, breast, colon CA; squamous cell carcinoma of the anus; NSCLC, head & neck, cervical; bladder CA (intravesically) **Acts:** Alkylating agent; generates oxygen-free radicals w/ DNA strand breaks **Dose:** (Per protocol) 20 mg/m² q6–8wk IV or 10 mg/m² combo w/ other myelosuppressive drugs q6–8wk. *Bladder CA:* 20–40 mg in 40 mL NS via a urethral catheter once/wk × 8 wk, followed by monthly × 12 mo for 1 y; ↓ in renal/hepatic impair **Caution:** [D, –] **CI:** ↓ Plt, ↓ WBC, coagulation disorders, Cr >1.7 mg/dL, ↑ cardiac tox w/ vinca alkaloids/doxorubicin **Disp:** Inj 5, 20, 40 mg **SE:** ↓ BM (persists for 3–8 wk, may be cumulative; minimize w/ lifetime dose <50–60 mg/m^2), N/V, anorexia, stomatitis, renal tox, microangiopathic hemolytic anemia w/ renal failure (hemolytic–uremic synd), venoocclusive liver Dz, interstitial pneumonia, alopecia, extrav Rxns, contact dermatitis; CHF

Mitoxantrone (Novantrone) **BOX:** Administer only by physician experienced in chemotherapy; except for acute leukemia, do not use w/ ANC count of <1500 cells/mm^3; severe neutropenia can result in Infxn, follow CBC; cardiotoxic (CHF), secondary AML reported **Uses:** *AML (w/ cytarabine), ALL, CML, PCA, MS, Lung CA* breast CA, & NHL **Acts:** DNA-intercalating agent; ↓ DNA synth by interacting w/ topoisomerase II **Dose:** Per protocol; ↓ w/ hepatic impair, leukopenia, thrombocytopenia **Caution:** [D, –] Reports of secondary AML, ↑ MS ↑ CV risk, do not treat MS pt w/ low LVEF **CI:** PRG, sig ↓ in LVEF **Disp:** Inj 2 mg/mL **SE:** ↓ BM, N/V, stomatitis, alopecia (infrequent), cardiotox, urine discoloration, secretions & scleras may be blue-green **Notes:** Maintain hydration; baseline CV evaluation w/ ECG & LVEF; cardiac monitoring prior to each dose; not for intrathecal use

Modafinil (Provigil) [C-IV] **Uses:** *Improve wakefulness in pts w/ excess daytime sleepiness (narcolepsy, sleep apnea, shift work sleep disorder)* **Acts:** Alters dopamine & norepinephrine release, ↓ GABA-mediated neurotransmission **Dose:** 200 mg PO q A.M.; ↓ dose 50% w/ elderly/hepatic impair **Caution:** [C, ?/–] CV Dz; ↑ effects of warfarin, diazepam, phenytoin; ↓ OCP, cyclosporine, & theophylline effects **CI:** Component allergy **Disp:** Tabs 100, 200 mg **SE:** Serious rash including SJS, HA, N, D, paresthesias, rhinitis, agitation, psychological Sx **Notes:** CV assessment before using

Moexipril (Univasc) **BOX:** ACE inhib can cause fatal injury/death in 2nd/3rd tri; D/C w/ PRG **Uses:** *HTN, post-MI*, DN **Acts:** ACE inhib **Dose:** 7.5–30 mg in 1–2 ÷ doses 1 h ac ↓ in renal impair **Caution:** [C (1st tri, D 2nd & 3rd tri), ?] **CI:** ACE inhib sensitivity **Disp:** Tabs 7.5, 15 mg; **SE:** ↓ BP, edema, angioedema, HA, dizziness, cough, ↑ K$^+$

Molindone (Moban) **Uses:** *Schizophrenia* **Acts:** Piperazine phenothiazine **Dose:** *Adults.* 50–75 mg/d PO, ↑ to max 225 mg/d q3–4d PRN. *Peds 3–5 y:* 1–2.5 mg/d PO in 4 ÷ doses. *5–12 y:* 0.5–1.0 mg/kg/d in 4 ÷ doses **Caution:** [C, ?] NAG **CI:** Drug/EtOH CNS depression, coma **Disp:** Tabs 5, 10, 25, 50 mg scored; **SE:** Drowsiness, depression, ↓ BP, tachycardia, arrhythmias, EPS, neuroleptic malignant synd, Szs, constipation, xerostomia, blurred vision **Notes:** ✓ lipid profile, fasting glucose, HgA$_{1c}$; may ↑ prolactin

Mometasone and Formoterol (DULERA) **BOX:** Increased risk of worsening wheezing or asthma-related death w/ long- acting β$_2$-adrenergic agonists; use only if asthma not controlled on agent such as inhaled steroid **Uses:** *Maint Rx for asthma* **Acts:** Corticosteroid (Mometasone) w/ LA bronchodilator β$_2$ agonist (formoterol) **Dose:** *Adults & Peds >12 y:* 2 Inh q12h **Caution:** [C, M] w/ P450 3A4 inhib (e.g. ritonavir), adrenergic/beta blockers, meds that ↑ QT interval; candida infection of mouth/throat, immunosuppression, adrenal suppression, ↓ bone density, w/glaucoma/cataracts, may ↑ glucose, ↓ K; other LABA should not be used **CI:** Acute asthma attack; component hypersensitivity **Disp:** MDI 120 inhal/canister (mg mometasone/mg formoterol) 100/5, 200/5 **SE:** Nasopharyngitis, sinusitis, HA, palpitations, chest pain, rapid heart rate, tremor or nervousness **Notes:** for pts not controlled on other meds (e.g., low-medium dose Inh steroids) or whose Dz severity warrants 2 maint therapies

Montelukast (Singulair) Uses: *Prevent/chronic Rx asthma ≥12 mo; seasonal allergic rhinitis ≥2 y; perennial allergic rhinitis ≥6 mo; prevent exercise induced bronchoconstriction (EIB) ≥15 y; prophylaxis & Rx of chronic asthma, seasonal allergic rhinitis* **Acts:** Leukotriene receptor antagonist **Dose:** *Asthma: Adults & Peds >15 y:* 10 mg/d PO in P.M. *6–23 mo:* 4-mg pack granules q day. *2–5 y:* 4 mg/d PO q P.M. *6–14 y:* 5 mg/d PO q P.M. **Caution:** [B, M] **CI:** Component allergy **Disp:** Tabs 10 mg; chew tabs 4, 5 mg; granules 4 mg/pack **SE:** HA, dizziness, fatigue, rash, GI upset, Churg-Strauss synd, flu, cough, neuropsych events (agitation, restlessness, suicidal ideation) **Notes:** Not for acute asthma; use w/in 15 min of opening package

Morphine (Avinza XR, Astramorph/PF, Duramorph, Infumorph, MS Contin, Kadian SR, Oramorph SR, Roxanol) [C-II] **BOX:** Do not crush/chew SR/CR forms; 100 and 200 mg for opioid-tolerant pt only; controlled release; not to be crushed or chewed **Uses:** *Rx severe pain* AMI, acute pulmonary edema **Acts:** Narcotic analgesic; SR/CR forms for chronic use **Dose:** *Adults.* *Short-term use PO:* 5–30 mg q4h PRN; *IV/IM:* 2.5–15 mg q2–6h; *supp:* 10–30 mg q4h. SR formulations 15–60 mg q8–12h (do not chew/crush). *IT/epidural* (Duramorph, Infumorph, Astramorph/PF): Per protocol in Inf device. *Peds >6 mo:* 0.1–0.2 mg/kg/dose IM/IV q2–4h PRN to 15 mg/dose max; 0.2–0.5 mg/kg PO q4–6h PRN; 0.3–0.6 mg/kg SR tabs PO q12h; 2–4 mg IV (over 1–5 min) q5–30 min *(ECC 2005)* **Caution:** [C, +/–] Severe resp depression possible; w/ head injury; chewing delayed release forms can cause severe rapid release of morphine **CI:** Severe asthma, resp depression, GI obst **Disp:** IR tabs 15, 30 mg; soln 10, 20, 100 mg/5 mL; supp 5, 10, 20, 30 mg; Inj 2, 4, 5, 8, 10, 15, 25, 50 mg/mL; *MS Contin CR* tabs 15, 30, 60, 100, 200 mg; *Oramorph SR* tabs 15, 30, 60, 100 mg; *Kadian SR caps* 10, 20, 30, 50, 60, 80, 100 mg; *Avinza XR* caps 30, 60, 90, 120 mg; *Duramorph/Astramorph PF:* Inj 0.5, 1 mg/mL; *Infumorph* 10, 25 mg/mL, **SE:** Narcotic SE (resp depression, sedation, constipation, N/V, pruritus, diaphoresis, urinary retention, biliary colic), granulomas w/ IT **Notes:** May require scheduled dosing to relieve severe chronic pain

Morphine Liposomal (DepoDur) Uses: *Long-lasting epidural analgesia* **Acts:** ER morphine analgesia **Dose:** 10–20 mg lumbar epidural Inj (C-section 10 mg after cord clamped) **Caution:** [C, +/–] Elderly, biliary Dz (sphincter of Oddi spasm) **CI:** Ileus, resp depression, asthma, obstructed airway, suspected/known head injury ↑ ICP, allergy to morphine **Disp:** Inj 10 mg/mL **SE:** Hypoxia, resp depression, ↓ BP, retention, N/V, constipation, flatulence, pruritus, pyrexia, anemia, HA, dizziness, tachycardia, insomnia, ileus **Notes:** Effect = 48 h; not for IT/IV/IM

Moxifloxacin (Avelox) **BOX:** ↑ Increase risk of tendon rupture and tendonitis. **Uses:** *Acute sinusitis & bronchitis, skin/soft-tissue/intra-Abd infxns, conjunctivitis, CAP* **Acts:** 4th-gen quinolone; ↓ DNA gyrase. *Spectrum:* Excellent gram(+) except MRSA & *E. faecium*; good gram(−) except *P. aeruginosa*, *Stenotrophomonas maltophilia*, & *Acinetobacter* sp; good anaerobic **Dose:** 400 mg/d PO/IV daily; avoid cation products, antacids. tid **Caution:** [C, ?/−] Quinolone sensitivity; interactions w/ Mg^{2+}, Ca^{2+}, Al^{2+}, Fe^{2+} containing products, & class IA & III antiarrhythmic agents (Table 9 p 279) **CI:** Quinolone/component sensitivity **Disp:** Tabs 400 mg, ABC Pak 5 tabs, Inj **SE:** Dizziness, N, QT prolongation, Szs, photosens, tendon rupture

Moxifloxacin ophthalmic (Vigamox Ophthalmic) **Uses:** *Bacterial conjunctivitis* **Acts:** See Moxifloxacin **Dose:** 1 gtt tid × 7 d **Caution:** [C, ?/−] **CI:** Quinolone/component sensitivity **Disp:** 4 mL ophthal 0.5% **SE:** ↓ Visual acuity, ocular pain, itching, tearing, conjunctivitis

Multivitamins, Oral [OTC] (Table 12, page 283)

Mupirocin (Bactroban, Bactroban Nasal) **Uses:** *Impetigo (oint); skin lesion infect w/ S. aureus or S. pyogenes; eradicate MRSA in nasal carriers* **Acts:** ↓ Bacterial protein synth **Dose:** *Topical:* Apply small amount 3×/d × 5–14 d. *Nasal:* Apply 1/2 single-use tube bid in nostrils × 5 d **Caution:** [B, ?] **CI:** Do not use w/ other nasal products **Disp:** Oint 2%; cream 2%; nasal oint 2% 1-g single-use tubes **SE:** Local irritation, rash **Notes:** Pt to contact health-care provider if no improvement in 3–5 d.

Muromonab-CD3 (Orthoclone OKT3) **BOX:** Can cause anaphylaxis; monitor fluid status; cytokine release synd **Uses:** *Acute rejection following organ transplantation* **Acts:** Murine Ab, blocks T-cell Fxn **Dose:** Per protocol **Adults.** 5 mg/d IV for 10–14 d. **Peds** *<30 kg:* 2.5 mg/d. *>30 kg:* 5 mg/d IV for 10–14 d **Caution:** [C, ?/−] w/ Hx of Szs, PRG, uncontrolled HTN **CI:** Murine sensitivity, fluid overload **Disp:** Inj 5 mg/5 mL **SE:** Anaphylaxis, pulm edema, fever/chills w/ 1st dose (premedicate w/ steroid/APAP/antihistamine); cytokine release synd (↓ BP, fever, rigors) **Notes:** Monitor during Inf; use 0.22-micron filter

Mycophenolic Acid (Myfortic) **BOX:** ↑ Risk of infxns, lymphoma, other CA's, progressive multifocal leukoencephalopathy PML), risk of PRG loss and malformation, female of childbearing potential must use contraception **Uses:** *Prevent rejection after renal transplant* **Acts:** Cytostatic to lymphocytes **Dose:** *Adults.* 720 mg PO bid. *Peds.* *BSA 1.19–1.58 m²:* 540 mg bid. *BSA >1.8 m²:* Adult dose; used w/ steroids & cyclosporine ↓ w/ renal Insuff/neutropenia; take on empty stomach **Caution:** [D, ?/−] **CI:** Component allergy **Disp:** Delayed release tabs 180, 360 mg **SE:** N/V/D, GI bleed, pain, fever, HA, Infxn, HTN, anemia, leukopenia, pure red cell aplasia, edema

Mycophenolate Mofetil (CellCept) BOX: ↑ Risk of infxns, lymphoma, other CAs, progressive multifocal leukoencephalopathy (PML); risk of PRG loss and malformation; female of childbearing potential must use contraception Uses: *Prevent organ rejection after transplant* Acts: Cytostatic to lymphocytes Dose: *Adults.* 1 g PO bid. *Peds. BSA 1.2–1.5 m²:* 750 mg PO bid. *BSA >1.5 m²:* 1 g PO bid; may taper up to 600 mg/m² PO bid; used w/ steroids & cyclosporine; ↓ in renal Insuff or neutropenia. *IV:* Infuse over >2 h. *PO:* Take on empty stomach, do not open caps Caution: [D, ?/–] CI: Component allergy; IV use in polysorbate 80 allergy Disp: Caps 250, 500 mg; susp 200 mg/mL, Inj 500 mg SE: N/V/D, pain, fever, HA, Infxn, HTN, anemia, leukopenia, edema

Nabilone (Cesamet) [CII] BOX: Psychotomimetic Rxns, may persist for 72 h following D/C; caregivers should be present during initial use or dosage modification; pts should not operate heavy machinery; avoid alcohol, sedatives, hypnotics, other psychoactive substances Uses: *Refractory chemotherapy-induced emesis* Acts: Synthetic cannabinoid Dose: *Adults.* 1–2 mg PO bid 1–3 h before chemotherapy, 6 mg/d max; may continue for 48 h beyond final chemotherapy dose Caution: [C, ?/–] Elderly, HTN, heart failure, w/ psychological illness, substance abuse; high protein binding w/ 1st-pass metabolism may lead to drug interactions Disp: Caps 1 mg SE: Drowsiness, vertigo, xerostomia, euphoria, ataxia, HA, difficulty concentrating, tachycardia, ↓ BP Notes: May require initial dose evening before chemotherapy; Rx only quantity for single treatment cycle

Nabumetone (Relafen) BOX: May ↑ risk of CV events & GI bleeding, perforation; CI w/ post-op coronary artery bypass graft Uses: *OA and RA*, pain Acts: NSAID; ↓ prostaglandins Dose: 1000–2000 mg/d ÷ daily-bid w/ food Caution: [C, –] Severe hepatic Dz CI: w/ Peptic ulcer, NSAID sensitivity, after coronary artery bypass graft surgery Disp: Tabs 500, 750 mg SE: Dizziness, rash, GI upset, edema, peptic ulcer, ↑ BP

Nadolol (Corgard) Uses: *HTN & angina* migraine prophylaxis Acts: Competitively blocks β-adrenergic receptors (β₁, β₂) Dose: 40–80 mg/d; ↑ to 240 mg/d (angina) or 320 mg/d (HTN) at 3–7-d intervals; ↓ in renal Insuff & elderly Caution: [C (1st tri; D if 2nd or 3rd tri), +] CI: Uncompensated CHF, shock, heart block, asthma Disp: Tabs 20, 40, 80, 120, 160 mg SE: Nightmares, paresthesias, ↓ BP, ↓ HR, fatigue

Nafcillin (Nallpen, Unipen) Uses: *infxns d/t susceptible strains of Staphylococcus & Streptococcus* Acts: Bactericidal; β-lactamase-resistant PCN; ↓ cell wall synth Spectrum: Good gram(+) except MRSA & enterococcus, no gram(–), poor anaerobe Dose: *Adults.* 1–2 g IV q4–6h. *Peds.* 50–200 mg/kg/d ÷ q4–6h Caution: [B, ?] CI: PCN allergy Disp: Inj powder l, 2 g SE: Interstitial nephritis, N/D, fever, rash, allergic Rxn Notes: No adjustment for renal Fxn

Naftifine (Naftin) Uses: *Tinea pedis, cruris, & corporis* Acts: Allylamine antifungal, ↓ cell membrane ergosterol synth Dose: Apply daily (cream) or bid (gel) Caution: [B, ?] CI: Component sensitivity Disp: 1% cream; gel SE: Local irritation

Nalbuphine (Nubain) Uses: *Mod–severe pain; pre-op & obstetric analgesia* Acts: Narcotic agonist–antagonist; ↓ ascending pain pathways Dose: *Adults. Pain:* 10 mg/70 kg IV/IM/SQ q3–6h; adjust PRN; 20 mg/dose or 160 mg/d max. *Anesthesia: Induction:* 0.3–3 mg/kg IV over 10–15 min; maint 0.25–0.5 mg/kg IV. *Peds.* 0.2 mg/kg IV or IM, 20 mg max; ↓ w/ renal/in hepatic impair Caution: [B, M] w/ Opiate use CI: Component sensitivity Disp: Inj 10, 20 mg/mL SE: CNS depression, drowsiness; caution, ↓ BP

Naloxone (Generic) Uses: *Opioid addiction (diagnosis) & OD* Acts: Competitive narcotic antagonist Dose: *Adults.* 0.4–2 mg IV, IM, or SQ q2–3 min; total dose 10 mg max. *Peds.* 0.01–0.1 mg/kg/dose IV, IM, or SQ; repeat IV q3min × 3 doses PRN Caution: [B, ?] May precipitate acute withdrawal in addicts Disp: Inj 0.4, 1 mg/mL SE: ↓ BP, tachycardia, irritability, GI upset, pulm edema Notes: If no response after 10 mg, suspect nonnarcotic cause

Naltrexone (Depade, ReVia, Vivitrol) BOX: Can cause hepatic injury, CI w/ active liver Dz Uses: *EtOH & narcotic addiction* Acts: Antagonizes opioid receptors Dose: *EtOH/narcotic addiction:* 50 mg/d PO; must be opioid-free for 7–10 d; *EtOH dependence:* 380 mg IM q4wk (*Vivitrol*) Caution: [C, M] Monitor for inj site reactions (*Vivitrol*) CI: Acute hep, liver failure, opioid use Disp: Tabs 50 mg; Inj 380 mg (*Vivitrol*) SE: Hepatotox; insomnia, GI upset, joint pain, HA, fatigue

Naphazoline (Albalon, Naphcon, Others), Naphazoline & Pheniramine Acetate (Naphcon A, Visine A) Uses: *Relieve ocular redness & itching caused by allergy* Acts: Sympathomimetic (α-adrenergic vasoconstrictor) & antihistamine (pheniramine) Dose: 1–2 gtt up to qid, 3 d max Caution: [C, +] CI: NAG, in children, w/ contact lenses, component allergy SE: CV stimulation, dizziness, local irritation Disp: Ophth 0.012, 0.025, 0.1%/15 mL; naphazoline & pheniramine 0.025%/0.3% soln

Naproxen (Aleve [OTC], Naprosyn, Anaprox) BOX: May ↑ risk of cardiovascular CV events & GI bleeding Uses: *Arthritis & pain* Acts: NSAID; ↓ prostaglandins Dose: *Adults & Peds >12 y:* 200–500 mg bid-tid to 1500 mg/d max. *>2 y: JRA* 5 mg/kg/dose bid; ↓ in hepatic impair Caution: [C, (D 3rd tri), +] CI: NSAID or ASA triad sensitivity, peptic ulcer, post coronary artery bypass graft pain, 3rd tri PRG Disp: *Tabs:* 220, 250, 375, 500 mg; *DR:* 375 mg, 500 mg; *CR:* 375 mg, 550 mg; susp 125 mL/5 mL SE: Dizziness, pruritus, GI upset, peptic ulcer, edema Note: Take w/ food to ↓ GI upset

Naratriptan (Amerge) Uses: *Acute migraine* Acts: Serotonin 5-HT$_1$ receptor agonist Dose: 1–2.5 mg PO once; repeat PRN in 4 h; 5 mg/24 h max; ↓ in mild renal/hepatic Insuff, take w/ fluids Caution: [C, M] CI: Severe renal/hepatic impair, avoid w/ angina, ischemic heart Dz, uncontrolled HTN, cerebrovascular synds, & ergot use Disp: Tabs 1, 2.5 mg SE: Dizziness, sedation, GI upset, paresthesias, ECG changes, coronary vasospasm, arrhythmias

Natalizumab (Tysabri) BOX: PML reported Uses: *Relapsing MS to delay disability and ↓ recurrences, Crohn Dz* Acts: Integrin receptor antagonist Dose: *Adults.* 300 mg IV q4wk; 2nd-line Tx only CI: PML; immune compromise or w/ immunosuppressant Caution: [C, ?/–] Baseline MRI to rule out PML Disp: Vial 300 mg SE: Infxn, immunosuppression; Inf Rxn precluding subsequent use; HA, fatigue, arthralgia Notes: Give slowly to ↓ Rxns; limited distribution (TOUCH Prescribing program); D/C immediately w/ signs of PML, weakness, paralysis, vision loss, impaired speech, cognitive ↓); evaluate at 3 and 6 mo, then q6mo thereafter

Nateglinide (Starlix) Uses: *Type 2 DM* Acts: ↑ Pancreatic insulin release Dose: 120 mg PO tid 1–30 min ac; ↓ to 60 mg tid if near target HbA$_{1c}$ Caution: [C, –] w/ CYP2C9 metabolized drug (Table 10 p 280) CI: DKA, type 1 DM Disp: Tabs 60, 120 mg SE: Hypoglycemia, URI; salicylates, nonselective β-blockers may enhance hypoglycemia

Nebivolol (Bystolic) Uses: *HTN* Acts: β$_1$-Selective blocker Dose: *Adults.* 5 mg PO daily, ↑ q2wk to 40 mg/d max, ↓ w/ CrCl <30 mL/min Caution: [D, +/–] w/ Bronchospastic Dz, DM, heart failure, pheochromocytoma, w/ CYP2D6 inhib CI: ↓ HR, cardiogenic shock, decompensated CHF, severe hepatic impair Disp: tabs 5, 10 mg SE: HA, fatigue, dizziness

Nefazodone BOX: Fatal hep & liver failure possible, D/C if LFTs >3× ULN, do not retreat; closely monitor for worsening depression or suicidality, particularly in ped pts Uses: *Depression* Acts: ↓ Neuronal uptake of serotonin & norepinephrine Dose: Initial 100 mg PO bid; usual 300–600 mg/d in 2 ÷ doses Caution: [C, M] CI: w/ MAOIs, pimozide, carbamazepine, alprazolam; active liver Dz Disp: Tabs 50, 100, 150, 200, 250 mg SE: Postural ↓ BP & allergic Rxns; HA, drowsiness, xerostomia, constipation, GI upset, liver failure Notes: Monitor LFTs, HR, BP

Nelarabine (Arranon) BOX: Fatal neurotox possible Uses: *T-cell ALL or T-cell lymphoblastic lymphoma unresponsive >2 other regimens* Acts: Nucleoside (deoxyguanosine) analog Dose: *Adults.* 1500 mg/m^2 IV over 2 h days 1, 3, 5 of 21-d cycle. *Peds.* 650 mg/m^2 IV over 1 h days 1–5 of 21-d cycle Caution: [D, ?/–] Disp: Vial 250 mg SE: Neuropathy, ataxia, Szs, coma, hematologic tox, GI upset, HA, blurred vision Notes: Prehydration, urinary alkalinization, allopurinol before dose; monitor CBC

Nelfinavir (Viracept) Uses: *HIV Infxn, other agents* Acts: Protease inhib causes immature, noninfectious virion production Dose: *Adults.* 750 mg PO tid or 1250 mg PO bid. *Peds.* 25–35 mg/kg PO tid or 45–55 mg/kg bid; take w/ food Caution: [B, –] Many drug interactions; do not use w/salmeterol, colchicine (w/renal/hepatic failure); adjust dose w/ bosentan, tadalafil for PAH CI: Phenylketonuria, w/ triazolam/midazolam use or drug dependent on CYP3A4 (Table 10 p 280); • alpha 1-adrenoreceptor antagonist (alfuzosin), PDE5 Inhibitor sildenafil Disp: Tabs 250, 625 mg; powder 50 mg/g; SE: Food ↑ absorption; interacts w/ St.

John's wort; dyslipidemia, lipodystrophy, D, rash **Notes:** PRG registry; tabs can be dissolved in water

Neomycin, Bacitracin, & Polymyxin B (Neosporin Ointment) (See Bacitracin, Neomycin, & Polymyxin B Topical, page 56)

Neomycin, Colistin, & Hydrocortisone (Cortisporin-TC Otic Drops); Neomycin, Colistin, Hydrocortisone, & Thonzonium (Cortisporin-TC Otic Susp)

Uses: *Otitis externa*, infxns of mastoid/fenestration cavities **Acts:** Antibiotic w/ anti-inflammatory **Dose:** *Adults.* 5 gtt in ear(s) tid-qid. *Peds.* 3–4 gtt in ear(s) tid-qid **CI:** component allergy; HSV, vaccinia, varicella **Caution:** [B, ?] **Disp:** Otic gtt & susp **SE:** Local irritation, rash **Notes:** Shake well, limit use to 10 d to minimize hearing loss

Neomycin & Dexamethasone (AK-Neo-Dex Ophthalmic, Neo-Decadron Ophthalmic)

Uses: *Steroid-responsive inflammatory conditions of the cornea, conjunctiva, lid, & anterior segment* **Acts:** Antibiotic w/ anti-inflammatory corticosteroid **Dose:** 1–2 gtt in eye(s) q3–4h or thin coat tid-qid until response, then ↓ to daily **Caution:** [C, ?] **Disp:** Cream: neomycin 0.5%/dexamethasone 0.1%; oint: neomycin 0.35%/dexamethasone 0.05%; soln: neomycin 0.35%/dexamethasone 0.1% **SE:** Local irritation **Notes:** Use under ophthalmologist's supervision

Neomycin & Polymyxin B (Neosporin Cream) [OTC]

Uses: *Infxn in minor cuts, scrapes, & burns* **Acts:** Bactericidal **Dose:** Apply bid-qid **Caution:** [C, ?] **CI:** Component allergy **Disp:** Cream: neomycin 3.5 mg/polymyxin B 10,000 units/g **SE:** Local irritation **Notes:** Different from *Neosporin oint*

Neomycin, Polymyxin B, & Dexamethasone (Maxitrol)

Uses: *Steroid-responsive ocular conditions w/ bacterial Infxn* **Acts:** Antibiotic w/ anti-inflammatory corticosteroid **Dose:** 1–2 gtt in eye(s) q3–4h; apply oint in eye(s) tid-qid **CI:** Component allergy; viral, fungal, TB eye Dz **Caution:** [C, ?] **Disp:** Oint: neomycin sulfate 3.5 mg/polymyxin B sulfate 10,000 units/dexamethasone 0.1%/g; susp: identical/5 mL **SE:** Local irritation **Notes:** Use under supervision of ophthalmologist

Neomycin-Polymyxin Bladder Irrigant [Neosporin GU Irrigant]

Uses: *Cont irrigant prevent bacteriuria & gram(–) bacteremia associated w/ indwelling catheter* **Acts:** Bactericidal; not for *Serratia* sp or streptococci **Dose:** 1 mL irrigant in 1 L of 0.9% NaCl; cont bladder irrigation w/ 1 L of soln/24 h 10 d max **Caution:** [D] **CI:** Component allergy **Disp:** Soln neomycin sulfate 40 mg & polymyxin B 200,000 units/mL; amp 1, 20 mL **SE:** Rash, neomycin ototox or nephrotox (rare) **Notes:** Potential for bacterial/fungal supper-Infxn; not for Inj; use only 3-way catheter for irrigation

Neomycin, Polymyxin, & Hydrocortisone Ophthalmic (Generic)

Uses: *Ocular bacterial infxns* **Acts:** Antibiotic w/ anti-inflammatory **Dose:** Apply a thin layer to the eye(s) or 1 gtt daily-qid **Caution:** [C, ?] **Disp:** Ophthal soln; ophthal oint **SE:** Local irritation

Neomycin, Polymyxin, & Hydrocortisone Otic (Cortisporin Otic Solution, Generic Susp) Uses: *Otitis externa and infected mastoidectomy and fenestration cavities* Acts: Antibiotic & anti-inflammatory Dose: *Adults.* 3–4 gtt in the ear(s) tid-qid *Peds.* >2 y: 3 gtt in the ear(s) tid-qid CI: Viral Infxn, hypersens to components Caution: [C, ?] Disp: Otic susp (generic); otic soln (Cortisporin) SE: Local irritation

Neomycin, Polymyxin B, & Prednisolone (Poly-Pred Ophthalmic) Uses: *Steroid-responsive ocular conditions w/ bacterial Infxn* Acts: Antibiotic & anti-inflammatory Dose: 1–2 gtt in eye(s) q4–6h; apply oint in eye(s) tid-qid Caution: [C, ?] Disp: Susp neomycin/polymyxin B/prednisolone 0.5%/mL SE: Irritation Notes: Use under supervision of ophthalmologist

Neomycin Sulfate (Neo-Fradin, Generic) BOX: Systemic absorption of oral route may cause neuro-/oto-/nephrotox; resp paralysis possible w/ any route of administration Uses: *Hepatic coma, bowel prep* Acts: Aminoglycoside, poorly absorbed PO; ↓ GI bacterial flora Dose: *Adults.* 3–12 g/24 h PO in 3–4 ÷ doses. *Peds.* 50–100 mg/kg/24 h PO in 3–4 ÷ doses Caution: [C, ?/–] Renal failure, neuromuscular disorders, hearing impair CI: Intestinal obst Disp: Tabs 500 mg; PO soln 125 mg/5 mL SE: Hearing loss w/ long-term use; rash, N/V Notes: Do not use parenterally (↑ tox); part of the Condon bowel prep; also topical form

Nepafenac (Nevanac) Uses: *Inflammation postcataract surgery* Acts: NSAID Dose: 1 gtt in eye(s) tid 1 d before, and continue 14 d after surgery CI: NSAID/ASA sensitivity Caution: [C, ?/–] May ↑ bleeding time, delay healing, causes keratitis Disp: Susp 3 mL SE: Capsular opacity, visual changes, foreign-body sensation, ↑ IOP Notes: Prolonged use ↑ risk of corneal damage; shake well before use; separate from other drops by >5 min

Nesiritide (Natrecor) Uses: *Acutely decompensated CHF* Acts: Human B-type natriuretic peptide Dose: 2 mcg/kg IV bolus, then 0.01 mcg/kg/min IV Caution: [C, ?/–] When vasodilators are not appropriate CI: SBP <90 mm Hg, cardiogenic shock Disp: Vials 1.5 mg SE: ↓ BP, HA, GI upset, arrhythmias, ↑ Cr Notes: Requires cont BP monitoring; some studies indicate ↑ in mortality

Nevirapine (Viramune) BOX: Reports of fatal hepatotox even w/ short-term use; severe life-threatening skin Rxns (SJS, toxic epidermal necrolysis, & allergic Rxns); monitor closely during 1st 8 wk of Rx Uses: *HIV Infxn* Acts: Nonnucleoside RT inhib Dose: *Adults.* Initial 200 mg/d PO × 14 d, then 200 mg bid. *Peds 2 mo–8 y:* 4 mg/kg/d × 14 d, then 7 mg/kg bid. *>8 y:* 4 mg/kg/d × 14 d, then 4 mg/kg bid max 200 mg/dose for peds (w/o regard to food) Caution: [B, –] OCP Disp: Tabs 200 mg; susp 50 mg/5 mL SE: Life-threatening rash; HA, fever, D, neutropenia, hep Notes: HIV resistance when used as monotherapy; use in combo w/ at least 2 additional antiretroviral agents. Not recommended if CD4 >250 microL in women or>400 microL in men unless benefit > risk of hepatotox

Niacin (Nicotinic Acid) (Niaspan, Slo-Niacin, Niacor, Nicolar) [some OTC forms] Uses: *Sig hyperlipidemia/hypercholesteremia, nutritional supl* **Acts:** Vit B_3; ↓ lipolysis; ↓ esterification of triglycerides; ↑ lipoprotein lipase **Dose:** *Hypercholesterolemia:* Start 500 mg PO qhs, ↑ 500 mg q4wk, maint 1–2 g/d; 2 g/d max; qhs w/ low fat snack; do not crush/chew; niacin supl 1 ER tab PO q day or 100 mg PO q day; *Pellagra:* Up to 500 mg/d **Caution:** [(C), +] **CI:** Liver Dz, peptic ulcer, arterial hemorrhage **Disp:** ER tabs (*Niaspan*) 500, 750, 1000 mg & (*Slo-Niacin*) 250, 500, 750 mg; tab 500 mg (Niacor); many OTC: tab 50, 100, 250, 500 mg, ER caps 125, 250, 400 mg, ER tab 250, 500 mg;, elixir 50 mg/5 mL **SE:** Upper body/facial flushing & warmth; hepatox, GI upset, flatulence, exacerbate peptic ulcer, HA, paresthesias, liver damage, gout, altered glucose control in DM **Notes:** ASA/NSAID 30–60 min prior to ↓ flushing; ✓ cholesterol, LFTs, if on statins (e.g., Lipitor, etc) also ✓ CPK and K^+; *RDA adults:* male 16 mg/d, female 14 mg/d

Niacin & Lovastatin (Advicor) Uses: *Hypercholesterolemia* Acts: Combo antilipemic agent w/ HMG-CoA reductase inhib Dose: **Adults.** Niacin 500 mg/lovastatin 20 mg, titrate q4wk, max niacin 2000 mg/lovastatin 40 mg **Caution:** [X, –] See individual agents, D/C w/ LFTs >3× ULN **CI:** PRG **Disp:** Niacin mg/lovastatin mg: 500/20, 750/20, 1000/20, 1000/40 tabs **SE:** Flushing, myopathy/ rhabdomyolysis, N, Abd pain, ↑ LFT's **Notes:** ↓ Flushing by taking ASA or NSAID 30 min before

Niacin & Simvastatin (Simcor) Uses: *Hypercholesterolemia* Acts: Combo antilipemic agent w/ HMG-CoA reductase inhib Dose: *Adults* Niacin 500 mg/simvastatin 20 mg, titrate q4wk not to exceed niacin 2000 mg/simvastatin 40 mg **Caution:** [X, –] See individual agents, discontinue Rx if LFTs >3× ULN **CI:** PRG **Disp:** Niacin mg/simvastatin mg: 500/20, 750/20, 1000/20 tabs **SE:** Flushing, myopathy/rhabdomyolysis, N, Abd pain, ↑ LFT's **Notes:** ↓ Flushing by taking ASA or NSAID 30 min before

Nicardipine (Cardene) Uses: *Chronic stable angina & HTN*; prophylaxis of migraine **Acts:** CCB **Dose:** *Adults.* PO: 20–40 mg PO bid. *SR:* 30–60 mg PO bid. *IV:* 5 mg/h IV cont Inf; ↑ by 2.5 mg/h q15min to max 15 mg/h. *Peds.* (Not established) *PO:* 20–30 mg PO q8h. *IV:* 0.5–5 mcg/kg/min; ↓ in renal/hepatic impair **Caution:** [C, ?/–] Heart block, CAD **CI:** Cardiogenic shock, aortic stenosis **Disp:** Caps 20, 30 mg; SR caps 30, 45, 60 mg; Inj 2.5 mg/mL **SE:** Flushing, tachycardia, ↓ BP, edema, HA **Notes:** *PO-to-IV conversion:* 20 mg tid = 0.5 mg/h, 30 mg tid = 1.2 mg/h, 40 mg tid = 2.2 mg/h; take w/ food (not high fat)

Nicotine Gum (Nicorette, others) [OTC] Uses: *Aid to smoking cessation, relieve nicotine withdrawal* **Acts:** Systemic delivery of nicotine **Dose:** Wk 1–6 one piece q1–2h PRN; wk 7–9 one piece q2–4h PRN; wk 10–12 one piece q4–8h PRN; max 24 pieces/d **Caution:** [C, ?] **CI:** Life-threatening arrhythmias, unstable angina **Disp:** 2 mg, 4 mg/piece; mint, orange, original flavors **SE:** Tachycardia, HA, GI upset, hiccups **Notes:** Must stop smoking & perform behavior modification for max effect; use at least 9 pieces first 1st 6 wk; >25 cigarettes/d use 4 mg; <25 cigarettes/d use 2 mg

Nicotine Nasal Spray (Nicotrol NS) Uses: *Aid to smoking cessation, relieve nicotine withdrawal* Acts: Systemic delivery of nicotine Dose: 0.5 mg/actuation; 1–2 doses/h, 5 doses/h max; 40 doses/d max Caution: [D, M] CI: Life-threatening arrhythmias, unstable angina Disp: Nasal inhaler 10 mg/mL SE: Local irritation, tachycardia, HA, taste perversion Notes: Must stop smoking & perform behavior modification for max effect; 1 dose = 1 spray each nostril = 1 mg

Nicotine Transdermal (Habitrol, NicoDerm CQ [OTC], others) Uses: *Aid to smoking cessation; relief of nicotine withdrawal* Acts: Systemic delivery of nicotine Dose: Individualized; 1 patch (14–21 mg/d) & taper over 6 wk Caution: [D, M] CI: Life-threatening arrhythmias, unstable angina Disp: *Habitrol & NicoDerm CQ:* 7, 14, 21 mg of nicotine/24 h SE: Insomnia, pruritus, erythema, local site Rxn, tachycardia, vivid dreams Notes: Wear patch 16–24 h; must stop smoking & perform behavior modification for max effect; >10 cigarettes/d start w/ 2-mg patch; <10 cigarettes/d 1-mg patch

Nifedipine (Procardia, Procardia XL, Adalat CC) Uses: *Vaso-spastic or chronic stable angina & HTN*; tocolytic Acts: CCB Dose: *Adults.* SR tabs 30–90 mg/d. *Tocolysis:* per local protocol. *Peds.* 0.25–0.9 mg/kg/24 h + tid-qid Caution: [C, +] Heart block, aortic stenosis CI: IR preparation for urgent or emergent HTN; acute MI Disp: Caps 10, 20 mg; SR tabs 30, 60, 90 mg SE: HA common on initial Rx; reflex tachycardia may occur w/ regular-release dose forms; peripheral edema, ↓ BP, flushing, dizziness Notes: Adalat CC & Procardia XL not interchangeable; SL administration not OK

Nilotinib (Tasigna) BOX: May ↑ QT interval; sudden deaths reported, use w/ caution in hepatic failure; administer on empty stomach Uses: *Ph(+) CML, refractory or at first diagnosis* Acts: TKI Dose: *Adults.* 400 mg bid, on empty stomach 1 h prior or 2 h post meal. Caution: [D, ?/–] Avoid w/ CYP3A4 inhib/inducers (Table 10 p 280), avoid w/ hepatic impair, heme tox, QT ↑, avoid QT-prolonging agents, w/Hx pancreatitis, ↓ absorption w/gastrectomy Disp: Bilirubin >3× ULN, AST/ALT >5× ULN, resume at 400 mg/d once levels return to normal Disp: 200 mg caps SE: ↓ WBC, ↓ plt, anemia, N/V/D, rash, edema, ↑ lipase Notes: Use chemotherapy precautions when handling

Nilutamide (Nilandron) BOX: Interstitial pneumonitis possible; most cases in 1st 3 mo; check CXR before and during Rx Uses: *Combo w/ surgical castration for metastatic PCa* Acts: Nonsteroidal antiandrogen Dose: 300 mg/d PO in ÷ doses × 30 d, then 150 mg/d Caution: [Not used in females] CI: Severe hepatic impair, resp Insuff Disp: Tabs 150 mg SE: Interstitial pneumonitis, hot flashes, ↓ libido, impotence, N/V/D, gynecomastia, hepatic dysfunction Notes: May cause Rxn when taken w/ EtOH, follow LFTs

Nimodipine (Nimotop) BOX: Do not give IV or by other parenteral routes can cause death Uses: *Prevent vasospasm following subarachnoid hemorrhage* Acts: CCB Dose: 60 mg PO q4h for 21 d; ↓ in hepatic failure Caution: [C, ?] CI:

Component allergy **Disp:** Caps 30 mg **SE:** ↓ BP, HA, constipation **Notes:** Give via NG tube if caps cannot be swallowed whole

Nisoldipine (Sular)   **Uses:** *HTN* **Acts:** CCB **Dose:** 8.5–34 mg/d PO; take on empty stomach; ↓ start doses w/ elderly or hepatic impair **Caution:** [C, –] **Disp:** ER tabs 8.5, 17, 25.5, 34 mg **SE:** Edema, HA, flushing, ↓ BP

Nitazoxanide (Alinia)   **Uses:** *Cryptosporidium* or *Giardia lamblia*-induced D* **Acts:** Antiprotozoal interferes w/ pyruvate ferredoxin oxidoreductase. *Spectrum: Cryptosporidium, Giardia* **Dose:** *Adults.* 500 mg PO q12h × 3 d. *Peds 1–3 y:* 100 mg PO q12h × 3 d. *4–11 y:* 200 mg PO q12h × 3 d. *>12 y:* 500 mg PO q12h × 3 d; take w/ food **Caution:** [B, ?] Not effective in HIV or immunocompromised **Disp:** 100 mg/5 mL PO susp, 500 tab **SE:** Abd pain **Notes:** Susp contains sucrose, interacts w/ highly protein-bound drugs

Nitrofurantoin (Furadantin, Macrodantin, Macrobid)   **BOX:** Pulm fibrosis possible **Uses:** *Prophylaxis & Rx UTI* **Acts:** Bacteriocidal; interferes w/ carbohydrate metabolism. *Spectrum:* Some gram(+) & (–) bacteria; *Pseudomonas, Serratia,* & most *Proteus* resistant **Dose:** *Adults.* Prophylaxis: 50–100 mg PO. *Rx:* 50–100 mg PO qid × 7 d; *Macrobid* 100 mg PO bid × 7 d. *Peds.* Prophylaxis: 1–2 mg/kg/d ÷ 1–2 doses, max 100 mg/d. *Rx:* 5–7 mg/kg/24 h in ÷ 4 doses w/ food/milk/antacid) **Caution:** [B, +/not OK if child <1 mo] Avoid w/ CrCl <60 mL/min **CI:** Renal failure, infants <1 mo, PRG at term **Disp:** Caps 25, 50, 100 mg; susp 25 mg/5 mL **SE:** GI effects, dyspnea, various acute/chronic pulm Rxns, peripheral neuropathy, hemolytic anemia w/ G6PD deficiency, rare aplastic anemia **Notes:** Macrocrystals (Macrodantin) < N than other forms; not for comp UTI; may turn urine brown

Nitroglycerin (Nitrostat, Nitrolingual, Nitro-Bid Ointment, Nitro-Bid IV, Nitrodisc, Transderm-Nitro, NitroMist, others)   **Uses:** *Angina pectoris, acute & prophylactic Rx, CHF, BP control* **Acts:** Relaxes vascular smooth muscle, dilates coronary arteries **Dose:** *Adults. SL:* 1 tab q5min SL PRN for 3 doses. *Translingual:* 1–2 metered-doses sprayed onto PO mucosa q3–5min, max 3 doses. *PO:* 2.5–9 mg tid. *IV:* 5–20 mcg/min, titrated to effect. *Topical:* Apply 1/2 inch of oint to chest wall tid, wipe off at night. *Transdermal:* 0.2–0.4 mg/h/patch daily; aerosol 1 spray at 5-min intervals, max 3 doses *(ECC 2005). Peds.* 0.25–0.5 mcg/kg/min IV, titrate **Caution:** [B, ?] Restrictive cardiomyopathy **CI:** w/ Sildenafil, tadalafil, vardenafil, head trauma, NAG, pericardial tamponade, constrictive pericarditis **Disp:** SL tabs 0.3, 0.4, 0.6 mg; translingual spray 0.4 mg/dose; SR caps 2.5, 6.5, 9 mg; Inj 0.5, 0.4 mg/mL (premixed); 5 mg/mL Inj soln; oint 2%; transdermal patches 0.1, 0.2, 0.4, 0.6 mg/h; aerosol (*NitroMist*) 0.4 mg/spray **SE:** HA, ↓ BP, light-headedness, GI upset **Notes:** Nitrate tolerance w/ chronic use after 1–2 wk; minimize by providing 10–12 h nitrate-free period daily, using shorter-acting nitrates tid, & removing LA patches & oint before sleep to ↓ tolerance

Nitroprusside (Nipride, Nitropress)   **Uses:** *Hypertensive crisis, CHF, controlled ↓ BP periop (↓ bleeding)*, aortic dissection, pulm edema* **Acts:** ↓

Systemic vascular resistance **Dose:** *Adults & Peds.* 0.5–10 mcg/kg/min IV Inf, titrate; usual dose 3 mcg/kg/min **Caution:** [C, ?] ↓ cerebral perfusion **CI:** High output failure, compensatory HTN **Disp:** Inj 25 mg/mL **SE:** Excessive hypotensive effects, palpitations, HA **Notes:** Thiocyanate (metabolite w/ renal excretion) w/ tox at 5–10 mg/dL, more likely if used for >2–3 d; w/ aortic dissection use w/ β-blocker

Nizatidine (Axid, Axid AR [OTC]) Uses: *Duodenal ulcers, GERD, heartburn* **Acts:** H₂-receptor antagonist **Dose:** *Adults. Active ulcer:* 150 mg PO bid or 300 mg PO hs; maint 150 mg PO hs. *GERD:* 150 mg PO bid. *Heartburn:* 75 mg PO bid. *Peds. GERD:* 10 mg/kg PO bid in ÷ doses, 150 mg bid max; ↓ in renal impair **Caution:** [B, ?] **CI:** H₂-receptor antagonist sensitivity **Disp:** Tab 75 mg [OTC]; caps 150, 300 mg; soln 15 mg/mL **SE:** Dizziness, HA, constipation, D

Norepinephrine (Levophed) Uses: *Acute ↓ BP, cardiac arrest (adjunct)* **Acts:** Peripheral vasoconstrictor of arterial/venous beds **Dose:** *Adults.* 8–30 mcg/min IV, titrate. *Peds.* 0.05–0.1 mcg/kg/min IV, titrate **Caution:** [C, ?] **CI:** ↓ BP d/t hypovolemia, vascular thrombosis, do not use w/ cyclopropane/halothane anesthetics **Disp:** Inj 1 mg/mL **SE:** ↑ HR, arrhythmia **Notes:** Correct vol depletion as much as possible before vasopressors; interaction w/ TCAs leads to severe HTN; use large vein to avoid extrav; phentolamine 5–10 mg/10 mL NS injected locally for extrav

Norethindrone Acetate/Ethinyl Estradiol Tablets (FemHRT) (See Estradiol/ Norethindrone Acetate)

Norfloxacin (Noroxin, Chibroxin ophthalmic) BOX: Use associated w/ tendon rupture and tendonitis (pending) Uses: *Comp & uncomp UTI d/t gram(−) bacteria, prostatitis, gonorrhea*, infectious D, conjunctivitis **Acts:** Quinolone, ↓ DNA gyrase, bactericidal *Spectrum:* Broad gram(+) and (−) *E. faecalis, E. coli, K. pneumoniae, P. mirabilis, P. aeruginosa, S. epidermidis, S. saprophyticus* **Dose:** *Uncomp UTI (E. coli, K. pneumoniae, P. mirabilis):* 400 mg PO bid × 3 d; other uncomp UTI Rx × 7–10 d. *Comp UTI:* 400 mg q12h for 10–21 d PO bid. *Gonorrhea:* 800 mg × 1 dose. *Prostatitis:* 400 mg PO bid × 28 d. *Gastroenteritis, traveler's D:* 400 mg PO × 1–3 d; take 1 h ac or 2 h pc. *Adults & Peds >1 y:* Ophthal: 1 gtt each eye qid for 7 d; CrCl <30 mL/min use 400 mg q day **Caution:** [C, −] Quinolone sensitivity, w/ some antiarrhythmics **CI:** Hx allergy or tendon problems **Disp:** Tabs 400 mg; ophthal 3 mg/mL **SE:** Photosens, HA, dizziness, asthenia, GI upset, pseudomembranous colitis; ocular burning w/ ophthal **Notes:** Interactions w/ antacids, theophylline, caffeine; good conc in the kidney & urine, poor blood levels; not for urosepsis; CDC suggests do not use for GC

Nortriptyline (Pamelor) BOX: ↑ Suicide risk in pts <24 y w/ major depressive/other psychological disorders especially during 1st month of Tx; risk ↓ pts >65 y; observe all pts for clinical Sxs; not for ped use Uses: *Endogenous depression* **Acts:** TCA; ↑ synaptic CNS levels of serotonin &/or norepinephrine **Dose:** *Adults.* 25 mg PO tid-qid; >150 mg/d not OK. *Elderly:* 10–25 mg hs. *Peds 6–7 y:*

10 mg/d. **8–11 y:** 10–20 mg/d. **>11 y:** 25–35 mg/d, ↓ w/ hepatic Insuff **Caution:** [D, –] NAG, CV Dz **CI:** TCA allergy, use w/ MAOI **Disp:** Caps 10, 25, 50, 75 mg; soln 10 mg/5 mL **SE:** Anticholinergic (blurred vision, retention, xerostomia, sedation) **Notes:** Max effect may take >2–3 wk

Nystatin (Mycostatin) Uses: *Mucocutaneous *Candida* infxns (oral, skin, vag)* **Acts:** Alters membrane permeability. *Spectrum:* Susceptible *Candida* sp **Dose:** *Adults & Peds. PO:* 400,000–600,000 units PO "swish & swallow" qid. *Vaginal:* 1 tab vaginally hs × 2 wk. *Topical:* Apply bid-tid to area. *Peds Infants:* 200,000 units PO q6h. **Caution:** [B (C PO), +] **Disp:** PO susp 100,000 units/mL; PO tabs 500,000 units; troches 200,000 units; vag tabs 100,000 units; topical cream/oint 100,000 units/g, powder 100,000 units/g **SE:** GI upset, SJS **Notes:** Not absorbed PO; not for systemic infxns

Octreotide (Sandostatin, Sandostatin LAR) Uses: *↓ Severe D associated w/ carcinoid & neuroendocrine GI tumors (e.g., vasoactive intestinal peptide-secreting tumor ([VIPoma]), ZE synd), acromegaly*; bleeding esophageal varices **Acts:** LA peptide; mimics natural somatostatin **Dose:** *Adults.* 100–600 mcg/d SQ/IV in 2–4 ÷ doses; start 50 mcg daily-bid. *Sandostatin LAR (depot):* 10–30 mg IM q4wk. *Peds.* 1–10 mcg/kg/24 h SQ in 2–4 ÷ doses **Caution:** [B, +] Hepatic/renal impair **Disp:** Inj 0.05, 0.1, 0.2, 0.5, 1 mg/mL; 10, 20, 30 mg/5 mL LAR depot **SE:** N/V, Abd discomfort, flushing, edema, fatigue, cholelithiasis, hyper-/hypoglycemia, hep, hypothyroidism **Notes:** Stabilize for at least 2 wk before changing to LAR form

Ofatumumab (Arzerra) BOX: Administer only by physician experienced in chemotherapy. Do not give IV push d/t severe inf rxn Uses: *Rx refractory CLL* **Action:** MoAb, binds CD20 molecule on B-lymphocytes w/ cell lysis **Dose:** *Adults.* 300 mg (0.3 mg/ml) IV week one, then 2000 mg (2 mg/ml) weekly × 7 doses, then 2000 mg q4wks × 4 doses. Titrate inf; start 12 ml/hr × 30 min, ↑ 25 ml/hr for 30 min, ↑ to 50 ml/hr × 30 min, ↑ to 100 ml/hr × 30 min, then 200 ml/hr for duration. **Caution:**[C,?] **Disp:** Inj 20 mg/ml (5 ml) **SE:** Infusion rxns (bronchospasm, pulmonary edema, ↑/↓ BP, syncope, cardiac ischemia, angioedema) ↓ WBC, anemia, fever, fatigue, rash, N/D, pneumonia, Infxns **Notes:** Premed w/ acetaminophen, antihistamine, and IV steroid.

Ofloxacin (Floxin) BOX: Use associated w/ tendon rupture and tendonitis Uses: *Lower resp tract, skin & skin structure, & UTI, prostatitis, uncomp gonorrhea, & Chlamydia infxns* **Acts:** Bactericidal; ↓ DNA gyrase. Broad spectrum gram(+) & (–): S. pneumoniae, S. aureus, S. pyogenes, H. influenzae, P. mirabilis, N. gonorrhoeae, C. trachomatis, E. coli **Dose:** *Adults.* 200–400 mg PO bid or IV q12h. *Adults & Peds >1 y: Ophthal:* 1–2 gtt in eye(s) q2–4h for 2 d, then qid × 5 more d. *Adults & Peds >12 y: Otic:* 10 gtt in ear(s) bid for 10 d. *Peds 1–12 y: Otic:* 5 gtt in ear(s) for 10 d; ↓ in renal impair, take on empty stomach **Caution:** [C, –] ↓ Absorption w/ antacids, sucralfate, Al²⁺, Ca²⁺, Mg²⁺, Fe²⁺, Zn⁺-containing drugs, Hx Szs **CI:** Quinolone allergy **Disp:** Tabs 200, 300, 400 mg; Inj 20, 40 mg/mL; ophthal & otic 0.3% **SE:** N/V/D, photosens, insomnia, HA, local irritation

Ofloxacin, Ophthalmic (Ocuflox Ophthalmic) Uses: *Bacterial conjunctivitis, corneal ulcer* Acts: See Ofloxacin Dose: *Adults & Peds >1 y:* 1–2 gtt in eye(s) q2–4h × 2 d, then qid × 5 more d Caution: [C, +/–] CI: Quinolone allergy Disp: Ophthal 0.3% soln SE: Burning, hyperemia, bitter taste, chemosis, photophobia

Ofloxacin, Otic (Floxin Otic, Floxin Otic Singles) Uses: *Otitis externa; chronic suppurative otitis media w/ perf drums; otitis media in peds w/ tubes* Acts: See Ofloxacin Dose: *Adults & Peds >13 y: Otitis externa:* 10 gtt in ear(s) × 7–14 d. *Peds 1–12 y: Otitis media* 5 gtt in ear(s) bid × 10 d Caution: [C, –] CI: Quinolone allergy Disp: Otic 0.3% soln 5/10 ml bottles; singles 0.25 mL foil pack SE: Local irritation Notes: OK w/ tubes/perforated drums; 10 gtt = 0.5 mL

Olanzapine (Zyprexa, Zydis) BOX: ↑ Mortality in elderly w/ dementia-related psychosis Uses: *Bipolar mania, schizophrenia*, psychotic disorders, acute agitation in schizophrenia Acts: Dopamine & serotonin antagonist Dose: *Bipolar/schizophrenia:* 5–10 mg/d, weekly PRN, 20 mg/d max. *Agitation:* 5–10 mg IM q2–4h PRN, 30 mg d/max Caution: [C, –] Disp: Tabs 2.5, 5, 7.5, 10, 15, 20 mg; PO disintegrating tabs (Zyprexa, Zydis) 5, 10, 15, 20 mg; Inj 10 mg SE: HA, somnolence, orthostatic ↓ BP, tachycardia, dystonia, xerostomia, constipation, hyperglycemia; wgt gain and sedation may be ↑ in peds Notes: Takes wk to titrate dose; smoking ↓ levels; may be confused w/ *Zyrtec*

Olopatadine, nasal (Patanase) Uses: *Seasonal allergic rhinitis* Acts: H₁-receptor antagonist Dose: 2 sprays each nostril bid Caution: [C, ?] Disp: 0.6% 240-Spray bottle SE: Epistasis, bitter taste somnolence, HA, rhinitis

Olopatadine, ophthalmic (Patanol, Pataday) Uses: *Allergic conjunctivitis* Acts: H₁-receptor antagonist Dose: *Patanol:* 1–2 gtt in eye(s) bid; *Pataday:* 1 gtt in eye(s) q day Caution: [C, ?] Disp: *Patanol:* Soln 0.1% 5 mL *Pataday:* 0.2% 2.5 mL SE: Local irritation, HA, rhinitis Notes: Wait 10 min after to insert contacts

Olsalazine (Dipentum) Uses: *Maintain remission in UC* Acts: Topical anti-inflammatory Dose: 500 mg PO bid (w/ food) Caution: [C, –] CI: Salicylate sensitivity Disp: Caps 250 mg SE: D, HA, blood dyscrasias, hep

Omalizumab (Xolair) BOX: Reports of anaphylaxis 2–24 h after administration, even in previously treated pts Uses: *Mod–severe asthma in ≥12 y w/ reactivity to an allergen & when Sxs inadequately controlled w/ inhaled steroids* Acts: Anti-IgE Ab Dose: 150–375 mg SQ q2–4wk (dose/frequency based on serum IgE level & body wgt; see PI) Caution: [B, ?/–] CI: Component allergy, acute bronchospasm Disp: 150-mg single-use 5-mL vial SE: Site Rxn, sinusitis, HA, anaphylaxis reported in 3% Notes: Continue other asthma meds as indicated

Omega-3 Fatty Acid [Fish Oil] (Lovaza) Uses: *Rx hypertriglyceridemia* Acts: Omega-3 acid ethyl esters, ↓ thrombus inflammation & triglycerides Dose: *Hypertriglyceridemia:* 4 g/d ÷ in 1–2 doses Caution: [C, –], Fish hypersens, PRG risk factor w/ anticoagulant use, w/ bleeding risk CI: Hypersens to components

Disp: 1000-mg gel caps **SE:** Dyspepsia, N, GI pain, rash, flu-like synd **Notes:** Only FDA-approved fish oil supl; not for exogenous hypertriglyceridemia (type 1 hyperchylomicronemia); many OTC products (page 264). D/C after 2 mo if triglyceride levels do not ↓; previously called "Omacor"

Omeprazole (Prilosec, Prilosec OTC) Uses: *Duodenal/gastric ulcers (adults), GERD and erosive gastritis (adults and children) *prevent NSAID ulcers, ZE synd, *H. pylori* infxns **Acts:** Proton pump inhib **Dose: Adults.** 20–40 mg PO daily-bid × 4–8 wk; *H. pylori* 20 mg PO bid × 10 d w/ amoxicillin & clarithromycin or 40 mg PO × 14 d w/ clarithromycin; pathologic hypersecretory cond 60 mg/d (varies); 80 mg/d max. *Peds (1–16 y)* **5–10 kg:** 5 mg/d; **10–20 kg:** 10 mg PO q day. *>20 kg:* 20 mg PO q day; 40 mg/d max **Caution:** [C, –/+]w/ drugs that rely on gastric acid (e.g., ampicillin); avoid w/atazanavir and nelfinavir; caution w/ warfarin, diazepam, phenytoin; do not use w/ clopidogrel (↓ effect); response does not R/O malignancy **Disp:** OTC tabs 20 mg; *Prilosec* DR caps 10, 20, 40 mg; *Prilosec* DR susp 2.5, 10 mg **SE:** HA, abd pain, N/V/D, flatulence **Notes:** Combo w/ antibiotic Rx for *H. pylori*; ? ↑ risk of fractures w/ all PPI

Omeprazole and sodium bicarbonate (Zegerid, Zegerid OTC) Uses: *Duodenal/gastric ulcers, GERD and erosive gastritis, (↓ GI bleed in critically ill patients)* prevent NSAID ulcers, ZE synd, *H. pylori* infxns **Acts:** Proton pump inhib w/ sodium bicarb **Dose:** *Duodenal ulcer:* 20 PO daily-bid × 4–8 wk; *Gastric ulcer:* 40 PO daily-bid × 4–8 wk; *GERD no erosions* 20 mg PO daily × 4 wks, w/erosions treat 4–6 wks; *UGI bleed prevention:* 40 mg Q 6–8h the 40 mg/d × 14 d **Caution:** [C, –/+]w/ drugs that rely on gastric acid (e.g., ampicillin); avoid w/Atazanavir and nelfinavir; w/ warfarin, diazepam, phenytoin; do not use w/ clopidogrel (↓ effect); response does not R/O malignancy **Disp:** omeprazole mg/sodium bicarb: *Zegerid* OTC caps 20/1100; *Zegerid* 20/1100, mg 40/1100; *Zegerid* powder packet for oral susp 20/1680, 40/1680 **SE:** HA, abd pain, N/V/D, flatulence **Notes:** not approved in Peds; take 1 h ac; mix powder in small cup w/ 2 tbsp H_2O (not food or other liq) refill and drink; do not open caps; possible ↑ risk of fractures w/ all PPI

Ondansetron (Zofran, Zofran ODT) Uses: *Prevent chemotherapy-associated & post-op N/V* **Acts:** Serotonin receptor ($5\text{-}HT_3$) antagonist **Dose: Adults & Peds.** *Chemotherapy:* 0.15 mg/kg/dose IV prior to chemotherapy, then 4 & 8 h after 1st dose or 4–8 mg PO tid; 1st dose 30 min prior to chemotherapy & give on schedule, not PRN. **Adults.** *Post-operation:* 4 mg IV immediately preanesthesia or post-operation. **Peds.** *Post-operation: <40 kg:* 0.1 mg/kg. *>40 kg:* 4 mg IV; ↓ w/ hepatic impair **Caution:** [B, +/–] **Disp:** Tabs 4, 8, 24 mg, soln 4 mg/5 mL, Inj 2 mg/mL, 32 mg/50 mL; *Zofran* ODT tabs 4, 8 mg **SE:** D, HA, constipation, dizziness

Oprelvekin (Neumega) BOX: Allergic Rxn w/ anaphylaxis reported; D/C w/ any allergic Rxn Uses: *Prevent ↓ plt w/ chemotherapy* **Acts:** ↑ Proliferation & maturation of megakaryocytes (IL-11) **Dose: Adults.** 50 mcg/kg/d SQ for

10–21 d. **Peds** *>12 y:* 75–100 mcg/kg/d SQ for 10–21 d. *<12 y:* Use only in clinical trials; ↓ w/ CrCl <30 mL/min 25 mcg/kg. **Caution:** [C, ?/–] **Disp:** 5 mg powder for Inj **SE:** Tachycardia, palpitations, arrhythmias, edema, HA, dizziness, visual disturbances, papilledema, insomnia, fatigue, fever, N, anemia, dyspnea, allergic Rxns including anaphylaxis

Oral Contraceptives (see Table 5 p 270) BOX: Cigarette smoking ↑ risk of serious CV SEs; ↑ risk w/ >15 cigarettes/d, >35 y; strongly advise women on OCP to not smoke. Pt should be counseled that these products do not protect against HIV and other STD **Uses:** *Birth control; regulation of anovulatory bleeding; dysmenorrhea; endometriosis; polycystic ovaries; acne* (FDA approvals vary widely, see PI) **Acts:** *Birth control:* Suppresses LH surge, prevents ovulation; progestins thicken cervical mucus; ↓ fallopian tubule cilia, ↓ endometrial thickness to ↓ chances of fertilization. *Anovulatory bleeding:* Cyclic hormones mimic body's natural cycle & regulate endometrial lining, results in regular bleeding q28d; may ↓ uterine bleeding & dysmenorrhea **Dose:** Start day 1 menstrual cycle or 1st Sunday after onset of menses; 28-d cycle pills take daily; 21-d cycle pills take daily, no pills during last 7 d of cycle (during menses); some available as transdermal patch **Caution:** [X, +] Migraine, HTN, DM, sickle cell Dz, gallbladder Dz; monitor for breast Dz, ✓ K⁺ if taking drugs w/ ↑ K⁺ risk **CI:** AUB, PRG, estrogen-dependent malignancy, ↑ hypercoagulation/liver Dz, hemiplegic migraine, smokers >35 y **Disp:** 28-d cycle pills (21 active pills + 7 placebo or Fe supl); 21-d cycle pills (21 active pills) **SE:** Intra-menstrual bleeding, oligomenorrhea, amenorrhea, ↑ appetite/wgt gain, ↓ libido, fatigue, depression, mood swings, mastalgia, HA, melasma, ↑ vag discharge, acne/greasy skin, corneal edema, N **Notes:** Taken correctly, 99.9% effective for contraception; no STDs prevention, use additional barrier contraceptive; long-term, can ↓ risk of ectopic PRG, benign breast Dz, ovarian & uterine CA.

- *Rx menstrual cycle control:* Start w/ monophasic × 3 mo before switching to another brand; w/ continued bleeding change to pill w/ ↑ estrogen
- *Rx birth control:* Choose pill w/lowest SE profile for particular pt; SEs numerous; d/t estrogenic excess or progesterone deficiency; each pill's SE profile can be unique (see PI); newer extended-cycle combos have shorter/fewer hormone-free intervals; ? ↓ PRG risk; OCP troubleshooting SE w/ suggested OCP.
  - *Absent menstrual flow:* ↑ Estrogen, ↓ progestin: Brevicon, Necon 1/35, Norinyl 1/35, Modicon, Necon 1/50, Norinyl 1/50, Ortho-Cyclen, Ortho-Novum 1/50, Ortho-Novum 1/35, Ovcon 35
  - *Acne:* Use ↑ estrogen, ↓ androgenic: Brevicon, Ortho-Cyclen, Demulen 1/50, Ortho Tri-Cyclen, Mircette, Modicon, Necon, Ortho Evra, Yasmin, Yaz
  - *Break-through bleed:* ↑ Estrogen, ↑ progestin, ↓ androgenic: Demulen 1/50, Desogen, Estrostep, Loestrin 1/20, Ortho-Cept, Ovcon 50, Yasmin, Zovia 1/50
  - *Breast tenderness or ↑ wgt:* ↓ Estrogen, ↓ progestin: Use ↓ estrogen pill rather than current; Alesse, Levlite, Loestrin 1/20 Fe, Ortho Evra, Yasmin, Yaz

- *Depression:* ↓ Progestin: Alesse, Brevicon, Levlite, Modicon, Necon, Ortho Evra, Ovcon 35, Ortho-Cyclen, Ortho Tri-Cyclen Tri-Levlen, Triphasil, Trivora
- *Endometriosis:* ↓ Estrogen, ↑ progestin: Demulen 1/35, Loestrin 1.5/30, Loestrin 1/20 Fe, Lo Ovral, Levlen, Levora, Nordette, Zovia 1/35; cont w/o placebo pills or w/ 4 d of placebo pills
- *HA:* ↓ Estrogen, ↓ progestin: Alesse, Levlite, Ortho Evra
- *Moodiness &/or irritability:* ↓ Progestin: Alesse, Brevicon, Levlite, Modicon, Necon 1/35, Ortho Evra, Ortho-Cyclen, Ortho Tri-Cyclen, Ovcon 35, Tri-Levlen, Triphasil, Trivora
- *Severe menstrual cramping:* ↑ Progestin: Demulen 1/50, Desogen, Loestrin 1.5/30, Mircette, Ortho-Cept, Yasmin, Yaz, Zovia 1/50E, Zovia 1/35E

Orlistat (Xenical, Alli [OTC]).

Uses: *Manage obesity w/ body mass index ≥30 kg/m² or ≥27 kg/m² w/ other risk factors; type 2 DM, dyslipidemia* Acts: Reversible inhib of gastric & pancreatic lipases. Dose: 120 mg PO tid w/ a fat-containing meal; Alli (OTC) 60 mg PO tid w/ fat-containing meals Caution: [B, ?] May ↓ cyclosporine & warfarin dose requirements; severe liver injury reported CI: Cholestasis, malabsorption, organ transplant Disp: *Xenical* caps 120 mg; *Alli OTC* caps 60 mg SE: Abd pain/discomfort, fatty stools, fecal urgency Notes: Do not use if meal contains no fat; GI effects ↑ w/ higher-fat meals; supl w/ fat-soluble vits; tell patients about S/Sx of liver injury (including itching, yellow eyes or skin, etc)

Orphenadrine (Norflex)

Uses: *Discomfort associated w/ painful musculoskeletal conditions* Acts: Central atropine-like effect; indirect skeletal muscle relaxation, euphoria, analgesia Dose: 100 mg PO bid, 60 mg IM/IV q12h Caution: [C, +/–] CI: NAG, GI/ or bladder obst, cardiospasm, MyG Disp: SR tabs 100 mg; Inj 30 mg/mL SE: Drowsiness, dizziness, blurred vision, flushing, tachycardia, constipation

Oseltamivir (Tamiflu)

Uses: *Prevention & Rx influenza A & B* Acts: ↓ Viral neuraminidase Dose: *Adults. Tx:* 75 mg PO bid for 5 d; *Prophylaxis:* 75 mg PO daily × 10 d. *Peds. Tx:* dose BID × 5 days: ≤33 lbs: 30 mg; 33-51 lbs 45 mg; 51-88 lbs: 60 mg; >88 lbs: 75 mg PO bid; dosing: *<15 kg:* 30 mg. *15–23 kg:* 45 mg. *23–40 kg:* 60 mg. *>40 kg:* adult dose. *Prophylaxis:* Same dosing but once daily for 10 days ↓ w/ renal impair Caution: [C, ?/–] CI: Component allergy Disp: Caps 30, 45, 75 mg, powder 12 mg/mL SE: N/V, insomnia, reports of neuropsychological events in children (self-injury, confusion, delirium) Notes: Start w/in 48 h of Sx onset or exposure; 2009 H1N1 strains susceptible; ✓ CDC updates http://www.cdc.gov/h1n1flu/guidance/

Oxacillin (Prostaphlin)

Uses: *↑infxns d/t susceptible S. aureus & Streptococcus* Acts: Bactericidal; ↓ cell wall synth. Spectrum: Excellent gram(+), poor gram(–)Dose: *Adults.* 250–500 mg (2 g severe) IM/IV q4–6h. *Peds.* 150–200 mg/kg/d IV ÷ q4–6h Caution: [B, M] CI: PCN sensitivity Disp: Powder for Inj 500 mg, 1, 2, 10 g SE: GI upset, interstitial nephritis, blood dyscrasias

Oxaliplatin (Eloxatin) BOX: Administer w/ supervision of physician experienced in chemotherapy. Appropriate management is possible only w/ adequate diagnostic & Rx facilities. Anaphylactic-like Rxns reported Uses: *Adjuvant Rx stage-III colon CA (primary resected) & metastatic colon CA w/ 5-FU* Acts: Metabolized to platinum derivatives, crosslinks DNA Dose: Per protocol; see PI. *Premedicate:* Antiemetic w/ or w/o dexamethasone Caution: [D, –] See Box CI: Allergy to components or platinum Disp: Inj 50, 100 mg SE: Anaphylaxis, granulocytopenia, paresthesia, N/V/D, stomatitis, fatigue, neuropathy, hepatotox, pulm tox Notes: 5-FU & leucovorin are given in combo; epi, corticosteroids, & antihistamines alleviate severe Rxns

Oxaprozin (Daypro, Daypro ALTA) BOX: May ↑ risk of cardiovascular CV events & GI bleeding Uses: *Arthritis & pain* Acts: NSAID; ↓ prostaglandin synth Dose: *Adults.* 600–1200 mg/daily (÷ dose helps GI tolerance); ↓ w/ renal/hepatic impair Peds. JRA (Daypro): 22–31 kg: 600 mg/d. 32–54 kg: 900 mg/d Caution: [C (D 3rd tri), ?] Peptic ulcer, bleeding disorders CI: ASA/NSAID sensitivity, perioperative pain w/ CABG Disp: *Daypro ALTA:* tabs 600 mg; caplets 600 mg SE: CNS inhibition, sleep disturbance, rash, GI upset, peptic ulcer, edema, renal failure, anaphylactoid Rxn w/ "ASA triad" (asthmatic w/ rhinitis, nasal polyps and bronchospasm w/ NSAID use)

Oxazepam [C-IV] Uses: *Anxiety, acute EtOH withdrawal*, anxiety w/ depressive Sxs Acts: Benzodiazepine; diazepam metabolite Dose: *Adults.* 10–15 mg PO tid-qid; severe anxiety & EtOH withdrawal may require up to 30 mg qid. Peds. 1 mg/kg/d ÷ doses Caution: [D, ?/–] CI: Component allergy, NAG Disp: Caps 10, 15, 30 mg; tabs 15 mg SE: Sedation, ataxia, dizziness, rash, blood dyscrasias, dependence Notes: Avoid abrupt D/C

Oxcarbazepine (Trileptal) Uses: *Partial Szs*, bipolar disorders Acts: Blocks voltage-sensitive Na⁺ channels, stabilization of hyperexcited neural membranes Dose: *Adults.* 300 mg PO bid, ↑ weekly to target maint 1200–2400 mg/d. Peds. 8–10 mg/kg bid, 600 mg/d max, ↑ weekly to target maint dose; ↓ w/ renal Insuff Caution: [C, –] Carbamazepine sensitivity; CI: Component sensitivity Disp: Tabs 150, 300, 600 mg; susp 300 mg/5 mL SE: ↓ Na⁺, HA, dizziness, fatigue, somnolence, GI upset, diplopia, concentration difficulties, fatal skin/multiorgan hypersens Rxns Notes: Do not abruptly D/C, √ Na⁺ if fatigued; advise about SJS and topic epidermal necrolysis

Oxiconazole (Oxistat) Uses: *Tinea cruris, tinea corporis, tinea pedis, tinea versicolor* Acts: ? ↓ Ergosterols in fungal cell membrane. *Spectrum:* Most *Epidermophyton floccosum, Trichophyton mentagrophytes, Trichophyton rubrum, Malassezia furfur* Dose: Apply thin layer daily-bid Caution: [B, M] CI: Component allergy Disp: Cream, lotion 1% SE: Local irritation

Oxybutynin (Ditropan, Ditropan XL) Uses: *Symptomatic relief of urgency, nocturia, incontinence w/ neurogenic or reflex neurogenic bladder* Acts: Anticholinergic, relaxes bladder smooth muscle, ↑ bladder capacity Dose: *Adults.*

5 mg bid-tid, 5 mg qid max. XL 5–10 mg/d, 30 mg/d max. *Peds >5 y:* 5 mg PO bid-tid; 15 mg/d max. *Peds 1–5 y:* 0.2 mg/kg/dose bid-qid (syrup 5 mg/5 mL); 15 mg/d max; ↓ in elderly; periodic drug holidays OK **Caution:** [B, ?] **CI:** NAG, MyG, GI/GU obst, ulcerative colitis, megacolon **Disp:** Tabs 5, 10, 15 mg; syrup 5 mg/5 mL **SE:** Anticholinergic (drowsiness, xerostomia, constipation, tachycardia), ↑ QT interval, memory impair; ER form empty shell expelled in stool

Oxybutynin Transdermal System (Oxytrol) **Uses:** *Rx OAB* **Acts:** Anticholinergic, relaxes bladder smooth muscle, ↑ bladder capacity **Dose:** One 3.9 mg/d system apply 2×/wk (q3–4d) to abd, hip, or buttock **Caution:** [B, ?/–] **CI:** GI/GU obst, NAG **Disp:** 3.9 mg/d transdermal patch **SE:** Anticholinergic, itching/redness at site **Notes:** Do not apply to same site w/in 7 d

Oxycodone [Dihydro hydroxycodone] (OxyContin, Roxicodone) [C-II] **BOX:** High abuse potential; controlled release only for extended chronic pain, not for PRN use; 60, 80-mg tab for opioid-tolerant pts; do not crush, break or chew **Uses:** *Mod–severe pain, usually in combo w/ nonnarcotic analgesics* **Acts:** Narcotic analgesic **Dose:** *Adults.* 5 mg PO q6h PRN (IR). *Mod–severe chronic pain:* 10–160 mg PO q12h (ER). *Peds 6–12 y:* 1.25 mg PO q6h PRN. *>12 y:* 2.5 mg q6h PRN; ↓ w/ severe liver/renal Dz, elderly; w/ food **Caution:** [B ✓ D if prolonged use/near term), M] **CI:** Allergy, resp depression, acute asthma, ileus w/ microsomal morphine **Disp:** IR caps (OxyIR) 5 mg; CR Roxicodone tabs 15, 30 mg; ER (OxyContin) 10, 15, 20, 30, 40, 60, 80 mg; liq 5 mg/5 mL; soln conc 20 mg/mL **SE:** BP, sedation, resp depression, dizziness, GI upset, constipation, risk of abuse **Notes:** *OxyContin* for chronic CA pain; do not crush/chew/cut ER product; sought after as drug of abuse; reformulated *OxyContin* is intended to prevent the opioid medication from being cut, broken, chewed, crushed or dissolved to release more medication

Oxycodone & Acetaminophen (Percocet, Tylox) [C-II] **Uses:** *Mod–severe pain* **Acts:** Narcotic analgesic **Dose:** *Adults.* 1–2 tabs/caps PO q4–6h PRN (acetaminophen max dose 4 g/d). *Peds.* Oxycodone 0.05–0.15 mg/kg/dose q 4–6h PRN, 5 mg/dose max **Caution:** [C (D prolonged use or near term), M] **CI:** Allergy, paralytic ileus, resp depression **Disp:** Percocet tabs, mg oxycodone/mg APAP: 2.5/325, 5/325, 7.5/325, 10/325, 7.5/500, 10/650; Tylox caps 5 mg oxycodone, 500 mg APAP; soln 5 mg oxycodone & 325 mg APAP/5 mL **SE:** ↓ BP, sedation, dizziness, GI upset, constipation

Oxycodone & Aspirin (Percodan) [C-II] **Uses:** *Mod–severe pain* **Acts:** Narcotic analgesic w/ NSAID **Dose:** *Adults.* 1–2 tabs/caps PO q4–6h PRN. *Peds.* Oxycodone 0.05–0.15 mg/kg/dose q 4–6h PRN, up to 5 mg/dose; ↓ in severe hepatic failure **Caution:** [D, –] w/peptic ulcer, CNS depression, elderly, hx Szs **CI:** Component allergy, children (<16 y) w/ viral Infxn (Reyes synd), resp depression, ileus, hemophilia **Disp:** *Generics:* 4.83 mg oxycodone hydrochloride, 0.38 mg oxycodone terephthalate, 325 mg ASA; *Percodan* 4.83 mg oxycodone hydrochloride, 325 mg ASA **SE:** Sedation, dizziness, GI upset/ulcer, constipation, allergy **Notes:** monitor for possible drug abuse

Oxycodone/Ibuprofen (Combunox) [C-II] BOX: May ↑ risk of serious CV events; CI in perioperative coronary artery bypass graft pain; ↑ risk of GI events such as bleeding Uses: *Short-term (not >7 d) management of acute mod–severe pain* Acts: Narcotic w/ NSAID Dose: 1 tab q6h PRN 4 tab max/24 h; 7 d max Caution: [C, –] w/ Impaired renal/hepatic Fxn; COPD, CNS depression, avoid in PRG CI: Paralytic ileus, 3rd tri PRG, allergy to ASA or NSAIDs, where opioids are CI Disp: Tabs 5 mg oxycodone/400 mg ibuprofen SE: N/V, somnolence, dizziness, sweating, flatulence, ↑ LFTs Notes: ✓ renal Fxn; abuse potential w/ oxycodone

Oxymorphone (Opana, Opana ER) [C-II] BOX: (Opana ER) Abuse potential, controlled release only for chronic pain; do not consume EtOH-containing beverages, may cause fatal OD Uses: *Mod/severe pain, sedative* Acts: Narcotic analgesic Dose: 10–20 mg PO q4–6h PRN if opioid-naïve or 1–1.5 mg SQ/IM q4–6h PRN or 0.5 mg IV q4–6h PRN; starting 20 mg/dose max PO; Chronic pain: ER 5 mg PO q12h; if opioid-naïve ↑ PRN 5–10 mg PO q12h q3–7d; take 1 h pc or 2 h ac; ↓ dose w/ elderly, renal/hepatic impair Caution: [B, ?] CI: ↑ ICP, severe resp depression, w/ EtOH or liposomal morphine, severe hepatic impair Disp: Tabs 5, 10 mg; ER 5, 10, 20, 40 mg SE: ↓ BP, sedation, GI upset, constipation, histamine release Notes: Related to hydromorphone

Oxytocin (Pitocin) Uses: *Induce labor, control postpartum hemorrhage* Acts: Stimulate muscular contractions of the uterus Dose: 0.0005–0.001 units/min IV Inf; titrate 0.001–0.002 units/min q30–60min Caution: [Uncategorized, +/–] CI: Where vag delivery not favorable, fetal distress Disp: Inj 10 units/mL SE: Uterine rupture, fetal death; arrhythmias, anaphylaxis, H_2O intoxication Notes: Monitor vital signs; nasal form for breast-feeding only

Paclitaxel (Taxol, Abraxane) BOX: Administration only by physician experienced in chemotherapy; fatal anaphylaxis and hypersens possible; severe myelosuppression possible Uses: *Ovarian & breast CA, PCa*, Kaposi sarcoma, NSCLC Acts: Mitotic spindle poison; promotes microtubule assembly & stabilization against depolymerization Dose: Per protocols; use glass or polyolefin containers (e.g., nitroglycerin tubing set); PVC sets leach plasticizer; ↓ in hepatic failure Caution: [D, –] CI: Neutropenia <1500 WBC/mm³; solid tumors, component allergy Disp: Inj 6 mg/mL, 5 mg/mL albumin bound (Abraxane) SE: ↓ BM, peripheral neuropathy, transient ileus, myalgia, ↓ HR, ↓ BP, mucositis, N/V/D, fever, rash, HA, phlebitis; hematologic tox schedule-dependent; leukopenia dose-limiting by 24-h Inf; neurotox limited w/ short (1–3 h) Inf; allergic Rxns (dyspnea, ↓ BP, urticaria, rash) Notes: Maintain hydration; allergic Rxn usually w/in 10 min of Inf; minimize w/ corticosteroid, antihistamine pretreatment

Palivizumab (Synagis) Uses: *Prevent RSV Infxn* Acts: MoAb Dose: Peds. 15 mg/kg IM monthly, typically Nov–Apr Caution: [C, ?] Renal/hepatic dysfunction CI: Component allergy Disp: Vials 50, 100 mg SE: hypersens Rxn, URI, rhinitis, cough, ↑ LFTs, local irritation

Palifermin (Kepivance)   Uses: *Oral mucositis w/ BMT* Acts: Synthetic keratinocyte GF Dose: *Phase 1:* 60 mcg/kg IV daily × 3, 3rd dose 24–48 h before chemotherapy. *Phase 2:* 60 mcg/kg IV daily × 3, immediately after stem cell Inf Caution: [C, ?/–] CI: N/A Disp: Inj 6.25 mg SE: Unusual mouth sensations, tongue thickening, rash, ↑ amylase & lipase Notes: *E. coli* –derived; separate phases by 4 d; safety unknown w/ nonhematologic malignancies

Paliperidone (Invega)   BOX: Not for dementia-related psychosis Uses: *Schizophrenia* Acts: Risperidone metabolite, antagonizes dopamine, and serotonin receptors Dose: 6 mg PO q A.M., 12 mg/d max; CrCl 50–79 mL/min: 6 mg/d max; CrCl 10–49 mL/min: 3 mg/d max Caution: [C:, ?/–] w/ ↓ HR, ↓ K/Mg²⁺, renal/hepatic impair CI: Risperidone hypersens, w/ phenothiazines, ranolazine, ziprasidone, prolonged QT, Hx arrhythmia Disp: ER tabs 3, 6, 9 mg SE: Impaired temperature regulation, ↑ QT & HR, HA, anxiety, dizziness, N, dry mouth, fatigue, EPS Notes: Do not chew/cut/crush pill

Palonosetron (Aloxi)   BOX: May ↑ QTc interval Uses: *Prevention acute & delayed N/V w/ emetogenic chemotherapy; prevent postoperative N/V* Acts: 5-HT₃-receptor antagonist Dose: *Chemotherapy:* 0.25 mg IV 30 min prior to chemotherapy. *Postoperative N/V:* 0.75 mg immediately before induction Caution: [B, ?] CI: Component allergy Disp: 0.25 mg/5 mL vial SE: HA, constipation, dizziness, Abd pain, anxiety

Pamidronate (Aredia)   Uses: *Hypercalcemia of malignancy, Paget Dz, palliate symptomatic bone metastases* Acts: Bisphosphonate; ↓ nl & abnormal bone resorption Dose: *Hypercalcemia:* 60–90 mg IV over 2–24 h or 90 mg IV over 24 h if severe; may repeat in 7 d. *Paget Dz:* 30 mg IV slow Inf over 4 h × 3 d. *Osteolytic bone mets in myeloma:* 90 mg IV over 4 h q mo. *Osteolytic bone mets breast CA:* 90 mg IV over 2 h q3–4wk; 90 mg/max single dose. Caution: [D, ?/–] Avoid invasive dental procedures w/ use CI: PRG, bisphosphonate sensitivity Disp: Inj 30, 60, 90 mg SE: Fever, malaise, convulsions, Inj site Rxn, uveitis, fluid overload, HTN, Abd pain, N/V, constipation, UTI, bone pain, ↓ K⁺, ↓ Ca²⁺, ↓ Mg²⁺, hypophosphatemia; jaw osteonecrosis (mostly CA pts; avoid dental work), renal tox Notes: Perform dental exam prethrapy; follow Cr, hold dose if Cr ↑ by 0.5 mg/dL w/ nl baseline or by 1 mg/dL w/ abnormal baseline; restart when Cr returns w/in 10% of baseline; may ↑ atypical subtrochanteric femur fractures

Pancrelipase (Pancrease, Cotazym, Creon, Ultrase)   Uses: *Exocrine pancreatic secretion deficiency (e.g., CF, chronic pancreatitis, pancreatic Insuff), steatorrhea of malabsorption* Acts: Pancreatic enzyme supl Dose: 1–3 caps (tabs) w/ meals & snacks; ↑ to 8 caps (tabs); do not crush or chew EC products; dose dependent on digestive requirements of pt; avoid antacids Caution: [C, ?/–] CI: Pork product allergy, acute pancreatitis Disp: Caps, tabs SE: N/V, Abd cramps Notes: Individualize Rx

Pancuronium (Pavulon)   BOX: Should only be administered by adequately trained individuals Uses: *Paralysis w/ mechanical ventilation* Acts: Nondepolarizing neuromuscular blocker Dose: *Adults & Peds >1 mo:* Initial 0.06–0.1 mg/kg; maint 0.01 mg/kg 60–100 min after, then 0.01 mg/kg q25–60min PRN; ↓ w/ renal/hepatic impair; intubate pt & keep on controlled ventilation; use adequate sedation or analgesia Caution: [C, ?/–] CI: Component or bromide sensitivity Disp: Inj 1, 2 mg/mL SE: Tachycardia, HTN, pruritus, other histamine Rxns

Panitumumab (Vectibix) BOX: Derm tox common (89%) and severe in 12%; can be associated w/ Infxn (sepsis, abscesses requiring I&D; w/ severe derm tox, hold or D/C and monitor for Infxn; severe inf Rxns (anaphylactic Rxn, bronchospasm, fever, chills, hypotension) in 1%; w/ severe Rxns, immediately D/C inf and possibly permanent D/C Uses: *Rx EGFR-expressing metastatic colon CA* Acts: Anti-EGFR MoAb Dose: 6 mg/kg IV Inf over 60 min q14d; doses >1000 mg over 90 min ↓ Inf rate by 50% w/ grade 1–2 Inf Rxn, D/C permanently w/ grade 3–4 Rxn. For derm tox, hold until <grade 2 tox. If improves <1 mo, restart 50% original dose. If tox recurs or resolution >1 mo permanently D/C. If ↓ dose tolerated, ↑ dose by 25% Caution: [C,; –] D/C nursing during, 2 mo after Disp: Vial 20 mg/mL SE: Rash, acneiform dermatitis, pruritus, paronychia, ↓ Mg²⁺, Abd pain, N/V/D, constipation, fatigue, dehydration, photosens, conjunctivitis, ocular hyperemia, ↑ lacrimation, stomatitis, mucositis, pulm fibrosis, severe derm tox, inf Rxns Notes: May impair female fertility; ✓ lytes; wear sunscreen/hats, limit sun exposure

Pantoprazole (Protonix) Uses: *GERD, erosive gastritis*, ZE synd, PUD Acts: Proton pump inhib Dose: 40 mg/d PO; do not crush/chew tabs; 40 mg IV/d (not >3 mg/min, use Protonix filter) Caution: [B, ?/–] do not use w/ clopidogrel (↓ effect) Disp: Tabs, DR 20, 40 mg; 40 mg powder for oral susp (mix in applesauce or juice, give immediately) Inj 40 mg SE: Chest pain, anxiety, GI upset, ↑ LFTs Notes: ? ↑ risk of fractures w/ all PPI

Paregoric [Camphorated Tincture of Opium] [C-III] Uses: *D*, pain & neonatal opiate withdrawal synd Acts: Narcotic Dose: *Adults.* 5–10 mL PO daily–qid PRN. *Peds.* 0.25–0.5 mL/kg daily–qid. *Neonatal withdrawal:* 3–6 gtt PO q3–6h PRN to relieve Sxs × 3–5 d, then taper over 2–4 wk Caution: [B (D w/ prolonged use/high dose near term, +] CI: Toxic D; convulsive disorder, morphine sensitivity Disp: Liq 2 mg morphine = 20 mg/equiv opium/5 mL SE: ↓ BP, sedation, constipation Notes: Contains anhydrous morphine from opium; short-term use only

Paroxetine (Paxil, Paxil CR, Pexeva) BOX: Closely monitor for worsening depression or emergence of suicidality, particularly in children, adolescents, and young adults; not for use in peds Uses: *Depression, OCD, panic disorder, social anxiety disorder*, PMDD Acts: SSRI Dose: 10–60 mg PO single daily dose in A.M.; CR 25 mg/d PO; ↑ 12.5 mg/wk (max range 26–62.5 mg/d) Caution: [D, ?/] ↑ Bleeding risk CI: w/ MAOI, thioridazine, pimozide Disp: Tabs 10, 20, 30, 40 mg; susp 10 mg/5mL; CR 12.5, 25, 37.5 mg SE: HA, somnolence, dizziness, GI upset, N/D, ↓ appetite, sweating, xerostomia, tachycardia, ↓ libido, ED, anrogasmia

Pazopanib hydrochloride (Votrient) BOX: Administer only by physician experienced in chemotherapy. Severe and fatal hepatotoxicity observed.

Uses: *Rx advanced RCC* **Action:** TKI **Dose:** *Adults.* 800 mg po once daily, ↓ to 200 mg daily if moderate hepatic impair, not recommended in severe hepatic disease (bili > 3x ULN) **Caution:** [D, -] Avoid w/CYP 3A4 inducers/inhibitors and QTc prolonging drugs, all SSRI. **CI:** Severe hepatic disease **Disp:** 200 mg tablet **SE:** ↑ BP, N/V/D, GI perf, anorexia, hair depigmentation, ↓ WBC, ↓ plt, ↑ bleeding, ↑ AST/ALT/bili, ↓ Na, chest pain, ↑ QT **Notes:** Hold for surgical procedures

Pegfilgrastim (Neulasta) **Uses:** *↓ Frequency of Infxn in pts w/ nonmyeloid malignancies receiving myelosuppressive anti-CA drugs that cause febrile neutropenia* **Acts:** Granulocyte and macrophage-stimulating factor **Dose:** *Adults.* 6 mg SQ × 1/chemotherapy cycle. **Caution:** [C, M] **CI:** Allergy to E. coli-derived proteins or filgrastim **Disp:** Syringes: 6 mg/0.6 mL **SE:** Splenic rupture, HA, fever, weakness, fatigue, dizziness, insomnia, edema, N/V/D, stomatitis, anorexia, constipation, taste perversion, dyspepsia, Abd pain, granulocytopenia, neutropenic fever, ↑ LFTs & uric acid, arthralgia, myalgia, bone pain, ARDS, alopecia, worsen sickle cell Dz **Notes:** Never give between 14 d before & 24 h after dose of cytotoxic chemotherapy

Peginterferon Alfa-2a [Pegylated interferon] (Pegasys) BOX: Can cause or aggravate fatal or life-threatening neuropsychological, autoimmune, ischemic, and infectious disorders. Monitor pts closely **Uses:** *Chronic hep C w/ compensated liver Dz* **Acts:** Immune modulator **Dose:** 180 mcg (1 mL) SQ q wk × 48 wk; ↓ in renal impair **Caution:** [C, ?/–] **CI:** Autoimmune hep, decompensated liver Dz **Disp:** 180 mcg/mL Inj **SE:** Depression, insomnia, suicidal behavior, GI upset, ↓ WBC and plt, alopecia, pruritus

Peginterferon Alfa-2b [Pegylated interferon] (PegIntron) BOX: Can cause or aggravate fatal or life-threatening neuropsychological, autoimmune, ischemic, and infectious disorders; monitor pts closely **Uses:** *Rx hep C* **Acts:** Immune modulator **Dose:** 1 mcg/kg/wk SQ; 1.5 mcg/kg/wk combo w/ ribavirin; ↓ w/ depression **Caution:** [C, ?/–] **CI:** Autoimmune hep, decompensated liver Dz, hemoglobinopathy **Disp:** Vials 50, 80, 120, 150 mcg/0.5 mL; Redipen 50, 80, 120, 150 mcg/5 mL; reconstitute w/ 0.7 mL w/ sterile water **SE:** Depression, insomnia, suicidal behavior, GI upset, neutropenia, thrombocytopenia, alopecia, pruritus **Notes:** Give hs or w/ APAP to ↓ flu-like Sxs; monitor CBC/plt; use immediately or store in refrigerator × 24 h; do not freeze

Pemetrexed (Alimta) **Uses:** *w/ Cisplatin in nonresectable mesothelioma*, NSCLC **Acts:** Antifolate antineoplastic **Dose:** 500 mg/m² IV over 10 min q3wk; hold if CrCl <45 mL/min; give w/ vit B₁₂ (1000 mcg IM q9wk) & folic acid (350–1000 mcg PO daily); start 1 wk before; dexamethasone 4 mg PO bid × 3, start 1 d before each Rx **Caution:** [D, –] w/ Renal/hepatic/BM impair **CI:** Component sensitivity **Disp:** 500-mg vial **SE:** Neutropenia, thrombocytopenia, N/V/D, anorexia, stomatitis, renal failure, neuropathy, fever, fatigue, mood changes, dyspnea, anaphylactic Rxns **Notes:** Avoid NSAIDs, follow CBC/plt; ↓ dose w/ grade 3–4 mucositis

Pemirolast (Alamast) Uses: *Allergic conjunctivitis* Acts: Mast cell stabilizer Dose: 1–2 gtt in each eye qid Caution: [C, ?/–] Disp: 0.1% (1 mg/mL) in 10-mL bottles SE: HA, rhinitis, cold/flu Sxs, local irritation Notes: Wait 10 min before inserting contacts

Penbutolol (Levatol) Uses: *HTN* Acts: β-Adrenergic receptor blocker, $β_1$, $β_2$ Dose: 20–40 mg/d; ↓ in hepatic Insuff Caution: [C 1st tri; D if 2nd/3rd tri, M] CI: Asthma, cardiogenic shock, cardiac failure, heart block, ↓ HR, COPD, pulm edema Disp: Tabs 20 mg SE: Flushing, ↓ BP, fatigue, hyperglycemia, GI upset, sexual dysfunction, bronchospasm

Penciclovir (Denavir) Uses: *Herpes simplex (herpes labialis/cold sores)* Acts: Competitive inhib of DNA polymerase Dose: Apply at 1st sign of lesions, then q2h while awake × 4 d Caution: [B, ?/–] CI: Allergy, previous Rxn to famciclovir Disp: Cream 1% SE: Erythema, HA Notes: Do not apply to mucous membranes

Penicillin G, Aqueous (Potassium or Sodium) (Pfizerpen, Pentids) Uses: *Bacteremia, endocarditis, pericarditis, resp tract infxns, meningitis, neurosyphilis, skin/skin structure infxns* Acts: Bactericidal; ↓ cell wall synth. *Spectrum:* Most gram(+) (not staphylococci), streptococci, *N. meningitidis*, syphilis, clostridia, & anaerobes (not *Bacteroides*) Dose: *Adults.* Based on indication range 0.6–24 mill units/d in ÷ doses q4h. *Peds Newborns <1 wk:* 25,000–50,000 units/kg/dose IV q12h. *Infants 1 wk–<1 mo:* 25,000–50,000 units/kg/dose IV q8h. *Children:* 100,000–300,000 units/kg/24h IV ÷ q4h; ↓ in renal impair Caution: [B, M] CI: Allergy Disp: Powder for Inj SE: Allergic Rxns; interstitial nephritis, D, Szs Notes: Contains 1.7 mEq of K^+/mill units

Penicillin G Benzathine (Bicillin) Uses: *Single-dose regimen for streptococcal pharyngitis, rheumatic fever, glomerulonephritis prophylaxis, & syphilis* Acts: Bactericidal; ↓ cell wall synth. Spectrum: See Penicillin G Dose: *Adults.* 1.2–2.4 mill units deep IM Inj q2–4wk. *Peds.* 50,000 units/kg/dose, 2.4 mill units/ dose max; deep IM Inj q2–4 wk Caution: [B, M] CI: Allergy Disp: Inj 300,000, 600,000 units/mL; Bicillin L-A benzathine salt only; Bicillin C-R combo of benzathine & procaine (300,000 units procaine w/ 300,000 units benzathine/mL or 900,000 units benzathine w/ 300,000 units procaine/2 mL) SE: Inj site pain, acute interstitial nephritis, anaphylaxis Notes: IM use only; sustained action, w/ levels up to 4 wk; drug of choice for noncongenital syphilis

Penicillin G Procaine (Wycillin, others) Uses: *Infxns of resp tract, skin/soft tissue, scarlet fever, syphilis* Acts: Bactericidal; ↓ cell wall synth. Spectrum: PCN G-sensitive organisms that respond to low, persistent serum levels Dose: *Adults.* 0.6–4.8 mill units/d in ÷ doses q12–24h; give probenecid at least 30 min prior to PCN to prolong action. *Peds.* 25,000–50,000 units/kg/d IM ÷ daily-bid Caution: [B, M] CI: Allergy Disp: Inj 300,000, 500,000, 600,000 units/mL SE: Pain at Inj site, interstitial nephritis, anaphylaxis Notes: LA parenteral PCN; levels up to 15 h

Penicillin V (Pen-Vee K, Veetids, others) Uses: Susceptible streptococcal infxns, otitis media, URIs, skin/soft-tissue infxns (PCN-sensitive staphylococci) **Acts:** Bactericidal; ↓ cell wall synth. *Spectrum:* Most gram(+), including streptococci **Dose:** *Adults.* 250–500 mg PO q6h, q8h, q12h. *Peds.* 25–50 mg/kg/25h PO in 4 doses; ↓ in renal impair; take on empty stomach **Caution:** [B, M] **CI:** Allergy **Disp:** Tabs 125, 250, 500 mg; susp 125, 250 mg/5 mL **SE:** GI upset, interstitial nephritis, anaphylaxis, convulsions **Notes:** Well-tolerated PO PCN; 250 mg = 400,000 units of PCN G

Pentamidine (Pentam 300, NebuPent) Uses: *Rx & prevention of PCP* **Acts:** ↓ DNA, RNA, phospholipid, & protein synth **Dose:** *Rx: Adults & Peds.* 4 mg/kg/24 h IV daily × 14–21 d. *Prevention: Adults & Peds >5 y:* 300 mg once q4wk, give via Respirgard II nebulizer; ↓ IV w/ renal impair **Caution:** [C, ?] **CI:** Component allergy, use w/ didanosine **Disp:** Inj 300 mg/vial; aerosol 300 mg **SE:** Pancreatic cell necrosis w/ hyperglycemia; pancreatitis, CP, fatigue, dizziness, rash, GI upset, renal impair, blood dyscrasias (leukopenia, thrombocytopenia) **Notes:** Follow CBC, glucose, pancreatic Fxn monthly for 1st 3 mo; monitor for ↓ BP following IV dose; prolonged use may ↑ Infxn risk

Pentazocine (Talwin, Talwin Compound, Talwin NX) [C-IV] BOX: Oral use only; severe and potentially lethal Rxns from misuse by Inj Uses: *Mod–severe pain* **Acts:** Partial narcotic agonist–antagonist **Dose:** *Adults.* 30 mg IM or IV; 50–100 mg PO q3–4h PRN. *Peds 5–8 y:* 15 mg IM q4h PRN. *8–14 y:* 30 mg IM q4h PRN; ↓ in renal/hepatic impair **Caution:** [C (1st tri, D w/ prolonged use/high dose near term), +/−] **CI:** Allergy, ↑ ICP (unless ventilated) **Disp:** Talwin Compound tab 12.5 mg + 325 mg ASA; Talwin NX 50 mg + 0.5 mg naloxone; Inj 30 mg/mL **SE:** Considerable dysphoria; drowsiness, GI upset, xerostomia, Szs **Notes:** 30–60 mg IM = 10 mg of morphine IM; Talwin NX has naloxone to curb abuse by nonoral route

Pentobarbital (Nembutal, others) [C-II] Uses: *Insomnia (short-term), convulsions*, sedation, induce coma w/ severe head injury **Acts:** Barbiturate **Dose:** *Adults. Sedative:* 150–200 mg IM × 1100 mg IV, repeat PRN to 500 mg/max. *Hypnotic:* 100–200 mg PO or PR hs PRN. *Induced coma:* Load 5–10 mg/kg IV, w/ maint 1–3 mg/kg/h IV. *Peds. Induced coma:* As adult **Caution:** [D, +/−] Severe hepatic impair **CI:** Allergy **Disp:** Caps 50, 100 mg; elixir 18.2 mg/5 mL (= 20 mg pentobarbital); supp 30, 60, 120, 200 mg; Inj 50 mg/mL **SE:** Resp depression, ↓ BP w/ aggressive IV use for cerebral edema; ↓ HR, ↓ BP, sedation, lethargy, resp ↓, hangover, rash, SJS, blood dyscrasias **Notes:** Tolerance to sedative–hypnotic effect w/in 1–2 wk

Pentosan Polysulfate Sodium (Elmiron) Uses: *Relieve pain/discomfort w/ interstitial cystitis* **Acts:** Bladder wall buffer **Dose:** 100 mg PO tid; on empty stomach w/ H_2O 1 h ac or 2 h pc **Caution:** [B, ?/−] **CI:** Allergy **Disp:** Caps 100 mg **SE:** Alopecia, N/D, HA, ↑ LFTs, anticoagulant effects, ↓ plts, rectal bleed **Notes:** Reassess after 3 mo

Pentoxifylline (Trental) Uses: *Rx Sxs of peripheral vascular Dz* **Acts:** ↓ Blood cell viscosity, restores RBC flexibility **Dose:** *Adults.* 400 mg PO tid pc; Rx min 8 wk for effect; ↓ to bid w/ GI/CNS SEs **Caution:** [C, +/–] **CI:** Cerebral/retinal hemorrhage, methylxanthine (caffeine) intolerance **Disp:** Tabs CR 400 mg; Tabs ER 400 mg **SE:** Dizziness, HA, GI upset

Perindopril Erbumine (Aceon) **BOX:** ACE inhib can cause death to developing fetus; D/C immediately w/ PRG **Uses:** *HTN*, CHF, DN, post-MI **Acts:** ACE inhib **Dose:** 4–8 mg/d ÷ dose; 16 mg/d max; avoid w/ food; ↓ w/ elderly/renal impair **Caution:** [C (1st tri, D 2nd & 3rd tri), ?/–] ACE inhib-induced angioedema **CI:** Bilateral RAS, primary hyperaldosteronism **Disp:** Tabs 2, 4, 8 mg **SE:** Weakness, HA, ↓ BP, dizziness, GI upset, cough **Notes:** OK w/ diuretics

Permethrin (Nix, Elimite) [OTC] **Uses:** *Rx lice/scabies* **Acts:** Pediculicide **Dose:** *Adults & Peds. Lice:* Saturate hair & scalp; allow 10 min before rinsing. *Scabies:* Apply cream head to toe; leave for 8–14 h, wash w/ H$_2$O **Caution:** [B, ?/–] Allergy **Disp:** Topical lotion 1%; cream 5% **SE:** Local irritation **Notes:** Sprays available (Rid, A200, Nix) to disinfect clothing, bedding, combs, & brushes; lotion not OK in peds <2 y; may repeat after 7 d

Perphenazine (Trilafon) **Uses:** *Psychotic disorders, severe N*, intractable hiccups **Acts:** Phenothiazine, blocks brain dopaminergic receptors **Dose:** *Adults. Antipsychotic:* 4–16 mg PO tid; max 64 mg/d. *Hiccups:* 5 mg IM q6h PRN or 1 mg IV at intervals not <1–2 mg/min, 5 mg max. *Peds 1–6 y:* 4–6 mg/d PO in ÷ doses. *6–12 y:* 6 mg/d PO in ÷ doses. *>12 y:* 4–16 mg PO bid-qid; ↓ in hepatic Insuff **Caution:** [C, ?/–] NAG, severe ↑/↓ BP **CI:** Phenothiazine sensitivity, BM depression, severe liver or cardiac Dz **Disp:** Tabs 2, 4, 8, 16 mg; PO conc 16 mg/5 mL; Inj 5 mg/mL **SE:** ↓ BP, ↑/↓ HR, EPS, drowsiness, Szs, photosens, skin discoloration, blood dyscrasias, constipation

Phenazopyridine (Pyridium, Azo-Standard, Urogesic, Many others) **Uses:** *Lower urinary tract irritation* **Acts:** Anesthetic on urinary tract mucosa **Dose:** *Adults.* 100–200 mg PO tid; 2 d max w/ antibiotics for UTI; ↓ w/ renal Insuff **Caution:** [B, ?] Hepatic Dz **CI:** Renal failure **Disp:** Tabs 100, 200 mg **SE:** GI disturbances, red-orange urine color (can stain clothing, contacts), HA, dizziness, acute renal failure, methemoglobinemia, tinting of sclera/skin **Notes:** Take w/ food

Phenelzine (Nardil) **BOX:** Antidepressants ↑ risk of suicidal thinking and behavior in children and adolescents w/ major depressive disorder and other psychological disorders; not for peds use **Uses:** *Depression*, bulimia **Acts:** MAOI **Dose:** *Adults.* 15 mg PO tid, ↑ to 60–90 mg/d ÷ doses. *Elderly.* 15–60 mg/d ÷ doses **Caution:** [C, –] Interacts w/ SSRI, ergots, triptans **CI:** CHF, Hx liver Dz, pheochromocytoma **Disp:** Tabs 15 mg **SE:** Postural ↓ BP; edema, dizziness, sedation, rash, sexual dysfunction, xerostomia, constipation, urinary retention **Notes:** 2–4 wk for effect; avoid tyramine-containing foods (e.g., cheeses)

Phenobarbital [C-IV] **Uses:** *Sz disorders*, insomnia, anxiety **Acts:** Barbiturate **Dose:** *Adults. Sedative–hypnotic:* 30–120 mg/d PO or IM PRN. *Anticonvulsant:* Load 10–12 mg/kg in 3 ÷ doses, then 1–3 mg/kg/24 h PO, IM, or IV. *Peds. Sedative–hypnotic:* 2–3 mg/kg/24 h PO or IM hs PRN. *Anticonvulsant:* Load

15–20 mg/kg ÷ in 2 equal doses 4 h apart, then 3–5 mg/kg/24h PO ÷ in 2–3 doses; ↓ w/ CrCl <10 mL/min **Caution:** [D, M] **CI:** Porphyria, hepatic impair, dyspnea, airway obst **Disp:** Tabs 15, 16, 30, 32, 60, 65, 100 mg; elixir 15, 20 mg/5 mL; Inj 30, 60, 65, 130 mg/mL **SE:** ↓ HR, ↓ BP, hangover, SJS, blood dyscrasias, resp depression **Notes:** Tolerance develops to sedation; paradoxic hyperactivity seen in ped pts; long 1/2 allows single daily dosing. Levels: *Trough:* Just before next dose. *Therapeutic: Trough:* 15–40 mcg/mL; *Toxic: Trough:* >40 mcg/mL *1/2Half-life:* 40–120 h

Phenylephrine, Nasal (Neo-Synephrine Nasal) (OTC) BOX: Not
for use in Peds <2 y **Uses:** *Nasal congestion* **Acts:** α-Adrenergic agonist **Dose:** *Adults.* 1–2 sprays/nostril q4h (usual 0.25%) PRN. *Peds 2–6 y:* 0.125% 1 drop/ nostril q2–4h. *6–12 y:* 1–2 sprays/nostril q4h 0.25% 2–3 drops **Caution:** [C, +/–] HTN, acute pancreatitis, hep, coronary Dz, NAG, hyperthyroidism **CI:** ↓ HR, arrhythmias **Disp:** Nasal soln 0.125, 0.25, 0.5, 1%; liq 7.5 mg/5 mL; drops 2.5 mg/mL **SE:** Arrhythmias, HTN, nasal irritation, dryness, sneezing, rebound congestion w/ prolonged use, HA **Notes:** Do not use >3 d

Phenylephrine, ophthalmic (Neo-Synephrine Ophthalmic, AK-
Dilate, Zincfrin [OTC]) **Uses:** *Mydriasis, ocular redness [OTC], perioperative mydriasis, posterior synechiae, uveitis w/ posterior synechiae* **Acts:** α-Adrenergic agonist **Dose:** *Adults.* Redness: 1 gtt 0.12% q3–4h PRN. *Exam mydriasis:* 1 gtt 2.5% (15 min–1 h for effect). *Pre-op:* 1 gtt 2.5–10% 30–60 min pre-op. *Ocular disorders:* 1 gtt 2.5–10% daily-tid *Peds.* As adult, only use 2.5% for exam, pre-op, and ocular conditions **Caution:** [C, May cause late-term fetal anoxia↓ HR, +/–] HTN, w/ elderly w/ CAD **CI:** NAG **Disp:** Ophthal soln 0.12% (Zincfrin OTC), 2.5, 10% **SE:** Tearing, HA, irritation, eye pain, photophobia, arrhythmia, tremor

Phenylephrine, oral (Sudafed PE, SudoGest PE, Nasop, Lusonal,
AH-chew D, Sudafed PE quick dissolve) (OTC) **BOX:** Not for use in peds <2 y **Uses:** *Nasal congestion* **Acts:** α-Adrenergic agonist **Dose:** *Adults.* 10–20 mg PO q4h PRN, max 60 mg/d. *Peds.* 5 mg PO q4h PRN, max 60 mg/d **Caution:** [C, +/–] HTN, acute pancreatitis, hep, coronary Dz, NAG, hyperthyroidism **CI:** MAOI w/in 14 d, NAG, severe ↑ BP or CAD, urinary retention **Disp:** Liq 7.5 mg/5 mL; drops 2.5 mg/mL; tabs 5, 10 mg; chew tabs 10 mg; tabs once daily 10 mg; strips 10 mg. **SE:** Arrhythmias, HTN, HA, agitation, anxiety, tremor, palpitations

Phenylephrine, systemic (Neo-Synephrine) BOX: Prescribers should
be aware of full prescribing information before use **Uses:** *Vascular failure in shock, allergy, or drug-induced ↓ BP* **Acts:** α-Adrenergic agonist **Dose:** *Adults. Mild–mod ↓ BP:* 2–5 mg IM or SQ ↑ BP for 2 h; 0.1–0.5 mg IV elevates BP for 15 min. *Severe ↓ BP/shock:* Cont Inf at 100–180 mcg/min; after BP stable, maint 40–60 mcg/min. *Peds. ↓ BP:* 5–20 mcg/kg/dose IV q10–15min or 0.1–0.5 mcg/kg/min IV Inf, titrate to effect **Caution:** [C, +/–] HTN, acute pancreatitis, hep, coronary Dz, NAG, hyperthy-

roidism **CI:** ↓ HR, arrhythmias **Disp:** Inj 10 mg/mL **SE:** Arrhythmias, HTN, peripheral vasoconstriction ↑ w/ oxytocin, MAOIs, & TCAs; HA, weakness, necrosis, ↓ renal perfusion **Notes:** Restore blood vol if loss has occurred; use large veins to avoid extrav; phentolamine 10 mg in 10–15 mL of NS for local Inj to Rx extrav

Phenytoin (Dilantin) **Uses:** *Sz disorders* **Acts:** ↓ Sz spread in the motor cortex **Dose: Adults & Peds. Load:** 15–20 mg/kg IV, 50 mg/min max sv or PO in 400-mg doses at 4-h intervals; *Adults.* **Maint:** Initial 200 mg PO or IV bid or 300 mg hs then follow slowly; alternatively 5–7 mg/kg/d based on IBW ÷ daily-tid, **Peds.** **Maint:** 4–7 mg/kg/24h PO or IV ÷ daily-bid; avoid PO susp (erratic absorption) **Caution:** [D, +] **CI:** Heart block, sinus bradycardia **Disp:** *Dilantin Infatab:* chew 50 mg. *Dilantin/Phenytek:* caps 100 mg; caps, ER 30, 100, 200, 300 mg; susp 125 mg/5 mL; Inj 50 mg/mL **SE:** Nystagmus/ataxia early signs of tox; gum hyperplasia w/ long-term use. *IV:* ↓ BP, ↓ HR, arrhythmias, phlebitis; peripheral neuropathy, rash, blood dyscrasias, SJS **Notes:** Levels: *Trough:* Just before next dose. *Therapeutic:* 10–20 mcg/mL *Toxic:* >20 mcg/mL Phenytoin albumin bound, levels = bound & free phenytoin; w/ ↓ albumin & azotemia, low levels may be therapeutic (nl free levels); do not change dosage at intervals <7–10 d; hold tube feeds 1 h before and after dose if using oral susp; avoid large dose

Physostigmine (Antilirium) **Uses:** *Antidote for TCA, atropine, & scopolamine OD; glaucoma* **Acts:** Reversible cholinesterase inhib **Dose: Adults.** 0.5–2 mg IV or IM q20 min **Peds.** 0.01–0.03 mg/kg/dose IV q5–10 min up to 2 mg total PRN **Caution:** [C, ?] **CI:** GI/GU obst, CV Dz, asthma **Disp:** Inj 1 mg/mL **SE:** Rapid IV administration associated w/ Szs; cholinergic SEs; sweating, salivation, lacrimation, GI upset, asystole, changes in HR **Notes:** Excessive readmintration can result in cholinergic crisis; crisis reversed w/ atropine

Phytonadione [Vitamin K] (AquaMEPHYTON, others) **Uses:** *Coagulation disorders d/t faulty formation of factors II, VII, IX, X*; hyperalimentation **Acts:** Cofactor for production of factors II, VII, IX, & X **Dose: Adults & Peds.** *Anticoagulant-induced prothrombin deficiency:* 1–10 mg PO or IV slowly. *Hyperalimentation:* 10 mg IM or IV q wk. **Infants.** 0.5–1 mg/dose IM, SQ, or PO **Caution:** [C, +] **CI:** Allergy **Disp:** Tabs 5 mg; Inj 2, 10 mg/mL **SE:** Anaphylaxis from IV dosage; give IV slowly; GI upset (PO), Inj site Rxns **Notes:** w/ Parenteral Rx, 1st change in PT/INR usually seen in 12–24 h; use makes re-warfarinization more difficult

Pimecrolimus (Elidel) **BOX:** Associated w/ rare skin malignancies and lymphoma, limit to area, not for age <2 y **Uses:** *Atopic dermatitis* refractory, severe perianal itching **Acts:** Inhibits T -lymphocytes **Dose: Adults & Peds >2 y:** Apply bid; use at least 1 wk following resolution **Caution:** [C, ?/–] w/ Local Infxn, lymphadenopathy; immunocompromised; avoid in pts <2 y **CI:** Allergy component, <2 y **Disp:** Cream 1% **SE:** Phototox, local irritation/burning, flu-like Sxs, may ↑ malignancy **Notes:** Use on dry skin only; wash hands after; 2nd-line/short-term use only

Pimozide (Orap)   BOX: ↑ Mortality in elderly w/ dementia-related psychosis
Uses: * Tourette Dz *agitation, psychosis **Action:** typical antipsychotic, dopamine antagonist **Dose:** 10 mg PO q day, ↓ to 5 mg w/ SE or hepatic impair **Caution:** [D, /−] NAG, elderly, hepatic impair, neurologic Dz's, **CI:** compound hypersens, CNS depression, coma, dysrhythmia, ↑QT syndrome, w/ QT prolonging drugs, ↓ K, ↓ Mg, w/ CYP3A4 inhib (Table 10 p 280) **Disp:** Tabs 1, 2 mg **SE:** CNS (somnolence, agitation, others), rash, xerostomia, weakness, rigidity, visual changes, constipation, ↑salivation, akathisia, tardive dyskinesia, neuroleptic malignant syndrome, ↑QT. **Notes:** ✓ ECG

Pindolol (Visken)   **Uses:** *HTN* **Acts:** β-Adrenergic receptor blocker, β₁, β₂, ISA **Dose:** 5–10 mg bid, 60 mg/d max; ↓ in hepatic/renal failure **Caution:** [B (1st tri; D 2nd/3rd tri), +/−] **CI:** Uncompensated CHF, cardiogenic shock, ↓ HR, heart block, asthma, COPD **Disp:** Tabs 5, 10 mg **SE:** Insomnia, dizziness, fatigue, edema, GI upset, dyspnea; fluid retention may exacerbate CHF

Pioglitazone (Actos)   BOX: May cause or worsen CHF **Uses:** *Type 2 DM* **Acts:** ↑ Insulin sensitivity **Dose:** 15–45 mg/d PO **Caution:** [C, −] **CI:** CHF, hepatic impair **Disp:** Tabs 15, 30, 45 mg **SE:** Wgt gain, myalgia, URI, HA, hypoglycemia, edema, ↑ fracture risk in women

Pioglitazone/Metformin (ACTOplus Met, ACTOplus MET XR)
BOX: Metformin can cause lactic acidosis, fatal in 50% of cases; pioglitazone may cause or worsen CHF **Uses:** *Type 2 DM as adjunct to diet and exercise* **Acts:** Combined ↑ insulin sensitivity w/ ↓ hepatic glucose release **Dose:** Initial 1 tab PO daily or bid, titrate; max daily pioglitazone 45 mg & metformin 2550 mg; XR: 1 tab PO daily w/ evening meal; max daily pioglitazone 45 mg & metformin IR 2550 mg, metformin ER 2000 mg; give w/ meals **Caution:** [C, −] Stop w/ radiologic IV contrast agents **CI:** CHF, renal impair, acidosis **Disp:** Tabs (pioglitazone mg/metformin mg): 15/500, 15/850; Tabs XR (pioglitazone mg/metformin ER mg) 15/1000, 30/1000, 30/1000 mg **SE:** Lactic acidosis, CHF, ↓ glucose, edema, wgt gain, myalgia, URI, HA, GI upset, liver damage **Notes:** Follow LFTs; ↑ fracture risk in women receiving pioglitazone

Piperacillin (Pipracil)   **Uses:** *Infxns of skin, bone, resp, & urinary tract, abd, sepsis* **Acts:** 4th-Gen PCN; bactericidal; ↓ cell wall synth. *Spectrum:* Primarily gram(+), better *Enterococcus, H. influenzae,* not staphylococci; gram(−) *E. coli, Proteus, Shigella, Pseudomonas,* not β-lactamase producing **Dose:** *Adults.* 2–4 g IV q4–6h. *Peds.* 200–300 mg/kg/d IV ÷ q4–6h; ↓ in renal failure **Caution:** [B, M] **CI:** PCN/β-lactam sensitivity **Disp:** Powder for Inj: 2, 3, 4, 40 g **SE:** ↓ Plt aggregation, interstitial nephritis, renal Insuff, anaphylaxis, hemolytic anemia **Notes:** Often used w/ aminoglycoside

Piperacillin–Tazobactam (Zosyn)   **Uses:** *Infxns of skin, bone, resp & urinary tract, abd, sepsis* **Acts:** 4th-Gen PCN plus β-lactamase inhib; bactericidal; ↓ cell wall synth. *Spectrum:* Good gram(+), excellent gram(−); anaerobes & β-lactamase producers **Dose:** *Adults.* 3.375–4.5 g IV q6h; ↓ in renal Insuff

Caution: [B, M] **CI:** PCN or β-lactam sensitivity **Disp:** *Powder for Inj:* Frozen, premix Inj 3.25, 3.375, 4.5 g **SE:** D, HA, insomnia, GI upset, serum sickness-like Rxn, pseudomembranous colitis **Notes:** Often used in combo w/ aminoglycoside

Pirbuterol (Maxair) **Uses:** *Prevention & Rx reversible bronchospasm* **Acts:** β₂-Adrenergic agonist **Dose:** 2 Inh q4–6h; max 12 Inh/d **Caution:** [C, ?/–] **Disp:** Aerosol 0.2 mg/actuation (contains ozone-depleting CFCs; will be gradually removed from US market) **SE:** Nervousness, restlessness, trembling, HA, taste changes, tachycardia **Note:** Teach pt proper inhaler technique

Piroxicam (Feldene) **BOX:** May ↑ risk of cardiovascular CV events & GI bleeding **Uses:** *Arthritis & pain* **Acts:** NSAID; ↓ prostaglandins **Dose:** 10–20 mg/d **Caution:** [B (1st tri; D if 3rd tri or near term), +] GI bleeding **CI:** ASA/NSAID sensitivity **Disp:** Caps 10, 20 mg **SE:** Dizziness, rash, GI upset, edema, acute renal failure, peptic ulcer

Pitavastatin (Livalo) **Uses:** *reduce elevated total cholesterol* **Action:** Statin, inhibits HMG Co-A reductase **Dose:** 1–4 mg once/d w/o regard to meals; Cr Cl 30–60 mg/min start 1 mg w/ 2 mg max **Caution:** [X, –] may cause myopathy and rhabdomyolysis **CI:** active liver dz, w/ lopinavir/ritonavir/cyclosporine, severe renal impair not on dialysis **Disp:** Tabs 1, 2, 4 mg **SE:** muscle pain, back pain, joint pain, and constipation, ↑ LFT's **Notes:** ✓ LFT's

Plasma Protein Fraction (Plasmanate, Others) **Uses:** *Shock & ↓ BP* **Acts:** Plasma vol expander **Dose:** *Adults. Initial:* 250–500 mL IV (not >10 mL/min); subsequent Inf based on response. *Peds.* 10–15 mL/kg/dose IV; subsequent Inf based on response **Caution:** [C, +] **CI:** Renal Insuff, CHF, cardiopulmonary bypass **Disp:** Inj 5% **SE:** ↓ BP w/ rapid Inf; hypocoagulability, metabolic acidosis, PE **Notes:** 130–160 mEq Na⁺²/L; not substitute for RBC

Plerixafor (Mozobil) **Uses:** *Mobilize stem cells for ABMT in lymphoma and myeloma in combo w/ G-CSF* **Action:** Hematopoietic stem cell mobilizer **Dose:** 0.24 mg/kg SQ daily; max 40 mg/d); CrCl < 50 mL/min: 0.16 mg/kg, max 27 mg/d) **Caution:** [D, /?] **CI: Disp:** IV: 20 mg/mL (1.2 mL) **SE:** HA, N/V/D, Inj site rxns, ↑ WBC, ↓ plt **Notes:** Give w/ filgrastim 10 mcg/kg

Pneumococcal 7-Valent Conjugate Vaccine (Prevnar) **Uses:** *Immunization against pneumococcal Infxns in infants & children* **Acts:** Active immunization **Dose:** 0.5 mL IM/dose; series of 3 doses; 1st dose age 2 mo; then doses q2mo, 4th dose at age 12–15 mo **CI:** Sensitivity to components or diphtheria toxoid, febrile illness **Disp:** Inj **SE:** Local Rxns, anorexia, arthralgia, D, fever, irritability, myalgia, V **Notes:** Keep epi (1:1000) available for Rxns. Does not replace Pneumovax-23 in age > 24 mo w/ immunosuppression

Pneumococcal Vaccine, Polyvalent (Pneumovax-23) **Uses:** *Immunization against pneumococcal Infxns in pts at high risk (all pts > 65 y, also asplenia, sickle cell dz, HIV and other immunocompromised and w/ chronic illnesses)* **Acts:** Active immunization **Dose:** 0.5 mL IM or SQ. **Caution:** [C, ?] **CI:** Do not vaccinate during immunosuppressive Rx **Disp:** Inj 0.5 mL **SE:** Fever,

Inj site Rxn also hemolytic anemia w/ other heme conditions, ↓ plt w/ stable ITP, anaphylaxis, Guillain-Barré synd **Notes:** Keep epi (1:1000) available for Rxns. Revaccinate Q q3-5 y if very high risk (e.g.eg, asplenia, nephrotic synd), consider revaccination if > 6 y since initial or if previously vaccinated w/ 14-valent vaccine.

Podophyllin (Podocon-25, Condylox Gel 0.5%, Condylox)
Uses: *Topical Rx of benign growths (genital & perianal warts [condylomata acuminata]*, papillomas, fibromas) **Acts:** Direct antimitotic effect; exact mechanism unknown **Dose:** *Condylox gel & Condylox:* Apply bid for 3 consecutive d/wk for 4 wk; 0.5 mL/d max; *Podocon-25:* Use sparingly on the lesion, leave on for 1–4 h, thoroughly wash off **Caution:** [X, ?] Immunosuppression **CI:** DM, bleeding lesions **Disp:** *Podocon-25* (w/ benzoin) 15-mL bottles; *Condylox gel* 0.5% 35-g clear gel; *Condylox soln* 0.5% 35-g clear **SE:** Local Rxns, sig absorption; anemias, tachycardia, paresthesias, GI upset, renal/hepatic damage **Notes:** Podocon-25 applied by the clinician; do not dispense directly to pt

Polyethylene Glycol [PEG]-Electrolyte Soln (GoLYTELY, Colyte)
Uses: *Bowel prep prior to examination or surgery* **Acts:** Osmotic cathartic **Dose:** *Adults.* Following 3–4-h fast, drink 240 mL of soln q10min until 4 L consumed or until BMs are clear. *Peds.* 25–40 mL/kg/h for 4–10 h **Caution:** [C, ?] GI obst, bowel perforation, megacolon, ulcerative colitis **Disp:** Powder for recons to 4 L **SE:** Cramping or N, bloating **Notes:** 1st BM should occur in approximately 1 h; chilled soln more palatable

Polyethylene Glycol [PEG] 3350 (MiraLAX)
Uses: *Occasional constipation* **Acts:** Osmotic laxative **Dose:** 17-g powder (1 heaping tsp) in 8 oz (1 cup) of H_2O & drink; max 14 d **Caution:** [C, ?] Rule out bowel obst before use **CI:** GI obst, allergy to PEG **Disp:** Powder for reconstitution; bottle cap holds 17 g **SE:** Upset stomach, bloating, cramping, gas, severe D, hives **Notes:** Can add to H_2O, juice, soda, coffee, or tea

Polymyxin B & Hydrocortisone (Otobiotic Otic)
Uses: *Superficial bacterial infxns of external ear canal* **Acts:** Antibiotic/anti-inflammatory combo **Dose:** 4 gtt in ear(s) tid-qid **Caution:** [B, ?] **CI:** Component sensitivity **Disp:** Soln polymyxin B 10,000 units/hydrocortisone 0.5%/mL **SE:** Local irritation **Notes:** Useful in neomycin allergy

Posaconazole (Noxafil)
Uses: *Prevent Aspergillus and Candida infxns in severely immunocompromised; Rx oropharyngeal candida* **Acts:** ↓ Cell membrane ergosterol synth **Dose:** *Adults. Invasive fungal prophylaxis:* 200 mg PO tid. *Oropharyngeal candidiasis:* 100 mg PO daily × 13 d, if refractory 400 mg PO bid *Peds >13 y:* 200 mg PO tid; take w/ meal **Caution:** [C.;?] Multiple drug interactions; ↑ QT, cardiac Dzs, severe renal/liver impair **CI:** Component hypersens; w/ many drugs including alfuzosin, astemizole, aprazolam, phenothiazines, terfenadine, triazolam, others **Disp:** Soln 40 mg/mL **SE:** ↑ QT, ↑ LFTs, hepatic failure, fever, N/V/D, HA, Abd pain, anemia, ↓ plt, ↓ K^+ rash, dyspnea, cough, anorexia, fatigue **Notes:** Monitor LFTs, CBC, lytes

Potassium Citrate (Urocit-K) Uses: *Alkalinize urine, prevention of urinary stones (uric acid, calcium stones if hypocitraturic)* Acts: Urinary alkalinizer Dose: 1 packet dissolved in H_2O or 15–30 mL pc & hs 10–20 mEq PO tid w/ meals, max 100 mEq/d Caution: [A, +] CI: Severe renal impair, dehydration, ↑ K^+, peptic ulcer; w/ K^+-sparing diuretics, salt substitutes Disp: 540, 1080 mg tabs SE: GI upset, ↓ Ca^{2+}, ↑ K^+, metabolic alkalosis Notes: Tabs 540 mg = 5 mEq, 1080 mg = 10 mEq

Potassium Citrate & Citric Acid (Polycitra-K) Uses: *Alkalinize urine, prevent urinary stones (uric acid, CA stones if hypocitraturic)* Acts: Urinary alkalinizer Dose: 10–20 mEq PO tid w/ meals, max 100 mEq/d Caution: [A, +] CI: Severe renal impair, dehydration, ↑ K^+, peptic ulcer; w/ use of K^+-sparing diuretics or salt substitutes Disp: Soln 10 mEq/5 mL; powder 30 mEq/packet SE: GI upset, ↓ Ca^{2+}, ↑ K^+, metabolic alkalosis

Potassium Iodide [Lugol Soln] (SSKI, Thyro-Block, ThyroSafe, ThyroShield) Uses: *Thyroid storm*, ↓ vascularity before thyroid surgery, block thyroid uptake of radioactive iodine, thin bronchial secretions Acts: Iodine supl Dose: *Adults & Peds >2 y: Pre-op thyroidectomy:* 50–250 mg PO tid (2–6 gtt strong iodine soln); give 10 d pre-op. *Protection:* 130 mg/d. Peds. *Protection: <1 y:* 16.25 mg q day. *1 mo–3y:* 32.5 mg q day. *3–12 y:* 1/2 adult dose Caution: [D, +] ↑ K^+, TB, PE, bronchitis, renal impair CI: Iodine sensitivity Disp: Tabs 65, 130 mg; soln (saturated soln of potassium iodide [SSKI]) 1 g/mL; Lugol Soln, strong iodine 100 mg/mL; syrup 325 mg/5 mL SE: Fever, HA, urticaria, angioedema, goiter, GI upset, eosinophilia Notes: w/ Nuclear radiation emergency, give until radiation exposure no longer exists

Potassium Supplements (Kaon, Kaochlor, K-Lor, Slow-K, Micro-K, Klorvess, others) Uses: *Prevention or Rx of ↓ K^+* (e.g., diuretic use) Acts: K^+ supl Dose: *Adults.* 20–100 mEq/d PO ÷ daily-bid; IV 10–20 mEq/h, max 40 mEq/d & 150 mEq/d (monitor K^+ levels frequently and in presence of continuous ECG monitoring w/ high-dose IV). Peds. Calculate K^+ deficit; 1–43 mEq/kg/d PO ÷ daily–qid; IV max dose 0.5–1 mEq/kg/× 1-2 h Caution: [A, +] Renal Insuff, use w/ NSAIDs & ACE inhib CI: ↑ K^+ Disp: PO forms (Table 6 p 276); Inj SE: GI irritation; ↓ HR, ↑ K^+, heart block Notes: Mix powder & liq w/ beverage (unsalted tomato juice, etc); swallow SR tabs must be swallowed whole; follow monitor K^+; Cl^- salt OK w/ alkalosis; w/ acidosis use acetate, bicarbonate, citrate, or gluconate salt; Do not administer IV K^+ undiluted

Pralatrexate (Folotyn) BOX: Administer only by physician experienced in chemotherapy. Uses: *Tx refractory T-cell lymphoma* Action: Folate analogue metabolic inhibitor; ↓ dihydrofolate reductase Dose: *Adults.* IV push over 3–5 min: 30 mg/m^2 once weekly for 6 wks Caution: [D, -] Disp: Inj 20 mg/ml (1 ml, 2ml) SE: ↓ plt, anemia, ↓ WBC, mucositis, N/V/D, edema, fever, fatigue, rash Notes: Give folic acid supplements prior to and during therapy

Pramipexole (Mirapex) Uses: *Parkinson Dz, restless leg synd* Acts: Dopamine agonist Dose: 1.5–4.5 mg/d PO, initial 0.375 mg/d in 3 ÷ doses; titrate slowly **Caution:** [C, ?/–] ↓ Renal impair **CI:** Component allergy **Disp:** Tabs 0.125, 0.25, 0.5, 1, 1.5 mg **SE:** Postural ↓ BP, asthenia, somnolence, abnormal dreams, GI upset, EPS, hallucinations (elderly)

Pramoxine (Anusol Ointment, ProctoFoam-NS, others) **Uses:** *Relief of pain & itching from hemorrhoids, anorectal surgery*; topical for burns & dermatosis **Acts:** Topical anesthetic **Dose:** Apply freely to anal area q3h **Caution:** [C, ?] **Disp:** [OTC] All 1%; foam (*ProctoFoam-NS*), cream, oint, lotion, gel, pads, spray **SE:** Contact dermatitis, mucosal thinning w/ chronic use

Pramoxine + Hydrocortisone (Enzone, ProctoFoam-HC) **Uses:** *Relief of pain & itching from hemorrhoids* **Acts:** Topical anesthetic & anti-inflammatory **Dose:** Apply freely to anal area tid-qid **Caution:** [C, ?/–] **Disp:** *Cream:* pramoxine 1% acetate 0.5/1%; *foam:* pramoxine 1% hydrocortisone 1%; *lotion:* pramoxine 1% hydrocortisone 0.25/1/2.5%, pramoxine 2.5% & hydrocortisone 1% **SE:** Contact dermatitis, mucosal thinning w/ chronic use

Prasugrel hydrochloride (Effient) **BOX:** Can cause significant, sometimes fatal, bleeding; not recommended in do not use w/planned CABG w/ active bleeding, HX TIA or stroke or pts > 75y **Uses:** * ↓ thrombotic CV events (e.g. stent thrombosis)* administer ASAP in ECC setting w/ high-risk ST depression or T-wave inversion w/planned PCI **Acts:** ↓ Plt aggregation **Dose:** 10 mg/d; wgt<60 kg, consider 5 mg/d; 60 mg PO loading dose in ECC; 2009 ACCF/AHA/SCAI joint STEMI/PCI guidelines: use at least 12 mo w/ cardiac stent (bare or drug eluting); consider >15 mos w/drug eluting stent **Caution:** [B, ?] Active bleeding; ↑ bleed risk; w/CYP3A4 substrates **CI:** Coag disorders, active intracranial bleeding or PUD; Hx TIA/stroke **Disp:** Tabs 5, 10 mg **SE:** ↑ bleeding time, ↑ BP, GI intolerance, HA, dizziness, rash, ↓ WBC **Notes:** Plt aggregation to baseline ~ 7 d after D/C, plt transfusion reverses acutely

Pravastatin (Pravachol) **Uses:** *↓ Cholesterol* **Acts:** HMG-CoA reductase inhibitor **Dose:** 10–80 mg PO hs; ↓ in sig renal/hepatic impair **Caution:** [X, –] w/ Gemfibrozil **CI:** Liver Dz or persistent LFTs ↑ **Disp:** Tabs 10, 20, 40, 80 mg **SE:** Use caution w/ concurrent gemfibrozil; HA, GI upset, hep, myopathy, renal failure

Prazosin (Minipress) **Uses:** *HTN* **Acts:** Peripherally acting α-adrenergic blocker **Dose:** *Adults.* 1 mg PO tid; can ↑ to 20 mg/d max PRN. *Peds.* 0.05–0.1 mg/kg/d in 3 ÷ doses; max 0.5 mg/kg/d **Caution:** [C, ?] use w/ phosphodiesterase-5 (PDE-5) inhib (e.g., sildenafil) can cause ↓ BP **CI:** Component allergy, concurrent use of PDE5 inhib **Disp:** Caps 1, 2, 5 mg; tabs ER 2.5, 5 mg **SE:** Dizziness, edema, palpitations, fatigue, GI upset **Notes:** Can cause orthostatic ↓ BP, take the 1st dose hs; tolerance develops to this effect; tachyphylaxis may result

Prednisolone [(See Steroids page 228 and Table 2, page 265)]
Prednisone [(See Steroids page 228 and Table 2, page 265)]
Pregabalin (Lyrica) **BOX:** Increased risk of suicidal behavior ideation **Uses:** *DM peripheral neuropathy pain; postherpetic neuralgia; fibromyalgia; adjunct w/

adult partial onset Szs* **Acts:** Nerve transmission modulator, antinociceptive, anti-seizure effect; mechanism ?; related to gabapentin **Dose:** *Neuropathic pain:* 50 mg PO tid, ↑ to 300 mg/d w/in 1 wk based on response, 300 mg/d max *Postherpetic neuralgia:* 75–150 mg bid, or 50–100 mg tid; start 75 mg bid or 50 mg tid; ↑ to 300 mg/d w/in 1 wk PRN; if pain persists after 2–4 wk, ↑ to 600 mg/d. *Epilepsy:* Start 150 mg/d (75 mg bid or 50 mg tid) may ↑ to max 600 mg/d; ↓ w/ renal Insuff; w/ or w/o food **Caution:** [C, –] w/ Sig renal impair (see PI), w/ elderly & severe CHF avoid abrupt D/C **CI:** PRG **Disp:** Caps 25, 50, 75, 100, 150, 200, 225, 300 mg **SE:** Dizziness, drowsiness, xerostomia, edema, blurred vision, wgt gain, difficulty concentrating **Notes:** w/ D/C, taper over at least 1 wk

Probenecid (Benemid, others) **Uses:** *Prevent gout & hyperuricemia; extends levels of PCNs & cephalosporins* **Acts:** Uricosuric, renal tubular blocker of organic anions **Dose:** *Adults. Gout:* 250 mg bid × 1 wk, then 0.5 g PO bid; can ↑ by 500 mg/mo up to 2–3 g/d. *Antibiotic effect:* 1–2 g PO 30 min before dose. *Peds >2 y:* 25 mg/kg, then 40 mg/kg/d PO ÷ qid **Caution:** [B, ?] **CI:** High-dose ASA, mod–severe renal impair, age <2 y **Disp:** Tabs 500 mg **SE:** HA, GI upset, rash, pruritus, dizziness, blood dyscrasias **Notes:** Do not use during acute gout attack

Procainamide (Pronestyl, Pronestyl SR, Procanbid) **BOX:** Positive ANA titer or SLE w/ prolonged use; only use in life-threatening arrhythmias; hematologic tox can be severe, follow CBC **Uses:** *Supraventricular/ventricular arrhythmias* **Acts:** Class 1A antiarrhythmic (Table 9 p 279) **Dose:** *Adults. Recurrent VF/VT:* 20 mg/min IV (total 17 mg/kg max). *Maint:* 1–4 mg/min. *Stable wide-complex tachycardia of unknown origin, AF w/ rapid rate in WPW:* 20 mg/min IV until in arrhythmia suppression, ↓ BP, or QRS widens >50%, then 1–4 mg/min. *Chronic dosing:* 50 mg/kg/d PO in ÷ doses q4–6h. *Recurrent VF/VT:* 20–50 mg/min IV; max total 17 mg/kg. *Others:* 20 mg/min IV until one these: arrhythmia stopped, ↓ hypotension, QRS widens >50%, total 17 mg/kg; then 1–4 mg/min *(ECC 2005).* *Peds. Chronic maint:* 15–50 mg/kg/24 h PO ÷ q3–6h; ↓ in renal/hepatic impair **Caution:** [C, +] **CI:** Complete heart block, 2nd/3rd-degree heart block w/o pacemaker, torsades de pointes, SLE **Disp:** Tabs & caps 250, 500 mg; SR tabs 500, 750, 1000 mg; Inj 100, 500 mg/mL **SE:** BP, lupus-like synd, GI upset, taste perversion, arrhythmias, tachycardia, heart block, angioneurotic edema, blood dyscrasias **Notes:** Levels: *Trough:* Just before next dose. *Therapeutic:* 4–10 mcg/mL; *N*-acetyl procainamide (NAPA) + procaine 5–30 mcg/mL *Toxic:* >10 mcg/mL; NAPA + procaine >30 mcg/mL *1/2-life:* procaine 3–5 h, NAPA 6–10 h

Procarbazine (Matulane) **BOX:** Highly toxic; handle w/ care **Uses:** *Hodgkin Dz*, NHL, brain & lung tumors **Acts:** Alkylating agent; ↓ DNA & RNA synth **Dose:** Per protocol **Caution:** [D, ?] w/ EtOH ingestion **CI:** Inadequate BM reserve **Disp:** Caps 50 mg **SE:** ↓ BM, hemolytic Rxns (w/ G6PD deficiency), N/V/D; disulfiram-like Rxn; cutaneous & constitutional Sxs, myalgia, arthralgia, CNS effects, azoospermia, cessation of menses

Prochlorperazine (Compazine) Uses: *N/V, agitation, & psychotic disorders* Acts: Phenothiazine; blocks postsynaptic dopaminergic CNS receptors Dose: *Adults.* Antiemetic: 5–10 mg PO tid-qid or 25 mg PR bid or 5–10 mg deep IM q4–6h. *Antipsychotic:* 10–20 mg IM acutely or 5–10 mg PO tid-qid for maint; ↑ doses may be required for antipsychotic effect. *Peds.* 0.1–0.15 mg/kg/dose IM q4–6h or 0.4 mg/kg/24 h PO ÷ tid-qid Caution: [C, +/–] NAG, severe liver/cardiac Dz CI: Phenothiazine sensitivity, BM suppression; age <2 y or wgt <9 kg Disp: Tabs 5, 10, 25 mg; SR caps 10, 15 mg; syrup 5 mg/5 mL; supp 2.5, 5, 25 mg; Inj 5 mg/mL SE: EPS common; Rx w/ diphenhydramine or benztropine

Promethazine (Phenergan) BOX: Do not use in pts < 2 yrs; resp depression risk; tissue damage, including gangrene w/ extravasation. Uses: *N/V, motion sickness, adjunct to post op analgesics, sedation, rhinitis* Acts: Phenothiazine; blocks CNS postsynaptic mesolimbic dopaminergic receptors Dose: *Adults.* 12.5–50 mg PO, PR, or IM bid-qid PRN. *Peds > 2 yrs.* 0.1–0.5 mg/kg/dose PO/ or IM q2–6h PRN Caution: [C, +/–] Use w/ agents w/ resp depressant effects CI: Component allergy, NAG, age <2 y Disp: Tabs 12.5, 25, 50 mg; syrup 6.25 mg/5 mL, 25 mg/5 mL; supp 12.5, 25, 50 mg; Inj 25, 50 mg/mL SE: Drowsiness, tardive dyskinesia, EPS, lowered Sz threshold, ↓ BP, GI upset, blood dyscrasias, photosens, resp depression in children Notes: IM/PO preferred route; not SQ or intra-arterial

Propafenone (Rythmol) BOX: Excess mortality or nonfatal cardiac arrest rate possible; avoid use w/ asymptomatic and symptomatic non–life-threatening ventricular arrhythmias Uses: *Life-threatening ventricular arrhythmias, AF* Acts: Class IC antiarrhythmic (Table 9 p 279) Dose: *Adults.* 150–300 mg PO q8h. Peds. 8–10 mg/kg/d ÷ in 3–4 doses; may ↑ 2 mg/kg/d, 20 mg/kg/d max Caution: [C, ?] w/ Fosamprenavir, ritonavir, MI w/in 2 y, w/ liver/renal impair CI: Uncontrolled CHF, bronchospasm, cardiogenic shock, AV block w/o pacer Disp: Tabs 150, 225, 300 mg; ER caps 225, 325, 425 mg SE: Dizziness, unusual taste, 1st-degree heart block, arrhythmias, prolongs QRS & QT intervals; fatigue, GI upset, blood dyscrasias

Propantheline (Pro-Banthine) Uses: *PUD*, symptomatic Rx of small intestine hypermotility, spastic colon, ureteral spasm, bladder spasm, pylorospasm* Acts: Antimuscarinic Dose: *Adults.* 15 mg PO ac & 30 mg PO hs; ↓ in elderly. *Peds.* 2–3 mg/kg/24 h PO ÷ tid-qid Caution: [C, ?] CI: NAG, ulcerative colitis, toxic megacolon, GI/GU obst Disp: Tabs 7.5, 15 mg SE: Anticholinergic (e.g., xerostomia, blurred vision)

Propofol (Diprivan) Uses: *Induction & maint of anesthesia; sedation in intubated pts* Acts: Sedative–hypnotic; mechanism unknown; acts in 40 s Dose: *Adults.* Anesthesia: 2–2.5 mg/kg dose (also *ECC 2005*), then 0.1–0.2 mg/kg/min Inf. *ICU sedation:* 5 mcg/kg/min IV × 5 min, ↑ PRN 5–10 mcg/kg/min q5–10 min, 5–50 mcg/kg/min cont Inf. *Peds. Anesthesia:* 2.5–3.5 mg/kg induction; then 125–300 mcg/kg/min; ↓ in elderly, debilitated, ASA II/IV pts Caution: [B, +] CI: If general anesthesia CI, sensitivity to egg, egg products, soybeans, soybean products **Disp:** Inj 10 mg/mL **SE:** May ↑ triglycerides w/ extended dosing; ↓ BP, pain at site, apnea, anaphylaxis **Notes:** 1 mL has 0.1 g fat

Propoxyphene (Darvon); Propoxyphene & Acetaminophen (Darvocet); Propoxyphene & Aspirin (Darvon Compound-65, Darvon-N + w/ Aspirin) [C-IV] **BOX:** Excessive doses alone or in combo w/ other CNS depressants can be cause of death; use w/ caution in depressed or suicidal pts Uses: *Mild–mod pain* **Acts:** Narcotic analgesic **Dose:** 1–2 PO q4h PRN; ↓ in hepatic impair, elderly **Caution:** [C (D if prolonged use), M] Hepatic impair (APAP), peptic ulcer (ASA); severe renal impair, Hx EtOH abuse **CI:** Allergy, suicide risk, Hx drug abuse **Disp:** *Darvon:* Propoxyphene HCl caps 65 mg. *Darvon-N:* Propoxyphene napsylate 100-mg tabs. *Darvocet-N:* Propoxyphene napsylate 50 mg/APAP 325 mg. *Darvocet-N 100:* Propoxyphene napsylate 100 mg/APAP 650 mg. *Darvon Compound-65:* Propoxyphene HCl caps 65-mg/ASA 389 mg/caffeine 32 mg. *Darvon-N w/ ASA:* Propoxyphene napsylate 100 mg/ASA 325 mg **SE:** OD can be lethal; ↓ BP, dizziness, sedation, GI upset, ↑ LFTs

Propranolol (Inderal) Uses: *HTN, angina, MI, hyperthyroidism, essential tremor, hypertrophic subaortic stenosis, pheochromocytoma; prevents migraines & atrial arrhythmias* **Acts:** β-Adrenergic receptor blocker, $β_1$, $β_2$; only β-blocker to block conversion of T_4 to T_3 **Dose:** *Adults. Angina:* 80–320 mg/d PO ÷ bid–qid or 80–160 mg/d SR. *Arrhythmia:* 10–80 mg PO tid-qid or 1 mg IV slowly, repeat q5min, 5 mg max. *HTN:* 40 mg PO bid or 60–80 mg/d SR, ↑ weekly to max 640 mg/d. *Hypertrophic subaortic stenosis:* 20–40 mg PO tid-qid. *MI:* 180–240 mg PO ÷ tid-qid. *Migraine prophylaxis:* 80 mg/d ÷ qid-tid, ↑ weekly 160–240 mg/d ÷ tid-qid max; wean if no response in 6 wk. *Pheochromocytoma:* 30–60 mg/d ÷ bid-qid. *Thyrotoxicosis:* 1–3 mg IV × 1; 10–40 mg PO q6h. *Tremor:* 40 mg PO bid, ↑ PRN 320 mg/d max; 0.1 mg/kg slow IV push, ÷ 3 equal doses q2–3min, max 1 mg/min; repeat in 2 min PRN (ECC 2005). *Peds. Arrhythmia:* 0.5–1.0 mg/kg/d ÷ tid-qid, ↑ PRN q3–7d to 60 mg/d max; 0.01–0.1 mg/kg IV over 10 min, 1 mg max. *HTN:* 0.5–1.0 mg/kg ÷ bid-qid, ↑ PRN q3–7d to 2 mg/d max; ↓ in renal impair **Caution:** [C (1st tri, D if 2nd or 3rd tri), +] **CI:** Uncompensated CHF, cardiogenic shock, ↓ HR, heart block, PE, severe resp Dz **Disp:** Tabs 10, 20, 40, 80 mg; SR caps 60, 80, 120, 160 mg; oral soln 4, 8, mg/mL; Inj 1 mg/mL **SE:** ↓ HR, ↓ BP, fatigue, GI upset, ED

Propylthiouracil [PTU] **BOX:** Severe liver failure reported; use only if pt cannot tolerate methimazole; d/t fetal anomalies w/ methimazole, PTU may be DOC in 1st tri Uses: *Hyperthyroidism* **Acts:** ↓ Production of T_3 & T_4 & conversion of T_4 to T_3 **Dose:** *Adults. Initial:* 100 mg PO q8h (may need up to 1200 mg/d); after pt euthyroid (6–8 wk), taper dose by 1/2 q4–6wk to maint, 50–150 mg/24 h; can usually PO in 2–3 y; ↓ in elderly. *Peds. Initial:* 5–7 mg/kg/24 h PO ÷ q8h. *Maint:* 1/3–2/3 of initial dose **Caution:** [D, −](See BOX) **CI:** Allergy **Disp:** Tabs 50 mg **SE:** Fever, rash, leukopenia, dizziness, GI upset, taste perversion, SLE-like synd, ↑ LFT, liver failure **Notes:** Monitor pt clinically; report any S/Sx of hepatic dysfunction, ✓ TFT and LFT

Protamine (generic) **Uses:** *Reverse heparin effect* **Acts:** Neutralize heparin by forming a stable complex **Dose:** Based on degree of heparin reversal; give IV slowly; 1 mg reverses ~ 100 units of heparin given in the preceding 3–4 h, 50 mg max **Caution:** [C, ?] **CI:** Allergy **Disp:** Inj 10 mg/mL **SE:** Follow coagulants; anticoagulant effect if given w/o heparin; ↓ BP, ↓ HR, dyspnea, hemorrhage **Notes:** ↑ aPTT ~ 15 min after use to assess response

Pseudoephedrine (Sudafed, Novafed, Afrinol, Others) [OTC] **BOX:** Not for use in peds <2 y **Uses:** *Decongestant* **Acts:** Stimulates α-adrenergic receptors w/ vasoconstriction **Dose:** *Adults.* 30–60 mg PO q6–8h. *Peds 2–5 y:* 15 mg q 4–6 h, 60 mg/24 h max. *6–12 y:* 30 mg q4–6h, 120 mg/24 h max; ↓ w/ renal Insuff **Caution:** [C, +] **CI:** Poorly controlled HTN or CAD, w/ MAOIs **Disp:** Tabs 30, 60 mg; caps 60 mg; SR tabs 120, 240 mg; liq 7.5 mg/0.8 mL, 15, 30 mg/5 mL **SE:** HTN, insomnia, tachycardia, arrhythmias, nervousness, tremor **Notes:** Found in many OTC cough/cold preparations; OTC restricted distribution

Psyllium (Metamucil, Serutan, Effer-Syllium) **Uses:** *Constipation & colonic diverticular Dz* **Acts:** Bulk laxative **Dose:** 1 tsp (7 g) in glass of H_2O PO daily–tid **Caution:** [B, ?] Effer-Syllium (effervescent psyllium) usually contains K^+, caution w/ renal failure; phenylketonuria (in products w/ aspartame) **CI:** Suspected bowel obst **Disp:** Granules 4, 25 g/tsp; powder 3.5 g/packet, caps 0.52g (3 g/6 caps), wafers 3.4 g/dose **SE:** D, Abd cramps, bowel obst, constipation, bronchospasm

Pyrazinamide (Generic) **Uses:** *Active TB in combo w/ other agents* **Acts:** Bacteriostatic; unknown mechanism **Dose:** *Adults.* 15–30 mg/kg/24 h PO ÷ tid-qid; max 2 g/d; dosing based on lean body wt; ↓ dose in renal/hepatic impair. *Peds.* 15–30 mg/kg/d PO ÷ daily-bid; ↓ w/ renal/hepatic impair **Caution:** [C, +/–] **CI:** Severe hepatic damage, acute gout **Disp:** Tabs 500 mg **SE:** Hepatotox, malaise, GI upset, arthralgia, myalgia, gout, photosens **Notes:** Use in combo w/ other anti-TB drugs; consult *MMWR* for latest TB recommendations; dosage regimen differs for "directly observed" Rx

Pyridoxine [Vitamin B₆] **Uses:** *Rx & prevention of vit B₆ deficiency* **Acts:** Vit B₆ supl **Dose:** *Adults. Deficiency:* 10–20 mg/d PO. *Drug-induced neuritis:* 100–200 mg/d; 25–100 mg/d prophylaxis. *Peds.* 5–25 mg/d × 3 wk **Caution:** [A (C if doses exceed RDA), +] **CI:** Component allergy **Disp:** Tabs 25, 50, 100 mg; Inj 100 mg/mL **SE:** Allergic Rxns, HA, N

Quetiapine (Seroquel, Seroquel XR) **BOX:** Closely monitor pts for worsening depression or emergence of suicidality, particularly in ped pts; not for use in peds; ↑ mortality in elderly w/ dementia-related psychosis **Uses:** *Acute exacerbations of schizophrenia* **Acts:** Serotonin & dopamine antagonist **Dose:** 150–750 mg/d; initiate at 25–100 mg bid-tid; slowly ↓ dose; *XR:* 400–800 mg PO q P.M.; start 300 mg/d, ↑ 300 mg/d, 800 mg d max ↓ dose w/ hepatic & geriatric pts **Caution:** [C, –] **CI:** Component allergy **Disp:** Tabs 25, 50, 100, 200, 300, 400 mg; 200, 300, 400 XR **SE:** Confusion w/ nefazodone; HA, somnolence, ↑ wgt,

↓ BP, dizziness, cataracts, neuroleptic malignant synd, tardive dyskinesia, ↑ QT internal

Quinapril (Accupril) **BOX:** ACE inhib used during PRG can cause fetal injury & death **Uses:** *HTN, CHF, DN, post-MI* **Acts:** ACE inhib **Dose:** 10–80 mg PO daily; ↓ in renal impair **Caution:** [D, +] w/ RAS, vol depletion **CI:** ACE inhib sensitivity, angioedema, PRG **Disp:** Tabs 5, 10, 20, 40 mg **SE:** Dizziness, HA, ↓ BP, impaired renal Fxn, angioedema, taste perversion, cough

Quinidine (Quinidex, Quinaglute) **BOX:** Mortality rates increased when used to treat non-life- threatening arrhythmias **Uses:** *Prevention of tachy dysrhythmias, malaria* **Acts:** Class IA antiarrhythmic **Dose:** *Adults.* *AF/A flutter conversion:* After digitalization, 200 mg q2–3h × 8 doses; ↑ daily to 3–4 g max or nl rhythm. *Peds.* 15–60 mg/kg/24 h PO in 4–5 ÷ doses; ↓ in renal impair **Caution:** [C, +] w/ Ritonavir **CI:** Digitalis tox & AV block; conduction disorders **Disp:** *Sulfate:* Tabs 200, 300 mg; SR tabs 300 mg. *Gluconate:* SR tabs 324 mg; Inj 80 mg/mL **SE:** Extreme ↓ BP w/ IV use; syncope, QT prolongation, GI upset, arrhythmias, fatigue, cinchonism (tinnitus, hearing loss, delirium, visual changes), fever, hemolytic anemia, thrombocytopenia, rash **Notes:** *Trough:* just before next dose. *Therapeutic:* 2–5 mcg/mL *Toxic:* >10 mcg/mL *1/2Half-life:* 6–8h; sulfate salt 83% quinidine; gluconate salt 62% quinidine; use w/ drug that slows AV conduction (e.g., digoxin, diltiazem, β-blocker)

Quinupristin–Dalfopristin (Synercid) **Uses:** *Vancomycin-resistant infxns d/t E. faecium & other gram(+)* **Acts:** ↓ Ribosomal protein synth. *Spectrum:* Vancomycin-resistant E. faecium, methicillin-susceptible S. aureus, S. pyogenes; not against E. faecalis **Dose:** *Adults & Peds.* 7.5 mg/kg IV q8–12h (central line preferred); incompatible w/ NS or heparin; flush IV w/ dextrose; ↓ w/ hepatic failure **Caution:** [B, M] Multiple drug interactions w/ drugs metabolized by CYP3A4 (e.g., cyclosporine) **CI:** Component allergy **Disp:** Inj 500 mg (150 mg quinupristin/350 mg dalfopristin) 600 mg (180 quinupristin/420 mg dalfopristin) **SE:** Hyperbilirubinemia, Inf site Rxns & pain, arthralgia, myalgia

Rabeprazole (AcipHex) **Uses:** *PUD, GERD, ZE* *H. pylori* **Acts:** Proton pump inhib **Dose:** 20 mg/d; may ↑ to 60 mg/d; *H. pylori* 20 mg PO bid × 7 d (w/ amoxicillin and clarithromycin); do not crush/chew tabs **Caution:** [B, ?/–] do not use w/ clopidogrel (↓ effect) **Disp:** Tabs 20 mg ER **SE:** HA, fatigue, GI upset **Notes:** ? ↑ risk of fractures w/ all PPI

Raloxifene (Evista) **BOX:** Increased risk of venous thromboembolism and death from stroke **Uses:** *Prevent osteoporosis, breast CA prevention* **Acts:** Partial antagonist of estrogen, behaves like estrogen **Dose:** 60 mg/d **Caution:** [X, –] **CI:** Thromboembolism, PRG **Disp:** Tabs 60 mg **SE:** Chest pain, insomnia, rash, hot flashes, GI upset, hepatic dysfunction, leg cramps

Raltegravir (Isentress) **BOX:** Development of immune reconstitution synd: ↑ CK, myopathy and rhabdomyolysis **Uses:** *HIV in combo w/ other antiretroviral agents* **Acts:** HIV-integrase strand transfer inhib **Dose:** 400 mg PO bid, 800 mg PO bid if w/ rifampin; w/ or w/o food **Caution:** [C, –] **CI:** None **Disp:** tabs 400 mg **SE:** N/D, HA, fever, ↑ cholesterol, paranoia and anxiety **Notes:** Monitor lipid profile; initial therapy may cause immune reconstitution synd (inflammatory response to residual opportunistic infections (e.g., *M. avium, Pneumocystis jiroveci*)

Ramipril (Altace) **BOX:** ACE inhib used during PRG can cause fetal injury & death **Uses:** *HTN, CHF, DN, post-MI* **Acts:** ACE inhib **Dose:** 2.5–20 mg/d PO ÷ daily-bid; ↓ in renal failure **Caution:** [D, +] **CI:** ACE inhib-induced angioedema **Disp:** Caps 1.25, 2.5, 5, 10 mg **SE:** Cough, HA, dizziness, ↓ BP, renal impair, angioedema **Notes:** OK in combo w/ diuretics

Ranibizumab (Lucentis) **Uses:** *Neovascular "wet" macular degeneration* **Acts:** VEGF inhib **Dose:** 0.5 mg intravitreal Inj q mo **Caution:** [C,; ?] Hx thromboembolism **CI:** periocular Infxn **Disp:** Inj **SE:** Endophthalmitis, retinal detachment/hemorrhage, cataract, intraocular inflammation, conjunctival hemorrhage, eye pain, floaters

Ranitidine Hydrochloride (Zantac, Zantac OTC, Zantac EFFERdose) **Uses:** *Duodenal ulcer, active benign ulcers, hypersecretory conditions, & GERD* **Acts:** H₂-receptor antagonist **Dose:** *Adults.* Ulcer: 150 mg PO bid, 300 mg PO hs, or 50 mg IV q6–8h; or 400 mg IV/d cont Inf, then maint of 150 mg PO hs. *Hypersecretion:* 150 mg PO bid, up to 600 mg/d. *GERD:* 300 mg PO bid; maint 300 mg PO hs. *Dyspepsia:* 75 mg PO daily-bid. *Peds.* 0.75–1.5 mg/kg/dose IV q6–8h or 1.25–2.5 mg/kg/dose PO q12h; ↓ in renal Insuff/failure **Caution:** [B, +] **CI:** Component allergy **Disp:** Tabs 75 [OTC], 150, 300 mg; caps 150, 300 mg; effervescent tabs 25 mg (contains phenylalanine); syrup 15 mg/mL; Inj 25 mg/mL **SE:** Dizziness, sedation, rash, GI upset **Notes:** PO & parenteral doses differ

Ranolazine (Ranexa) **Uses:** *Chronic angina* **Acts:** ↓ Ischemia-related Na⁺ entry into myocardium **Dose:** *Adults.* 500 mg bid-1000 mg PO bid **CI:** w/ Hepatic impair, CYP3A inhib (Table 10 p 280); w/ agents that ↑ QT interval; ↓ K⁺ **Caution:** [C, ?/–] HTN may develop w/ renal impair **Disp:** SR tabs 500 mg **SE:** Dizziness, HA, constipation, arrhythmias **Notes:** Not first 1st line; use w/ amlodipine, nitrates, β-blockers

Rasagiline mesylate (Azilect) **Uses:** *Early Parkinson Dz monotherapy; levodopa adjunct w/ advanced Dz* **Acts:** MAO B inhib **Dose:** *Adults.* Early Dz: 1 mg PO daily, start 0.5 mg PO daily w/ levodopa; ↓ w/ CYP1A2 inhib or hepatic impair **CI:** MAOIs, sympathomimetic amines, meperidine, methadone, tramadol, propoxyphene, dextromethorphan, mirtazapine, cyclobenzaprine, St. John's wort, sympathomimetic vasoconstrictors, general anesthetics, SSRIs **Caution:** [C, ?] Avoid tyramine-containing foods; mod/severe hepatic impair **Disp:** Tabs 0.5, 1 mg **SE:** Arthralgia, indigestion, dyskinesia, hallucinations, ↓ wgt, postural ↓ BP, N/, V, constipation, xerostomia, rash, sedation, CV conduction disturbances **Notes:** Rare melanoma reported; periodic skin exams (skin cancer risk); D/C 14 d prior to elective surgery; initial ↓ levodopa dose OK

Rasburicase (Elitek) BOX: Anaphylaxis possible; do not use in G6PD deficiency and hemolysis; can cause methemoglobinemia; can interfere w/uric acid assays; collect blood samples and store on ice Uses: *Reduce ↑ uric acid d/t tumor lysis* Acts: Catalyzes uric acid Dose: Adult & Peds. 0.20 mg/kg IV over 30 min, daily × 5; do not bolus Caution: [C, ?/–] Falsely ↓ uric acid values CI: Anaphylaxis, screen for G6PD deficiency to avoid hemolysis, methemoglobinemia Disp: 1.5, 7.5 mg powder Inj SE: Fever, neutropenia, GI upset, HA, rash Note: Place blood test tube for uric acid level on ice to stop enzymatic Rxn; removed by dialysis

Repaglinide (Prandin) Uses: *Type 2 DM* Acts: ↑ Pancreatic insulin release Dose: 0.5–4 mg ac, PO start 1–2 mg, ↑ to 16 mg/d max; take pc Caution: [C, ?/–] CI: DKA, type 1 DM Disp: Tabs 0.5, 1, 2 mg SE: HA, hyper-/hypoglycemia, GI upset

Retapamulin (Altabax) Uses: *Topical Rx impetigo in pts >9 mo* Acts: Pleuromutilin antibiotic, bacteriostatic, ↓ bacteria protein synth; *Spectrum: S. aureus* (not MRSA), *S. pyogenes* Dose: Apply bid × 5 d Caution: [B, ?] Disp: 10 mg/1 g SE: Local irritation

Reteplase (Retavase) Uses: *Post-AMI* Acts: Thrombolytic Dose: 10 units IV over 2 min, 2nd dose in 30 min, 10 units IV over 2 min; 10 units IV bolus over 2 min; 30 min later, 10 units IV bolus over 2 min NS flush before and after each dose [ECC 2005] Caution: [C, ?/–] CI: Internal bleeding, spinal surgery/trauma, Hx CNS AVM/CVA, bleeding diathesis, severe uncontrolled ↑ BP, sensitivity to thrombolytics Disp: Inj 10.8 units/2 mL SE: Bleeding including CNS, allergic Rxns

Ribavirin (Virazole, Copegus) BOX: Monotherapy for chronic hep C ineffective; hemolytic anemia possible, teratogenic and embryocidal; use 2 forms of birth control for up to 6 mo after D/C drug; decrease in resp fxn when used in infants as Inh Uses: *RSV Infxn in infants [Virazole]; hep C (in combo w/ interferon- αalfa-2b [Copegus])* Acts: Unknown Dose: *RSV:* 6 g in 300 mL sterile H₂O, inhale over 12–18 h. *Hep C:* 600 mg PO bid in combo w/ interferon-α₂ᵦ alfa-2b (see Rebetron) Caution: [X, ?] May accumulate on soft contacts lenses CI: PRG, autoimmune hep, CrCl <50 mL/min Disp: Powder for aerosol 6 g; tabs 200, 400, 600 mg, caps 200 mg, soln 40 mg/mL SE: Fatigue, HA, GI upset, anemia, myalgia, alopecia, bronchospasm, ↓ HCT; pancytopenia reported Notes: Virazole aerosolized by a SPAG, monitor resp Fxn closely; ✓ Hgb/Hct; PRG test monthly; hep C viral genotyping may modify dose

Rifabutin (Mycobutin) Uses: *Prevent MAC Infxn in AIDS pts w/ CD4 count <100 microL* Acts: ↓ DNA-dependent RNA polymerase activity Dose: *Adults.* 150–300 mg/d PO. *Peds 1 y:* 15–25 mg/kg/d PO. *2–10 y:* 4.4–18.8 mg/kg/d PO. *14–16 y:* 2.8–5.4 mg/kg/d PO Caution: [B,; ?/–] WBC <1000 cells/mm³ or plts <50,000 cells/mm³; ritonavir CI: Allergy Disp: Caps 150 mg SE: Discolored urine, rash, neutropenia, leukopenia, myalgia, ↑ LFTs **Notes:** SE/interactions similar to rifampin

Rifampin (Rifadin) **Uses:** *TB & Rx & prophylaxis of *N. meningitidis, H. influenzae,* or *S. aureus* carriers* **Acts:** ↓ DNA-dependent RNA polymerase **Dose:** *Adults. N. meningitidis* & *H. influenzae* carrier: 600 mg/d PO for 4 d. *TB:* 600 mg PO or IV daily or 2×/wk w/ combo regimen. *Peds.* 10–20 mg/kg/dose PO or IV daily-bid; ↓ in hepatic failure **Caution:** [C, +] w/ Fosamprenavir, multiple drug interactions **CI:** Allergy, active *N. meningitidis* Infxn, w/ saquinavir/ritonavir **Disp:** Caps 150, 300 mg; Inj 600 mg **SE:** Red-orange-colored bodily fluids, ↑ LFTs, flushing, HA **Notes:** Never use as single agent w/ active TB

Rifapentine (Priftin) **Uses:** *Pulm TB* **Acts:** ↓ DNA-dependent RNA polymerase. *Spectrum: Mycobacterium tuberculosis* **Dose:** *Intensive phase:* 600 mg PO 2×/wk for 2 mo; separate doses by >3 d. *Continuation phase:* 600 mg/wk for 4 mo; part of 3–4 drug regimen **Caution:** [C, +/− red-orange breast milk] Strong CYP450 inducer, ↓ protease inhib efficacy, antiepileptics, β-blockers, CCBs **CI:** Rifamycins allergy **Disp:** 150-mg tabs **SE:** Neutropenia, hyperuricemia, HTN, HA, dizziness, rash, GI upset, blood dyscrasias, ↑ LFTs, hematuria, discolored secretions **Notes:** Monitor LFTs

Rifaximin (Xifaxan) **Uses:** *Traveler's D (noninvasive strains of *E. coli*) in pts >12 y* **Acts:** Not absorbed, derivative of rifamycin. *Spectrum: E. coli* **Dose:** 1 tab PO daily × 3 d **Caution:** [C, ?/−) Hx allergy; pseudomembranous colitis **CI:** Allergy to rifamycins **Disp:** Tabs 200 mg **SE:** Flatulence, HA, Abd pain, GI distress, fever **Notes:** D/C if Sx worsen or persist >24–48 h, or w/ fever or blood in stool

Rimantadine (Flumadine) **Uses:** *Prophylaxis & Rx of influenza A viral infxns* **Acts:** Antiviral **Dose:** *Adults & Peds >9 y:* 100 mg PO bid. *Peds 1–9 y:* 5 mg/kg/d PO, 150 mg/d max; daily w/ severe renal/hepatic impair & elderly; initiate w/in 48 h of Sx onset **Caution:** [C, −] w/ Cimetidine; avoid w/ PRG, breastfeeding **CI:** Component & amantadine allergy **Disp:** Tabs 100 mg; syrup 50 mg/5 mL **SE:** Orthostatic ↓ BP, edema, dizziness, GI upset, ↓ Sz threshold **Note:** See CDC (*MMWR*) for current Influenza A guidelines

Rimexolone (Vexol Ophthalmic) **Uses:** *Post-op inflammation & uveitis* **Acts:** Steroid **Dose:** *Adults & Peds >2 y: Uveitis:* 1–2 gtt/h daytime & q2h at night, taper to 1 gtt q4h. *Post-op:* 1–2 gtt qid × 2 wk **Caution:** [C, ?/−] Ocular infxns **Disp:** Susp 1% **SE:** Blurred vision, local irritation **Notes:** Taper dose

Risedronate (Actonel, Actonel w/ calcium) **Uses:** *Paget Dz; Rx/prevention glucocorticoid-induced/postmenopausal osteoporosis, ↑ bone mass in osteoporotic men; w/ calcium only FDA approved for female osteoporosis* **Acts:** Bisphosphonate; ↓ osteoclast-mediated bone resorption **Dose:** *Paget Dz:* 30 mg/d PO for 2 mo. *Osteoporosis Rx/prevention:* 5 mg daily or 35 mg q wk; 30 min before 1st food/drink of the d; stay upright for at least 30 min after dose **Caution:** [C, ?/−] Ca²⁺ supls & antacids ↓ absorption; jaw osteonecrosis, avoid dental work

CI: Component allergy, ↓ Ca^{2+}, esophageal abnormalities, unable to stand/sit for 30 min, CrCl <30 mL/min **Disp:** Tabs 5, 30, 35, 75 mg; Risedronate 35 mg (4 tabs)/ calcium carbonate 1250 mg (24 tabs) **SE:** Back pain, HA, Abd pain, dyspepsia, arthralgia; flu-like Sxs, hypersensitivity (rash, etc), esophagitis, bone pain, eye inflammation **Notes:** Monitor LFTs, Ca^{2+}, PO^{3+}, K^+; may ↑ atypical subtrochanteric femur fractures

Risperidone, Oral (Risperdal, Risperdal M-Tab) **BOX:** ↑ Mortality in elderly w/ dementia-related psychosis **Uses:** *Psychotic disorders (schizophrenia)*, dementia of the elderly, bipolar disorder, mania, Tourette disorder, autism **Acts:** Benzisoxazole antipsychotic **Dose:** *Adults.* 0.5–6 mg PO bid; *M-Tab:* 1–6 mg/d start 1–2 mg/d, titrate q3–7d. *Peds.* 0.25 mg PO bid, ↑ q5–7d; ↓ start dose w/ elderly, renal/hepatic impair **Caution:** [C, –], ↓ BP w/ antihypertensives, clozapine **CI:** Component allergy **Disp:** Tabs 0.25, 0.5, 1, 2, 3, 4 mg; soln 1 mg/mL, *M-Tab* (ODT) tabs 0.5, 1, 2, 3, 4 mg **SE:** Orthostatic ↓ BP, EPS w/ high dose, tachycardia, arrhythmias, sedation, dystonias, neuroleptic malignant synd, sexual dysfunction, constipation, xerostomia, ↓ WBC, neutropenia and agranulocytosis, cholestatic jaundice **Notes:** Several wk for effect

Risperidone, Parenteral (Risperdal Consta) **BOX:** Not approved for dementia-related psychosis; ↑ mortality risk in elderly dementia pts on atypical antipsychotics; most deaths d/t CV or infectious events **Uses:** Schizophrenia **Acts:** Benzisoxazole antipsychotic **Dose:** 25 mg q2wk IM may ↑ to max 50 mg q2wk; w/ renal/hepatic impair start PO Risperdal 0.5 mg PO bid × 1 wk titrate weekly **Caution:** [C, –], ↑ BP w/ antihypertensives, clozapine **CI:** Component allergy **Disp:** Inj 25, 37.5, 50 mg/vial **SE:** See Risperidone, oral **Note:** Long-acting Inj

Ritonavir (Norvir) **BOX:** Life-threatening adverse events when used w/ certain nonsedating antihistamines, sedative hypnotics, antiarrhythmics, or ergot alkaloids d/t inhibited drug metabolism **Uses:** *HIV* **Actions:** Protease inhib; ↓ maturation of immature noninfectious virions to mature infectious virus **Dose:** *Adults.* Initial 300 mg PO bid, titrate over 1 wk to 600 mg PO bid (titration will ↓ GI SE). *Peds >1 mo:* 250 mg/m² titrate to 400 mg bid (adjust w/ fosamprenavir, indinavir, nelfinavir, & saquinavir); take w/ food **Caution:** [B, +] w/ Ergotamine, amiodarone, bepridil, flecainide, propafenone, quinidine, pimozide, midazolam, triazolam **CI:** Component allergy **Disp:** Caps 100 mg; soln 80 mg/mL **SE:** ↑ Triglycerides, ↑ LFTs, N/V/D/C, Abd pain, taste perversion, anemia, weakness, HA, fever, malaise, rash, paresthesias **Notes:** Refrigerate

Rivastigmine (Exelon) **Uses:** *Mild–mod dementia in Alzheimer Dz* **Acts:** Enhances cholinergic activity **Dose:** 1.5 mg bid; ↑ to 6 mg bid, w/ ↑ at 2-wk intervals (take w/ food) **Caution:** [B, ?] w/ β-Blockers, CCBs, smoking, neuromuscular blockade, digoxin **CI:** Rivastigmine or carbamate allergy **Disp:** Caps 1.5, 3, 4.5, 6 mg; soln 2 mg/mL **SE:** Dose-related GI effects, N/V/D, dizziness, insomnia, fatigue, tremor, diaphoresis, HA, wgt loss (in 18–26%) **Notes:** Swallow caps whole, do not break/chew/crush; avoid EtOH

Rivastigmine, Transdermal (Exelon Patch) Uses: *Mild/mod Alzheimer and Parkinson Dz dementia* Acts: Acetylcholinesterase inhib Dose: *Initial:* 4.6-mg patch/d applied to back, chest, upper arm, ↑ 9.5 mg after 4 wk if tolerated Caution: [?/ ?] Sick sinus synd, conduction defects, asthma, COPD, urinary obst, Szs CI: Hypersens to rivastigmine, other carbamates Disp: Transdermal patch 5 cm² (4.6 mg/24 h), 10 cm² (9.5 mg/24 h) SE: N/V/D

Rizatriptan (Maxalt, Maxalt MLT) Uses: *Rx acute migraine* Acts: Vascular serotonin receptor agonist Dose: 5–10 mg PO, repeat in 2 h, PRN, 30 mg/d max Caution: [C, M] CI: Angina, ischemic heart Dz, ischemic bowel Dz, hemiplegic/basilar migraine, uncontrolled HTN, ergot or serotonin 5-HT₁ agonist use w/in 24 h, MAOI use w/in 14 d Disp: Tab 5, 10 mg; *Maxalt MLT:* OD tabs 5, 10 mg. SE: Chest pain, palpitations, N, V, asthenia, dizziness, somnolence, fatigue

Rocuronium (Zemuron) Uses: *Skeletal muscle relaxation during rapid-sequence intubation, surgery, or mechanical ventilation* Acts: Nondepolarizing neuromuscular blocker Dose: *Rapid sequence intubation:* 0.6–1.2 mg/kg IV. *Continuous Inf:* 5–12.5 mcg/kg/min IV; adjust/titrate based on monitoring; ↓ in hepatic impair Caution: [C, ?] Aminoglycosides, vancomycin, tetracycline, polymyxins enhance blockade CI: Component or pancuronium allergy Disp: Inj preservative-free 10 mg/mL SE: BP changes, tachycardia

Romidepsin (Istodax) Uses: *Rx cutaneous T-cell lymphoma in pts who have received at least one prior systemic therapy* Action: Histone deacetylase (HDAC) inhibitor Dose: 14 mg/m² IV over 4h days 1, 8 and 15 of a 28-day cycle; repeat cycles every 28 days if tolerated; treatment d/c or interruption w/ or w/o dose reduction to 10 mg/m² to manage adverse drug reactions Caution: [D, ?] risk of ↑QT, hematologic toxicity; strong CYP3A4 inhibitors may ↑ conc Disp: Inj 10 mg SE: N, V, fatigue, infxn, anorexia, ↓ plt Notes: Hazardous agent, precautions for handling and disposal

Romiplostim (Nplate) BOX: ↑ risk for heme malignancies and thromboembolism. D/C may worsen ↓ plt Uses: *Rx ↓ Plt d/t ITP w/poor response to other therapies* Action: Thrombopoietic, thrombopoietin receptor agonist Dose: *Adults.* 1 mcg/kg SQ weekly, adjust 1 mcg/kg/week to plt count > 50,000/mm³; max 10 mcg/kg/wk Caution: [C, /?] CI: None Disp: 500 mcg/mL (250- mcg vial) SE: HA, fatigue, dizziness, N/V/D, myalgia, epistaxis Notes: ✓ CBC/diff/Plt weekly; plt ↑ 4–9 d, peak 12-16 d; D/C if no ↑ plt after 4 wks max dose; ↓ dose w/ plt count >200,000/mm³.

Ropinirole (Requip) Uses: *Rx of Parkinson Dz, restless leg synd (RLS)* Acts: Dopamine agonist Dose: Initial 0.25 mg PO tid, weekly ↑ 0.25 mg/dose, to 3 mg max, max 4 mg for RLS Caution: [C, ?/–] Severe CV/renal/hepatic impair CI: Component allergy Disp: Tabs 0.25, 0.5, 1, 2, 3, 4, 5 mg SE: Syncope, postural ↓ BP, N/V, HA, somnolence, dosed-related hallucinations, dyskinesias, dizziness Notes: D/C w/ 7-d taper

Rosiglitazone (Avandia) BOX: May cause or worsen CHF; may increase myocardial ischemia Uses: *Type 2 DM* Acts: Thiazolidinedione; ↑ insulin sensitivity **Dose:** 4–8 mg/d PO or in 2 ÷ doses (w/o regard to meals) **Caution:** [C, –] w/ ESRD, CHF, edema, **CI:** DKA, severe CHF (NYHA class III), ALT >2.5 ULN **Disp:** Tabs 2, 4, 8 mg **SE:** May ↑ CV, CHF & ? CA risk; wgt gain, hyperlipidemia, HA, edema, fluid retention, worsen CHF, hepatic damage w/ ↑ LFTs **Notes:** Not OK in class III, IV heart Dz; ? increased MI risk

Rosuvastatin (Crestor) **Uses:** *Rx primary hypercholesterolemia & mixed dyslipidemia* **Acts:** HMG-CoA reductase inhib **Dose:** 5–40 mg PO daily; max 5 mg/d w/ cyclosporine, 10 mg/d w/ gemfibrozil or CrCl <30 mL/min (avoid Al-/Mg-based antacids for 2 h after) **Caution:** [X, ?/–] **CI:** Active liver Dz, unexplained ↑ LFTs **Disp:** Tabs 5, 10, 20, 40 mg **SE:** Myalgia, constipation, asthenia, Abd pain, N, myopathy, rarely rhabdomyolysis **Notes:** May ↑ warfarin effect; monitor LFTs at baseline, 12 wk, then q6mo; ↓ dose in Asian pts

Rotavirus Vaccine, Live, Oral, Monovalent (Rotarix) **Uses:** *Prevent rotavirus gastroenteritis in peds* **Acts:** Active immunization w/ live attenuated rotavirus **Dose:** *Peds 6–14 wk:* 1st dose PO at 6 wk of age, wait at least 4 wk then a 2nd dose by 24 wk of age. **Caution:** [C, ?] **CI:** Component sensitivity, uncorrected congenital GI malformation, chronic GI illness, acute mod-severe D illness, fever **Disp:** single -dose vial **SE:** Irritability, cough, runny nose, fever, ↓ appetite, V **Notes:** Begin series by age 12 wk, conclude by age 24 wk; can be given to infant in house w/ immunosuppressed family member or mother who is breast feeding. Safety and effectiveness not studied in immunocompromised infants.

Rotavirus Vaccine, Live, Oral, Pentavalent (RotaTeq) **Uses:** *Prevent rotavirus gastroenteritis in peds* **Acts:** Active immunization w/ live attenuated rotavirus **Dose:** *Peds 6–14 wk:* Single dose PO at 2, 4, & 6 mo **Caution:** [?, ?] **CI:** Uncorrected congenital GI malformation, chronic GI illness, acute diarrheal illness, fever **Disp:** Oral susp 2-mL single-use tubes **SE:** Fever, D/V **Notes:** Begin series by age 12 wk and conclude by age 32 wk; can be given to infant in house w/ immunosuppressed family member or mother who is breast-feeding. Safety and effectiveness not studied in immunocompromised infants.

Rufinamide (Banzel) **BOX:** Antiepileptics associated w/ ↑ risk of suicide ideation. Severe hypersens rxns reported **Uses:** *Adjunct Lennox-Gastaut seizures* **Action:** Anticonvulsant **Dose:** *Adults.* *Initial:* 400-800 mg/d ÷ bid (max 3200 mg/d ÷ bid) *Peds.≥4 yrs:* *Initial:* 10 mg/kg/day ÷ bid, target 45 mg/kg/day ÷ bid; 3200 mg/d MAX **Caution:** [C, –/] **CI:** familial short QT synd **Disp:** Tab: 200, 400 mg **SE:** ↑ QT, HA, somnolence, N/V, ataxia, rash **Notes:** Monitor for rash; use w/ OCP may lead to contraceptive failure

Salmeterol (Serevent Diskus) **BOX:** Long-acting β_2-agonists, such as salmeterol, may ↑ risk of asthma-related death. Do not use alone, only as additional Rx for pts not controlled on other asthma meds **Uses:** *Asthma, exercise-induced asthma, COPD* **Acts:** Sympathomimetic bronchodilator, long acting β_2-agonist **Dose:** *Adults & Peds >12 y:* 1 Diskus-dose inhaled bid **Caution:** [C, ?/–] **CI:** Acute asthma; w/in 14 d of MAOI; w/o concomitant use of inhaled steroid **Disp:** 50 mcg/dose, dry powder discus, metered-dose inhaler, 21 mcg/activation **SE:** HA, pharyngitis, tachycardia, arrhythmias, nervousness, GI upset, tremors **Notes:** Not for acute attacks; must use w/ steroid or short-acting β-agonist

Saquinavir (Fortovase, Invirase) **BOX:** Invirase and Fortovase not bioequivalent/interchangeable; must use Invirase in combo w/ ritonavir, which provides saquinavir plasma levels = to those w/ Fortovase **Uses:** *HIV Infxn* **Acts:** HIV protease inhib **Dose:** 1200 mg PO tid w/in 2 h pc (dose adjust w/ ritonavir, delavirdine, lopinavir, & nelfinavir) **Caution:** [B, +] w/ Ketoconazole, statins, sildenafil **CI:** w/ Rifampin, severe hepatic impair, allergy, sun exposure w/o sunscreen/clothing, triazolam, midazolam, ergots, **Disp:** Caps 200 mg:, tabs 500 mg **SE:** Dyslipidemia, lipodystrophy, rash, hyperglycemia, GI upset, weakness **Notes:** Take 2 h after meal, avoid direct sunlight

Sargramostim [GM-CSF] (Leukine) **Uses:** *Myeloid recovery following BMT or chemotherapy* **Acts:** Recombinant GF, activates mature granulocytes & macrophages **Dose:** *Adults & Peds.* 250 mcg/m^2/d IV for 21 d (BMT) **Caution:** [C, ?/–] Li, corticosteroids **CI:** >10% blasts, allergy to yeast, concurrent chemotherapy/RT **Disp:** Inj 250, 500 mcg **SE:** Bone pain, fever, ↓ BP, tachycardia, flushing, GI upset, myalgia **Notes:** Rotate Inj sites; use APAP PRN for pain

Saxagliptin (Onglyza) **Uses:** * Monotherapy/combo for Type 2 DM* **Action:** Dipeptidyl peptidase-4 (DDP-4) inhibitor, ↑insulin synth/release **Dose:** 2.5 or 5 mg once/d w/o regard to meals; 2.5 mg once/d w/ CrCl < 50 ml/min or w/ strong CYP 3A4/5 inhibitor (e.g. atazanavir, clarithromycin, indinavir, itraconazole, ketoconazole, nefazodone, nelfinavir, ritonavir, saquinavir, and telithromycin) **Caution:** [B, ?] may ↓ glucose when used w/ insulin secretagogues (e.g., sulfonylureas) **CI:** w/ insulin or to treat DKA **Disp:** Tabs 2.5,5 mg **SE:** URI, nasopharyngitis, UTI, HA, **Notes:** No evidence for ↑ CV risk

Scopolamine, Scopolamine transdermal & ophthalmic (Scopace, Transderm-Scop) **Uses:** *Prevent N/V associated w/ motion sickness, anesthesia, opiates; mydriatic*, cycloplegic, Rx uveitis & iridocyclitis **Acts:** Anticholinergic, inhibits iris & ciliary bodies, antiemetic **Dose:** 1 mg/72 h, 1 patch behind ear q3d; apply >4 h before exposure; cycloplegic 1–2 gtt 1 h preprocedure, uveitis 1–2 gtt up to qid max; ↓ in elderly **Caution:** [C, +] w/ APAP, levodopa, ketoconazole, digitalis, KCl **CI:** NAG, GI or GU obst, thyrotoxicosis, paralytic ileus **Disp:** Patch 1.5 mg, (releases 1 mg over 72 h), ophthal 0.25% **SE:** Xerostomia, drowsiness, blurred vision, tachycardia, constipation **Notes:** Do not blink excessively after dose, wait 5 min before dosing other eye; antiemetic activity w/ patch requires several hours

Secobarbital (Seconal) [C-II] **Uses:** *Insomnia, short-term use *, preanesthetic agent **Acts:** Rapid-acting barbiturate **Dose:** *Adults.* 100–200 mg hs, 100–300 mg pre-op. *Peds.* 2–6 mg/kg/dose, 100 mg/max, ↓ in elderly **Caution:**

[D, +] w/ CYP2C9, 3A3/4, 3A5/7 inducer (Table 10 p 280); ↑ tox w/ other CNS depressants CI: Porphyria, w/ voriconazole, PRG Disp: Caps 50, 100 mg SE: Tolerance in 1–2 wk; resp depression, CNS depression, porphyria, photosens

Selegiline, Oral (Eldepryl, Zelapar) BOX: Closely monitor for worsening depression or emergence of suicidality, particularly in ped pts Uses: *Parkinson Dz* Acts: MAOI Dose: 5 mg PO bid; 1.25–2.5 once daily tabs PO q A.M. (before breakfast w/o liq) 2.5 mg/d max; ↓ in elderly Caution: [C, ?] w/ Drugs that induce CYP3A4 (Table 10 p 280) (e.g., phenytoin, carbamazepine, nafcillin, phenobarbital, & rifampin); avoid w/ antidepressants CI: w/ Meperidine, MAOI, dextromethorphan, general anesthesia w/in 10 d, pheochromocytoma Disp: Tabs/caps 5 mg; once-daily tabs 1.25 mg SE: N, dizziness, orthostatic ↓ BP, arrhythmias, tachycardia, edema, confusion, xerostomia Notes: ↓ Carbidopa/levodopa if used in combo; see transdermal form

Selegiline, Transdermal (Emsam) BOX: May ↑ risk of suicidal thinking and behavior in children and adolescents w/ major depression disorder Uses: *Depression* Acts: MAOI Dose: *Adults.* Apply patch daily to upper torso, upper thigh, or outer upper arm CI: Tyramine-containing foods w/ 9 or 12-mg doses; serotonin-sparing agents Caution: [C, –] ↑ Carbamazepine and oxcarbazepine levels Disp: ER Patches 6, 9, 12 mg SE: Local Rxns requiring topical steroids; HA, insomnia, orthostatic, ↓ BP, serotonin synd, suicide risk Notes: Rotate site; see oral form

Selenium Sulfide (Exsel Shampoo, Selsun Blue Shampoo, Selsun Shampoo) Uses: *Scalp seborrheic dermatitis*, scalp itching & flaking d/t *dandruff*; tinea versicolor Acts: Antiseborrheic Dose: *Dandruff, seborrhea:* Massage 5–10 mL into wet scalp, leave on 2–3 min, rinse, repeat; use 2× wk, then once q1–4wk PRN. *Tinea versicolor:* Apply 2.5% daily on area & lather w/ small amounts of water; leave on 10 min, then rinse Caution: [C, ?] CI: Open wounds Disp: Shampoo [OTC]; 2.5% lotion SE: Dry or oily scalp, lethargy, hair discoloration, local irritation Notes: Do not use more than 2×/wk

Sertaconazole (Ertaczo) Uses: *Topical Rx interdigital tinea pedis* Acts: Imidazole antifungal. *Spectrum: Trichophyton rubrum, Trichophyton mentagrophytes, Epidermophyton floccosum* Dose: *Adults & Peds >12:* Apply between toes & immediate surrounding healthy skin bid × 4 wk Caution: [C, ?] CI: Component allergy Disp: 2% Cream SE: Contact dermatitis, dry/burning skin, tenderness Notes: Use in immunocompetent pts; not for oral, intravag, ophthal use

Sertraline (Zoloft) BOX: Closely monitor pts for worsening depression or emergence of suicidality, particularly in ped pts Uses: *Depression, panic disorders, OCD,PTSD)*, * social anxiety disorder, eating disorders, premenstrual disorders Acts: ↓ Neuronal uptake of serotonin Dose: *Adults. Depression:* 50–200 mg/d PO. *PTSD:* 25 mg PO daily × 1 wk, then 50 mg PO daily, 200 mg/d max. *Peds 6–12 y:* 25 mg PO daily. *13–17 y:* 50 mg PO daily Caution: [C, ?/–] w/ Haloperidol (serotonin synd), sumatriptan, linezolid, hepatic impair CI: MAOI use w/in 14 d;

concomitant pimozide **Disp:** Tabs 25, 50, 100, 150, 200 mg; 20 mg/mL oral **SE:** Activate manic/hypomanic state, ↓ wgt, insomnia, somnolence, fatigue, tremor, xerostomia, N/D, dyspepsia, ejaculatory dysfunction, ↓ libido, hepatotox

Sevelamer carbonate (Renvela) **Uses:** *Control ↑ PO_4^{3-} in ESRD* **Acts:** Phosphate binder **Dose:** *Initial:* PO_4^{3-} >5.5 and <7.5 mg/dL: 800 mg PO; ≥7.5 mg/dL: 1600 mg PO tid. *Switching from Sevelamer HCl:* g/-per-g basis; titrate ↑/↓ 1 tab/meal 2-wk intervals PRN; take w/ food **Caution:** [C, ?] w/ Swallow disorders, bowel problems, may ↓ absorption of vits D, E, K, ↓ ciprofloxacin & other medicine levels **CI:** ↓ PO_4^{3-}, bowel obst **Disp:** Tab 800 mg **SE:** N/V/D, dyspepsia, Abd pain, flatulence, constipation **Notes:** Separate other meds 1 h before or 3 h after

Sevelamer HCl (Renagel) **Uses:** *↓ PO_4^{3-} in ESRD* **Acts:** Binds intestinal PO_4^{3-} **Dose:** 2–4 caps PO tid w/ meals; adjust based on PO_4^{3-}; max 4 g/dose **Caution:** [C, ?] May ↓ absorption of vits D, E, K, ↓ ciprofloxacin & other medicine levels **CI:** ↓ PO_4^{3-}, bowel obst **Disp:** Tab 400, 800 mg **SE:** BP changes, N/V/D, dyspepsia, thrombosis **Notes:** Do not open/chew caps; separate other meds 1 h before or 3 h after; 800 mg sevelamer = 667 mg Ca acetate

Sibutramine (Meridia) [C-IV] **Uses:** *Obesity* **Acts:** Blocks uptake of norepinephrine, serotonin, dopamine **Dose:** 10 mg/d PO, may ↑ mg/d after 4 wk **Caution:** [C, –] w/ SSRIs, Li, dextromethorphan, opioids **CI:** MAOI w/in 14 d, uncontrolled HTN, arrhythmias, tachycardia, HTN **SE:** HA, insomnia, xerostomia, constipation, tachycardia, HTN **Notes:** Use w/ low-calorie diet, monitor BP; only for BMI >30 kg/m² or >27 kg/m² w/ CV risk factors; recent FDA review over possible ↑CV events

Sildenafil (Viagra, Revatio) **Uses:** *Viagra:* *ED*; *Revatio:* *Pulm artery HTN* **Acts:** ↓ Phosphodiesterase type 5 (PDE5) (responsible for cGMP breakdown); ↑ cGMP activity to relax smooth muscles & ↑ flow to corpus cavernosum and pulm vasculature; ? antiproliferative on pulm artery smooth muscle **Dose:** *ED:* 25–100 mg PO 1 h before sexual activity, max 1/d; ↓ if >65 y; avoid fatty foods w/ dose; *Revatio: Pulm HTN:* 20 mg PO tid **Caution:** [B, ?] w/ CYP3A4 inhib (Table 10 p 280), ↓ dose w/ ritonavir; retinitis pigmentosa; hepatic/severe renal impair; w/ sig hypo-/hypertension **CI:** w/ Nitrates or w/ sex not advised; w/protease inhibitors for HIV **Disp:** Tabs *Viagra:* 25, 50, 100 mg, tabs *Revatio:* 20 mg **SE:** HA; flushing; dizziness; blue haze visual change, hearing loss, priapism **Notes:** Cardiac events in presence of nitrates debatable; transient global amnesia reports

Silodosin (Rapaflo) **Uses:** *BPH* **Acts:** α-blockers of prostatic $α_{1a}$ **Dose:** 8 mg/d; 4 mg/d w/ CrCl 30–50 mL/min; take w/ food **Caution:** [B, ?], not for use in females; do not use w/ other α-blockers or w/ cyclosporine; R/O PCa before use; IFIS possible w/ cataract surgery **CI:** Severe hepatic/renal impair (CrCl <30 mL/min), w/ CYP3A4 inhib (e.g., ketoconazole, clarithromycin, itraconazole, ritonavir) **Disp:** Caps 4, 8 mg **SE:** Retrograde ejaculation, dizziness, D, syncope, somnolence, orthostatic ↓ BP, nasopharyngitis, nasal congestion **Notes:** Not for use as antihypertensive; no effect on QT interval

Silver Nitrate (Dey-Drop, Others) Uses: *Removal of granulation tissue & warts; prophylaxis in burns* Acts: Caustic antiseptic & astringent Dose: *Adults & Peds.* Apply to moist surface 2–3× wk for several wk or until effect Caution: [C, ?] CI: Do not use on broken skin Disp: Topical impregnated applicator sticks, soln 0.5, 10, 25, 50%; ophthal 1% amp; topical ointment 10% SE: May stain tissue black, usually resolves; local irritation, methemoglobinemia Notes: D/C if redness or irritation develop; no longer used in US for newborn prevention of gonococcus conjunctivitis

Silver Sulfadiazine (Silvadene, Others) Uses: *Prevention & Rx of Infxn in 2nd- & 3rd-degree burns* Acts: Bactericidal Dose: *Adults & Peds.* Aseptically cover the area w/ 1/16-inch coating bid Caution: [B unless near term, ?/–] CI: Infants <2 mo, PRG near term Disp: Cream 1% SE: Itching, rash, skin discoloration, blood dyscrasias, hep, allergy Notes: Systemic absorption w/ extensive application

Simethicone (Mylicon, Others) [OTC] Uses: Flatulence Acts: Defoaming, alters gas bubble surface tension action Dose: *Adults & Peds >12 y:* 40–125 mg PO pc & hs PRN; 500 mg/d max. *Peds <2 y:* 20 mg PO qid PRN. *2–12 y:* 40 mg PO qid PRN Caution: [C, ?] CI: GI Intestinal perforation or obst Disp: [OTC] Tabs 80, 125 mg; caps 125 mg; softgels 125, 166, 180 mg; susp 40 mg/0.6 mL; chew tabs 80, 125 mg SE: N/D Notes: Available in combo products OTC

Simvastatin (Zocor) Uses: ↓ Cholesterol Acts: HMG-CoA reductase inhib Dose: *Adults.* 5–80 mg PO; w/ meals; ↓ in renal Insuff. *Peds 10–17 y:* 10 mg, 40 mg/d max Caution: [X, –] Avoid w/gemfibrozil; avoid high dose w/diltiazem; w/Chinese pt on lipid modifying meds CI: PRG, liver Dz Disp: Tabs 5, 10, 20, 40, 80 mg SE: HA, GI upset, myalgia, myopathy (muscle pain, tenderness or weakness w/creatine kinase 10× ULN) and rhabdomyolysis, hep Notes: Combo w/ ezetimibe/simvastatin; follow LFTs; pt to report muscle pain

Sipuleucel-T (Provenge) Uses: *Asymptomatic/minimally symptomatic metastatic CRPC (hormone refractory) prostate cancer* Acts: Autologous cellular immunotherapy Dose: 3 doses IV over 60 min at approx 2 wk intervals (premed w/ acetaminophen and diphenhydramine) Caution: [D, +/–] do not use expired product or in line filter; verify patient identity to specific product; observe for acute infusion Rxn CI: None Disp: Patient-specific infusion bag 250 mL LR w/min 50 mill autologous CD54+ cells activated w/PAP GM-CSF SE: chills, fatigue, fever, back pain, N, joint ache, HA Notes: pt blood mononuclear cells are obtained by leukapheresis 3 days before infusion. Autologous peripheral blood mononuclear cells, including antigen presenting cells (APCs) are cultured w/recombinant human protein, PAP-GM-CSF and reinfused.

Sirolimus [Rapamycin] (Rapamune) BOX: Use only by physicians experienced in immunosuppression; immunosuppression associated w/ lymphoma, ↑ Infxn risk; do not use in lung transplant (fatal bronchial anastomotic dehiscence) Uses: *Prevent organ rejection in new Tx pts* Acts: ↓ T-lymphocyte activation **Dose:** *Adults >40 kg:* 6 mg PO on day 1, then 2 mg/d PO. *Peds: <40 kg & ≥13 y:* 3 mg/m² load, then 1 mg/m²/d (in H₂O/orange juice; no grapefruit juice w/ sirolimus); take 4 h after cyclosporine; ↓ in hepatic impair **Caution:** [C, ?/–] Grapefruit juice, ketoconazole **CI:** Component allergy **Disp:** Soln 1 mg/mL, tab 1, 2 mg **SE:** HTN, edema, CP, fever, HA, insomnia, acne, rash, ↑ cholesterol, GI upset, ↑/↓ K⁺, infxns, blood dyscrasias, arthralgia, tachycardia, renal impair, graft loss & death in liver transplant (hepatic artery thrombosis), ascites, delayed healing **Notes:** Levels: *Trough:* 4–20 ng/mL; varies w/assay method

Sitagliptin (Januvia) **Uses:** * monotherapy or combo for Type 2 DM* **Action:** Dipeptidyl peptidase-4 (DDP-4) inhib, ↑ insulin synth/release **Dose:** 2.5 or 5 mg once/d w/o regard to meals; 2.5 mg once/d w/ CrCl < 50 mL ml/min or w/ strong CYP 3A4/5 inhib (e.g., atazanavir, clarithromycin, indinavir, itraconazole, ketoconazole, nefazodone, nelfinavir, ritonavir, saquinavir, and telithromycin) **Caution:** [?,/ ?] may cause ↓ blood sugar when used w/ insulin secretagogues such as sulfonylureas **CI:** w/ insulin or to treat DKA **Disp:** Tabs 2.5, 5 mg **SE:** URI, nasopharyngitis, UTI, HA, **Notes:** no evidence for ↑ CV risk

Sitagliptin/Metformin (Janumet) **WARNING:** Associated w/ lactic acidosis **Uses:** *Adjunct to diet and exercise in type 2 DM* **Action:** See individual agents **Dose:** 1 tab PO bid, titrate; 100 mg sitagliptin & 2000 mg metformin/d max; take w/ meals **Caution:** [B, ?/–] **CI:** Type 1 DM, DKA, male Cr >15; female Cr >1.4 mg/dL **Disp:** Tabs 50/500, 50 mg/1000 mg **SE:** Nasopharyngitis, N/V/D, flatulence, Abd discomfort, dyspepsia, asthenia, HA **Notes:** Hold w/ contrast study;✓ Cr, CBC

Smallpox Vaccine (Dryvax) **BOX:** Acute myocarditis and other infectious complications possible; CI in immunocompromised, eczema or exfoliative skin conditions, infants <1 y **Uses:** Immunization against smallpox (variola virus) **Acts:** Active immunization (live attenuated cowpox virus) **Dose:** *Adults (routine nonemergency) or all ages (emergency):* 2–3 Punctures w/ bifurcated needle dipped in vaccine into deltoid, posterior triceps muscle; ✓ site for Rxn in 6–8 d; if major Rxn, site scabs & heals, leaving scar; if mild/equivocal Rxn, repeat w/ 15 punctures **Caution:** [X, N/A] **CI:** *Nonemergency use:* febrile illness, immunosuppression, Hx eczema & in household contacts. *Emergency:* No absolute CI **Disp:** Vial for reconstitution: 100 million pock-forming units/mL **SE:** Malaise, fever, regional lymphadenopathy, encephalopathy, rashes, spread of inoculation to other sites; SJS, eczema vaccinatum w/ severe disability **Notes:** Avoid infants for 14 d; intradermal use only; restricted distribution

Sodium Bicarbonate [NaHCO₃] **Uses:** *Alkalinization of urine, RTA, *metabolic acidosis, ↑ K⁺, TCA OD* **Acts:** Alkalinizing agent **Dose:** *Adults. Cardiac arrest:* Initiate ventilation, 1 mEq/kg IV bolus; repeat 1/2 dose q10min PRN *(ECC 2005). Metabolic acidosis:* 2–5 mEq/kg IV over 8 h & PRN based on acid–base status. ↑ K⁺: 1 mg/kg IV over 5 min. *Alkalinize urine:* 4 g (48 mEq) PO, then 1–2 g q4h; adjust based on urine pH; 2 amp (100 mEq/1 L D₅W at 100–250 mL/h IV, monitor urine pH & serum bicarbonate. *Chronic renal failure:* 1–3 mEq/

kg/d. *Distal RTA:* 1 mEq/kg/d PO. *Peds >1 y: Cardiac arrest:* See Adults dosage. *Peds <1 y: ECC 2005:* Initiate ventilation, 1:1 dilution 1 mEq/mL dosed 1 mEq/kg IV; can repeat w/ 0.5 mEq/kg in 10 min ×1 or based on acid–base status. *Chronic renal failure:* See Adults dosage. *Distal RTA:* 2–3 mEq/kg/d PO. *Proximal RTA:* 5–10 mEq/kg/d; titrate based on serum bicarbonate. *Urine alkalinization:* 84–840 mg/kg/d (1–10 mEq/kg/d) in ÷ doses; adjust based on urine pH **Caution:** [C, ?] **CI:** Alkalosis, ↑ Na^+, severe pulm edema, ↓ Ca^{2+} **Disp:** Powder, tabs; 300 mg = 3.6 mEq; 325 mg = 3.8 mEq; 520 mg = 6.3 mEq; 600 mg = 7.3 mEq; 650 mg = 7.6 mEq; Inj 1 mEq/1 mL, 4.2% (5 mEq/10 mL), 7.5% (8.92 mEq/mL), 8.4% (10 mEq/10 mL) vial or amp **SE:** Belching, edema, flatulence, ↑ Na^+, metabolic alkalosis **Notes:** 1 g neutralizes 12 mEq of acid; 50 mEq bicarbonate = 50 mEq Na; can make 3 amps in 1 L D_5W to = D_5NS w/ 150 mEq bicarbonate

Sodium Citrate/Citric Acid (Bicitra, Oracit) **Uses:** *Chronic metabolic acidosis, alkalinize urine; dissolve uric acid & cysteine stones* **Acts:** Urinary alkalinizer **Dose:** *Adults.* 10–30 mL in 1–3 oz H_2O pc & hs. *Peds.* 5–15 mL in 1–3 oz H_2O pc & hs; best after meals **Caution:** [C, +] **CI:** Al-based antacids; severe renal impair or Na-restricted diets **Disp:** 15- or 30-mL unit dose: 16 (473 mL) or 4 (118 mL) fl oz **SE:** Tetany, metabolic alkalosis, ↑ K^+, GI upset; avoid use of multiple 50-mL amps; can cause ↑ Na^+/hyperosmolality **Notes:** 1 mL = 1 mEq Na & 1 mEq bicarbonate

Sodium Oxybate (Xyrem) [C-III] **BOX:** Known drug of abuse even at recommended doses; confusion, depression, resp depression may occur **Uses:** *Narcolepsy-associated cataplexy* **Acts:** Inhibitory neurotransmitter **Dose:** *Adults & Peds >16 y:* 2.25 g PO qhs, 2nd dose 2.5–4 h later; may ↑ 9 g/d max **Caution:** [B, ?/–] **CI:** Succinic semialdehyde dehydrogenase deficiency; potentiates EtOH **Disp:** 500 mg/mL (180-mL) PO soln **SE:** Confusion, depression, ↓ diminished level of consciousness, incontinence, sig V, resp depression, psychological Sxs **Notes:** May lead to dependence; synonym for γ-hydroxybutyrate (GHB), abused as a "date rape drug"; controlled distribution (prescriber & pt registration); must be administered when pt in bed

Sodium Phosphate (Visicol) **Uses:** *Bowel prep prior to colonoscopy*, short-term constipation **Acts:** Hyperosmotic laxative **Dose:** 3 Tabs PO w/ at least 8 oz clear liq q15min (20 tabs total night before procedure; 3–5 h before colonoscopy, repeat) **Caution:** [C, ?] Renal impair, electrolyte disturbances **CI:** Megacolon, bowel obst, CHF, ascites, unstable angina, gastric retention, bowel perforation, colitis, hypomotility **Disp:** Tabs 0.398, 1.102 g **SE:** ↑ QT, ↑ PO^{3-}, ↓ K^+, Na^{1+}, D, flatulence, cramps, Abd bloating/pain

Sodium Polystyrene Sulfonate (Kayexalate) **Uses:** *Rx of ↑ K^+* **Acts:** Na^+/K^+ ion-exchange resin **Dose:** *Adults.* 15–60 g PO or 30–60 g PR q6h based on serum K^+. *Peds.* 1 g/kg/dose PO or PR q6h based on serum K^+ (given w/ agent, e.g., sorbitol, to promote movement through the bowel) **Caution:** [C, M] **CI:** ↑ Na^+ **Disp:** Powder; susp 15 g/60 mL sorbitol **SE:** ↑ Na^+, ↓ K^+, Na retention,

GI upset, fecal impaction **Notes:** Enema acts more quickly than PO; PO most effective, onset action >2 h

Solifenacin (Vesicare) **Uses:** *OAB* **Acts:** Antimuscarinic, ↓ detrusor contractions **Dose:** 5 mg PO daily, 10 mg/d max; ↓ w/ renal/hepatic impair **Caution:** [C, ?/–] BOO or GI obst, ulcerative colitis, MyG, renal/hepatic impair, QT prolongation risk **CI:** NAG, urinary/gastric retention **Disp:** Tabs 5, 10 mg **SE:** Constipation, xerostomia, dyspepsia, blurred vision, drowsiness **Notes:** CYP3A4 substrate; azole antifungals ↑ levels; recent concern over cognitive effects

Sorafenib (Nexavar) **Uses:** *Advanced RCC* metastatic liver CA **Acts:** Kinase inhib **Dose:** *Adults.* 400 mg PO bid on empty stomach **Caution:** [D, –] w/ Irinotecan, doxorubicin, warfarin; avoid conception (male/female) **Disp:** Tabs 200 mg **SE:** Hand–foot synd; Tx-emergent hypertension; bleeding, ↑ INR, cardiac infarction/ischemia; ↑ pancreatic enzymes, hypophosphatemia, lymphopenia, anemia, fatigue, alopecia, pruritus, D, GI upset, HA, neuropathy **Notes:** Monitor BP 1st 6 wk; may require ↓ dose (daily or q other day); impaired metabolism w/Asian descent; may effect wound healing, D/C before major surgery

Sorbitol (Generic) **Uses:** *Constipation* **Acts:** Laxative **Dose:** 30–60 mL PO of a 20–70% soln PRN **Caution:** [B, +] **CI:** Anuria **Disp:** Liq 70% **SE:** Edema, electrolyte loss, lactic acidosis, GI upset, xerostomia **Notes:** Vehicle for many liq formulations (e.g., zinc, Kayexalate)

Sotalol (Betapace) **BOX:** To minimize risk of induced arrhythmia, pts initiated/reinitiated on *Betapace AF* should be placed for a minimum of 3 d (on their maint) in a facility that can provide cardiac resuscitation, cont ECG monitoring, & calculations of CrCl. *Betapace* should not be substituted for *Betapace AF* because of labeling **Uses:** *Ventricular arrhythmias, AF* **Acts:** β-Adrenergic-blocking agent **Dose:** *Adults. CrCl >60 mL/min:* 80 mg PO bid, may ↑ to 240–320 mg/d. CrCl 30–60 mL/min: 80 mg q24h. CrCl 10–30 mL/min: Dose q36–48h 80 mg PO bid. *Peds Neonates:* 9 mg/m² bid. *1–19 mo:* 20.4 mg/m² tid. *20–23 mo:* 29.1 mg/m² tid. *≥2 y:* 30 mg/m² tid; to max dose of 90 mg/m² tid; ↓ w/ renal impair **Caution:** [B (1st tri) (D if 2nd or 3rd tri), +] **CI:** Asthma, COPD, ↓ HR, ↑ prolonged QT interval, 2nd-/3rd-degree heart block w/o pacemaker, cardiogenic shock, uncontrolled CHF **Disp:** Tabs 80, 120, 160, 240 mg **SE:** ↓ HR, CP, palpitations, fatigue, dizziness, weakness, dyspnea

Sotalol (Betapace AF) **BOX:** See sotalol (*Betapace*) **Uses:** *Maintain sinus rhythm for symptomatic AF/A flutter* **Acts:** β-Adrenergic-blocking agent **Dose:** *Adults. CrCl >60 mL/min:* 80 mg PO q12h. *CrCl 40–60 mL/min:* 80 mg PO q24h; ↑ to 120 mg during hospitalization; monitor QT interval 2–4 h after each dose, dose reduction or D/C if QT interval ≥500 msec. *Peds Neonates:* 9 mg/m² bid. *1–19 mo:* 20 mg/m² tid. *20–23 mo:* 29.1 mg/m² tid. *≥2 y:* 30 mg/m² tid; can double all doses as max daily dose; allow ~36 h between changes **Caution:** [B (1st tri; D if 2nd or 3rd tri), +] when converting from other antiarrhythmic **CI:** Asthma, ↓ HR, ↑ QT interval, 2nd/3rd-degree heart block w/o pacemaker, cardiogenic shock, uncontrolled

CHF, CrCl <40 mL/min **Disp:** Tabs 80, 120, 160 mg **SE:** ↓ HR, CP, palpitations, fatigue, dizziness, weakness, dyspnea **Notes:** Follow renal Fxn & QT interval; Betapace should not be substituted for Betapace AF because of differences in labeling

Spironolactone (Aldactone) **BOX:** Tumorogenic in anmial studies; avoid unnecessary use **Uses:** *Hyperaldosteronism, HTN, Class III/IV CHF, ascites from cirrhosis* **Acts:** Aldosterone antagonist; K⁺-sparing diuretic **Dose:** *Adults.* CHF (NYHA class III–IV) 12.5–25 mg/d (w/ ACE and loop diuretic); *Ascites:* 100–400 mg Q AM with 40–160 mg of furosemide, start w 100 mg/40 mg, wait at least 3 d before ↑ dose *Peds.* 1–3.3 mg/kg/24 h PO ÷ bid-qid. *Neonates:* 0.5–1 mg/kg/dose q8h; take w/ food **Caution:** [D, +] **CI:** ↑ K⁺, acute renal failure, anuria **Disp:** Tabs 25, 50, 100 mg **SE:** ↑ K⁺ & gynecomastia, arrhythmia, sexual dysfunction, confusion, dizziness, D/N/V, abnormal menstruation

Starch, Topical, Rectal (Tucks Suppositories [OTC]) **Uses:** *Temporary relief of anorectal disorders (itching, etc)* **Acts:** Topical protectant **Dose:** Adults & Peds ≥12 y: Cleanse, rinse and dry, insert 1 sup rectally 6×/d × 7 d max. **Caution:** [?, ?] **CI:** None **Disp:** Supp **SE:** D/C w/ or if rectal bleeding occurs or if condition worsens or does not improve w/n 7 d

Stavudine (Zerit) **BOX:** Lactic acidosis & severe hepatomegaly w/ steatosis & pancreatitis reported **Uses:** *HIV in combo w/ other antiretrovirals* **Acts:** Reverse transcriptase inhib **Dose:** *Adults >60 kg:* 40 mg bid. *<60 kg:* 30 mg bid. *Peds Bbirth–13 d:* 0.5 mg/kg q12h. *>14 d & <30 kg:* 1 mg/kg q12h. *≥30 kg:* Adult dose; ↓ w/ renal Insuff **Caution:** [C, +] **CI:** Allergy **Disp:** Caps 15, 20, 30, 40 mg; soln 1 mg/mL **SE:** Peripheral neuropathy, HA, chills, fever, malaise, rash, GI upset, anemias, lactic acidosis, ↑ LFTs, pancreatitis **Notes:** Take w/ plenty of H₂O

Steroids, Systemic (See Table 2 p 265) The following relates only to the commonly used systemic glucocorticoids **Uses:** *Endocrine disorders (adrenal insuff), *rheumatoid disorders, collagen–vascular Dzs, derm Dzs, allergic states, cerebral edema*, nephritis, nephrotic synd, immunosuppression for transplantation, ↑ Ca²⁺, malignancies (breast, lymphomas), pre-op (pt who has been on steroids in past year, known hypoadrenalism, pre-op for adrenalectomy); Inj into joints/tissue **Acts:** Glucocorticoid **Dose:** Varies w/ use & institutional protocols.

- *Adrenal Insuff, acute: Adults. Hydrocortisone:* 100 mg IV; then 300 mg/d ÷ q6h; convert to 50 mg PO q8h × 6 doses, taper to 30–50 mg/d ÷ bid. *Peds. Hydrocortisone:* 1–2 mg/kg IV, then 150–250 mg/d ÷ tid.
- *Adrenal Insuff, chronic (physiologic replacement):* May need mineralocorticoid supl such as Florinef. *Adults. Hydrocortisone:* 20 mg PO q A.M., 10 mg PO q P.M.; *cortisone:* 0.5–0.75 mg/kg/d ÷ bid; *cortisone:* 0.25–0.35 mg/kg/d IM; *dexamethasone:* 0.03–0.15 mg/kg/d or 0.6–0.75 mg/m²/d ÷ q6–12h PO, IM, IV. *Peds. Hydrocortisone:* 0.5–0.75 mg/kg/d PO tid; *hydrocortisone succinate:* 0.25–0.35 mg/kg/d IM.
- *Asthma, acute: Adults. Methylprednisolone* 60 mg PO/IV q6h or *dexamethasone* 12 mg IV q6h. *Peds. Prednisolone* 1–2 mg/kg/d or *prednisone* 1–2 mg/kg/d ÷

daily-bid for up to 5 d; *methylprednisolone* 2–4 mg/kg/d IV ÷ tid; *dexamethasone* 0.1–0.3 mg/kg/d ÷ q6h.

- *Congenital adrenal hyperplasia:* **Peds.** Initial *hydrocortisone* 30–36 mg/m²/d PO ÷ 1/3 dose q A.M., 2/3 dose q P.M.; maint 20–25 mg/m²/d ÷ bid.
- *Extubation/airway edema:* **Adults.** *Dexamethasone:* 0.5–1 mg/kg/d IM/IV ÷ q6h (start 24 h prior to extubation; continue × 4 more doses). **Peds.** *Dexamethasone:* 0.1–0.3 mg/kg/d ÷ q6h × 3–5 d (start 48–72 h before extubation)
- *Immunosuppressive/anti-inflammatory:* **Adults & Older Peds.** Hydrocortisone: 15–240 mg PO, IM, IV q12h; *methylprednisolone:* 4–48 mg/d PO, taper to lowest effective dose; *methylprednisolone Na succinate:* 10–80 mg/d IM. **Adults.** *Prednisone or prednisolone:* 5–60 mg/d PO ÷ daily-qid. **Infants & Younger Children.** Hydrocortisone: 2.5–10 mg/kg/d PO ÷ q6–8h; 1–5 mg/kg/d IM/IV ÷ bid.
- *Nephrotic synd:* **Peds.** *Prednisolone or prednisone:* 2 mg/kg/d PO tid-qid until urine is protein-free for 5 d, use up to 28 d; for persistent proteinuria, 4 mg/kg/dose PO q other day max 120 mg/d for an additional 28 d; maint 2 mg/kg/dose q other day for 28 d; taper over 4–6 wk (max 80 mg/d).
- *Septic shock (controversial):* **Adults.** Hydrocortisone: 500 mg–1 g IM/IV q2–6h. **Peds.** Hydrocortisone: 50 mg/kg IM/IV, repeat q4–24 h PRN.
- *Status asthmaticus:* **Adults & Peds.** Hydrocortisone: 1–2 mg/kg/dose IV q6h; then ↓ by 0.5–1 mg/kg q6h.
- *Rheumatic Dz:* **Adults.** *Intra-articular:* Hydrocortisone acetate: 25–37.5 mg large joint, 10–25 mg small joint *Methylprednisolone acetate:* 20–80 mg large joint, 4–10 mg small joint. *Intrabursal:* Hydrocortisone acetate: 25–37.5 mg. *Intra-ganglial:* Hydrocortisone acetate: 25–37.5 mg. *Tendon sheath:* Hydrocortisone acetate: 5–12.5 mg.
- *Perioperative steroid coverage:* Hydrocortisone: 100 mg IV night before surgery, 1 h pre-op, intraoperative, & 4, 8, & 12 h post-op; post-op day No. 1 100 mg IV q6h; post-op day No. 2 100 mg IV q8h; post-op day No. 3 100 mg IV q12h; post-op day No. 4 50 mg IV q12h; post-op day No. 5 25 mg IV q12h; resume prior PO dosing if chronic use or D/C if only perioperative coverage required.
- *Cerebral edema:* Dexamethasone: 10 mg IV; then 4 mg IV q4–6h

Caution: [C, ?/–] **CI:** Active varicella Infxn, serious Infxn except TB, fungal infxns **Disp:** Table 2 p 265 **SE:** ↑ Appetite, hyperglycemia, ↓ K⁺, osteoporosis, nervousness, insomnia, "steroid psychosis," adrenal suppression **Notes:** Hydrocortisone succinate for systemic, acetate for intraarticular; never abruptly D/C steroids, taper dose; also used for bacterial and TB meningitis

Steroids, Topical (See Table 3 p 266) **Uses:** * Steroid-responsive dermatoses (seborrheic/atopic dermatitis, neurodermatitis, anogenital pruritus, psoriasis) * **Action:** glucocorticoid; ↓ capillary permeability, stabilizes lysosomes to control inflammation; controls protein synthesis; ↓ migration of leukocytes, fibroblasts; **Dose:** Use lowest potency produce for shortest period for effect (See

Table 3 p 266) **Caution:** [C, +] Do not use occlusive dressings; high potency topical products not for rosacea, perioral dermatitis; not for use on face, groin, axillae; none for use in a diapered area. **CI:** component hypersens **Disp:** See Table 3 p 266 **SE:** Skin atrophy w/ chronic use; chronic administration or application over large area may cause adrenal suppression or hyperglycemia

Streptokinase (Streptase, Kabikinase) **Uses:** *Coronary artery thrombosis, acute massive PE, DVT, & some occluded vascular grafts* **Acts:** Activates plasminogen to plasmin that degrades fibrin **Dose:** *Adults.* PE: Load 250,000 units peripheral IV over 30 min, then 100,000 units/h IV for 24–72 h. *Coronary artery thrombosis:* 1.5 mill units IV over 60 min. *DVT or arterial embolism:* Load as w/ PE, then 100,000 units/h for 72 h; 1.5 mill Int Units in a 1-h Inf *(ECC 2005).* Peds. 3500–4000 units/kg over 30 min, then 1000–1500 units/kg/h. *Occluded catheter (controversial):* 10,000–25,000 units in NS to final vol of catheter (leave in for 1 h, aspirate & flush w/ NS) **Caution:** [C, +] **CI:** Streptococcal Infxn or streptokinase in last 6 mo, active bleeding, CVA, TIA, spinal surgery/trauma in last month, vascular anomalies, severe hepatic/renal Dz, endocarditis, pericarditis, severe uncontrolled HTN **Disp:** Powder for Inj 250,000, 750,000, 1,500,000 units **SE:** Bleeding, ↓ BP, fever, bruising, rash, GI upset, hemorrhage, anaphylaxis **Notes:** If Inf inadequate to keep clotting time 2–5× control, see PI for adjustments; antibodies remain 3–6 mo following dose

Streptomycin **BOX:** Neuro/oto/renal tox possible; neuromuscular blockage w/ resp paralysis possible **Uses:** *TB combo Rx therapy* streptococcal or enterococcal endocarditis **Acts:** Aminoglycoside; ↓ protein synth **Dose:** *Adults. Endocarditis:* 1 g q12h 1–2 wk, then 500 mg q12h 1–4 wk; *TB:* 15 mg/kg/d (up to 1 g), directly observed therapy (DOT) 2× wk 20–30 mg/kg/dose (max 1.5 g), DOT 3× wk 25–30 mg/kg/dose (max 1 g). *Peds.* 15 mg/kg/d; DOT 2× wk 20–40 mg/kg/dose (max 1 g); DOT 3× wk 25–30 mg/kg/dose (max 1 g); ↓ w/ renal Insuff, either IM or IV over 30–60 min **Caution:** [D, +] **CI:** PRG **Disp:** Inj 400 mg/mL (1-g vial) **SE:** ↑ Incidence of vestibular & auditory tox, ↑ neurotox risk in pts w/ impaired renal fxn **Notes:** Monitor levels: *Peak:* 20–30 mcg/mL; *Trough:* <5 mcg/mL; *Toxic peak:* >50 mcg/mL, *Trough:* >10 mcg/mL; IV over 30–60 min

Streptozocin (Zanosar) **Uses:** *Pancreatic islet cell tumors* & carcinoid tumors **Acts:** DNA–DNA (intrastrand) cross-linking; DNA, RNA, & protein synth inhib **Dose:** Per protocol; ↓ in renal failure **Caution:** w/ Renal failure [D, ?/–] **CI:** w/ Rotavirus vaccine, PRG **Disp:** Inj 1 g **SE:** N/V/D, duodenal ulcers, depression, ↓ BM rare (20%) & mild; nephrotox (proteinuria & azotemia dose related), hypophosphatemia dose limiting; hypo-/hyperglycemia; Inj site Rxns **Notes:** Monitor Cr

Succimer (Chemet) **Uses:** *Lead poisoning (levels >45 mcg/mL)* **Acts:** Heavy metal-chelating agent **Dose:** *Adults & Peds.* 10 mg/kg/dose q8h × 5 d, then 10 mg/kg/dose q12h for 14 d; ↓ in renal Insuff **Caution:** [C, ?] **CI:** Allergy **Disp:** Caps 100 mg **SE:** Rash, fever, GI upset, hemorrhoids, metallic taste, drowsiness, ↑ LFTs **Notes:** Monitor lead levels, maintain hydration, may open caps

Succinylcholine (Anectine, Quelicin, Sucostrin, others) BOX: Risk of cardiac arrest from hyperkalemic rhabdomyolysis Uses: *Adjunct to general anesthesia, facilitates ET intubation; induce skeletal muscle relaxation during surgery or mechanical ventilation* Acts: Depolarizing neuromuscular blocker; rapid onset, short duration (3–5 min) Dose: *Adults.* Rapid sequence intubation 1–2 mg/kg IV over 10–30 s or 2–4 mg/kg IM (*ECC 2005*). *Peds.* 1–2 mg/kg/dose IV, then by 0.3–0.6 mg/kg/dose q5min; ↓ w/ severe renal/hepatic impair Caution: See Box [C, M] CI: w/ Malignant hyperthermia risk, myopathy, recent major burn, multiple trauma, extensive skeletal muscle denervation, NAG, pseudocholinesterase deficiency Disp: Inj 20, 50, 100 mg/mL SE: Fasciculations, ↑ IOP, ICP, intragastric pressure, salivation, myoglobinuria, malignant hyperthermia, resp depression, prolonged apnea; multiple drugs potentiate CV effects (arrhythmias, ↓ BP, brady/tachycardia) Notes: May be given IV push/Inf/IM deltoid; hyperkalemic rhabdomyolysis in children w/ undiagnosed myopathy such as Duchenne muscular dystrophy

Sucralfate (Carafate) Uses: *Duodenal ulcer, gastric ulcers, stomatitis, GERD, preventing stress ulcers, esophagitis* Acts: Forms ulcer-adherent complex that protects against acid, pepsin, & bile acid Dose: *Adults.* 1 g PO qid, 1 h prior to meals & hs. *Peds.* 40–80 mg/kg/d ÷ q6h; continue 4–8 wk unless healing demonstrated by x-ray or endoscopy; separate from other drugs by 2 h; take on empty stomach ac Caution: [B, +] CI: Component allergy Disp: Tabs 1 g; susp 1 g/10 mL SE: Constipation; D, dizziness, xerostomia Notes: Al may accumulate in renal failure

Sulfacetamide (Bleph-10, Cetamide, Sodium Sulamyd) Uses: *Conjunctival infxns* Acts: Sulfonamide antibiotic Dose: 10% oint apply qid & hs; soln for keratitis apply q2–3h based on severity Caution: [C, M] CI: Sulfonamide sensitivity; age <2 mo Disp: Oint 10%; soln 10, 15, 30%; topical cream 10%; foam, gel, lotion, pad all 10% SE: Irritation, burning, blurred vision, brow ache, SJS, photosens

Sulfacetamide & Prednisolone (Blephamide, Others) Uses: *Steroid-responsive inflammatory ocular conditions w/ Infxn or a risk of Infxn* Acts: Antibiotic & anti-inflammatory Dose: *Adults & Peds >2 y:* Apply oint lower conjunctival sac daily-qid; soln 1–3 gtt 2–3 h while awake Caution: [C, ?/–] Sulfonamide sensitivity; age <2 mo Disp: *Oint:* sulfacetamide 10%/prednisolone 0.5%, sulfacetamide 10%/prednisolone 0.2%, sulfacetamide 10%/prednisolone 0.25%. *Susp:* sulfacetamide 10%/prednisolone 0.25%, sulfacetamide 10%/prednisolone 0.5%, sulfacetamide 10%/prednisolone 0.2% SE: Irritation, burning, blurred vision, brow ache, SJS, photosens Notes: OK ophthal susp use as otic agent

Sulfasalazine (Azulfidine, Azulfidine EN) Uses: *Ulcerative colitis, RA, juvenile RA*, active Crohn Dz, ankylosing spondylitis, psoriasis* Acts: Sulfonamide; actions unclear Dose: *Adults. Ulcerative colitis:* Initial, 1 g PO tid-qid; ↑ to a max of 8 g/d in 3–4 ÷ doses; maint 500 mg PO qid. *RA:* (EC tab) 0.5–1 g/d, ↑ weekly to maint 2 g/ ÷ bid. *Peds. Ulcerative colitis:* Initial: 40–60 mg/kg/24 h PO ÷ q4–6h; maint: 20–30 mg/kg/24 h PO ÷ q6h. *RA >6 y:* 30–50 mg/kg/d in

2 doses, start w/ 1/4–1/3 maint dose, ↑ weekly until dose reached at 1 mo, 2 g/d max; ↓ w/ renal Insuff **Caution:** [B (D if near term), M] **CI:** Sulfonamide or salicylate sensitivity, porphyria, GI or GU obst; avoid in hepatic impair **Disp:** Tabs 500 mg; EC DR tabs 500 mg **SE:** GI upset; discolors urine; dizziness, HA, photosens, oligospermia, anemias, SJS **Notes:** May cause yellow-orange skin/contact lens discoloration; avoid sunlight exposure

Sulfinpyrazone   **Uses:** *Acute & chronic gout* **Acts:** ↓ Renal tubular absorption of uric acid **Dose:** 100–200 mg PO bid for 1 wk, ↑ PRN to maint of 200–400 mg bid; max 800 mg/d; take w/ food or antacids, & plenty of fluids; avoid salicylates **Caution:** [C (D if near term), ?/–] CI: Renal impair, avoid salicylates; peptic ulcer; blood dyscrasias, near -term PRG, allergy **Disp:** Tabs 100 mg; caps 200 mg **SE:** N/V, stomach pain, urolithiasis, leukopenia **Notes:** Take w/ plenty of H_2O

Sulindac (Clinoril)   **BOX:** May ↑ risk of cardiovascular CV events & GI bleeding; do not use for post CABG pain control **Uses:** *Arthritis & pain* **Acts:** NSAID; ↓ prostaglandins **Dose:** 150–200 mg bid, 400 mg max; w/ food **Caution:** [B (D if 3rd tri or near term), ?] **CI:** NSAID or ASA sensitivity, w/ ketorolac, ulcer, GI bleeding, post-op pain in coronary artery bypass graft **Disp:** Tabs 150, 200 mg **SE:** Dizziness, rash, GI upset, pruritus, edema, ↓ renal blood flow, renal failure (? fewer renal effects than other NSAIDs), peptic ulcer, GI bleeding

Sumatriptan (Imitrex)   **Uses:** *Rx acute migraine* **Acts:** Vascular serotonin receptor agonist **Dose:** *Adults. SQ:* 6 mg SQ as a single-dose PRN; repeat PRN in 1 h to a max of 12 mg/24 h. *PO:* 25 mg, repeat in 2 h, PRN, 100 mg/d max PO dose; max 300 mg/d. *Nasal spray:* 1 spray into 1 nostril, repeat in 2 h to 40 mg/24 h max. *Peds. Nasal spray:* **6–9 y:** 5–20 mg/d. **12–17 y:** 5–20 mg, up to 40 mg/d **Caution:** [C, M] **CI:** Angina, ischemic heart Dz, uncontrolled HTN, severe hepatic impair, ergot use, MAOI use w/in 14 d **Disp:** OD tabs 25, 50, 100 mg; Inj 6, 8, 12 mg/mL; OD tabs 25, 50, 100 mg, ODTs 25, 50, 100 mg; nasal spray 5, 10, 20 mg/spray **SE:** Pain & bruising at site; dizziness, hot flashes, paresthesias, CP, weakness, numbness, coronary vasospasm, HTN

Sumatriptan & Naproxen Sodium (Treximet)   **BOX:** ↑ Risk of serious CV (MI, stroke) serious GI events (bleeding, ulceration, perforation) of the stomach or intestines **Uses:** *Prevent migraines* **Acts:** Anti-inflammatory NSAID w/ 5-HT$_1$ receptor agonist, constricts CNS vessels **Dose:** *Adults.* 1 tab PO; repeat PRN after 2 h; max 2 tabs/24 h, w/ or w/o food **Caution:** [C, –] **CI:** CV Dz, severe hepatic impair, severe ↑ BP **Disp:** Tab naproxen/sumatriptan 500 mg/85 mg **SE:** Dizziness, somnolence, paresthesia, N, dyspepsia, dry mouth, chest/neck/throat/jaw pain, tightness, pressure **Notes:** Do not split/crush/chew

Sunitinib (Sutent)   **Uses:** *Advanced GI stromal tumor (GIST) refractory/intolerant of imatinib; advanced RCC* **Acts:** Multi-TKI **Dose:** *Adults.* 50 mg PO daily × 4 wk, followed by 2 wk holiday = 1 cycle; ↓ to 37.5 mg w/ CYP3A4 inhib (Table 10 p 280), to ↑ 87.5 mg w/ CYP3A4 inducers **CI:** w/ Atazanavir **Caution:** [D, –] Multiple interactions require dose modification (e.g., St. John's wort)

Disp: Caps 12.5, 25, 50 mg **SE:** ↓ WBC & plt, bleeding, ↑ BP, ↓ ejection fraction, ↑ QT interval, pancreatitis, DVT, Szs, adrenal insufficiency, N/V/D, skin discoloration, oral ulcers, taste perversion, hypothyroidism **Notes:** Monitor left ventricular ejection fraction, ECG, CBC/plts, chemistries (K+/Mg²+/phosphate), TFT & LFTs periodically; ↓ dose in 12.5-mg increments if not tolerated

Tacrine (Cognex) **Uses:** *Mild–mod Alzheimer dementia* **Acts:** Cholinesterase inhib **Dose:** 10–40 mg PO qid to 160 mg/d; separate doses from food **Caution:** [C, ?] **CI:** Previous tacrine-induced jaundice **Disp:** Caps 10, 20, 30, 40 mg **SE:** ↑ LFTs, HA, dizziness, GI upset, flushing, confusion, ataxia, myalgia, ↓ HR **Notes:** Serum conc >20 ng/mL have more SE; monitor LFTs

Tacrolimus [FK506] (Prograf, Protopic) **BOX:** ↑ Risk of Infxn and lymphoma **Uses:** *Prevent organ rejection *, eczema **Acts:** Macrolide immunosuppressant **Dose:** *Adults.* IV: 0.05–0.1 mg/kg/d cont Inf. PO: 0.1–0.2 mg/kg/d ÷ 2 doses. *Peds.* IV: 0.03–0.05 mg/kg/d as cont Inf. PO: 0.15–0.2 mg/kg/d PO ÷ q 12 h. *Adults & Peds. Eczema:* Apply bid, continue 1 wk after clearing; take on empty stomach; ↓ w/ hepatic/renal impair **Caution:** [C, −] w/ Cyclosporine; avoid topical if <2 y of age **CI:** Component allergy, castor oil allergy w/ IV form **Disp:** Caps 0.5, 1, 5 mg; Inj 5 mg/mL; oint 0.03, 0.1% **SE:** Neuro- & nephrotox, HTN, edema, HA, insomnia, fever, pruritus, ↓/↑ K+, hyperglycemia, GI upset, anemia, leukocytosis, tremors, paresthesias, pleural effusion, Szs, lymphoma **Notes:** Monitor levels; *Trough:* 5–20 ng/mL based on indication and time since transplant; reports of ↑ CA risk; topical use for short-term/2nd-line

Tadalafil (Cialis) **Uses:** *ED dysfunction* **Acts:** PDE5 inhib, ↑ cyclic guanosine monophosphate & NO levels; relaxes smooth muscles, dilates cavernosal arteries **Dose:** *Adults.* PRN: 10 mg PO before sexual activity (5–20 mg max) 1 dose/72 h. *Daily dosing:* 2.5 mg q day w/o regard to timing of sex, may ↑ to 5 mg q day; w/o regard to meals; ↓ w/ renal/hepatic Insuff **Caution:** [B, −] w/ α-Blockers (except tamsulosin); use w/ CYP3A4 inhib (Table 10 p 280)(e.g., ritonavir, ketoconazole, itraconazole) 2.5 mg/daily dose or 5 mg PRN dose; CrCl <30 mL/min/hemodialysis/severe hepatic impair do not use daily dosing **CI:** Nitrates, severe hepatic impair **Disp:** Tabs 5-, 10-, 20- mg **SE:** HA, flushing, dyspepsia, back/limb pain, myalgia, nasal congestion, urticaria, SJS, dermatitis, visual field defect, NIAON, sudden ↓/loss of hearing, tinnitus **Notes:** Longest acting of class (36 h); daily dosing may ↑ drug interactions; excessive EtOH may ↑ orthostasis; transient global amnesia reports

Talc (Sterile Talc Powder) **Uses:** *↓ Recurrence of malignant pleural effusions (pleurodesis)* **Acts:** Sclerosing agent **Dose:** Mix slurry: 50 mL NS w/ 5-g vial, mix, distribute 25 mL into two 60-mL syringes, vol to 50 mL/syringe w/ NS. Infuse each into chest tube, flush w/ 25 mL NS. Keep tube clamped; have pt change positions q15min for 2 h, unclamp tube **Caution:** [X, −] **CI:** Planned further surgery on site **Disp:** 5- g powder **SE:** Pain, Infxn **Notes:** May add 10–20 mL 1% lidocaine/syringe; must have chest tube placed, monitor closely while tube clamped (tension pneumothorax), not antineoplastic

Tamoxifen (Generic) BOX: CA of the uterus, stroke, and blood clots can occur Uses: *Breast CA [postmenopausal, estrogen receptor(+)], ↓ risk of breast CA in high-risk, met male breast CA*, ductal carcinoma in situ, mastalgia, pancreatic CA, gynecomastia, ovulation induction Acts: Nonsteroidal antiestrogen; mixed agonist–antagonist effect Dose: 20–40 mg/d; doses >20 mg ÷ bid. *Prevention:* 20 mg PO/d × 5 y Caution: [D, –] w/ ↓ WBC, ↓ plts, hyperlipidemia CI: PRG, undiagnosed vag bleeding, Hx thromboembolism Disp: Tabs 10, 20 mg; oral soln 10 mg/5 mL SE: Uterine malignancy & thrombosis events seen in breast CA prevention trials; menopausal Sxs (hot flashes, N/V) in premenopausal pts; vag bleeding & menstrual irregularities; skin rash, pruritus vulvae, dizziness, HA, peripheral edema; acute flare of bone metastasis pain & ↑ Ca^{2+}; retinopathy reported (high dose) Notes: ↑ Risk of PRG in premenopausal women (induces ovulation); brand Nolvadex suspended in US

Tamsulosin (Flomax, generic) Uses: *BPH* Acts: Antagonist of prostatic α-receptors Dose: 0.4 mg/d, may ↑ to 0.8 mg PO daily Caution: [B, ?] CI: Female gender Disp: Caps 0.4 mg SE: HA, dizziness, syncope, somnolence, ↓ libido, GI upset, retrograde ejaculation, rhinitis, rash, angioedema, IFIS Notes: Not for use as antihypertensive; do not open/crush/chew; approved for use w/ dutasteride for BPH

Tapentadol (Nucynta) [C-II] Uses: *Mod/severe acute pain * Acts: Mu-opioid agonist and norepinephrine reuptake inhib Dose: 50-100 mg PO q 4-6 hrs PRN (max 600 mg/d); w/ mod hepatic impair: 50 mg q 8h PRN (max 3 doses/24 hr) Caution: [C, –] Hx of seizures, CNS depression; ↑ ICP, severe renal impair, biliary tract Dz, elderly, serotonin synd w/ concomitant serotonergic agents CI: ↓ pulm fxn, use w/ or w/in 14 d of MAOI Disp: Tabs 50, 75, 100 mg SE: N/V, dizziness, somnolence, headache Notes: Taper dose w/ D/C

Tazarotene (Tazorac, Avage) Uses: *Facial acne vulgaris; stable plaque psoriasis up to 20% BSA* Acts: Keratolytic Dose: *Adults & Peds >12 y: Acne:* Cleanse face, dry, apply thin film qhs lesions. *Psoriasis:* Apply qhs Caution: [X, ?/–] CI: Retinoid sensitivity Disp: Gel 0.05, 0.1%; cream 0.05, 0.1% SE: Burning, erythema, irritation, rash, photosens, desquamation, bleeding, skin discoloration Notes: D/C w/ excessive pruritus, burning, skin redness, or peeling until Sxs resolve

Telavancin (Vibativ) BOX: Fetal risk; must have pregnancy test prior to use in childbearing age Uses: *Complicated skin/skin structure infxns d/t susceptible Gram-positive bacteria* Acts: lipoglycopeptide antibacterial; *Spectrum:* Good gram(+) aerobic and anaerobic include MRSA,MSSA some VRE; poor gram(−) Dose: 10 mg/kg IV q24h; 7.5 mg/kg q24h w/CrCl 30-50 mL/min; 10 mg/kg q48h w/CrCl 10-30 mL/min; Caution: [C/?] Nephrotoxicity, *C.difficile*-associated disease, ↑ QTc, interferes w/coag tests: CI: Pregnancy Disp: Inj 250, 750 mg SE: taste disturbance, N, V, foamy urine Notes: ↓ efficacy w/mod/severe renal impair

Telbivudine (Tyzeka) BOX: May cause lactic acidosis and severe hepatomegaly w/ steatosis when used alone or w/ antiretrovirals; D/C of the drug may lead to exacerbations of hep B; monitor LFTs **Uses:** *Rx chronic hep B* **Acts:** Nucleoside RT inhib **Dose:** *CrCl >50 mL/min:* 600 mg PO daily; *CrCl 30–49 mL/min:* 600 mg q 48 h; *CrCl <30 mL/min:* 600 mg q 72 h; *ESRD:* 600 mg q96h; dose after hemodialysis **Caution:** [B, ?/–]; may cause myopathy; follow closely w/ other myopathy causing drugs **Disp:** Tabs 600 mg **SE:** Fatigue, Abd pain, N/V/D, HA, URI, nasopharyngitis, ↑ LFTs/creatine phosphokinase, myalgia/myopathy, flu-like Sxs, dizziness, insomnia, dyspepsia **Notes:** Use w/ PEG-interferon may ↑ peripheral neuropathy risk

Telithromycin (Ketek) **BOX:** CI in myasthenia MyG **Uses:** *Mild–mod CAP* **Acts:** Unique macrolide, blocks ↑ protein synth; bactericidal. *Spectrum:* S. *aureus, S. pneumoniae, H. influenzae, M. catarrhalis, C. pneumoniae, M. pneumoniae* **Dose:** *CAP:* 800 mg (2 tabs) PO daily × 7–10 d **Caution:** [C, M] Pseudomembranous colitis, ↑ QTc interval, visual disturbances, hepatic dysfunction; dosing in renal impair unknown **CI:** Macrolide allergy, w/ pimozide; allergy **Disp:** Tabs 300, 400 mg **SE:** N/V/D, dizziness, blurred vision **Notes:** A CYP450 inhib; multiple drug interactions; hold statins d/t ↑ risk of myopathy

Telmisartan (Micardis) **Uses:** *HTN, CHF* **Acts:** Angiotensin II receptor antagonist **Dose:** 40–80 mg/d **Caution:** [C (1st tri; D 2nd & 3rd tri), ?/–] **CI:** Angiotensin II receptor antagonist sensitivity **Disp:** Tabs 20, 40, 80 mg **SE:** Edema, GI upset, HA, angioedema, renal impair, orthostatic ↓ BP

Temazepam (Restoril) [C-IV] **Uses:** *Insomnia*, anxiety, depression, panic attacks **Acts:** Benzodiazepine **Dose:** 15–30 mg PO hs PRN; ↓ in elderly **Caution:** [X, ?/–] Potentiates CNS depressive effects of opioids, barbs, EtOH, antihistamines, MAOIs, TCAs **CI:** NAG **Disp:** Caps 7.5, 15, 22.5, 30 mg **SE:** Confusion, dizziness, drowsiness, hangover **Notes:** Abrupt D/C after >10 d use may cause withdrawal

Temozolomide (Temodar) **Uses:** *Glioblastoma multiforme (GBM), refractory anaplastic astrocytoma* **Acts:** Alkylating agent **Dose:** *GBM, new:* 75 mg/m²
PO/IV/d × 42 days w/ RT, maint 150 mg/m²/d days 1-5 of 28 day cycle × 6 cycles; may ↑ to 200 mg/m²/day X 5 days every 28 days in cycle 2; *Refractory astrocytoma:* 150 mg/m² PO/IV/day X 5 days per 28- day cycle; Adjust dose based on ANC and plt count (per PI and local protocols). **Caution:** [D, ?/–] w/ Severe renal/hepatic impair, myelosuppression (monitor ANC & plt), myelodysplastic synd, secondary malignancies, PCP pneumonia (PCP prophylaxis required) **CI:** Hypersens to components or dacarbazine **Disp:** Caps 5, 20, 100, 140, 180, & 250 mg; Powder for Inj 100 mg **SE:** N/V/D, fatigue, HA, asthenia, seizure, hemiparesis, fever, dizziness, coordination abnormality, alopecia, rash, constipation, anorexia, amnesia, insomnia, viral infxn, ↓ WBC, plt **Notes:** Infuse over 90 min; swallow caps whole; if caps open avoid inhalation and contact w/ skin/mucous membranes.

Temsirolimus (Torisel) **Uses:** *Advanced RCC* **Acts:** Multikinase inhib, ↓ mTOR (mammalian target of rapamycin), ↓ hypoxic-induced factors, ↓ VEGF **Dose:** 25 mg IV 30–60 min 1×/wk. Hold w/ ANC <1000 cells/microL, plt <75,000 cells/microL, or NCI grade 3 tox. Resume when tox grade 2 or less, restart w/ dose ↓ 5 mg/wk not <15 mg/wk. w/ CYP3A4 Inhib: ↓ 12.5 mg/wk. w/ CYP3A4 Inducers ↑ 50 mg/wk **Caution:** [D, –] Avoid live vaccines, ↓ wound healing, avoid periop **CI:** None **Disp:** Inj 25 mg/mL w/ 250 mL diluent **SE:** Rash, asthenia, mucositis, N, bowel perforation, anorexia, edema, ↑ lipids, ↓ glucose, ↑ triglycerides, ↑ LFTs, ↑ Cr, ↑ WBC, ↓ HCT, ↓ plt, ↓ PO₄ **Notes:** Premedicate w/ antihistamine; ✓ lipids, CBC, plt, Cr, glucose; w/ sunitinib dose-limiting tox likely; females use w/ contraception

Tenecteplase (TNKase) **Uses:** *Restore perfusion & ↓ mortality w/ AMI* **Acts:** Thrombolytic; TPA **Dose:** 30–50 mg; see Table below **Caution:** [C, ?], ↑ Bleeding w/ NSAIDs, ticlopidine, clopidogrel, GPIIb/IIIa antagonists **CI:** Bleeding, CVA, CNS neoplasm, uncontrolled ↑ BP, major surgery (intracranial, intraspinal) or trauma w/in 2 mo **Disp:** Inj 50 mg, reconstitute w/ 10 mL sterile H₂O only **SE:** Bleeding, allergy **Notes:** Do not shake w/ reconstitution; start ASA ASAP, IV heparin ASAP w/ aPTT 50–70 s

Tenecteplase Dosing (From one vial of reconstituted TNKase)

Weight (kg)	TNKase (mg)	TNKase Volume (mL)
<60	30	6
60–69	35	7
70–79	40	8
80–89	45	9
≥90	50	10

Tenofovir (Viread) **BOX:** Lactic acidosis & severe hepatomegaly w/ steatosis, including fatal cases, have been reported w/ the use of nucleoside analogs alone or in combo w/ other antiretrovirals. Not OK w/ chronic hep; effects in pts co infected w/ hep B & HIV unknown **Uses:** *HIV Infxn* **Acts:** HIV RT inhib **Dose:** 300 mg PO daily w/ or w/o meal; CrCl ≥50 mL/min Δ q24h, CrCl 30–49 mL/min q48H, CrCl 10–29 mL/min 2×/wk **Caution:** [B, ?/–] Didanosine (separate administration times), lopinavir, ritonavir w/ known risk factors for liver Dz **CI:** Hypersens **Disp:** Tabs 300 mg **SE:** GI upset, metabolic synd, hepatotox; separate didanosine doses by 2 h **Notes:** Combo product w/ emtricitabine is Truvada

Tenofovir/Emtricitabine (Truvada) **BOX:** Lactic acidosis & severe hepatomegaly w/ steatosis, including fatal cases, have been reported w/ the use of nucleoside analogs alone or in combo w/ other antiretrovirals. Not OK w/ chronic hep; effects in pts co infected w/ hep B & HIV unknown **Uses:** *HIV Infxn* **Acts:** Dual nucleotide RT inhib **Dose:** 1 PO daily w/ or w/o a meal; adjust w/ renal impair **Caution:** [B, ?/–] w/ Known risk factors for liver Dz **CI:** CrCl <30 mL/min; **Disp:** Tabs 200 mg emtricitabine/300 mg tenofovir **SE:** GI upset, rash, metabolic synd, hepatotox

Terazosin (Hytrin) **Uses:** *BPH & HTN* **Acts:** α₁-Blocker (blood vessel & bladder neck/prostate) **Dose:** Initial, 1 mg PO hs; ↑ 20 mg/d max; may ↓ w/

diuretic or other BP medicine **Caution:** [C, ?] w/ β- Blocker, CCB, ACE inhib; use w/ phosphodiesterase-5 (PDE-5) inhib (e.g., sildenafil) can cause ↓ BP **CI:** α-Antagonist sensitivity **Disp:** Tabs 1, 2, 5, 10 mg; caps 1, 2, 5, 10 mg **SE:** ↓ BP, & syncope following 1st dose or w/ PDE-5 inhib; dizziness, weakness, nasal congestion, peripheral edema, palpitations, GI upset **Notes:** Caution w/ 1st dose syncope; if for HTN, combine w/ thiazide diuretic

Terbinafine (Lamisil, Lamisil AT, others [OTC]) **Uses:** *Onychomycosis, athlete's foot, jock itch, ringworm*, cutaneous candidiasis, pityriasis versicolor **Acts:** ↓ Squalene epoxidase resulting in fungal death **Dose:** *PO:* 250 mg/d PO for 6–12 wk. *Topical:* Apply to area tinea pedis bid, tinea cruris & corporus q day-bid, tinea versicolor soln bid; ↓ PO in renal/hepatic impair **Caution:** [B, −] PO ↑ effects of drug metabolism by CYP2D6, w/ liver/renal impair **CI:** CrCl <50 mL/min, WBC <1000/mm³, severe liver Dz **Disp:** Tabs 250 mg; *Lamisil AT* [OTC] cream, gel, soln 1% **SE:** HA, dizziness, rash, pruritus, alopecia, GI upset, taste perversion, neutropenia, retinal damage, SJS, ↑ LFTs **Notes:** Effect may take months d/t need for new nail growth; topical not for nails; do not use occlusive dressings; PO follow CBC/LFTs

Terbutaline (Brethine) **Uses:** *Reversible bronchospasm (asthma, COPD); inhibit labor* **Acts:** Sympathomimetic; tocolytic **Dose:** *Adults. Bronchodilator:* 2.5–5 mg PO qid or 0.25 mg SQ; repeat in 15 min PRN; max 0.5 mg in 4 h. *Metered-dose inhaler:* 2 Inh q4–6h. *Premature labor:* Acutely 2.5–10 mg/min/IV, gradually ↑ as tolerated q10–20min; maint 2.5–5 mg PO q4–6h until term. *Peds. PO:* 0.05–0.15 mg/kg/dose PO tid; max 5 mg/24h; ↓ in renal failure **Caution:** [B, +] ↑ Tox w/ MAOIs, TCAs; DM, HTN, hyperthyroidism, CV Dz, convulsive disorders, ↓ K⁺ **CI:** Component allergy **Disp:** Tabs 2.5, 5 mg; Inj 1 mg/mL; metered-dose inhaler **SE:** HTN, hyperthyroidism, β₁-adrenergic effects w/ high dose, nervousness, trembling, tachycardia, HTN, dizziness

Terconazole (Terazol 7) **Uses:** *Vag fungal infxns* **Acts:** Topical triazole antifungal **Dose:** 1 applicator-full or 1 supp intravag hs × 3–7 d **Caution:** [C, ?] **CI:** Component allergy **Disp:** Vag cream 0.4, 0.8%, vag supp 80 mg **SE:** Vulvar/vag burning **Notes:** Insert high into vagina

Teriparatide (Forteo) **BOX:** ↑ Osteosarcoma risk in animals, therefore only use in pts for whom the potential benefits outweigh risks **Uses:** *Severe/refractory osteoporosis* **Acts:** PTH (recombinant) **Dose:** 20 mcg SQ daily in thigh or Abd **Caution:** [C, ?/−] **CI:** w/ Paget Dz, prior radiation, bone metastases, ↑ Ca²⁺; caution in urolithiasis **Disp:** 3-mL Prefilled device (discard after 28 d) **SE:** Orthostatic ↓ BP on administration, N/D, ↑ Ca²⁺; leg cramps **Notes:** 2 yrs Max use; osteosarcoma in animals

Testosterone (AndroGel, Androderm, Striant, Testim) [CIII] **Uses:** *Male hypogonadism* **Acts:** Testosterone replacement; ↑ lean body mass, libido **Dose:** All daily *AndroGel:* 5-g gel. *Androderm:* Two 2.5-mg or one 5-mg patch daily. *Striant:* 30-mg Buccal tabs bid. *Testim:* One 5-g gel tube. **Caution:** [N/A, N/A] **CI:** PCa, male breast CA **Disp:** *AndroGel, Testim:* 5-g gel (50-mg test); *Androderm:* 2.5-, 5-mg patches; *Striant:* 30-mg buccal tabs **SE:** Site Rxns, acne, edema, wgt gain, gynecomastia, HTN, ↑ sleep apnea, prostate enlargement **Notes:** IM testosterone enanthate (*Delatestryl; Testro-L.A.*) & cypionate (*Depo-Testosterone*) dose q14–28d w/ highly variable serum levels; PO agents (methyltestosterone & oxandrolone) associated w/ hep/hepatic tumors; transdermal/mucosal forms preferred

Tetanus Immune Globulin **Uses:** Prophylaxis *passive tetanus immunization* (suspected contaminated wound w/ unknown immunization status, see Table 7 p 277), or Tx of tetanus **Acts:** Passive immunization **Dose:** *Adults & Peds. Prophylaxis:* 250–500 units IM (<7 y 4 unit/kg) 500 units if tx delayed; *Tx:* children 500-3,000 units, adults 3,000-6,000 units **Caution:** [C, ?] **CI:** Thimerosal sensitivity **Disp:** Inj 250-unit vial/syringe **SE:** Pain, tenderness, erythema at site; fever, angioedema, anaphylaxis **Notes:** May begin active immunization series at different Inj site if required

Tetanus Toxoid (TT) **Uses:** *Tetanus prophylaxis* **Acts:** Active immunization **Dose:** Based on previous immunization, Table 7 p 277 **Caution:** [C, ?/–] **CI:** Chloramphenicol use, neurologic Sxs w/ previous use, active Infxn w/ recurrent primary immunization **Disp:** Inj tetanus toxoid fluid, 4–5 Lf units/0.5 mL; tetanus toxoid adsorbed, 5, Lf units/0.5 mL **SE:** Inj site erythema, induration, sterile abscess; arthralgias, fever, malaise, neurologic disturbances **Notes:** DTaP rather than TT or Td all adults 19-64 y who have not previously received one dose of DTaP (protection adult pertussis); also use DT or Td instead of TT to maintain diphtheria immunity; if IM, use only preservative-free Inj; Do not confuse Td (for adults) w/ DT (for children)

Tetracycline (Achromycin V, Sumycin) **Uses:** *Broad-spectrum antibiotic* **Acts:** Bacteriostatic; ↓ protein synth. *Spectrum:* Gram(+): *Staphylococcus, Streptococcus.* Gram(–): *H. pylori.* Atypicals: *Chlamydia, Rickettsia, & Mycoplasma* **Dose:** *Adults.* 250–500 mg PO bid-qid. *Peds >8 y:* 25–50 mg/kg/24 h PO q6–12h; ↓ w/ renal/hepatic impair, w/o food preferred **Caution:** [D, +] **CI:** PRG, antacids, w/ dairy products, children <8 y **Disp:** Caps 100, 250, 500 mg; tabs 250, 500 mg; PO susp 250 mg/5 mL **SE:** Photosens, GI upset, renal failure, pseudotumor cerebri, hepatic impair **Notes:** Can stain tooth enamel & depress bone formation in children

Thalidomide (Thalomid) **BOX:** Restricted use; use associated w/ severe birth defects and ↑ risk of venous thromboembolism **Uses:** *Erythema nodosum leprosum (ENL)*, GVHD, aphthous ulceration in HIV(+) **Acts:** ↓ Neutrophil chemotaxis, ↓ monocyte phagocytosis **Dose:** *GVHD:* 100–1600 mg PO daily. *Stomatitis:* 200 mg bid for 5 d, then 200 mg daily up to 8 wk. *Erythema nodosum leprosum:* 100–300 mg PO qhs **Cautions:** [X, –] May ↑ HIV viral load; Hx Szs **CI:** PRG; sexually active males not using latex condoms, or females not using 2 forms of contraception **Disp:** 50-, 100-, 200-mg caps **SE:** Dizziness, drowsiness, rash, fever, orthostasis, SJS, peripheral neuropathy, Szs **Notes:** MD must register w/ STEPS risk-management program; informed consent necessary; immediately D/C if rash develops

Theophylline (Theo24, Theochron) **Uses:** *Asthma, bronchospasm* **Acts:** Relaxes smooth muscle of the bronchi & pulm blood vessels **Dose:** *Adults.* 900 mg PO ÷ q6h; SR products may be ÷ q8–12h (maint). *Peds.* 16–22 mg/kg/24 h

PO ÷ q6h; SR products may be ÷ q8–12h (maint); ↓ in hepatic failure **Caution:** [C, +] Multiple interactions (e.g., caffeine, smoking, carbamazepine, barbiturates, β-blockers, ciprofloxacin, E-mycin, INH, loop diuretics) **CI:** Arrhythmia, hyperthyroidism, uncontrolled Szs **Disp:** Elixir 80, 15 mL; soln 80 mg/15 mL; syrup 80, 150 mg/15 mL; caps 100, 200, 250 mg; tabs 100, 125, 200, 250, 300 mg; SR caps 100, 125, 200, 250, 260, 300 mg; SR tabs 100, 200, 300, 400, 450, 600 mg **SE:** N/V, tachycardia, Szs, nervousness, arrhythmias **Notes:** IV Levels: Sample 12–24 h after Inf started; *Therapeutic:* 5–15 mcg/mL; *Toxic:* >20 mcg/mL. PO Levels: *Trough:* just before next dose; *Therapeutic:* 5–15 mcg/mL

Thiamine [Vitamin B₁] Uses: *Thiamine deficiency (beriberi), alcoholic neuritis, Wernicke encephalopathy* **Acts:** Dietary supl **Dose:** *Adults. Deficiency:* 100 mg/d IM for 2 wk, then 5–10 mg/d PO for 1 mo. *Wernicke encephalopathy:* 100 mg IV single dose, then 100 mg/d IM for 2 wk. *Peds.* 10–25 mg/d IM for 2 wk, then 5–10 mg/24 h PO for 1 mo **Caution:** [A (C if doses exceed RDA), +] **CI:** Component allergy **Disp:** Tabs 5, 10, 25, 50, 100, 250, 500 mg; Inj 100, 200 mg/mL **SE:** Angioedema, paresthesias, rash, anaphylaxis w/ rapid IV **Notes:** IV use associated w/ anaphylactic Rxn; give IV slowly

Thiethylperazine (Torecan) Uses: *N/V* **Acts:** Antidopaminergic antiemetic **Dose:** 10 mg PO, PR, or IM daily-tid; ↓ in hepatic failure **Caution:** [X, ?] **CI:** Phenothiazine & sulfite sensitivity, PRG **Disp:** Tabs 10 mg; supp 10 mg; Inj 5 mg/mL **SE:** EPS, xerostomia, drowsiness, orthostatic ↓ BP, tachycardia, constipation

6-Thioguanine [6-TG] (Tabloid) Uses: *AML, ALL, CML* **Acts:** Purine-based antimetabolite (substitutes for natural purines interfering w/ nucleotide synth) **Dose:** 2 mg/kg/d; ↓ in severe renal/hepatic impair **CI:** Resistance to mercaptopurine **Disp:** Tabs 40 mg **SE:** ↓ BM (leucopenia/thrombocytopenia), N/V/D, anorexia, stomatitis, rash, hyperuricemia, rare hepatotox

Thioridazine (Mellaril) BOX: Dose-related QT prolongation Uses: *Schizophrenia*, psychosis **Acts:** Phenothiazine antipsychotic **Dose:** *Adults.* Initial, 50–100 mg PO tid; maint 200–800 mg/24 h PO in 2–4 ÷ doses **Peds** *>2 y:* 0.5–3 mg/kg/24 h PO in 2–3 ÷ doses **Caution:** [C, ?] Phenothiazines, QTc-prolonging agents, Al **CI:** Phenothiazine sensitivity **Disp:** Tabs 10, 15, 25, 50, 100, 150, 200 mg; PO conc 30, 100 mg/mL **SE:** Low incidence of EPS; ventricular arrhythmias; ↓ BP, dizziness, drowsiness, neuroleptic malignant synd, Szs, skin discoloration, photoses, constipation, sexual dysfunction, blood dyscrasias, pigmentary retinopathy, hepatic impair **Notes:** Avoid EtOH, dilute PO conc in 2–4 oz liq

Thiothixene (Navane) BOX: Not for dementia-related psychosis; increased mortality risk in elderly on antipsychotics Uses: *Psychosis* **Acts:** ? may Antagonize dopamine receptors **Dose:** *Adults & Peds >12 y: Mild–mod psychosis:* 2 mg PO tid, up to 20–30 mg/d. *Severe psychosis:* 5 mg PO bid; ↑ to max of 60 mg/24 h PRN. *IM use:* 16–20 mg/24 h ÷ bid-qid; max 30 mg/d. *Peds <12 y:* 0.25 mg/kg/24 h PO ÷ q6–12h **Caution:** [C, ?] Avoid w/ ↑ QT interval or meds that can ↑ QT **CI:** Phenothiazine sensitivity **Disp:** Caps 1, 2, 5, 10, 20 mg; PO conc 5 mg/mL; Inj

10 mg/mL SE: Drowsiness, EPS most common; ↓ BP, dizziness, drowsiness, neuroleptic malignant synd, Szs, skin discoloration, photosens, constipation, sexual dysfunction, leukopenia, neutropenia and agranulocytosis, pigmented retinopathy, hepatic impair Notes: Dilute PO conc immediately before use

Tiagabine (Gabitril) Uses: *Adjunct in partial Szs*, bipolar disorder Acts: Antiepileptic, enhances activity of GABA Dose: Adults & Peds ≥12 y: Initial 4 mg/d PO, ↑ by 4 mg during 2nd wk; ↑ PRN by 4–8 mg/d based on response, 56 mg/d max; take w/ food Caution: [C, M] May ↑ suicidal risk CI: Component allergy Disp: Tabs 2, 4, 12, 16, 20 mg SE: Dizziness, HA, somnolence, memory impair, tremors Notes: Use gradual withdrawal; used in combo w/ other anticonvulsants

Ticarcillin/Potassium Clavulanate (Timentin) Uses: *Infxns of the skin, bone, resp & urinary tract, Abd, sepsis* Acts: Carboxy-PCN; bactericidal; ↓ cell wall synth; clavulanic acid blocks β-lactamase. Spectrum: Good gram(+), not MRSA; good gram(−) & anaerobes Dose: Adults. 3.1 g IV q4–6h max 24 g ticarcillin component/d. Peds. 200–300 mg/kg/d IV ÷ q4–6h; ↓ in renal failure Caution: [B, +/−] PCN sensitivity Disp: Inj ticarcillin/clavulanate acid 3.1 g/0.1 g vial SE: Hemolytic anemia, false(+) proteinuria Notes: Often used in combo w/ aminoglycosides; penetrates CNS w/ meningeal irritation

Ticlopidine (Ticlid) BOX: Neutropenia/agranulocytosis, TTP, aplastic anemia reported Uses: *↓ Risk of thrombotic stroke*, protect grafts status post-coronary artery bypass graft, diabetic microangiopathy, ischemic heart Dz, DVT prophylaxis, graft prophylaxis after renal transplant Acts: Plt aggregation inhibitor Dose: 250 mg PO bid w/ food Caution: [B, ?/−], ↑ Tox of ASA, anticoagulation, NSAIDs, theophylline; do not use w/ clopidogrel (↓ effect) CI: Bleeding, hepatic impair, neutropenia, ↓ plt Disp: Tabs 250 mg SE: Bleeding, GI upset, rash, ↑ LFTs Notes: ✓CBC 1st 3 mo

Tigecycline (Tygacil) Uses: *Rx complicated skin & soft-tissue infxns, & complicated intra-Abd infxns* Acts: New class: related to tetracycline; Spectrum: Broad gram(+), gram(−), anaerobic, some mycobacterial; E. coli, E. faecalis (vancomycin-susceptible isolates), S. aureus (methicillin-susceptible/resistant), Streptococcus (agalactiae, anginosus grp, pyogenes), Citrobacter freundii, Enterobacter cloacae, B. fragilis group, C. perfringens, Peptostreptococcus Dose:100 mg, then 50 mg q12h IV over 30–60 min q12h Caution: [D, ?] Hepatic impair, monotherapy w/ intestinal perforation, not OK in peds, w/ tetracycline allergy CI: Component sensitivity Disp: Inj 50 mg vial SE: N/V, Inj site Rxn

Timolol (Blocadren) BOX: Exacerbation of ischemic heart Dz w/ abrupt D/C Uses: *HTN & MI* Acts: β-Adrenergic receptor blocker, β₁, β₂ Dose: HTN: 10–20 mg bid, up to 60 mg/d. MI: 10 mg bid Caution: [C (1st tri; D if 2nd or 3rd tri), +] CI: CHF, cardiogenic shock, ↓ HR, heart block, COPD, asthma Disp: Tabs 5, 10, 20 mg SE: Sexual dysfunction, arrhythmia, dizziness, fatigue, CHF

Timolol, Ophthalmic (Timoptic) Uses: *Glaucoma* Acts: β-Blocker Dose: 0.25% 1 gt bid; ↓ to daily when controlled; use 0.5% if needed; 1-gtt/d gel

Caution: [C (1st tri; D 2nd or 3rd), ?/+] **Disp:** Soln 0.25/0.5%; Timoptic XE (0.25, 0.5%) gel-forming soln **SE:** Local irritation

Tinidazole (Tindamax) **BOX:** Off-label use discouraged (animal carcinogenicity w/ other drugs in class) **Uses:** *Adults/children >3 y:* *Trichomoniasis & giardiasis; intestinal amebiasis or amebic liver abscess* **Acts:** Antiprotozoal nitroimidazole; *Spectrum:* Trichomonas vaginalis, Giardia duodenalis, Entamoeba histolytica **Dose:** *Adults.* *Trichomoniasis:* 2 g PO; Rx partner. *Giardiasis:* 2 g PO. *Amebiasis:* 2 g PO daily × 3 d. *Amebic liver abscess:* 2 g PO daily × 3–5 d. *Peds.* *Trichomoniasis:* 50 mg/kg PO, 2 g/d max. *Giardiasis:* 50 mg/kg PO, 2 g max. *Amebiasis:* 50 mg/kg PO daily × 3 d, 2 g/d max. *Amebic liver abscess:* 50 mg/kg PO daily × 3–5 d, 2 g/d max; take w/ food **Caution:** [C, D in 1st tri,; −] May be cross-resistant w/ metronidazole; Sz/peripheral neuropathy may require D/C; w/ CNS/hepatic impair **CI:** Metronidazole allergy, 1st tri PRG, w/ EtOH use **Disp:** Tabs 250, 500 **SE:** CNS disturbances; blood dyscrasias, taste disturbances, N/V, darkens urine **Notes:** D/C EtOH during & 3 d after Rx; potentiates warfarin & Li; clearance ↓ w/ other drugs; crush & disperse in cherry syrup for peds; removed by HD

Tinzaparin (Innohep) **BOX:** Risk of spinal/epidural hematomas development w/ spinal anesthesia or lumbar puncture **Uses:** *Rx of DVT w/ or w/o PE* **Acts:** LMW heparin **Dose:** 175 units/kg SQ daily at least 6 d until warfarin dose stabilized **Caution:** [B, ?] Pork allergy, active bleeding, mild–mod renal impair, morbid obesity **CI:** Allergy to sulfites, heparin, benzyl alcohol; HIT **Disp:** Inj 20,000 units/mL **SE:** Bleeding, bruising, ↓ plts, Inj site pain, ↑ LFTs **Notes:** Monitor via anti-Xa levels; no effect on bleeding time, plt Fxn, PT, aPTT

Tioconazole (Vagistat) **Uses:** *Vag fungal infxns* **Acts:** Topical antifungal **Dose:** 1 Applicator-full Intravag hs (single dose) **Caution:** [C, ?] **CI:** Component allergy **Disp:** Vag oint 6.5% **SE:** Local burning, itching, soreness, polyuria **Notes:** Insert high into vagina; may damage condom or diaphragm

Tiotropium (Spiriva) **Uses:** *Bronchospasm w/ COPD, bronchitis, emphysema* **Acts:** Synthetic anticholinergic like atropine **Dose:** 1 Caps/d inhaled using HandiHaler, *do not* use w/ spacer **Caution:** [C, ?/−] BPH, NAG, MyG, renal impair **CI:** Acute bronchospasm **Disp:** Inh caps 18 mcg **SE:** URI, xerostomia **Notes:** Monitor FEV1 or peak flow

Tirofiban (Aggrastat) **Uses:** *Acute coronary synd* **Acts:** Glycoprotein IIB/IIIa inhib **Dose:** Initial 0.4 mcg/kg/min for 30 min, followed by 0.1 mcg/kg/min 12–24h; use in combo w/ heparin; *ACS or PCI:* 0.4 mcg/kg/min IV for 30 min, then 0.1 mcg/kg/min *(ECC 2005);* ↓ in renal Insuff **Caution:** [B, ?/−] **CI:** Bleeding, intracranial neoplasm, vascular malformation, stroke/surgery/trauma w/in last 30 d, severe HTN **Disp:** Inj 50, 250 mcg/mL **SE:** Bleeding, ↓ HR, coronary dissection, pelvic pain, rash

Tobramycin (Nebcin) **Uses:** *Serious gram(−) infxns* **Acts:** Aminoglycoside; ↓ protein synth. *Spectrum:* Gram(−) bacteria (including *Pseudomonas*) **Dose:** *Adults.* Conventional dosing: 1–2.5 mg/kg/dose IV q8–12h. Once-daily dosing: 5–7 mg/kg/dose q24h. *Peds.* 2.5 mg/kg/dose IV q8h; ↓ w/ renal Insuff **Caution:**

[C, M] **CI:** Aminoglycoside sensitivity **Disp:** Inj 10, 40 mg/mL **SE:** Nephro/ototox **Notes:** Follow CrCl & levels. Levels: *Peak:* 30 min after Inf; *Trough:* <0.5 h before next dose; *Therapeutic Conventional: Peak:* 5-10 mcg/mL, *Trough:* <2 mcg/mL

Tobramycin Ophthalmic (AKTob, Tobrex) **Uses:** *Ocular bacterial infxns* **Acts:** Aminoglycoside **Dose:** 1–2 gtt q4h; oint bid–tid; if severe, use oint q3–4h, or 2 gtt q30–60 min, then less frequently **Caution:** [C, M] **CI:** Aminoglycoside sensitivity **Disp:** Oint & soln tobramycin 0.3% **SE:** Ocular irritation

Tobramycin & Dexamethasone Ophthalmic (TobraDex) **Uses:** *Ocular bacterial infxns associated w/ sig inflammation* **Acts:** Antibiotic w/ anti-inflammatory **Dose:** 0.3% Oint apply q3–8h or soln 0.3% apply 1–2 gtt q1–4h **Caution:** [C, M] **CI:** Aminoglycoside sensitivity **Disp:** Oint & susp 2.5, 5, & 10 mL tobramycin 0.3% & dexamethasone 0.1% **SE:** Local irritation/edema **Notes:** Use under ophthalmologist's direction

Tolazamide (Tolinase) **Uses:** *Type 2 DM* **Acts:** Sulfonylurea; ↑ pancreatic insulin release; ↑ peripheral insulin sensitivity; ↓ hepatic glucose output **Dose:** 100–500 mg/d (no benefit >1 g/d) **Caution:** [C, +/–] Elderly, hepatic or renal impair **Disp:** Tabs 100, 250, 500 mg **SE:** HA, dizziness, GI upset, rash, hyperglycemia, photosens, blood dyscrasias

Tolazoline (Priscoline) **Uses:** *Peripheral vasospastic disorders, persistent pulm hypertension of newborn* **Acts:** Competitively blocks α-adrenergic receptors **Dose:** *Adults.* 10–50 mg IM/IV/SQ qid. *Neonates.* 1–2 mg/kg IV over 10–15 min, then 1–2 mg/kg/h (adjust w/ ↓ renal Fxn) **Caution:** [C, ?] Avoid alcohol, w/ CAD, renal impair, CVA, PUD, ↓ BP **CI:** CAD **Disp:** Inj 25 mg/mL **SE:** ↓ BP, peripheral vasodilation, tachycardia, arrhythmias, GI upset & bleeding, blood dyscrasias, renal failure

Tolbutamide (Orinase) **Uses:** *Type 2 DM* **Acts:** Sulfonylurea; ↑ pancreatic insulin release; ↑ peripheral insulin sensitivity; ↓ hepatic glucose output **Dose:** 500–1000 mg bid; 3 g/d max; ↓ in hepatic failure **Caution:** [C, +] **CI:** Sulfonylurea sensitivity **Disp:** Tabs 250, 500 mg **SE:** HA, dizziness, GI upset, rash, photosens, blood dyscrasias, hypoglycemia, heartburn

Tolcapone (Tasmar) **BOX:** Cases of fulminant liver failure resulting in death have occurred **Uses:** *Adjunct to carbidopa/levodopa in Parkinson Dz* **Acts:** Catechol-*O*-methyltransferase inhib slows levodopa metabolism **Dose:** 100 mg PO tid w/ first 1st daily levodopa/carbidopa dose, then dose 6 & 12 h later; ↓ /w/ renal Insuff **Caution:** [C, ?] **CI:** Hepatic impair; w/ nonselective MAOI **Disp:** Tabs 100 mg, 200 mg **SE:** Constipation, xerostomia, vivid dreams, hallucinations, anorexia, N/D, orthostasis, liver failure, rhabdomyolysis **Notes:** Do not abruptly D/C or ↓ dose; monitor LFTs

Tolmetin (Tolectin) **BOX:** May ↑ risk of cardiovascular CV events & GI bleeding **Uses:** *Arthritis & pain* **Acts:** NSAID; ↓ prostaglandins **Dose:** 200–600 mg PO tid; 2000 mg/d max **Caution:** [C (D in 3rd tri or near term), +] **CI:** NSAID or ASA sensitivity; use for pain post-coronary artery bypass graft **Disp:** Tabs 200, 600 mg; caps 400 mg **SE:** Dizziness, rash, GI upset, edema, GI bleeding, renal failure

Tolnaftate (Tinactin) [OTC] Uses: *Tinea pedis, cruris, corporis, manus, versicolor* Acts: Topical antifungal Dose: Apply to area bid for 2–4 wk Caution: [C, ?] CI: Nail & scalp infxns Disp: OTC 1% liq; gel; powder; topical cream; ointment, powder, spray soln SE: Local irritation Notes: Avoid ocular contact, Infxn should improve in 7–10 d

Tolterodine (Detrol, Detrol LA) Uses: *OAB (frequency, urgency, incontinence)* Acts: Anticholinergic Dose: *Detrol:* 1–2 mg PO bid; *Detrol LA:* 2–4 mg/d Caution: [C, ?/–] w/ CYP2D6 & 3A3/4 inhib (Table 10 p 280) CI: Urinary retention, gastric retention, or uncontrolled NAG Disp: Tabs 1, 2 mg; *Detrol LA* tabs 2, 4 mg SE: Xerostomia, blurred vision, headache, constipation Notes: LA form may see "intact" pill in stool

Tolvaptan (Samsca) BOX: Hospital use only w/ close monitoring of Na^+ Uses: *Hypervolemic or euvolemic $\downarrow Na^+$* Acts: Vasopressin V_2-receptor antagonist Dose: *Adults.* 15 mg PO daily; after ≥24 hrs, may $\uparrow$ to 30 mg × 1 daily; max 60 mg X daily; titrate at 24-hr intervals to Na^+ goal Caution: [C, –] Monitor Na^+, volume, neurologic status; GI bleed risk w/ cirrhosis, avoid w/ CYP3A inducers and moderate inhib, $\downarrow$ dose w/ P-gp inhib, $\uparrow K^+$ CI: Hypovolemic hyponatremia; urgent need to raise Na^+; in pts incapable of sensing/reacting to thirst; anuria; w/ strong CYP3A inhib Disp: Tabs 15, 30 mg SE: N, xerostomia, pollakiuria, polyuria, thirst, weakness, constipation, hyperglycemia Notes: monitor K^+

Topiramate (Topamax) Uses: *Adjunctive Rx for complex partial Szs & tonic–clonic Szs*, bipolar disorder, neuropathic pain, migraine prophylaxis Acts: Anticonvulsant Dose: *Adults:* neuropathic pain. *Seizures:* Total dose 400 mg/d; see PI for 8-wk titration schedule. *Migraine prophylaxis:* titrate 100 m/d total. *Peds 2–16 y:* Initial: 1–3 mg/kg/d PO qhs; titrate per insert to 5–9 mg/kg/d; $\downarrow$ w/ renal impair Caution: [C, ?/–] CI: Component allergy Disp: Tabs 25, 50, 100, 200 mg; caps sprinkles 15, 25, 50 mg SE: Wgt loss, memory impair, metabolic acidosis, kidney stones, fatigue, dizziness, psychomotor slowing, paresthesias, GI upset, tremor, nystagmus, acute glaucoma requiring D/C Notes: Metabolic acidosis responsive to $\downarrow$ dose or D/C; D/C w/ taper

Topotecan (Hycamtin) BOX: Chemotherapy precautions, for use by physicians familiar w/ chemotherapeutic agents, BM suppression possible Uses: *Ovarian CA (cisplatin-refractory), cervical CA, NSCLC*, sarcoma, ped NSCLC Acts: Topoisomerase I inhib; $\downarrow$ DNA synth Dose: 1.5 mg/m²/d as a 1-h IV Inf × 5 d, repeat q3wk; $\downarrow$ w/ renal impair Caution: [D, –] CI: PRG, breast-feeding Disp: Inj 4-mg vials SE: $\downarrow$ BM, N/V/D, drug fever, skin rash, interstitial lung disease

Torsemide (Demadex) Uses: *Edema, HTN, CHF, & hepatic cirrhosis* Acts: Loop diuretic; $\downarrow$ reabsorption of Na^+ & Cl^- in ascending loop of Henle & distal tubule Dose: 5–20 mg/d PO or IV; 200 mg/d max Caution: [B, ?] CI: Sulfonylurea sensitivity Disp: Tabs 5, 10, 20, 100 mg; Inj 10 mg/mL SE: Orthostatic $\downarrow$ BP, HA, dizziness, photosens, electrolyte imbalance, blurred vision, renal impair Notes: 10–20 mg torsemide = 40 mg furosemide = 1 mg bumetanide

Tramadol (Ultram, Ultram ER) Uses: *Mod–severe pain* Acts: Centrally acting synthetic opioid analgesic Dose: *Adults.* 50–100 mg PO q4–6h PRN, start 25 mg PO q A.M., ↑ q3d to 25 mg PO qid; ↑ 50 mg q3d, 400 mg/d max (300 mg if >75 y); ER 100–300 mg PO daily. *Peds.* 0.5–1 mg/kg PO q4–6h PRN; ↓ w/ renal Insuff Caution: [C, ?/–]Suicide risk in addiction prone, w/tranquilizers or antidepressants CI: Opioid dependency; w/ MAOIs; sensitivity to codeine Disp: Tabs 50 mg; ER 10, 20, 30 mg SE: Dizziness, HA, somnolence, GI upset, resp depression, anaphylaxis Notes: ↓ Sz threshold; tolerance/dependence may develop; abuse potential d/t mu-opioid agonist activity; Avoid EtOH

Tramadol/Acetaminophen (Ultracet) Uses: *Short-term Rx acute pain (<5 d)* Acts: Centrally acting analgesic; nonnarcotic analgesic Dose: 2 tabs PO q4–6h PRN; 8 tabs/d max. *Elderly/renal impair:* Lowest possible dose; 2 tabs q12h max if CrCl <30 mL/min Caution: [C, –] Szs, hepatic/renal impair, suicide risk in addiction prone, w/tranquilizers or antidepressants CI: Acute intoxication Disp: Tab 37.5 mg tramadol/325 mg APAP SE: SSRIs, TCAs, opioids, MAOIs ↑ risk of Szs; dizziness, somnolence, tremor, HA, N/V/D, constipation, xerostomia, liver tox, rash, pruritus, ↑ sweating, physical dependence Notes: Avoid EtOH; abuse potential mu-opioid agonist activity (tramadol)

Trandolapril (Mavik) BOX: Use in PRG in 2nd/3rd tri can result in fetal death Uses: *HTN*, heart failure, LVD, post-AMI Acts: ACE inhib Dose: *HTN:* 1–4 mg/d. *Heart failure/LVD:* Start 1 mg/d, titrate to 4 mg/d; ↓ w/ severe renal/hepatic impair Caution: [D, +] ACE inhib sensitivity, angioedema w/ ACE inhib Disp: Tabs 1, 2, 4 mg SE: ↓ BP, ↓ HR, dizziness, ↑ K+, GI upset, renal impair, cough, angioedema Notes: African Americans minimum dose is 2 mg vs 1 mg in caucasians

Trastuzumab (Herceptin) BOX: Can cause cardiomyopathy and ventricular dysfunction; Inf Rxns and pulm tox reported Uses: *Met breast CA that over express the HER2/neu protein*, breast CA adjuvant, w/ doxorubicin, cyclophosphamide, and paclitaxel if pt HER2/neu(+) Acts: MoAb; binds human epidermal growth factor receptor 2 protein (HER2); mediates cellular cytotoxicity Dose: Per protocol, typical 2 mg/kg/IV/wk Caution: [B, ?] CV dysfunction, allergy/Inf Rxns CI: Live vaccines Disp: Inj 21 mg/mL SE: Anemia, cardiomyopathy, nephric synd, pneumonitis Notes: Inf-related Rxns minimized w/ acetaminophen, diphenhydramine, & meperidine

Trazodone (Desyrel) BOX: Closely monitor for worsening depression or emergence of suicidality, particularly in pts <24 y Uses: *Depression*, hypnotic, augment other antidepressants Acts: Antidepressant; ↓ reuptake of serotonin & norepinephrine Dose: *Adults & Adolescents.* 50–150 mg PO daily–qid; max 600 mg/d. *Sleep:* 50 mg PO, qhs, PRN Caution: [C, ?/–] CI: Component allergy Disp: Tabs 50, 100, 150, 300 mg SE: Dizziness, HA, sedation, N, xerostomia, syncope, confusion, tremor, hep, EPS Notes: Takes 1–2 wk for Sx improvement; may interact w/ CYP3A4 inhib to ↑ trazodone concentrations, carbamazepine to ↓ trazodone concentrations

Treprostinil (Remodulin, Tyvaso) Uses: *NYHA class II–IV pulm arterial HTN* Acts: Vasodilation, ↓ plt aggregation Dose: *Remodulin* 0.625–1.25 ng/kg/min cont Inf/SQ (preferred), titrate to effect; *Tyvaso:* Initial: 18 mcg (3 inhal) Q4H 4 times/day; if not tolerated, ↓ to 1-2 inhalations, then ↑ to 3 inhal; Maint: ↑ additional 3 inhal 1-2 wk intervals; 54 mcg (or 9 inhal) 4 X/day MAX **Caution:** [B, ?/–] **Component allergy Disp:** *Remodulin* Inj 1, 2.5, 5, 10 mg/mL; *Tyvaso:* 0.6 mg/mL (2.9 mL) ~6 mcg/inhal **SE:** Additive effects w/ anticoagulants, antihypertensives; Inf site Rxns; D, N, HA, ↓ BP **Notes:** Initiate in monitored setting; do not D/C or ↓ dose abruptly

Tretinoin, Topical [Retinoic Acid] (Avita, Retin-A, Renova, Retin-A Micro) **Uses:** *Acne vulgaris, sun-damaged skin, wrinkles* (photo aging), some skin CAs **Acts:** Exfoliant retinoic acid derivative **Dose:** *Adults & Peds >12 y:* Apply daily hs (w/ irritation, ↓ frequency). *Photoaging:* Start w/ 0.025%, ↑ to 0.1% over several mo (apply only q3d on neck area; dark skin may require bid use) **Caution:** [C, ?] **CI:** Retinoid sensitivity **Disp:** Cream 0.02, 0.025, 0.05, 0.1%; gel 0.01, 0.025, micro formulation gel 0.1, 0.04%; liq 0.05% **SE:** Avoid sunlight; edema; skin dryness, erythema, scaling, changes in pigmentation, stinging, photosens

Triamcinolone (Azmacort) **Uses:** *Chronic asthma* **Actions:** Topical steroid **Dose:** 2-Inhs tid-qid or 4 Inh bid **Caution:** [C, ?] **CI:** Component allergy **Disp:** Aerosol, metered inhaler 100-mcg spray **SE:** Cough, oral candidiasis **Notes:** Instruct pts to rinse mouth after use; not for acute asthma; contains ozone-depleting CFCs; will be gradually removed from US market

Triamcinolone & Nystatin (Mycolog-II) **Uses:** *Cutaneous candidiasis* **Acts:** Antifungal & anti-inflammatory **Dose:** Apply lightly to area bid; max 25 mg/d **Caution:** [C, ?] **CI:** Varicella; systemic fungal infxns **Disp:** Cream & oint 15, 30, 60, 120 mg **SE:** Local irritation, hypertrichosis, pigmentation changes **Notes:** For short-term use (<7 d)

Triamterene (Dyrenium) **Uses:** *Edema associated w/ CHF, cirrhosis* **Acts:** K⁺-sparing diuretic **Dose:** *Adults.* 100–300 mg/24 h PO ÷ daily-bid. *Peds. HTN:* 2–4 mg/kg/d in 1–2 ÷ doses; ↓ w/ renal/hepatic impair **Caution:** [B (manufacturer; D ed. opinion), ?/–] **CI:** ↑ renal impair; caution w/ other K⁺-sparing diuretics **Disp:** Caps 50, 100 mg **SE:** ↓ K⁺, blood dyscrasias, liver damage, other Rxns

Triazolam (Halcion) [C-IV] **Uses:** *Short-term management of insomnia* **Acts:** Benzodiazepine **Dose:** 0.125–0.25 mg/d PO hs PRN; ↓ in elderly **Caution:** [X, ?/–] **CI:** NAG; cirrhosis; concurrent fosamprenavir, ritonavir, nelfinavir, itraconazole, ketoconazole, nefazodone **Disp:** Tabs 0.125, 0.25 mg **SE:** Tachycardia, CP, drowsiness, fatigue, memory impair, GI upset **Notes:** Additive CNS depression w/ EtOH & other CNS depressants, avoid abrupt D/C, do not prescribe >1 mo supply

Triethanolamine (Cerumenex) [OTC] **Uses:** *Cerumen (ear wax) removal* **Acts:** Ceruminolytic agent **Dose:** Fill ear canal & insert cotton plug; irrigate w/ H₂O after 15 min; repeat PRN **Caution:** [C, ?] **CI:** Perforated tympanic membrane, otitis media **Disp:** Soln 6,12 mL **SE:** Local dermatitis, pain, erythema, pruritus

Triethylenethiophosphoramide (Thiotepa, Thioplex, Tespa, TSPA) **Uses:** *Hodgkin Dz & NHLs; leukemia; breast, ovarian CAs, preparative regimens for allogeneic & ABMT w/ high doses, intravesical for bladder CA* **Acts:** Polyfunctional alkylating agent **Dose:** 0.5 mg/kg q1–4wk, 6 mg/m² IM or IV × 4 d q2–4wk, 15–35 mg/m² by cont IV Inf over 48 h; 60 mg into the bladder & retained 2 h q1–4wk; 900–125 mg/m² in ABMT regimens (highest dose w/o ABMT is 180 mg/m²); 1–10 mg/m² (typically 15 mg) IT 1 or 2×/wk; 0.8 mg/kg in 1–2 L of soln may be instilled intraperitoneally; ↓ in renal failure **Caution:** [D, –] **CI:** Component allergy **Disp:** Inj 15, 30 mg **SE:** ↓ BM, N/V, dizziness, HA, allergy, paresthesias, alopecia **Notes:** Intravesical use in bladder CA infrequent today

Trifluoperazine (Stelazine) **Uses:** *Psychotic disorders* **Acts:** Phenothiazine; blocks postsynaptic CNS dopaminergic receptors **Dose:** *Adults.* 2–10 mg PO bid. *Peds 6–12 y:* 1 mg PO daily-bid initial, gradually ↑ to 15 mg/d; ↓ in elderly/debilitated pts **Caution:** [C, ?/–] **CI:** Hx blood dyscrasias; phenothiazine sensitivity **Disp:** Tabs 1, 2, 5, 10 mg; PO conc 10 mg/mL; Inj 2 mg/mL **SE:** Orthostatic ↓ BP, EPS, dizziness, neuroleptic malignant synd, skin discoloration, lowered Sz threshold, photosens, blood dyscrasias **Notes:** PO conc must be diluted to 60 mL or more prior to administration; requires several wk for onset of effects

Trifluridine Ophthalmic (Viroptic) **Uses:** *Herpes simplex keratitis & conjunctivitis* **Acts:** Antiviral **Dose:** 1 gtt q2h, max 9 gtt/d; ↓ to 1 gtt q4h after healing begins; Rx up to 21 d **Caution:** [C, M] **CI:** Component allergy **Disp:** Soln 1% **SE:** Local burning, stinging

Trihexyphenidyl (Artane) **Uses:** *Parkinson Dz* **Acts:** Blocks excess acetylcholine at cerebral synapses **Dose:** 2–5 mg PO daily-qid **Caution:** [C, +] **CI:** NAG, GI obst, MyG, BOO **Disp:** Tabs 2, 5 mg; elixir 2 mg/5 mL **SE:** Dry skin, constipation, xerostomia, photosens, tachycardia, arrhythmias

Trimethobenzamide (Tigan) **Uses:** *N/V* **Acts:** ↓ Medullary chemoreceptor trigger zone **Dose:** *Adults.* 300 mg PO or 200 mg IM tid-qid PRN. *Peds.* 20 mg/kg/24 h PO in 3–4 ÷ doses **Caution:** [C, ?] **CI:** Benzocaine sensitivity **Disp:** Caps 300 mg; Inj 100 mg/mL **SE:** Drowsiness, ↓ BP, dizziness; hepatic impair, blood dyscrasias, Szs, parkinsonian-like synd **Notes:** In the presence of viral infxns, may mask emesis or mimic CNS effects of Reye synd

Trimethoprim (Primsol, Proloprim, Trimpex) **Uses:** *UTI d/t susceptible gram(+) & gram(–) organisms; Rx PCP w/ dapsone* **Suppression of UTI** **Acts:** ↓ Dihydrofolate reductase. **Spectrum:** Many gram(+) & (–) except *Bacteroides, Branhamella, Brucella, Chlamydia, Clostridium, Mycobacterium, Mycoplasma, Nocardia, Neisseria, Pseudomonas,* & *Treponema* **Dose:** *Adults.* 100 mg PO bid or 200 mg PO q day; PCP 5 mg/kg tid × 21 d w/ dapsone. *Peds.* 4 mg/kg/d in 2 ÷ doses; ↓ w/ renal failure **Caution:** [C, +] **CI:** Megaloblastic anemia d/t folate deficiency **Disp:** Tabs 100 mg; PO soln 50 mg/5 mL **SE:** Rash, pruritus, megaloblastic anemia, hepatic impair, blood dyscrasias **Notes:** Take w/ plenty of H₂O

Trimethoprim (TMP)–Sulfamethoxazole (SMX) [Co-Trimoxazole, TMP-SMX] (Bactrim, Septra) **Uses:** *UTI Rx & prophylaxis, otitis media, sinusitis, bronchitis, prevent PCP pneumonia (w/CD4 count < 200 cells/mm3)* **Acts:** SMX ↓ synth of dihydrofolic acid, TMP ↓ dihydrofolate reductase to impair protein synth. *Spectrum:* Includes *Shigella*, PCP, & *Nocardia* infxns, *Mycoplasma*, *Enterobacter* sp, *Staphylococcus*, *Streptococcus*, & more **Dose:** *Adults.* 1 DS tab PO bid or 5–20 mg/kg/24 h (based on TMP) IV in 3–4 ÷ doses. *PCP:* 15–20 mg/kg/d IV or PO (TMP) in 4 ÷ doses. *Nocardia:* 10–15 mg/kg/d IV or PO (TMP) in 4 ÷ doses. PCP prophylaxis: 1 reg tab daily or DS tab 3 X wk *UTI prophylaxis:* 1 PO daily. *Peds.* 8–10 mg/kg/24 h (TMP) PO ÷ into 2 doses or 3–4 doses IV; do not use in newborns; ↓ in renal failure; maintain hydration **Caution:** [B (D if near term), +] **CI:** Sulfonamide sensitivity, porphyria, megaloblastic anemia w/ folate deficiency, sig hepatic impair **Disp:** Regular tabs 80 mg TMP/400 mg SMX; DS tabs 160 mg TMP/800 mg SMX; PO susp 40 mg TMP/200 mg SMX/5 mL; Inj 80 mg TMP/400 mg SMX/5 mL **SE:** Allergic skin Rxns, photosens, GI upset, SJS, blood dyscrasias, hep **Notes:** Synergistic combo, interacts w/ warfarin

Trimetrexate (NeuTrexin)   **BOX:** Must be used w/ leucovorin to avoid tox **Uses:** *Mod–severe PCP* **Acts:** ↓ Dihydrofolate reductase **Dose:** 45 mg/m² IV q24h for 21 d; administer w/ leucovorin 20 mg/m² IV q6h for 24 d; ↓ in hepatic impair **Caution:** [D, ?/–] **CI:** MTX sensitivity **Disp:** Inj 25, 200 mg/vial **SE:** Sz, fever, rash, GI upset, anemias, ↑ LFTs, peripheral neuropathy, renal impair **Notes:** Use cytotoxic cautions; Inf over 60 min

Triptorelin (Trelstar 3.75, Trelstar 11.25, Trelstar 22.5) **Uses:** *Palliation of advanced PCa* **Acts:** LHRH analog; ↓ GNRH w/ cont dosing; transient ↑ in LH, FSH, testosterone, & estradiol 7–10 d after 1st dose; w/ chronic use (usually 2–4 wk), sustained ↓ LH & FSH w/ ↓ testicular & ovarian steroidogenesis similar to surgical castration **Dose:** 3.75 mg IM q 4 wk; or 11.25 mg IM q12 wk or 22.5 mg q 24 wk **Caution:** [X, N/A] **CI:** Not indicated in females **Disp:** Inj Depot 3.75 mg;11.25 mg; 22.5 mg **SE:** Dizziness, emotional lability, fatigue, HA, insomnia, HTN, D, V, ED, retention, UTI, pruritus, anemia, Inj site pain, musculoskeletal pain, osteoporosis, allergic Rxns **Notes:** only 6 month formulation, ✓periodic testosterone levels

Trospium (Sanctura, Sanctura XR) **Uses:** *OAB w/ Sx of urge incontinence, urgency, frequency* **Acts:** Muscarinic antagonist, ↓ bladder smooth muscle tone **Dose:** 20 mg tab PO bid; 60 mg ER caps PO q day A.M., 1 h ac or on empty stomach. ↓ w/ CrCl <30 mL/min and elderly **Caution:** [C, +/–] w/ EtOH use, in hot environments, ulcerative colitis, MyG, renal/hepatic impair **CI:** Urinary/gastric retention, NAG **Disp:** Tab 20 mg; caps ER 60 mg **SE:** Dry mouth, constipation, HA, rash

Urokinase (Abbokinase) **Uses:** *PE, DVT, restore patency to IV catheters* **Acts:** Converts plasminogen to plasmin; causes clot lysis **Dose:** *Adults & Peds. Systemic effect:* 4400 units/kg IV over 10 min, then 4400–6000 units/kg/h for 12 h. *Restore catheter patency:* Inject 5000 units into catheter & aspirate up to 2 doses **Caution:** [B, +] **CI:** Do not use w/in 10 d of surgery, delivery, or organ biopsy; bleeding, CVA, vascular malformation **Disp:** Powder for Inj, 250,000-unit vial **SE:** Bleeding, ↓ BP, dyspnea, bronchospasm, anaphylaxis, cholesterol embolism **Notes:** aPTT should be <2× nl before use and before starting anticoagulants after

Ustekinumab (Stelara) **Uses:** *Moderate-to-severe plaque psoriasis * **Action:** Human IL-12 and -23 antagonist **Dose:** Wgt <100 kg, 45 mg SQ initial and 4 wks later, then 45 mg q 12 wks. Wgt >100 kg, 90 mg SQ initially and 4 wks later, then 90 mg q 12 wks. **Caution:** [B/?] **Disp:** Prefilled syringe and single dose vial 45 mg/0.5 mL, 90 mg/1 mL **SE:** Nasopharyngitis, URI, HA, fatigue **Notes:** Do not use with live vaccines

Valacyclovir (Valtrex) **Uses:** *Herpes zoster; genital herpes; herpes labialis* **Acts:** Prodrug of acyclovir; ↓ viral DNA replication. *Spectrum:* Herpes simplex I & II **Dose:** *Zoster:* 1 g PO tid × 7 d. *Genital herpes(initial episode):* 1 g PO bid × 7–10 d, *(recurrent)* 500 mg PO bid × 3 d or 1 g PO q day × 5 d. *Herpes prophylaxis:* 500–1000 mg/d. *Herpes labialis:* 2 g PO q12h × 1 d ↓ w/ renal failure **Caution:** [B, +] ↑ CNS effects in elderly **Disp:** Caplets 500, 1000 mg **SE:** HA, GI upset, dizziness, pruritus, photophobia

Valganciclovir (Valcyte) **BOX:** Granulocytopenia, anemia, and thrombocytopenia reported. Carcinogenic, teratogenic, and may cause aspermatogenesis **Uses:** *CMV retinitis and CMV prophylaxis in solid-organ transplantation* **Acts:** Ganciclovir prodrug; ↓ viral DNA synth **Dose:** *CMV Retinitis induction:* 900 mg PO bid w/ food × 21 d, then 900 mg PO daily; *CMV prevention:* 900 mg PO q day × 100 d posttransplant, ↓ w/ renal dysfunction **Caution:** [C, ?/–] Use w/ imipenem/cilastatin, nephrotoxic drugs **CI:** Allergy to acyclovir, ganciclovir, valganciclovir; ANC <500 cells/mcL; plt <25,000 cells/mcL K; Hgb <8 g/dL **Disp:** Tabs 450 mg **SE:** BM suppression, headache, GI upset **Notes:** Monitor CBC & Cr

Valproic Acid (Depakene, Depakote, Stavzor) **BOX:** Fatal hepatic failure (usually during 1st 6 mo of tx, peds < 2 yrs high risk, monitor LFTs at baseline and frequent intervals), teratogenic effects, and life-threatening pancreatitis reported **Uses:** *Rx epilepsy, mania; prophylaxis of migraines*, Alzheimer behavior disorder **Acts:** Anticonvulsant; ↑ availability of GABA **Dose:** *Adults & Peds. Szs:* 30–60 mg/kg/24 h PO ÷ tid (after initiation of 10–15 mg/kg/24 h). *Mania:* 750 mg in 3 ÷ doses, ↑ 60 mg/kg/d max. *Migraines:* 250 mg bid, ↑ 1000 mg/d max; ↓ w/ hepatic impair **Caution:** [D, +] Multiple drug interactions **CI:** Severe hepatic impair, urea cycle disorder **Disp:** Caps 250 mg; caps w/ coated particles 125 mg; tabs DR 125, 250, 500 mg; tabs ER 250, 500 mg; Caps DR (Stavzor) 125, 250,500 mg; syrup 250 mg/5 mL; Inj 100 mg/mL **SE:** Somnolence, dizziness, GI upset, diplopia, ataxia, rash, thrombocytopenia↓, plt, hep, pancreatitis, ↑ bleeding times, alopecia, ↑ wgt ↑, hyperammonemic encephalopathy in pts w/ urea cycle disorders **Notes:** Monitor LFTs & levels: *Trough:* Just before next dose; *Therapeutic: Peak:* 50–100 mcg/mL; *Toxic Trough:* >100 mcg/mL. *Half-life:* 5–20 h; phenobarbital & phenytoin may alter levels

Valsartan (Diovan) **BOX:** Use during 2nd/3rd tri of PRG can cause fetal harm **Uses:** HTN, CHF, DN **Acts:** Angiotensin II receptor antagonist **Dose:** 80–160 mg/d, max 320 mg/d **Caution:** [D, ?/–] w/ K⁺-sparing diuretics or K⁺ supls

CI: Severe hepatic impair, biliary cirrhosis/obst, primary hyperaldosteronism, bilateral RAS **Disp:** Tabs 40, 80, 160, 320 mg **SE:** ↓ BP, dizziness, HA, viral Infxn, fatigue, Abd pain, D, arthralgia, fatigue, back pain, hyperkalemia, cough, ↑ Cr

Vancomycin (Vancocin, Vancoled) **Uses:** *Serious MRSA infxns; enterococcal infxns; PO Rx of *S. aureus* and *C. difficile* pseudomembranous colitis* **Acts:** ↓ Cell wall synth. *Spectrum:* Gram(+) bacteria & some anaerobes (includes MRSA, *Staphylococcus, Enterococcus, Streptococcus* sp, *C. difficile*) **Dose:** *Adults.* 1 g IV q12h or 15–20 mg/kg/dose; *C. difficile:* 125–500 mg PO q6h × 7–10 d. *Peds.* 40–60 mg/kg/d IV in ÷ doses q6–12 h; *C. difficile:* 40–60 mg/kg/d PO × 7-10 d. *Neonates.* 10–15 mg/kg/dose q12h; ↓ w/ renal Insuff **Caution:** [C, M] **CI:** Component allergy; avoid in Hx hearing loss **Disp:** Caps 125, 250 mg; powder 250 mg/5 mL, 500 mg/6 mL for PO soln; powder for Inj 500 mg, 1000 mg, 10 g/vial **SE:** Oto-/nephrotoxic, GI upset (PO), ↓ WBC **Notes:** Not absorbed PO, effect in gut only; give IV slowly (over 1–3 h) to prevent "red-man synd" (flushing of head/neck/upper torso); IV product used PO for colitis. *Levels: Peak:* 1 h after Inf; *Trough:* <0.5 h before next dose; *Therapeutic: Peak:* 20–40 mcg/mL; *Trough:* 10–20 mcg/mL; *Toxic Peak:* >50 mcg/mL; *Trough:* >20 mcg/mL. *1/2:* 6–8 h

Vardenafil (Levitra, Staxyn) **Uses:** *ED* **Acts:** PDE5 inhib, increases cyclic guanosine monophosphate (cGMP) and NO levels; relaxes smooth muscles, dilates cavernosal arteries **Dose:** *Levitra* 10 mg PO 60 min before sexual activity; titrate; max × 1 = 20 mg; 2.5 mg w/ CYP3A4 inhib (Table 10 p 280); *Staxyn* 1 (10 mg) ODT 60 min before sex **Caution:** [B, −] w/ CV, hepatic, or renal Dz or if sex activity not advisable; potentiate the hypotensive effects of nitrates, alpha-blockers, and antihypertensives **CI:** w/ nitrates, **Disp:** *Levitra* Tabs 2.5, 5, 10, 20 mg tabs; *Staxyn* 10 mg ODT (contains phenylalanine) **SE:** ↑ QT interval ↓ BP, HA, dyspepsia, priapism, flushing, rhinitis, sinusitis, flu synd, sudden ↓/loss of hearing, tinnitus, NIAON. **Notes:** Concomitant α-blockers may cause ↓ BP; transient global amnesia reports

Varenicline (Chantix) **BOX:** Serious neuropsychiatric events (depression, suicidal ideation/attempt) reported. **Uses:** *Smoking cessation* **Acts:** Nicotine receptor partial agonist **Dose:** *Adults.* 0.5 mg PO daily × 3 d, 0.5 mg bid × 4 d, then 1 mg PO bid for 12 wk total; after meal w/ glass of water **Caution:** [C, ?/−] ↓ Dose w/ renal impair **Disp:** Tabs 0.5, 1 mg **SE:** Serious psychological disturbances, N, V, insomnia, flatulence, unusual dreams **Notes:** Slowly ↑ dose to ↓ N; initiate 1 wk before desired smoking cessation date; monitor for changes in behavior

Varicella Immune Globulin (VarZIG) ([investigational, call (800)843-7477]) **Uses:** Post-exposure prophylaxis for persons w/o immunity, exposure likely to result in Infxn (household contact, > 5 min) and ↑ risk for severe Dz (immunosuppression, PRG) **Acts:** Passive immunization **Dose:** 125 Units/10 kg up to 625 Units IV (over 3–5 min) or IM (deltoid or proximal thigh); give w/in 4–5 days (best < 72 hr) of exposure **Caution:** [?,-]indicated for PRG women exposed to varicella **CI:** IgA deficiency **Disp:** Inj, 125-mg unit vials **SE:** Inj site Rxn, dizziness, fever, HA, N; ARF, thrombosis rare **Notes:** Wait 5 mo before varicella vaccination after varicella immune globulin; may ↓ vaccine effectiveness; observe for varicella for 28 d; if *VariZIG* admin not possible w/in 96 hours of exposure consider admin of IGIV (400 mg/Kg)

Varicella Virus Vaccine (Varivax) Uses: *Prevent varicella (chicken-pox)* **Acts:** Active immunization w/ live attenuated virus **Dose:** *Adults & Peds (>12 mo).* 0.5 mL SQ, repeat 4–8 wk **Caution:** [C, M] **CI:** Immunosuppression; PRG, fever, untreated TB, neomycin-anaphylactoid Rxn; **Disp:** Powder for Inj **SE:** Varicella rash, generalized or at Inj site, arthralgias/myalgias, fatigue, fever, HA, irritability, GI upset **Notes:** For all children & adults who have not had chick-enpox; avoid PRG for 3 mo after; do not give w/in 3 mo of immunoglobulin (IgG) and no IgG w/in 2 mo of vaccination; avoid ASA for 6 wks; avoid high- risk people for 6 wk after vaccination

Vasopressin [Antidiuretic Hormone, ADH] (Pitressin) Uses: *DI; Rx post-op Abd distention*; adjunct Rx of GI bleeding & esophageal varices; asys-tole, PEA, pulseless VT & VF, adjunct systemic vasopressor (IV drip) **Acts:** Poste-rior pituitary hormone, potent GI, and peripheral vasoconstrictor **Dose:** *Adults & Peds. DI:* 2.5–10 units SQ or IM tid-qid. *GI hemorrhage:* 0.2–0.4 units/min; ↓ in cirrhosis; caution in vascular Dz. *VT/VF:* 40 units IV push × 1. *Vasopressor:* 0.01–0.04 units/min **Caution:** [B, +] w/ Vascular Dz **CI:** Allergy **Disp:** Inj 20 units/mL **SE:** HTN, arrhythmias, fever, vertigo, GI upset, tremor **Notes:** Addition of vaso-pressor to concurrent norepinephrine or epi infusions

Vecuronium (Norcuron) BOX: to be administered only by appropriately trained individuals Uses: *Skeletal muscle relaxation* **Acts:** Nondepolarizing neu-romuscular blocker; onset 2–3 min **Dose:** *Adults & Peds.* 0.1–0.2 mg/kg IV bolus (also rapid intubation *(ECC 2005)*); maint 0.010–0.015 mg/kg after 25–40 min; ad-ditional doses q12–15 min PRN; ↓ w/ in severe renal/hepatic impair **Caution:** [C, ?] Drug interactions cause ↑ effect (e.g., aminoglycosides, tetracycline, succi-nylcholine) **Disp:** Powder for Inj 10, 20 mg **SE:** ↓ HR, ↓ BP, itching, rash, tachy-cardia, CV collapse **Notes:** Fewer cardiac effects than succinylcholine

Venlafaxine (Effexor, Effexor XR) BOX: Monitor for worsening depres-sion or emergence of suicidality, particularly in ped pts Uses: *Depression, gener-alized anxiety*, social anxiety disorder; panic disorder*, OCD, chronic fatigue synd, ADHD, autism **Acts:** Potentiation of CNS neurotransmitter activity **Dose:** 75–225 mg/d ÷ into 2–3 equal doses (IR) or q day (ER); 375 mg IR or 225 mg ER max/d ↓ w/ renal/hepatic impair **Caution:** [C, ?/–] **CI:** MAOIs **Disp:** Tabs IR 25, 37.5, 50, 75, 100 mg; ER caps 37.5, 75, 150 mg **SE:** HTN, ↑ HR, HA, somnolence, GI upset, sexual dysfunction; causes mania or Szs **Notes:** Avoid EtOH

Verapamil (Calan, Covera HS, Isoptin, Verelan) Uses: *Angina, HTN, PSVT, AF, atrial flutter*, migraine prophylaxis, hypertrophic cardiomyopa-thy, bipolar Dz **Acts:** CCB **Dose:** *Adults. Arrhythmias:* 2nd line for PSVT w/ narrow QRS complex & adequate BP 2.5–5 mg IV over 1–2 min; repeat

5–10 mg in 15–30 min PRN (30 mg max). *Angina:* 80–120 mg PO tid, ↑ 480 mg/24 h max. *HTN:* 80–180 mg PO tid or SR tabs 120–240 mg PO daily to 240 mg bid; 2.5–5.0 mg IV over 1–2 min; repeat 5–10 mg, in 5–30 min PRN; or 5-mg bolus q15min (max 30 mg) (*ECC 2005*). *Peds <1 y:* 0.1–0.2 mg/kg IV over 2 min (may repeat in 30 min). *1–16 y:* 0.1–0.3 mg/kg IV over 2 min (may repeat in 30 min); 5 mg max. *PO: 1–5 y:* 4–8 mg/kg/d in 3 ÷ doses. >*5 y:* 80 mg q6–8h; ↓ in renal/hepatic impair **Caution:** [C, +] Amiodarone/β-blockers/flecainide can cause ↓ HR; statins, midazolam, tacrolimus, theophylline levels may be ↑; use w/cloni-dine may cause severe ↓ HR w/ elderly pts **CI:** Conduction disorders, cardiogenic shock; β-blocker/thiazide combo, dofetilide, pimozide, ranolazine **Disp:** *Calan SR:* Caps 120, 180, 240 mg; *Verelan SR:* Caps 120, 180, 240, 360 mg *Verelan PM:* caps (ER) 100, 200, 300 mg; *Calan:* Tabs 40, 80, 120 mg; *Covera HS* tabs ER/con-trolled release 180, 240 mg; *Isoptin SR* 24-h 120, 180, 240 mg; Inj 2.5 mg/mL **SE:** Gingival hyperplasia, constipation, ↓ BP, bronchospasm, HR or conduction distur-bances; ↓ BP and bradyarrhythmias taken w/ telithromycin

Vigabatrin (Sabril) BOX: Vision loss reported **Uses:** * Refractory complex partial sz disorder, infantile spasms* **Action:** ↓ gamma-aminobutyric acid transam-inase (GABA-T) to ↑ levels of brain GABA **Dose:** *Adults.* Initially 500 mg 2X/d, then ↑ daily dose by 500 mg at weekly intervals based on response and tolerability; *Peds. Seizures:* 10–15 kg: 0.5–1 g/day divided 2X/d; 16–30 kg: 1–1.5 g/day di-vided 2X/d; 31–50 kg: 1.5–3 g/day divided 2X/d; >50 kg: 2–3 g/day divided 2X/d; *Infantile spasms:* Initially 50 mg/kg/day twice daily, ↑ 150 mg/kg/day max **Caution:** [C/±] ↓ dose by 25% w/ CrCl >50–80 mL/min, ↓ dose 50% w/ CrCl >30–50 mL/min, ↓ dose 75% w/ CrCl >10–30 mL/min; MRI signal changes re-ported in some infants **Disp:** Tabs 500mg, powder/oral soln 500mg/packet, **SE:** vi-sion loss/blurring, anemia, periph neuropathy, fatigue, somnolence, nystagmus, tremor, memory impairment, ↑wgt, arthralgia, abnormal coordination, confusion **Notes:** ↓ phenytoin levels reported; taper slowly to avoid withdrawal szs

Vinblastine (Velban, Velbe) BOX: Chemotherapeutic agent; handle w/ caution **Uses:** *Hodgkin Dz & NHLs, mycosis fungoides, CAs (testis, renal cell, breast, NSCLC), AIDS-related Kaposi sarcoma*, choriocarcinoma, histiocytosis **Acts:** ↓ Microtubule assembly **Dose:** 0.1–0.5 mg/kg/wk (4–20 mg/m²); ↓ in he-patic failure **Caution:** [D, ?] **CI:** Intrathecal IT use **Disp:** Inj 1 mg/mL in 10 mg vial **SE:** ↓ BM (especially leukopenia), N/V, constipation, neurotox, alopecia, rash, myalgia, tumor pain

Vincristine (Oncovin, Vincasar PFS) BOX: Chemotherapeutic agent; handle w/ caution; fatal if administered intrathecally **Uses:** *ALL, breast & small-cell lung CA, sarcoma (e.g., Ewing tumor, rhabdomyosarcoma), Wilms tumor, Hodgkin Dz & NHLs, neuroblastoma, multiple myeloma* **Acts:** Promotes disas-sembly of mitotic spindle, causing metaphase arrest **Dose:** 0.4–1.4 mg/m² (single doses 2 mg/max); ↓ in hepatic failure **Caution:** [D, ?] **CI:** Intrathecal IT use **Disp:** Inj 1 mg/mL, 5 mg vial **SE:** Neurotox commonly dose limiting, jaw pain (trigeminal neuralgia; fever, fatigue, anorexia, constipation & paralytic ileus, bladder atony; no sig ↓ BM w/ standard doses; tissue necrosis w/ extrav

Vinorelbine (Navelbine) BOX: Chemotherapeutic agent; handle w/ caution **Uses:** *Breast CA & NSCLC* (alone or w/ cisplatin) **Acts:** ↓ Polymerization of microtubules, impairing mitotic spindle formation; semisynthetic vinca alkaloid **Dose:** 30 mg/m²/wk; ↓ in hepatic failure **Caution:** [D, ?] **CI:** Intrathecal IT use, granulocytopenia (<1000/mm³) **Disp:** Inj 10 mg **SE:** ↓ BM (leukopenia), mild GI, neurotox (6–29%); constipation/paresthesias (rare); tissue damage from extrav

Vitamin B₁ See Thiamine (page 240)

Vitamin B₆ See Pyridoxine (page 214)

Vitamin B₁₂ See Cyanocobalamin (page 84)

Vitamin K See Phytonadione (page 205)

Vitamin, muti See Multivitamins (Table 12 p 283)

Voriconazole (VFEND) **Uses:** *Invasive aspergillosis, candidemia, serious fungal infxns* **Acts:** ↓ Ergosterol synth. *Spectrum: Candida, Aspergillus, Scedosporium, Fusarium* sp **Dose:** *Adults & Peds >12 y: IV:* 6 mg/kg q12h × 2, then 4 mg/kg bid; may ↓ to 3 mg/kg/dose. *PO: <40 kg:* 100 mg q12h, up to 150 mg; *>40 kg:* 200 mg q12h, up to 300 mg; ↓ w/ mild–mod hepatic impair; IV w/ renal CYP3A4 substrates (Table 10 p 280); do not use w/ clopidogrel (↓ effect) **Disp:** Tabs 50, 200 mg; susp 200 mg/5 mL; 200 mg Inj **SE:** Visual changes, fever, rash, GI upset, ↑ LFTs **Notes:** ✓ for multiple drug interactions (e.g., ↑ dose w/ phenytoin)

Vorinostat (Zolinza) **Uses:** *Rx cutaneous manifestations in cutaneous T-cell lymphoma* **Acts:** Histone deacetylase inhib **Dose:** 400 mg PO daily w/ food; if intolerant ↓ 300 mg PO d × 5 consecutive days each wk **Caution:** [D;, ?/−] w/ Warfarin (↑ INR) **Disp:** Caps 100 mg **SE:** N/V/D, dehydration, fatigue, anorexia, dysgeusia, DVT, PE, ↓ plt, anemia, hyperglycemia, QTc prolongation, **Notes:** Monitor CBC, lytes (K, Mg, Ca), glucose, & SCr q2wk × 2 mo then monthly; baseline & periodic ECGs; drink 2 L fluid/d

Warfarin (Coumadin) BOX: Can cause major or fatal bleeding **Uses:** *Prophylaxis & Rx of PE & DVT, AF w/ embolization*, other post-op indications **Acts:** ↓ Vit K–dependent clotting factors in this order: VII-IX-X-II **Dose:** *Adults.* Titrate, INR 2.0–3.0 for most; mechanical valves INR is 2.5–3.5. *American College of Chest Physicians guidelines:* 5 mg initial, may use 7.5–10 mg; ↓ if pt elderly or w/ other bleeding risk factors; maint 2–10 mg/d PO, follow daily INR initial to adjust dosage (Table 8 p 278). *Peds.* 0.05–0.34 mg/kg/24 h PO or IV; follow PT/INR to adjust dosage; monitor vit K intake; ↓ w/ hepatic impair/elderly **Caution:** [X, +] **CI:** Severe hepatic/renal Dz, bleeding, peptic ulcer, PRG **Disp:** Tabs 1, 2, 2.5, 3, 4, 5, 6, 7.5, 10 mg; Inj **SE:** Bleeding d/t over-anticoagulation or injury & therapeutic INR; bleeding, alopecia, skin necrosis, purple toe synd **Notes:** Monitor vit K intake (↓ effect); INR preferred test; to rapidly correct over-anticoagulation: vit K, fresh-frozen plasma, or both; highly teratogenic. Caution pt on taking w/ other meds, especially ASA. *Common warfarin interactions: Potentiated by:* APAP, EtOH (w/ liver Dz), amiodarone, cimetidine, ciprofloxacin, cotrimoxazole, erythromycin, fluconazole, flu vaccine, isoniazid, itraconazole, metronidazole, omeprazole, phenytoin, propranolol, quinidine, tetracycline. *Inhibited by:* barbiturates, carbamazepine, chlordiazepoxide, cholestyramine, dicloxacillin, nafcillin, rifampin, sucralfate, high–vit K foods. Consider genotyping for VKORC1 & CYP2C9

Witch Hazel (Tucks Pads, Others [OTC]) Uses: After bowel movement cleansing to decrease local irritation or relieve hemorrhoids; after anorectal surgery, episiotomy, vag hygiene **Acts:** Astringent; shrinks blood vessels locally **Dose:** Apply PRN **Caution:** [?, ?] External use only **CI:** None **Supplied:** Presoaked pads **SE:** Mild itching or burning

Zafirlukast (Accolate) Uses: *Adjunctive Rx of asthma* **Acts:** Selective & competitive inhib of leukotrienes *Dose: Adults & Peds >12 y:* 20 mg bid. *Peds 5–11 y:* 10 mg PO bid (empty stomach) **Caution:** [B, –] Interacts w/ warfarin, ↑ INR **CI:** Component allergy **Disp:** Tabs 10, 20 mg **SE:** Hepatic dysfunction, usually reversible on D/C; HA, dizziness, GI upset; Churg-Strauss synd, neuropsych events (agitation, restlessness, suicidal ideation) **Notes:** Not for acute asthma

Zaleplon (Sonata) [C-IV] Uses: *Insomnia* **Acts:** A nonbenzodiazepine sedative/hypnotic, a pyrazolopyrimidine **Dose:** 5–20 mg hs PRN; not w/ high-fat meal; ↓ w/ renal/hepatic Insuff, elderly **Caution:** [C, ?/–] w/ Mental/psychological conditions **CI:** Component allergy **Disp:** Caps 5, 10 mg **SE:** HA, edema, amnesia, somnolence, photosens **Notes:** Take immediately before desired onset

Zanamivir (Relenza) Uses: *Influenza A & B w/ Sxs <2 d; prophylaxis for influenza* **Acts:** ↓ Viral neuraminidase **Dose:** *Adults & Peds >7 y:* 2 Inh (10 mg) bid × 10 d, initiate w/in 48 h of Sxs. *Prophylaxis household:* 10 mg q day × 10 d. *Adults & Peds >12 y: Prophylaxis Community:* 10 mg q day × 28 d **Caution:** [C, M] Not OK for pt w/ airway Dz **CI:** Pulm Dz **Disp:** Powder for Inh 5 mg **SE:** Bronchospasm, HA, GI upset, allergic Rxn, abnormal behavior, ear, nose, throat Sx **Notes:** Uses a Disk-haler for administration; dose same time each day; 2009 H1N1 strains susceptible

Ziconotide (Prialt) **BOX:** Psychological, cognitive, neurologic impair may develop over several wk; monitor frequently; may necessitate D/C **Uses:** *IT Rx of severe, refractory, chronic pain* **Acts:** N-type CCB in spinal cord **Dose:** 2.4 mcg/d IT at 0.1 mcg/h; may ↑ 2.4 mcg/d 2–3×/wk to max 19.2 mcg/d (0.8 mcg/h) by day 21 **Caution:** [C, ?/–] w/ Neuro-/psychological impair **CI:** Psychosis **Disp:** Inj 25, 100 mcg/mL **SE:** Dizziness, N/V, confusion, psych disturbances, abnormal vision, meningitis; may require dosage adjustment **Notes:** May D/C abruptly; uses specific pumps; do not ↑ more frequently than 2–3×/wk

Zidovudine (Retrovir) **BOX:** Neutropenia, anemia, lactic acidosis, myopathy & hepatomegaly w/ steatosis **Uses:** *HIV Infxn, prevent maternal HIV transmission* **Acts:** ↓ RT **Dose:** *Adults.* 200 mg PO tid or 300 mg PO bid or 1 mg/kg/dose IV q4h. *PRG:* 100 mg PO 5×/d until labor; during labor 2 mg/kg IV over 1 h then 1 mg/kg/h until cord clamped. *Peds.4 weeks-18 yrs* 160 mg/m²/dose TID or see table below; ↓ in renal failure **Caution:** [C, ?/–] w/ganciclovir, interferon alfa,ribavirin; may alter many other meds (see PI) **CI:** Allergy **Disp:** Caps 100 mg; tabs 300 mg; syrup 50 mg/5 mL; Inj 10 mg/mL **SE:** Hematologic tox, HA, fever, rash, GI upset, malaise, myopathy, fat redistribution **Notes:** w/severe anemia/neutropenia dosage interruption may be needed

Recommended Pediatric Dosage of Retrovir

Body Weight (kg)	Total Daily Dose	Dosage Regimen and Dose	
		b.i.d.	t.i.d.
4 to <9	24 mg/kg/day	12 mg/kg	8 mg/kg
≥9 to <30	18 mg/kg/day	9 mg/kg	6 mg/kg
≥30	600 mg/day	300 mg	200 mg

Zidovudine & Lamivudine (Combivir) **BOX:** Neutropenia, anemia, lactic acidosis, myopathy & hepatomegaly w/ steatosis **Uses:** *HIV Infxn* **Acts:** Combo of RT inhib **Dose:** *Adults & Peds >12 y:* 1 tab PO bid; ↓ in renal failure **Caution:** [C, ?/–] **CI:** Component allergy **Disp:** Tab zidovudine 300 mg/lamivudine 150 mg **SE:** Hematologic tox, HA, fever, rash, GI upset, malaise, pancreatitis **Notes:** Combo product ↓ daily pill burden

Zileuton (Zyflo, Zyflo CR) **Uses:** *Chronic Rx asthma* **Acts:** Leuko-triene inhib (↓ 5-lipoxygenase) **Dose:** *Adults & Peds >12 y:* 600 mg PO qid; CR 1200 mg bid w/in 1 h of A.M./P.M. meal **Caution:** [C, ?/–] **CI:** Hepatic impair **Disp:** Tabs 600 mg; CR tabs 600 mg **SE:** Hepatic damage, HA, GI upset, leukopenia, neuropsych events (agitation, restlessness, suicidal ideation) **Notes:** Monitor LFTs q mo × 3, then q2–3mo; take regularly; not for acute asthma; do not chew/crush CR

Ziprasidone (Geodon) **BOX:** ↑ Mortality in elderly w/ dementia-related psychosis **Uses:** *Schizophrenia, acute agitation* **Acts:** Atypical antipsychotic **Dose:** 20 mg PO bid, may ↑ in 2-d intervals up to 80 mg bid; agitation 10–20 mg IM PRN up to 40 mg/d; separate 10 mg doses by 2 h & 20 mg doses by 4 h (w/ food) **Caution:** [C, –] w/ ↓ Mg²⁺; ↓ K⁺ **CI:** QT prolongation, recent MI, uncompensated heart failure, meds that ↑ QT interval **Disp:** Caps 20, 40, 60, 80 mg; susp 10 mg/mL; Inj 20 mg/mL **SE:** ↓ HR; rash, somnolence, resp disorder, EPS, wgt gain, orthostatic ↓ BP **Notes:** ✓ Lytes

Zoledronic Acid (Zometa, Reclast) **Uses:** *↑ Ca²⁺ of malignancy (HCM), ↓ skeletal-related events in CAP, multiple myeloma, & metastatic bone lesions (Zometa)*; *postmenopausal osteoporosis, Paget Dz (Reclast)* **Acts:** Bisphosphonate; ↓ osteoclastic bone resorption **Dose:** *Zometa HCM:* 4 mg IV over ≥15 min; may retreat in 7 d w/ adequate renal Fxn. *Zometa bone lesions/myeloma:* 4 mg IV over >15 min, repeat q3–4wk PRN; extend w/ ↑ Cr. *Reclast:* 5 mg IV annually **Caution:** [C, ?/–] Diuretics, aminoglycosides; ASA-sensitive asthmatics;

avoid invasive dental procedures **CI:** Bisphosphonate allergy; urticaria, angioedema, w/ dental procedures **Disp:** Vial 4 mg, 5 mg **SE:** All ↑ w/ renal dysfunction; fever, flu-like synd, GI upset, insomnia, anemia; electrolyte abnormalities, bone, joint, muscle pain, AF, osteonecrosis of jaw **Notes:** Requires vigorous prehydration; do not exceed recommended doses/Inf duration to ↓ renal dysfunction; follow Cr; effect prolonged w/ Cr ↑; avoid oral surgery; dental exam recommended prior to Rx; ↓ dose w/ renal dysfunction; give Ca²⁺ and vit D supls; may ↑ atypical subtrochanteric femur fractures

Zolmitriptan (Zomig, Zomig XMT, Zomig Nasal) **Uses:** *Acute Rx migraine* **Acts:** Selective serotonin agonist; causes vasoconstriction **Dose:** Initial 2.5 mg PO, may repeat after 2 h, 10 mg max in 24 h; if HA returns, repeat after 2 h, 10 mg max 24 h **Caution:** [C, ?/−] **CI:** Ischemic heart Dz, Prinzmetal angina, uncontrolled HTN, accessory conduction pathway disorders, ergots, MAOIs **Disp:** Tabs 2.5, 5 mg; rapid tabs (XMT) 2.5, 5 mg; nasal 5 mg, **SE:** Dizziness, hot flashes, paresthesias, chest tightness, myalgia, diaphoresis

Zolpidem (Ambien IR, Ambien CR, Edluar, ZolpiMist) [C-IV] **Uses:** *Short-term Tx of insomnia; Ambien and Edluar w/ difficulty of sleep onset; Ambien CR w/difficulty of sleep maint and/or sleep maint* **Acts:** Hypnotic agent **Dose:** *Adults. Ambien:* 5–10 mg or 12.5 mg *CR* PO qhs; *Edluar:* 10 mg SL q hs; *Zolpimist:* 10 mg spray qhs; ↓ dose in elderly, debilitated, & hepatic impair (5 mg or 6.25 mg CR) **Caution:** [C, −] may cause anaphylaxis, angioedema, abnormal thinking, CNS depression, withdrawal; evaluate for other comorbid conditions **CI:** None **Disp:** *Ambien IR:* Tabs 5, 10 mg; *Ambien CR* 6.25, 12.5 mg; *Edluar:* SL tabs 5, 10 mg; *Zolpimist:* oral soln 5 mg/spray (60 actuations/unit) **SE:** Drowsiness, dizziness, D, drugged feeling, HA, dry mouth, depression **Notes:** Take tabs on empty stomach; be able to sleep 7–8 hrs; *Zolpimist:* Prime w/ 5 sprays initially, and w/ 1 spray if not used in 14 days; store upright.

Zonisamide (Zonegran) **BOX:** ↑ Risk of suicidal thoughts or behavior **Uses:** *Adjunct Rx complex partial Szs* **Acts:** Anticonvulsant **Dose:** Initial 100 mg/d PO; may ↑ to 400 mg/d **Caution:** [C, −] ↑ tox w/ CYP3A4 inhib; ↓ levels w/ carbamazepine, phenytoin, phenobarbital, valproic acid **CI:** Allergy to sulfonamides; oligohidrosis & hyperthermia in peds **Disp:** Caps 25, 50, 100 mg **SE:** Metabolic acidosis, dizziness, drowsiness, confusion, ataxia, memory impair, paresthesias, psychosis, nystagmus, diplopia, tremor, anemia, leukopenia; GI upset, nephrolithiasis (↑ d/t metabolic acidosis), SJS ; monitor for ↓ sweating & ↑ body temperature **Notes:** Swallow caps whole

Zoster Vaccine, live (Zostavax) **Uses:** *Prevent varicella zoster in adults >60 y* **Acts:** Active immunization (live attenuated varicella) virus **Dose:** *Adults.* 0.65 mL SQ × 1 **CI:** Gelatin, neomycin anaphylaxis; fever, untreated TB, immunosuppression **Caution:** [C, ?/−] **Disp:** single dose vial **SE:** Inj site Rxn, HA **Notes:** may be used if previous Hx of zoster; do not use in place of Varicella Virus Vaccine in children; contact precautions not necessary; antivirals and immune globulins may ↓ effectiveness

NATURAL AND HERBAL AGENTS

The following is a guide to some common herbal products. These may be sold separately or in combo with other products. According to the FDA, "Manufacturers of dietary supplements can make claims about how their products affect the structure or function of the body, but they may not claim to prevent, treat, cure, mitigate, or diagnose a disease without prior FDA approval." The table on page 261 summarize some of the common dangerous aspects of natural and herbal agents.

Black Cohosh **Uses:** Sx of menopause (e.g., hot flashes), PMS, hypercholesterolemia, peripheral arterial Dz; has anti-inflammatory & sedative effects **Efficacy:** May have short-term benefit on menopausal Sx **Dose:** 20–40 mg bid **Caution:** May further ↓ lipids &/or BP w/ prescription meds **CI:** PRG (miscarriage, prematurity reports); lactation **SE:** w/ OD, N/V, dizziness, nervous system & visual changes, ↓ HR, & (possibly) Szs, liver damage/failure

Chamomile **Uses:** Antispasmodic, sedative, anti-inflammatory, astringent, antibacterial. **Dose:** 10–15 g PO daily (3 g dried flower heads tid-qid between meals; can steep in 250 mL hot H$_2$O) **Caution:** w/ Allergy to chrysanthemums, ragweed, asters (family *Compositae*) **SE:** Contact dermatitis; allergy, anaphylaxis **Interactions:** w/ Anticoagulants, additive w/ sedatives (benzodiazepines); delayed ↓ gastric absorption of meds if taken together (↓ GI motility)

Cranberry (*Vaccinium macrocarpon*) **Uses:** Prevention & Rx UTI. **Efficacy:** Possibly effective **Dose:** 300–400 mg bid in 6- oz. juice qid; tincture 1/2–1 tsp up to 3×/d, tea 2–3 tsps of dried flowers/cup; creams apply topically 2–3×/d PO **Caution:** May ↑ kidney stones in some susceptible individuals, V **SE:** None known **Interactions:** May potentiate warfarin

Dong Quai (*Angelica polymorpha, sinensis*) **Uses:** Uterine stimulant; anemia, menstrual cramps, irregular menses, & menopausal Sx; anti-inflammatory, vasodilator, CNS stimulant, immunosuppressant, analgesic, antipyretic, antiasthmatic **Efficacy:** Possibly effective for menopausal Sx **Dose:** 3–15 g daily, 9–12 g PO tab bid. **Caution:** Avoid in PRG & lactation **SE:** D, photosens, skin CA **Interactions:** Anticoagulants (↑ INR w/ warfarin)

Echinacea (*Echinacea purpurea*) **Uses:** Immune system stimulant; prevention/Rx URI of colds, flu; supportive care in chronic infxns of the resp/lower urinary tract **Efficacy:** Not established; may ↓ severity & duration of URI **Dose:** Caps 500 mg, 6–9 mL expressed juice or 2–5 g dried root PO **Caution:** Do not use w/ progressive systemic or immune Dzs (e.g., TB, collagen–vascular disorders, MS); may interfere w/ immunosuppressive Rx, not OK w/ PRG; do not use >8 consecutive wk; possible immunosuppression; 3 different commercial forms

SE: N; rash **Interactions:** Anabolic steroids, amiodarone, MTX, corticosteroids, cyclosporine

Ephedra/Ma Huang   **Uses:** Stimulant, aid in wgt loss, bronchial dilation. **Dose:** Not OK d/t reported deaths (>100 mg/d can be life-threatening); US sales banned by FDA in 2004; bitter orange w/ similar properties has replaced this compound in most wgt-loss supls **Caution:** Adverse cardiac events, strokes, death **SE:** Nervousness, HA, insomnia, palpitations, V, hyperglycemia **Interactions:** Digoxin, antihypertensives, antidepressants, diabetic meds

Fish Oil Supplements (Omega-3 Polyunsaturated Fatty acid) **Uses:** CAD, hypercholesterolemia, hypertriglyceridemia, type 2 DM, arthritis **Efficacy:** No definitive data on ↓ cardiac risk in general population; may ↓ lipids and help w/ secondary MI prevention **Dose:** One FDA approved (see Lovaza, page 196); OTC 1500–3000 mg/d; AHA rec: 1 g/d **Caution:** Mercury contamination possible, some studies suggest ↑ cardiac events **SE:** ↑ Bleeding risk, dyspepsia, belching, aftertaste **Interactions:** Anticoagulants

Evening Primrose Oil   **Uses:** PMS, diabetic neuropathy, ADHD **Efficacy:** Possibly for PMS, not for menopausal Sx **Dose:** 2–4 g/d PO SE: Indigestion, N, soft stools, HA **Interactions:** ↑ Phenobarbital metabolism, ↓ Sz threshold

Feverfew (Tanacetum parthenium)   **Uses:** Prevent/Rx migraine; fever; menstrual disorders; arthritis; toothache; insect bites **Efficacy:** Weak for migraine prevention **Dose:** 125 mg PO of dried leaf (standardized to 0.2% of parthenolide) PO **Caution:** Do not use in PRG **SE:** Oral ulcers, gastric disturbance, swollen lips, Abd pain; long-term SE unknown **Interactions:** ASA, warfarin

Garlic (Allium sativum)   **Uses:** Antioxidant; hyperlipidemia, HTN; anti-infective (antibacterial, antifungal); tick repellant (oral) **Efficacy:** ↓ Cholesterol by 4–6%; soln ↓ BP; possible ↓ GI/CAP risk **Dose:** 2–5 g, fresh garlic; 0.4–1.2 g of dried powder; 2–5 mg oil; 300–1000 mg extract or other formulations = to 2–5 mg of allicin daily, 400–1200 mg powder (2–5 mg allicin) PO **Caution:** Do not use in PRG (abortifacient); D/C 7 d pre-op (bleeding risk) **SE:** ↑ Insulin levels, ↑ insulin/lipid/cholesterol levels, anemia, oral burning sensation, N/V/D **Interactions:** Warfarin & ASA (↓ plt aggregation), additive w/ DM agents (↑ hypoglycemia). CYP 3A4 inducer (may ↑ cyclosporine, HIV antivirals, oral contraceptives)

Ginger (Zingiber officinale)   **Uses:** Prevent motion sickness; N/V d/t anesthesia **Efficacy:** Benefit in ↓ N/V w/ motion or PRG; weak for post-op or chemotherapy **Dose:** 1–4 g rhizome or 0.5–2 g powder PO daily **Caution:** Pt w/ gallstones; excessive dose (↑ depression, & may interfere w/ cardiac Fxn or anticoagulants) **SE:** Heartburn **Interactions:** Excessive consumption may interfere w/ cardiac, DM, or anticoagulant meds (↓ plt aggregation) **Dose:** Ginger powder tabs or caps or fresh-cut ginger in doses of 1–4 g daily PO, ÷ into smaller doses

Ginkgo Biloba   **Uses:** Memory deficits, dementia, anxiety, improvement Sx peripheral vascular Dz, vertigo, tinnitus, asthma/bronchospasm, antioxidant, premenstrual Sx (especially breast tenderness), impotence, SSRI-induced sexual dysfunction **Dose:** 60–80 mg standardized dry extract PO bid-tid **Efficacy:** Small cognition benefit w/ dementia; no other demonstrated benefit in healthy adults **Caution:** ↑ Bleeding risk (antagonism of plt-activating factor), concerning w/ anti-platlet agents (D/C 3 d pre-op); reports of ↑ Sz risk **SE:** GI upset, HA, dizziness, heart palpitations, rash **Interactions:** ASA, salicylates, warfarin

Ginseng **Uses:** "Energy booster" general; also for pt undergoing chemotherapy, stress reduction, enhance brain activity & physical endurance (adaptogenic), anti-oxidant, aid to control type 2 DM; Panax ginseng being studied for ED **Efficacy:** Not established **Dose:** 1–2 g of root or 100–300 mg of extract (7% ginsenosides) PO tid **Caution:** w/ Cardiac Dz, DM, ↓ BP, HTN, mania, schizophrenia, w/ corti-costeroids; avoid in PRG; D/C 7 d pre-op (bleeding risk) **SE:** Controversial "gin-seng abuse synd" w/ high dose (nervousness, excitation, HA, insomnia); palpitations, vag bleeding, breast nodules, hypoglycemia **Interactions:** Warfarin, antidepressants, & caffeine (↑ stimulant effect), DM meds (↑ hypoglycemia)

Glucosamine Sulfate (Chitosamine) and Chondroitin Sulfate **Uses:** Osteoarthritis (glucosamine: rate-limiting step in glycosaminoglycan synth), ↑ cartilage rebuilding; *Chondroitin:* biological polymer, flexible matrix between protein filaments in cartilage; draws fluids/nutrients into joint, "shock absorption" **Efficacy:** Controversial **Dose:** Glucosamine 500 PO tid, chondroitin 400 mg PO tid **Caution:** Many forms come from shellfish, so avoid if have shellfish allergy **SE:** ↑ Insulin resistance in DM; concentrated in cartilage, theoretically unlikely to cause toxic/teratogenic effects **Interactions:** *Glucosamine:* None. *Chondroitin:* Monitor anticoagulant Rx

Kava Kava (Kava Kava Root Extract, *Piper methysticum*) **Uses:** Anxiety, stress, restlessness, insomnia **Efficacy:** Possible mild anxiolytic **Dose:** Standardized extract (70% kavalactones) 100 mg PO bid-tid **Caution:** Hepatotox risk, banned in Europe/Canada. Not OK in PRG, lactation. D/C 24 h pre-op (may ↑ sedative effect of anesthetics) **SE:** Mild GI disturbances; rare allergic skin/rash Rxns, may ↑ cholesterol; ↑ LFTs/jaundice; vision changes, red eyes, puffy face, muscle weakness **Interactions:** Avoid w/ sedatives, alcohol, stimulants, barbiturates (may potentiate CNS effect)

Melatonin **Uses:** Insomnia, jet lag, antioxidant, immunostimulant **Efficacy:** Sedation most pronounced w/ elderly pts w/ ↑ endogenous melatonin levels; some evidence for jet lag **Dose:** 1–3 mg 20 min before HS (w/ CR 2 h before hs) **Caution:** Use synthetic rather than animal pineal gland, "heavy head," HA, depression, daytime sedation, dizziness **Interactions:** β-Blockers, steroids, NSAIDs, benzodi-azepines

Milk Thistle (*Silybum marianum*) **Uses:** Prevent/Rx liver damage (e.g., from alcohol, toxins, cirrhosis, chronic hep); preventive w/ chronic toxin exposure (painters, chemical workers, etc) **Efficacy:** Use before exposure more effective than use after damage has occurred **Dose:** 80–200 mg PO tid **SE:** GI intolerance **Interactions:** None

Saw Palmetto (*Serenoa repens*) **Uses:** Rx BPH, hair tonic, PCa prevention (weak 5α-reductase inhib like finasteride, dutasteride) **Efficacy:** Small, no sig benefit for prostatic Sx **Dose:** 320 mg daily **Caution:** Possible hormonal effects, avoid in PRG, w/ women of childbearing years **SE:** Mild GI upset, mild HA, D w/ large amounts **Interactions:** ↑ Iron absorption; ↑ estrogen replacement effects

St. John's Wort (*Hypericum perforatum*) **Uses:** Mild–mod depression, anxiety, gastritis, insomnia, vitiligo; anti-inflammatory; immune stimulant/anti-HIV/antiviral **Efficacy:** Variable; benefit w/ mild–mod depression in several trials, but not always seen in clinical practice **Dose:** 2–4 g of herb or 0.2–1 mg of total hypericin (standardized extract) daily. *Common preparations:* 300 mg PO tid (0.3% hypericin) **Caution:** Excess doses may potentiate MAOI, cause allergic Rxn, not OK in PRG **SE:** Photosens, xerostomia, dizziness, constipation, confusion, fluctuating mood w/ chronic use **Interactions:** CYP 3A enzyme inducer; do not use w/ Rx antidepressants(especially MAOI); ↓ cyclosporine efficacy (may cause rejection), digoxin (may ↑ CHF), protease inhib, theophylline, OCP; potency varies between products/batches

Valerian (*Valeriana officinalis*) **Uses:** Anxiolytic, sedative, restlessness, dysmenorrhea **Efficacy:** Probably effective sedative (reduces sleep latency) **Dose:** 2–3 g in extract PO daily-bid added to 2/3 cup boiling H_2O, tincture 15–20 drops in H_2O, oral 400–900 mg hs (combined w/ OTC sleep product Alluna) **Caution:** None known **SE:** Sedation, hangover effect, HA, cardiac disturbances, GI upset **Interactions:** Caution w/ other sedating agents (e.g., alcohol, or prescription sedatives): may cause drowsiness w/ impaired Fxn

Yohimbine (*Pausinystalia yohimbe*) Yocon, Yohimex **Uses:** Improve sexual vigor, Rx ED **Efficacy:** Variable **Dose:** 1 tab = 5.4 mg PO tid (use w/ physician supervision) **Caution:** Do not use w/ renal/hepatic Dz; may exacerbate schizophrenia/mania (if pt predisposed). $α_2$-Adrenergic antagonist (↓ BP, Abd distress, weakness w/ high doses), OD can be fatal; salivation, dilated pupils, arrhythmias **SE:** Anxiety, tremors, dizziness, ↑ BP, ↑ HR **Interactions:** Do not use w/ antidepressants (e.g., MAOIs or similar agents)

(Adapted from Haist SA and Robbins JB: *Internal Medicine on Call*, 4th ed., 2005 McGraw-Hill; and the FDA @ http://dietarysupplements.nlm.nih.gov/dietary/index.jsp (Accessed July 2010)).

Unsafe Herbs with Known Toxicity

Agent	Toxicities
Aconite	Salivation, N/V, blurred vision, cardiac arrhythmias
Aristolochic acid	Nephrotox
Calamus	Possible carcinogenicity
Chaparral	Hepatotox, possible carcinogenicity, nephrotox
"Chinese herbal mixtures"	May contain ma Huang or other dangerous herbs
Coltsfoot	Hepatotox, possibly carcinogenic
Comfrey	Hepatotox, carcinogenic
Ephedra/Ma huang	Adverse cardiac events, stroke, Sz
Juniper	High allergy potential, D, Sz, nephrotox
Kava kava	Hepatotox
Licorice	Chronic daily amounts (>30 g/mo) can result in increased K$^+$, Na/fluid retention w/HTN, myoglobinuria, hyporeflexia
Life root	Hepatotox, liver CA
Ma huang/ephedra	Adverse cardiac events, stroke, Sz
Pokeweed	GI cramping, N/D/V, labored breathing, increased BP, Sz
Sassafras	V, stupor, hallucinations, dermatitis, abortion, hypothermia, liver CA
Usnic acid	Hepatotox
Yohimbine	Hypotension, Abd distress, CNS stimulation (mania/& psychosis in predisposed individuals)

Based on data in Haist SA and Robbins JB: *Internal Medicine On Call*, 4th ed, 2005 McGraw-Hill) and www.fda.gov.

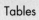
Tables

TABLE 1
Local Anesthetic Comparison Chart for Commonly Used Injectable Agents

Agent	Proprietary Names	Onset	Duration	Maximum Dose mg/kg	Maximum Dose Volume in 70-kg Adult[a]
Bupivacaine	Marcaine	7–30 min	5–7 h	3	70 mL of 0.25% solution
Lidocaine	Xylocaine, Anestacon	5–30 min	2 h	4	28 mL of 1% solution
Lidocaine with epinephrine (1:200,000)		5–30 min	2–3 h	7	50 mL of 1% solution
Mepivacaine	Carbocaine	5–30 min	2–3 h	7	50 mL of 1% solution
Procaine	Novocaine	Rapid	30 min–1 h	10–15	70–105 mL of 1% solution

[a] To calculate the maximum dose if not a 70-kg adult, use the fact that a 1% solution has 10 mg/ml drug.

264

TABLE 2
Comparison of Systemic Steroids (See also page 229)

AU: Please provide the page number

Drug	Relative Equivalent Dose (mg)	Relative Mineralo-corticoid Activity	Duration (h)	Route
Betamethasone	0.75	0	36–72	PO, IM
Cortisone (Cortone)	25	2	8–12	PO, IM
Dexamethasone (Decadron)	0.75	0	36–72	PO, IV
Hydrocortisone (Solu-Cortef, Hydrocortone)	20	2	8–12	PO, IM, IV
Methylprednisolone acetate (Depo-Medrol)	4	0	36–72	PO, IM, IV
Methylprednisolone succinate (Solu-Medrol)	4	0	8–12	PO, IM, IV
Prednisone (Deltasone)	5	1	12–36	PO
Prednisolone (Delta-Cortef)	5	1	12–36	PO, IM, IV

TABLE 3
Topical Steroid Preparations (see also page 230)

Agent	Common Trade Names	Potency	Apply
Alclometasone dipropionate	Aclovate, cream, oint 0.05%	Low	bid/tid
Amcinonide	Cyclocort, cream, lotion, oint 0.1%	High	bid/tid
Betamethasone			
Betamethasone valerate	Valisone cream, lotion 0.01%	Low	q day/bid
Betamethasone valerate	Valisone cream 0.01, 0.1%, oint, lotion 0.1%	Intermediate	q day/bid
Betamethasone dipropionate	Diprosone cream 0.05%	High	q day/bid
Betamethasone dipropionate	Diprosone aerosol 0.1%		
Betamethasone dipropionate, augmented	Diprolene oint, gel 0.05%	Ultrahigh	q day/bid
Clobetasol propionate	Temovate cream, gel, oint, scalp, soln 0.05%	Ultrahigh	bid (2 wk max)
Clocortolone pivalate	Cloderm cream 0.1%	Intermediate	q day–qid
Desonide	DesOwen, cream, oint, lotion 0.05%	Low	bid–qid
Desoximetasone			
Desoximetasone 0.05%	Topicort LP cream, gel 0.05%	Intermediate	q day–qid
Desoximetasone 0.25%	Topicort cream, oint	High	q day–bid
Dexamethasone base	Aeroseb-Dex aerosol 0.01%	Low	bid-qid
	Decadron cream 0.1%		
Diflorasone diacetate	Psorcon cream, oint 0.05%	Ultrahigh	bid/qid
Fluocinolone			
Fluocinolone acetonide 0.01%	Synalar cream, soln 0.01%	Low	bid/tid
Fluocinolone acetonide 0.025%	Synalar oint, cream 0.025%	Intermediate	bid/tid

Fluocinolone acetonide 0.2%	Synalar-HP cream 0.2%	High	bid/tid
Fluocinonide 0.05%	Lidex, anhydrous cream, gel, oint, soln 0.05%	High	bid/tid
	Lidex-E aqueous cream 0.05%		
Flurandrenolide	Cordran cream, oint 0.025%	Intermediate	bid/tid
	cream, lotion, oint 0.05%	Intermediate	bid/tid
	tape, 4 mcg/cm²	Intermediate	q day
Fluticasone propionate	Cutivate cream 0.05%, oint 0.005%	Intermediate	bid
Halobetasol	Ultravate cream, oint 0.05%	Very high	bid
Halcinonide	Halog cream 0.025%, emollient base 0.1% cream, oint, soln 0.1%	High	q day/tid
Hydrocortisone			
Hydrocortisone	Cortizone, Caldecort, Hycort, Hytone, etc—aerosol 1%, cream 0.5, 1, 2.5%, gel 0.5%, oint 0.5, 1, 2.5%, lotion 0.5, 1, 2.5%, paste 0.5%, soln 1%	Low	tid/qid
Hydrocortisone acetate	Corticaine cream, oint 0.5, 1%	Low	tid/qid
Hydrocortisone butyrate	Locoid oint, soln 0.1%	Intermediate	bid/tid
Hydrocortisone valerate	Westcort cream, oint 0.2%	Intermediate	bid/tid

TABLE 3 (continued)
Topical Steroid Preparations (see also page XXX)

Agent	Common Trade Names	Potency	Apply
Mometasone furoate	Elocon 0.1% cream, oint, lotion	Intermediate	q day
Prednicarbate	Dermatop 0.1% cream	Intermediate	bid
Triamcinolone			
Triamcinolone acetonide 0.025%	Aristocort, Kenalog cream, oint, lotion 0.025%	Low	tid/qid
Triamcinolone acetonide 0.1%	Aristocort, Kenalog cream, oint, lotion 0.1%	Intermediate	tid/qid
	Aerosol 0.2-mg/2-sec spray		
Triamcinolone acetonide 0.5%	Aristocort, Kenalog cream, oint 0.5%	High	tid/qid

TABLE 4
Comparison of Insulins (See also page 144)

Type of Insulin	Onset (h)	Peak (h)	Duration (h)
Ultra Rapid			
Apidra (glulisine)	<0.25	0.5–1.5	3–4
Humalog (lispro)	<0.25	0.5–1.5	3–4
NovoLog (aspart)	<0.25	0.5–1.5	3–4
Rapid (regular insulin)			
Humulin R, Novolin R	0.5–1	2–3	4–6
Intermediate			
Humulin N, Novolin L	1–4	6–10	10–16
Prolonged			
Lantus (insulin glargine)	1–4	No peak	24
Levemir (insulin detemir)	1–4	No peak	24
Combination Insulins			
Humalog Mix 75/25 (lispro protamine/lispro)	<0.25	Dual	Up to 10–6
Humalog Mix 50/50 (lispro protamine/lispro)	<0.25	Dual	Up to 10–16
NovoLog Mix 70/30 (Aspart protamine/aspart)	<0.25	Dual	Up to 10–16
Humulin 70/30, Novolin 70/30 (NPH/regular)	0.5–1	Dual	Up to 10–16

Note: Do not confuse Humalog, NovoLog, Humalog Mix, and NovoLog Mix with each other or with other agents as serious medication errors can result.

TABLE 5
Oral Contraceptives (See also page 193)
(Note: 21 = 21 Active pills; 24 = 24 Active pills; Standard for most products is 28 [unless specified] = 21 Active pills + 7 Placebo[a])

Drug (Manufacturer)	Estrogen (mcg)	Progestin (mg)	Iron/Other (d = days)
Monophasics			
Alesse 21, 28 (Wyeth)	Ethinyl estradiol (20)	Levonorgestrel (0.1)	
Apri (Barr)	Ethinyl estradiol (30)	Desogestrel (0.15)	
Aviane (Barr)	Ethinyl estradiol (20)	Levonorgestrel (0.1)	
Balziva (Barr)	Ethinyl estradiol (35)	Norethindrone (0.4)	
Brevicon (Watson)	Ethinyl estradiol (35)	Norethindrone (0.5)	
Cryselle (Barr)	Ethinyl estradiol (30)	Norgestrel (0.3)	
Demulen 1/35 21, 28 (Pfizer)	Ethinyl estradiol (35)	Ethynodiol diacetate (1)	
Demulen 1/50 21, 28 (Pfizer)	Ethinyl estradiol (50)	Ethynodiol diacetate (1)	
Desogen (Organon)	Ethinyl estradiol (30)	Desogestrel (0.15)	
Femcon Fe (Warner-Chilcott)	Ethinyl estradiol (35)	Norethindrone (0.4)	75 mg × 7 d
Junel Fe 1/20, 21, 28 (Barr)	Ethinyl estradiol (20)	Norethindrone acetate (1)	75 mg × 7 d
Junel Fe 1.5/30, 28 (Barr)	Ethinyl estradiol (30)	Norethindrone acetate (1.5)	75 mg × 7 d
Kariva (Barr)	Ethinyl estradiol (20, 0, 10)	Desogestrel (0.15)	2 inert; 2 ethinyl estradiol (10)
Kelnor 1/35 (Barr)	Ethinyl estradiol (35)	Ethynodiol Diacetate (1)	
Lessina (Barr)	Ethinyl estradiol (20)	Levonorgestrel (0.1)	
Levlen 21, 28 (Bayer)	Ethinyl estradiol (30)	Levonorgestrel (0.15)	
Levlite (Bayer)	Ethinyl estradiol (20)	Levonorgestrel (0.1)	
Levora (Watson)	Ethinyl estradiol (30)	Levonorgestrel (0.15)	
Loestrin 24 Fe (Warner-Chilcott)	Ethinyl estradiol (20)	Norethindrone (1)	75 mg × 4 d

Brand (Manufacturer)	Estrogen (µg)	Progestin (mg)	
Loestrin Fe 1.5/30 21, 28 (Warner-Chilcott)	Ethinyl estradiol (30)	Norethindrone acetate (1.5)	75 mg × 7 d in 28 d
Loestrin Fe 1/20 21, 28 (Warner-Chilcott)	Ethinyl estradiol (20)	Norethindrone acetate (1)	75 mg × 7 d in 28 d
Loestrin 1/20 21 (Warner-Chilcott)	Ethinyl estradiol (20)	Norethindrone acetate (1)	
Loestrin 1.5/20 21 (Warner-Chilcott)	Ethinyl estradiol (20)	Norethindrone acetate (1.5)	
Lo/Ovral 21, 28 (Wyeth)	Ethinyl estradiol (30)	Norgestrel (0.3)	
Low-Ogestrel (Watson)	Ethinyl estradiol (30)	Norgestrel (0.3)	
Lutera (Watson)	Ethinyl estradiol (20)	Levonorgestrel (0.1)	
Microgestin 1/20 21, 28 (Watson)	Ethinyl estradiol (20)	Norethindrone acetate (1)	
Microgestin 1.5/30 21, 28 (Watson)	Ethinyl estradiol (30)	Norethindrone acetate (1.5)	
Microgestin Fe 1/20 21, 28 (Watson)	Ethinyl estradiol (20)	Norethindrone acetate (1)	75 mg × 7 d in 28 d
Microgestin Fe 1.5/30 21, 28 (Watson)	Ethinyl estradiol (30)	Norethindrone acetate (1.5)	75 mg × 7 d in 28 d
Mircette (Organon)	Ethinyl estradiol (20, 0, 10)	Desogestrel (0.15)	2 inert; 2 ethinyl estradiol (10)
Modicon (Ortho-McNeil)	Ethinyl estradiol (35)	Norethindrone (0.5)	
MonoNessa (Watson)	Ethinyl estradiol (35)	Norgestimate (0.25)	
Necon 0.5/35 (Watson)	Mestranol (35)	Norethindrone (0.5)	
Necon 1/50 (Watson)	Mestranol (50)	Norethindrone (1)	
Necon 1/35 (Watson)	Ethinyl estradiol (35)	Norethindrone (0.5)	
Necon 1/35 (Watson)	Ethinyl estradiol (35)	Norethindrone (1)	
Nordette 21, 28 (King)	Ethinyl estradiol (30)	Levonorgestrel (0.15)	
Norinyl 1/35 (Watson)	Ethinyl estradiol (35)	Norethindrone (1)	

TABLE 5 (continued)
Oral Contraceptives (See also page 193)

[Note: 21 = 21 Active pills; 24 = 24 Active pills; Standard for most products is 28 [unless specified] = 21 Active pills + 7 Placebo[a]]

Drug (Manufacturer)	Estrogen (mcg)	Progestin (mg)	Iron/Other (d = days)
Monophasics			
Norinyl 1/50 (Watson)	Mestranol (50)	Norethindrone (1)	
Nortrel 0.5/35 (Barr)	Ethinyl estradiol (35)	Norethindrone (0.5)	
Nortrel 1/35 21, 28 (Barr)	Ethinyl estradiol (35)	Norethindrone (1)	
Ocella (Barr)	Ethinyl estradiol (30)	Drospirenone (3)	
Ogestrel 0.5/50 (Watson)	Ethinyl estradiol (50)	Norgestrel (0.5)	
Ortho-Cept (Ortho-McNeil)	Ethinyl estradiol (30)	Desogestrel (0.15)	
Ortho-Cyclen (Ortho-McNeil)	Ethinyl estradiol (35)	Norgestimate (0.25)	
Ortho-Novum 1/35 (Ortho-McNeil)	Ethinyl estradiol (35)	Norethindrone (1)	
Ortho-Novum 1/50 2 (Ortho-McNeil)	Mestranol (50)	Norethindrone (1)	
Ovcon 35 21, 28 (Warner-Chilcott)	Ethinyl estradiol (35)	Norethindrone (0.4)	
Ovcon 35 FE (Warner-Chilcott)	Ethinyl estradiol (35)	Norethindrone (0.4)	75 mg × 7 d in 28 d
Ovcon 50 (Warner-Chilcott)	Ethinyl estradiol (50)	Norethindrone (1)	
Ovral 21, 28 (Wyeth-Ayerst)	Ethinyl estradiol (50)	Norgestrel (0.5)	
Portia (Barr)	Ethinyl estradiol (30)	Levonorgestrel (0.15)	
Reclipsen (Watson)	Ethinyl estradiol (30)	Desogestrel (0.15)	
Solia (Prasco)	Ethinyl estradiol (30)	Desogestrel (0.15)	

Drug	Estrogen (mg)	Progestin (mcg)	Additional pills
Sprintec (Barr)	Ethinyl estradiol (35)	Norgestimate (0.25)	
Sronyx (Watson)	Ethinyl estradiol (20)	Levonorgestrel (0.1)	
Yasmin (Bayer)[e]	Ethinyl estradiol (30)	Drospirenone (3.0)	
Yaz (Bayer) 28 day[b,d,e]	Ethinyl estradiol (20)	Drospirenone (3.0)	4 inert in 28 d
Zenchent (Watson)	Ethinyl estradiol (35)	Ethynodiol diacetate (0.4)	
Zovia 1/35 (Watson)	Ethinyl estradiol (35)	Ethynodiol diacetate (1)	

Multiphasics

Drug	Estrogen (mg)	Progestin (mcg)	Additional pills
Aranelle (Barr)	Ethinyl estradiol (35)	Norethindrone (0.5, 1, 0.5)	
Cesia (Prasco)	Ethinyl estradiol (25)	Desogestrel (0.1, 0.125, 0.15)	
Cyclessa (Organon)	Ethinyl estradiol (25)	Desogestrel (0.1, 0.125, 0.15)	
Enpresse (Barr)	Ethinyl estradiol (30, 40, 30)	Levonorgestrel (0.05, 0.075, 0.125)	
Estrostep (Warner-Chilcott)[b]	Ethinyl estradiol (20, 30, 35)	Norethindrone acetate (1)	
Estrostep Fe (Warner-Chilcott)[b]	Ethinyl estradiol (20, 30, 35)	Norethindrone acetate (1)	75 mg Fe × 7 d in 28 d
Leena (Watson)	Ethinyl estradiol (35)	Norethindrone (0.5, 1, 0.5)	
Lessina (Watson)	Ethinyl estradiol (20)	Levonorgestrel (0.1)	
Lutera (Watson)	Ethinyl estradiol (20)	Levonorgestrel (0.1)	
Necon 10/11 21, 28 (Watson)	Ethinyl estradiol (35)	Norethindrone (0.5, 1)	
Necon 7/7/7 (Watson)	Ethinyl estradiol (35)	Norethindrone (0.5, 0.75, 1)	
Nortrel 7/7/7 (Barr)	Ethinyl estradiol (35)	Norethindrone (0.5, 0.75, 1)	
Ortho-Novum 10/11 (Ortho-McNeil)	Ethinyl estradiol (35)	Norethindrone (0.5, 1)	
Ortho-Novum 7/7/7 21 (Ortho-McNeil)	Ethinyl estradiol (35, 35, 35)	Norethindrone (0.5, 0.75, 1)	
Ortho Tri-Cyclen 21, 28 (Ortho-McNeil)[b]	Ethinyl estradiol (25)	Norgestimate (0.18, 0.215, 0.25)	

TABLE 5 (continued)
Oral Contraceptives (See also page 193)
[Note: 21 = 21 Active pills; 24 = 24 Active pills; Standard for most products is 28 [unless specified] = 21 Active pills + 7 Placebo[a]]

Drug	Estrogen (mg)	Progestin (mcg)	Additional pills
Multiphasics			
Ortho Tri-Cyclen Lo 21, 28 (Ortho-McNeil)	Ethinyl estradiol (35, 35, 35)	Norgestimate (0.18, 0.215, 0.25)	
Previfem (Teva)	Ethinyl estradiol (35)	Norgestimate (0.25)	
Tilia Fe (Watson)	Ethinyl estradiol (20, 30, 35)	Norethindrone (1)	75 mg Fe × 7 d in 28 d
Tri-Legest (Barr)	Ethinyl estradiol (20, 30, 35)	Norethindrone (1)	
Tri-Legest Fe (Barr)	Ethinyl estradiol (20, 30, 35)	Norethindrone (1)	75 mg Fe × 7 d in 28 d
Tri-Levlen (Bayer)	Ethinyl estradiol (30, 40, 30)	Levonorgestrel (0.05, 0.075, 0.125)	
Tri-Nessa (Watson)	Ethinyl estradiol (35)	Norgestimate (0.18, 0.215, 0.25)	
Tri-Norinyl 21, 28 (Watson)	Ethinyl estradiol (35, 35, 35)	Norethindrone (0.5, 1, 0.5)	
Tri-Previfem (Teva)	Ethinyl estradiol (35)	Norgestimate (0.18, 0.215, 0.25)	
Tri-Sprintec (Barr)	Ethinyl estradiol (35)	Norgestimate (0.18, 0.215, 0.25)	
Triphasil 21 (Wyeth)	Ethinyl estradiol (30, 40, 30)	Levonorgestrel (0.05, 0.075, 0.125)	
Trivora 28 (Watson)	Ethinyl estradiol (30, 40, 30)	Levonorgestrel (0.05, 0.075, 0.125)	
Velivet (Barr)	Ethinyl estradiol (25)	Desogestrel (0.1, 0.125, 0.15)	

274

Drug	Estrogen (mg)	Progestin (mcg)	Additional pills
Progestin Only (aka "mini-pills")			
Camila (Barr)	None	Norethindrone (0.35)	
Errin (Barr)	None	Norethindrone (0.35)	
Jolivette 28 (Watson)	None	Norethindrone (0.35)	
Micronor (Ortho-McNeil)	None	Norethindrone (0.35)	
Nor-QD (Watson)	None	Norethindrone (0.35)	
Nora-BE (Ortho-McNeil)	None	Norethindrone (0.35)	

Drug	Estrogen (mg)	Progestin (mcg)	Additional pills
Extended-Cycle Combination (aka COCP [combined oral contraceptive pills])			
Jolessa (Barr) 91-d pack	Ethinyl estradiol (30)	Levonorgestrel (0.15)	7 inert
Lybrel (Wyeth) 28-d pack[c]	Ethinyl estradiol (20)	Levonorgestrel (0.09)	None
Quasense (Watson)	Ethinyl estradiol (30)	Levonorgestrel (0.15)	7 inert
Seasonique (Duramed) 91-d pack	Ethinyl estradiol (30)	Levonorgestrel (0.15)	7 (10 mcg ethinyl estradiol)
Seasonale (Duramed) 91-d pack	Ethinyl estradiol (30)	Levonorgestrel (0.15)	7 inert

[a] The designations 21 and 28 refer to number of days in regimen available.

[b] Also approved for acne.

[c] First FDA-approved pill for 365 d dosing.

[d] Approved for premenstrual dysphoric disorder (PMDD) in women who use contraception for birth control.

[e] Avoid in patients with hyperkalemia risk.

Based in part on data published in the *Medical Letter*, Volume 49 (Issue 1266) 2007, manufacturers insert and web sites as of August 29, 2009.

TABLE 6
Oral Potassium Supplements

Brand Name	Salt	Form	mEq Potassium/ Dosing Unit
Glu-K	Gluconate	Tablet	2 mEq/tablet
Kaon elixir	Gluconate	Liquid	20 mEq/15 mL
Kaon-Cl 10	KCl	Tablet, SR	10 mEq/tablet
Kaon-Cl 20%	KCl	Liquid	40 mEq/15 mL
K-Dur 20	KCl	Tablet, SR	20 mEq/tablet
KayCiel	KCl	Liquid	20 mEq/15 mL
K-Lor	KCl	Powder	20 mEq/packet
K-lyte/Cl	KCl/bicarbonate	Effervescent tablet	25 mEq/tablet
Klorvess	KCl/bicarbonate	Effervescent tablet	20 mEq/tablet
Klotrix	KCl	Tablet, SR	10 mEq/tablet
K-Lyte	Bicarbonate/ citrate	Effervescent tablet	25 mEq/tablet
Klor-Con/EF	Bicarbonate/ citrate	Effervescent tablet	25 mEq/tablet
K-Tab	KCl	Tablet, SR	10 mEq/tablet
Micro-K	KCl	Capsule, SR	8 mEq/capsule
Potassium Chloride 10%	KCl	Liquid	20 mEq/15 mL
Potassium Chloride 20%	KCl	Liquid	40 mEq/15 mL
Slow-K	KCl	Tablet, SR	8 mEq/tablet
Tri-K	Acetate/ bicarbonate and citrate	Liquid	45 mEq/15 mL
Twin-K	Citrate/gluconate	Liquid	20 mEq/5 mL

SR = sustained release.

Note: Alcohol and sugar content vary between preparations.

TABLE 7
Tetanus Prophylaxis (See also page 239)

History of Absorbed Tetanus Toxoid Immunization	Clean, Minor Wounds		All Other Wounds[a]	
	Td[b]	TIG[c]	Td[d]	TIG[c]
Unknown or <3 doses	Yes	No	Yes	Yes
≥3 doses	No[e]	No	No[f]	No

[a] Such as, but not limited to, wounds contaminated with dirt, feces, soil, saliva, etc; puncture wounds; avulsions; and wounds resulting from missiles, crushing, burns, and frostbite.

[b] Td = tetanus-diphtheria toxoid (adult type), 0.5 mL IM.
  • For children <7 y, DPT (DT, if pertussis vaccine is contraindicated) is preferred to tetanus toxoid alone.
  • For persons >7 y, Td is preferred to tetanus toxoid alone.
  • DT = diphtheria-tetanus toxoid (pediatric), used for those who cannot receive pertussis.

[c] TIG = tetanus immune globulin, 250 units IM.

[d] If only 3 doses of fluid toxoid have been received, then a fourth dose of toxoid, preferably an adsorbed toxoid, should be given.

[e] Yes, if >10 y since last dose.

[f] Yes, if >5 y since last dose.

Based on guidelines from the Centers for Disease Control and Prevention and reported in *MMWR* (MMWR, December 1, 2006; 55(RR-15):1-48).

TABLE 8
Oral Anticoagulant Standards of Practice (See also warfarin page 253)

Thromboembolic Disorder	INR	Duration
Deep Venous Thrombosis & Pulmonary Embolism		
Treatment single episode		
Transient risk factor	2–3	3 mo
Idiopathic	2–3	6–12 mo
Recurrent systemic embolism	2–3	Indefinite
Prevention of Systemic Embolism		
Atrial fibrillation (AF)[a]	2–3	Indefinite
AF: cardioversion	2–3	3 wk prior; 4 wk post sinus rhythm
Valvular heart disease	2–3	Indefinite
Cardiomyopathy	2–3	Indefinite
Acute Myocardial Infarction		
High-risk patients[c]	2–3 + low-dose aspirin	3 mo
Prosthetic Valves		
Tissue heart valves	2–3	3 mo
Bileaflet mechanical valves in aortic position	2–3	Indefinite
Other mechanical prosthetic valves[b]	2.5–3.5	Indefinite

[a] With high-risk factors or multiple moderate risk factors.

[b] May add aspirin 81 mg to warfarin in patients with caged ball or caged disk valves or with additional risk factors.

[c] Large anterior MI, significant heart failure, intracardiac thrombus, and/or history of thromboembolic event.

INR = international normalized ratio.

Based on data published in Chest. 2004 Sep;126 (Suppl):163S–696S.

TABLE 9
Antiarrhythmics: Vaughn Williams Classification

Class I: Sodium Channel Blockade

A. **Class Ia:** Lengthens duration of action potential (↑ the refractory period in atrial and ventricular muscle, in SA and AV conduction systems, and Purkinje fibers)
   1. Amiodarone (also classes II, III, IV)
   2. Disopyramide (Norpace)
   3. Imipramine (MAO inhibitor)
   4. Procainamide (Pronestyl)
   5. Quinidine
B. **Class Ib:** No effect on action potential
   1. Lidocaine (Xylocaine)
   2. Mexiletine (Mexitil)
   3. Phenytoin (Dilantin)
   4. Tocainide (Tonocard)
C. **Class Ic:** Greater sodium current depression (blocks the fast inward Na$^+$ current in heart muscle and Purkinje fibers, and slows the rate of ↑ of phase 0 of the action potential)
   1. Flecainide (Tambocor)
   2. Propafenone

Class II: β-Blocker

D. Amiodarone (also classes Ia, III, IV)
E. Esmolol (Brevibloc)
F. Sotalol (also class III)

Class III: Prolong Refractory Period via Action Potential

G. Amiodarone (also classes Ia, II, IV)
H. Sotalol

Class IV: Calcium Channel Blocker

I. Amiodarone (also classes Ia, II, III)
J. Diltiazem (Cardizem)
K. Verapamil (Calan)

TABLE 10
Cytochrome P-450 Isoenzymes and Common Drugs
They Metabolize, Inhibit, and Induce[a]

CYP1A2

Substrates:	Acetaminophen, caffeine, cyclobenzaprine, clozapine, imipramine, mexiletine, naproxen, theophylline, propranolol
Inhibitors:	Cimetidine, most fluoroquinolone antibiotics, fluvoxamine, verapamil
Inducers:	Tobacco smoking, charcoal-broiled foods, cruciferous vegetables, omeprazole

CYP2C9

Substrates:	Most NSAIDs (including COX-2), glipizide, irbesartan, losartan, phenytoin, warfarin
Inhibitors:	Amiodarone, fluconazole, ketoconazole, metronidazole
Inducers:	Barbiturates, rifampin

CYP2C19

Substrates:	Diazepam, amitriptyline, lansoprazole, omeprazole, phenytoin, pantoprazole, rabeprazole, clopidogrel
Inhibitors:	Omeprazole, lansoprazole, isoniazid, ketoconazole, fluoxetine, fluvoxamine
Inducers:	Barbiturates, rifampin

CYP2D6

Substrates:	**Antidepressants:** Most tricyclic antidepressants, clomipramine, fluoxetine, paroxetine, venlafaxine **Antipsychotics:** Aripiprazole, clozapine, haloperidol, risperidone, thioridazine **Beta blockers:** Carvedilol, metoprolol, propranolol, timolol **Opioids:** Codeine, hydrocodone, oxycodone, propoxyphene, tramadol **Others:** Amphetamine, dextromethorphan, duloxetine, encainide, flecainide, mexiletine, ondansetron, propafenone, selegiline tamoxifen
Inhibitors:	Amiodarone, bupropion, cimetidine, clomipramine, doxepin, duloxetine, fluoxetine, haloperidol, methadone, paroxetine, quinidine, ritonavir
Inducers:	Unknown

CYP3A

Substrates:
Anticholinergics: Darifenacin, oxybutynin, solifenacin, tolterodine

Benzodiazepines: Alprazolam, diazepam, midazolam, triazolam

Ca channel blockers: Amlodipine, diltiazem, felodipine, nimodipine, nifedipine, nisoldipine, verapamil

Chemotherapy: Cyclophosphamide, erlotinib, ifosfamide, paclitaxel, tamoxifen, vinblastine, vincristine

HIV protease inhibitors: Amprenavir, atazanavir, indinavir, nelfinavir, ritonavir, saquinavir

HMG-CoA reductase inhibitors: Atorvastatin, lovastatin, simvastatin

Immunosuppressive agents: Cyclosporine, tacrolimus

Macrolide-type antibiotics: Clarithromycin, erythromycin, telithromycin, troleandomycin

Opioids: Alfentanil, cocaine, fentanyl, methadone, sufentanil

Steroids: Budesonide, cortisol, 17-®-estradiol, progesterone

Others: Acetaminophen, amiodarone, carbamazepine, delavirdine, efavirenz, nevirapine, quinidine, repaglinide, sildenafil, tadalafil, trazodone, vardenafil

Inhibitors:
Amiodarone, amprenavir, aprepitant, atazanavir, ciprofloxacin, cisapride, clarithromycin, diltiazem, erythromycin, fluconazole, fluvoxamine, grapefruit juice (in high ingestion), indinavir, itraconazole, ketoconazole, nefazodone, nelfinavir, norfloxacin, ritonavir, saquinavir, telithromycin, troleandomycin, verapamil, voriconazole

Inducers:
Carbamazepine, efavirenz, glucocorticoids, modafinil, nevirapine, phenytoin, phenobarbital, rifabutin, rifapentine, rifampin, St. John's wort

---

a Increased or decreased (primarily hepatic cytochrome P-450) metabolism of medications may influence the effectiveness of drugs or result in significant drug-drug interactions. Understanding the common cytochrome P-450 isoforms (e.g., CYP2C9, CYP2D9, CYP2C19, CYP3A4) and common drugs that are metabolized by (aka "substrates"), inhibit, or induce activity of the isoform helps minimize significant drug interactions. CYP3A is involved in the metabolism of >50% of drugs metabolized by the liver.

Based on data from Katzung B (ed): Basic and Clinical Pharmacology, 11th ed. McGraw-Hill, New York, 2009; The Medical Letter, Volume 47, July 4, 2004; N Engl J Med 2005:352:2211-21

TABLE 11
SSRIs/SNRI/Triptan and Serotonin Syndrome

A life-threatening condition, when selective serotonin reuptake inhibitors (SSRIs) and 5-hydroxytryptamine receptor agonists (triptans) are used together. However, many other drugs have been implicated (see below). Signs and symptoms of serotonin syndrome include the following:

Restlessness, coma, N/V/D, hallucinations, loss of coordination, overactive reflexes, ↑ HR/temperature, rapid changes in BP, increased body temperature

Class	Drugs
Antidepressants	MAOIs, TCAs, SSRIs, SNRIs, mirtazapine, venlafaxine
CNS stimulants	Amphetamines, phentermine, methylphenidate, sibutramine
5-HT₁ agonists	Triptans
Illicit drugs	Cocaine, methylenedioxymethamphetamine (ecstasy), lysergic acid diethylamide (LSD)
Opioids	Tramadol, pethidine, oxycodone, morphine, meperidine
Others	Buspirone, chlorpheniramine, dextromethorphan, linezolid, lithium, selegiline, tryptophan, St. John's wort

Management includes removal of the precipitating drugs and supportive care. To control agitation serotonin antagonists (cyproheptadine or methysergide) can be used. When symptoms are mild, discontinuation of the medication or medications and the control of agitation with benzodiazepines may be needed. Critically ill patients may require sedation and mechanical ventilation as well as control of hyperthermia. (Boyer EW, Shanon M. The serotonin syndrome. *N Engl J Med.* 2005;352(11):1112–1120.)

MOAI = monoamine oxidase inhibitor
TCA = tricyclic antidepressant
SNRI = serotonin-norepinephrine reuptake inhibitors

TABLE 12
Multivitamins, Oral OTC

Composition of Selected Multivitamins and Multivitamins with Mineral and Trace Element Supplements. Listings Show Vitamin Content (Part 1) and then the Mineral Trace Element and other Components (Part 2) of Popular US Brands. Values Listed are a Percentage of Daily Value. (See also page 285)

Part 1. Vitamins

	Fat Soluble				Water Soluble								
	A	D	E	K	C	B_1	B_2	B_3	B_6	Folate	B_{12}	Biotin	B_5
Centrum[a]	70	100	100	31	150	100	100	100	100	125	100	10	100
Centrum Performance[a]	70	100	200	31	200	300	300	200	300	100	300	17	100
Centrum Silver[a]	50	125	167	38	150	100	100	100	150	125	417	10	100
Nature Made Multi Complete	50	250	167	100	300	100	100	100	100	100	100	10	100
Nature Made Multi Daily	60	100	100	0	100	100	100	100	100	100	100	0	100
Nature Made Multi Max	60	100	500	50	500	3333	2941	250	2500	100	833	17	500
Nature Made Multi 50+	60	100	200	13	200	200	200	100	200	100	417	10	100
One-A-Day 50 Plus	50	100	110	25	200	300	200	100	300	100	417	10	150
One-A-Day Essential	60	100	100	0	100	100	100	100	100	100	100	0	100

283

TABLE 12 (continued)
Multivitamins, Oral OTC

One-A-Day Maximum[b]	50	100	100	31	100	100	100	100	100	100	100	10	100
Therapeutic Vitamin	100	100	100	0	150	200	200	100	100	100	150	10	100
Theragran-M Advanced High Protein	100	200	200	35	150	200	200	100	300	100	200	10	100
Theragran-M Premier High Potency	70	200	200	31	200	235	267	125	200	100	150	10	100
Theragran-M Premier 50 Plus High Potency	70	200	200	13	125	176	200	125	300	100	500	12	150
Therapeutic Vitamin + Minerals[b]	100	200	200	0	200	100	100	100	100	100	100	10	100
Unicap M	100	100	100	0	100	100	100	100	100	100	100	0	100
Unicap Sr.	100	50	50	NA	100	80	82	80	110	100	50	0	100
Unicap T	100	100	100	0	833	667	588	500	300	100	300	0	250

Part 2. Minerals, trace elements, and other components

	Minerals						Trace Elements						Other
	Ca	P	Mg	Fe	Zn	I	Se	K	Mn	Cu	Cr	Mo	
Centrum[a]	20	11	25	100	73	100	79	2	115	45	29	60	Lutein, lycopene
Centrum Performance[a]	10	5	10	100	73	100	100	2	200	45	100	100	Gingko, ginseng
Centrum Silver[a]	22	11	13	0	73	100	79	2	115	45	38	60	Lutein, lycopene
Nature Made Multi Complete	16	NA	25	100	100	100	35	NA	200	100	100	100	Lutein
Nature Made Multi Daily	45	0	0	100	100	0	0	0	0	0	0	0	
Nature Made Multi Max	10	4	6	50	100	100	100	1	100	100	100	0	Lutein
Nature Made Multi 50+	20	5	25		100	100	71	2	100	100	100	33	Lutein
One-A-Day 50 Plus	12	0	25	0	150	100	150	1	200	100	150	120	Lutein
One-A-Day Essential	5	0	0	0	0	100	0	0	0	0	0	0	
One-A-Day Maximum	16	11	25	100	100	100	29	2	175	100	54	213	
Therapeutic Vitamin[b]	0	0	0	100	100	100	0	0	0	0	0	0	
Theragran-M Advanced High Potency	4	3	25	50	100	100	100	1	100	100	42	100	

TABLE 12 (continued)
Multivitamins, Oral OTC

Theragran-M Premier High Protein	17	11	25	100	100	100	286	2	100	175	100	107	Lutein, lycopene, coenzyme Q10
Theragran-M Premier 50 Plus High Potency	20	5	25	0	113	100	286	2	100	100	21	100	Lutein, coenzyme Q10
Therapeutic Vitamin + Minerals[b]	4	3	10	50	50	36	<1	100	100	42	100		
Unicap M	6	5	0	100	100	0	<1	50	100	0			
Unicap Sr.	10	8	8	56	100	0	<1	50	100	0			
Unicap T	0	0	0	100	100	14		50	100	0			

Common multivitamins available without a prescription are listed. Most chain drug stores have generic versions of many of the multivitamin supplements listed above; thus, specific generic brands are not listed. Many specialty vitamin combinations are available, but not included in this list (examples are B vitamins plus C, supplements for a specific condition or organ, pediatric and infant formulations, and prenatal vitamins). Values are listed as percentages of the Daily Value (also known as %DV) based on Recommended Dietary Allowances of vitamins and minerals based on Dietary Reference Intakes (Food and Nutrition Board, Institute of Medicine, National Academy of Science). Additional information may be available for many other supplements from the NIH Dietary Supplements labels Database http://dietarysupplements.nlm.nih.gov/dietary

[a] New formulation October 2007.

[b] Formulations may vary. Consult with pharmacy for current product.

[c] Common generic brands (when other than the store name itself) are: Osco Drug Central-Vite (Albertson's); Kirkland Signature Daily Multivitamin (Costco); Whole Source, PharmAssure (Rite Aid); Central-Vite (Safeway); Member's Mark (Sam's Club); Vitasmart (Kmart); Century (Target); A thru Z Select, Super Ayinal, Ultra Choice (Walgreens), Equate Complete or Spring Valley Sentury-Vite (Wal-Mart).

Vitamins: B_1 = Thiamine; B_2 = Riboflavin; B_3 = Niacin; B_5 = Pantothenic Acid; B_6 = Pyridoxine; B_{12} = Cyanocobalamin. Elements: Ca = calcium; Cr = chromium; Cu = copper; Fe = iron; I = Iodine; K = potassium; Mg = magnesium; Mn = manganese; Mo = Molybdenum; P = phosphorus; Se = selenium; Zn = zinc; 0 = not applicable or not available.

Index

Page numbers followed by *t* indicate tables.

Generic (Trade) — Adult Dose (Continued)

Generic (Trade)	Adult Dose (Continued)
Magnesium Sulfate	**VF/pulseless VT arrest with torsade de pointes:** 1–2 g IV push (2–4 mL 5% solution) in 10 mL D₅W. If pulse present then 1–2 g in 50–100 mL D₅W over 5–60 min.
Metoprolol	5 mg slow IV q5min, total 15 mg.
Morphine	2–4 mg IV (over 1–5 min) then give 2–8 mg q5–15min as needed.
Nitroglycerin	IV bolus: infuse at 10–20 mcg/min every 3–5 min, ↑ by 5–10 mcg/min PRN; SL: 0.3–0.4 mg, repeat q5min. Aerosol spray: Spray 0.5–1 s at 5-min intervals.
Nitroprusside	0.1–0.3 mcg/kg/min start, titrate max dose (10 mcg/kg/min).
Procainamide	20 mg/min IV until one of these: arrhythmia stopped, hypotension, QRS widens >50%, total 17 mg/kg; then maintenance infusion of 1–4 mg/min.
Propranolol (Inderal)	0.1 mg/kg slow IV push, ÷ 3 equal doses q2–3min, max 1 mg/min; repeat in 2 min PRN.
Reteplase recombinant (Retavase)	10 Units IV bolus over 2 min: 30 min later, 10 units IV bolus over 2 min NS flush before and after each dose.
Sodium Bicarbonate	1 mEq/kg IV bolus; repeat ½ dose q10min PRN.
Sotalol (Betapace)	1–1.5 mg/kg IV over 5 min then 10 mg/min.
Streptokinase	**AMI:** 1.5 million Int Units over 1 h.
Tirofiban (Aggrastat)	**ACS or PCI:** 0.4 mcg/kg/min IV for 30 min, then 0.1 mcg/kg/min.
Verapamil	2.5–5 mg IV over 1–2 min; repeat 5–10 mg, in 15–30 min PRN max of 20 mg; or 5 mg bolus q15min (max 30 mg).

Based on 2005 American Heart Association Guidelines for Cardiopulmonary Resuscitation and Emergency Cardiovascular Care. *Circulation* 2005;112(24 Suppl). Available online at: http://circ.ahajournals.org/content/vol112/24_suppl (accessed July 4, 2010)

Generic (Trade)	Adult Dose
Calcium Chloride	**Hyperkalemia/hypermagnesemia/CCB overdose:** 8–16 mg/kg; 10% solution, 5–10 mL over 2–5 min.
Clopidogrel	**ACS:** 300-mg loading dose then 75 mg/d.
Diltiazem (Cardizem)	**Acute rate control:** 0.25 mg/kg (15–20 mg) over 2 min followed in 15 min by 0.35 mg/kg (20–25 mg) over 2 min maint inf 5–15 mg/h.
Dobutamine (Dobutrex)	0.5–1.0 mcg/kg/min; titrate to HR not >10% of baseline.
Dopamine	2–20 mcg/kg/min. **Bradycardia:** 2–10 mcg/kg/min. **Hypotension:** 10–20 mcg/kg/min.
Epinephrine	1-mg IV push, repeat q3–5min (0.2 mg/kg max) if 1 mg dose fails. Inf: 30 mg (30 mL of 1:1000 solution) in 250 mL NS or D5W, at 100 mL/h, titrate. ET 2–2.5 mg in 20 mL NS. **Profound bradycardia/hypotension:** 2–10 mg/min (1 mg of 1:1000; in 500 mL NS, infuse 1–5 mL/min).
Eptifibatide (Integrilin)	**ACS:** 180 mcg/kg/min IV bolus over 1–2 min then 2 mcg/kg/min.
Esmolol (Brevibloc)	0.5 mg/kg over 1 min, then 0.05 mg/kg/min for 4 min; if no response 2nd bolus of 0.5 mg/kg with maintenance of 0.1 mg/kg/min with maximum of 0.3 mg/kg/min.
Glucagon	**β-Blocker or CCB overdose:** 3 mg initially followed by 3 mg/h: **Hypoglycemia:** 1 mg IV, IM, or sub Q
Heparin (Unfractionated)	Bolus 80 Int Units/kg (max 4000 Int Units); then 18 Int Units/kg/h (max 1000 Int Units/h for patients >70 kg) round to nearest 50 IU; keep PTT 1.5–2 × control 48 h or until angiography. If adjunct with fibrin specific lytics then 60 IU/kg bolus then 12 Int Units/kg/h. Adults ≥60 kg, 1 mg (10 mL) over 10 min: a second dose may be used; <60 kg 0.01 mg/kg.
Ibutilide	10 mg IV over 1–2 min: repeat or double dose q10min (150 mg max); or initial bolus, then 2–8 mg/min.
Labetalol (Trandate)	**Cardiac arrest from VF/VT refractory VF:** Initial: 1–1.5 mg/kg IV, additional 0.5–0.75 mg/kg IV push, repeat in 3–5 min, max total 3 mg/kg. ET: 2–4 mg/kg.
Lidocaine	**Reperfusing stable VT, wide complex tachycardia or ectopy:** (up to 1–1.5 mg/kg may be used) IV push; repeat 0.5–0.75 mg/kg q5–10min; max total 3 mg/kg. Maint: 1–4 mg/min (30–50 mcg/min).

(continued)